AUTONOMIC TESTING

AUTONOMIC TESTING

Peter Novak, MD, PhD

DIVISION CHIEF, AUTONOMIC NEUROLOGY
DIRECTOR, AUTONOMIC LABORATORY
DEPARTMENT OF NEUROLOGY, BRIGHAM AND WOMEN'S HOSPITAL
ASSISTANT PROFESSOR OF NEUROLOGY, HARVARD MEDICAL SCHOOL
BOSTON, MA

OXFORD
UNIVERSITY PRESS

OXFORD
UNIVERSITY PRESS

Oxford University Press is a department of the University of Oxford. It furthers the University's objective of excellence in research, scholarship, and education by publishing worldwide. Oxford is a registered trade mark of Oxford University Press in the UK and certain other countries.

Published in the United States of America by Oxford University Press
198 Madison Avenue, New York, NY 10016, United States of America.

Library of Congress Cataloging-in-Publication Data
Names: Novak, Peter (Neurologist), author.
Title: Autonomic testing / by Peter Novak.
Description: New York, NY : Oxford University Press, [2019] |
Includes bibliographical references and index.
Identifiers: LCCN 2018036552 | ISBN 9780190889227
Subjects: | MESH: Autonomic Nervous System Diseases—diagnosis |
Autonomic Nervous System Diseases—physiopathology | Case Reports
Classification: LCC RC407 | NLM WL 600 | DDC 616.85/69—dc23
LC record available at https://lccn.loc.gov/2018036552

Dedicated to my family
Vera, Lukas, Laura, Leo, Kujo, Elf, Onslow

CONTENTS

PREFACE

Disorders associated with dysfunction of the autonomic nervous system are quite common yet frequently unrecognized. Quantitative autonomic testing can be an invaluable tool for the evaluation of these disorders. While there are many excellent general clinical textbooks of autonomic disorders, only a few texts are available to provide detailed guidelines on how to perform and interpret autonomic testing. This manual fills the gap and deals mainly with practical aspects of autonomic testing. In accord with the maxim that "a good picture is worth a thousand words," signal drawings are heavily used throughout the text.

Autonomic neurology is a relatively new subspecialty of neurology, and the field is still evolving. This text is intended to be a guide for autonomic fellows; residents in neurology, general medicine, and other specialties; or for everybody who is interested in performing and interpreting autonomic tests. A unique aspect of this book is the use of skin biopsies for the assessment of small autonomic and sensory fibers as a routine part of autonomic testing. Another important feature of this book is the use of continuous cerebral blood flow velocity and end tidal carbon dioxide (CO_2) monitoring in addition to standard heart rate and blood pressure recordings during autonomic testing. Some of the data were edited for clarity.

The author thanks Camilia Ellis, Christine Leonard, Natalie Cyprian, Jennifer Efstathiou, and Philp Gorman for their help in data collection.

PART I

AUTONOMIC TESTING BASICS

1.

CLASSIFICATION OF PATTERNS AND SYNDROMES ON AUTONOMIC TESTING

This chapter lists the main patterns seen during autonomic testing.[1,2] The classification is based on physiology and/or functional anatomy. Although the classification is arbitrary, the main goal of the pattern list is to assist in the correct interpretation of the test results. However, often more than one pattern can be detected simultaneously. For example, postural tachycardia syndrome (POTS) can be associated with orthostatic hypertension. Syncope can be superimposed on any pattern. Small fiber neuropathy seen in the skin biopsy may be associated with autonomic failure or with orthostatic intolerance syndromes.

- Orthostatic Intolerance Syndromes
  - Presyncope
  - Syncope: Neurally mediated: vasovagal, vasodepressor, mixed cardiac
  - Postural tachycardia syndrome (POTS)
    - Neuropathic
    - Hyperadrenergic
    - Due to deconditioning
    - Due to hypovolemia
  - Paroxysmal sinus tachycardia (PST)
  - Inappropriate sinus tachycardia (IST)
  - Orthostatic hypotension (OH)
    - Neurogenic
    - Nonneurogenic: Volume depletion
    - Nonneurogenic: Cardiac
    - Due to medication effect
  - Orthostatic hypertension (OHTN)
  - Orthostatic cerebral hypoperfusion syndrome (OCHOS)
  - Hypocapnic cerebral hypoperfusion (HYCH)
  - Psychogenic pseudosyncope
- Autonomic Failure (Underactivity)
  - Generalized or diffuse (affecting sudomotor, cardiovagal, and adrenergic system)
  - Restricted: Subset of generalized failure
  - Adrenergic (abnormal blood pressure responses to tilt and Valsalva maneuver)
  - Cholinergic (abnormal deep breathing test and sudomotor test)
  - Sudomotor (abnormal sudomotor test)
- Autonomic Overactivity
  - Adrenergic
  - Cholinergic
- Paroxysmal Dysautonomia
  - Paroxysmal overactivity
  - Paroxysmal autonomic failure (underactivity)
- Hypovolemia
- Cerebral Autoregulatory Failure
- Small Fiber Neuropathy
  - Based on the skin biopsy results
  - Type:
    - Mixed sensory and autonomic (sudomotor): Abnormal epidermal nerve fiber density (ENFD) and sweat gland nerve fiber density (SGNFD)
    - Sensory: Abnormal ENFD
    - Autonomic (sudomotor): Abnormal SGNFD
  - Distribution:
    - Length-dependent
    - Non–length dependent
  - Based on the sudomotor testing:
    - Abnormal quantitative sudomotor axon reflex test (QSART): May further stratify the pattern into length-dependent pattern, non–length dependent, and patchy
    - Abnormal electrochemical skin conductance (ESC)

REFERENCES

1. Novak P. Cerebral blood flow, heart rate, and blood pressure patterns during the tilt test in common orthostatic syndromes. *Neurosci J.* 2016:6127340. doi:10.1155/2016/6127340.
2. Novak P. Hypocapnic cerebral hypoperfusion: A biomarker of orthostatic intolerance. *PloS One.* 2018;*13*(9):e0204419. doi:10.1371/journal.pone.0204419

2.

FUNCTIONAL NEUROANATOMY OF AUTONOMIC NERVOUS SYSTEM

INTRODUCTION

The autonomic nervous system (ANS) has a unique physiologic role since it integrates and synchronizes the activities of many organs. Historically, the ANS has been divided into the *central autonomic system* (CAN), also called the preganglionic system, and the *peripheral autonomic system*, or postganglionic system, which includes the parasympathetic, sympathetic, and enteric systems.[1] The CAN is also called the *central autonomic network*[2] since many centers are defined by function rather than by anatomy.

CENTRAL AUTONOMIC NETWORK

The CAN is a neuronal substrate for autonomic reflexes aiming to preserve homeostasis. The main structures of the CAN are dispersed throughout the central nervous system (Figure 2.1). The CAN controls autonomic functions and, at the same time, modulates several vital and integrative functions including emotional, attentional, behavioral, endocrine, respiratory, vestibular, sexual, and pain perception. The CAN modulates activity of all organs through direct innervations by the parasympathetic and sympathetic nerves or neurohumoral signaling.

The most distinct characteristics of the CAN are:

1. *The network structure.* Many autonomic centers are defined by their function rather than by distinct anatomical or histological landmarks. A typical example is the reticular formation in the brainstem that forms clusters of neurons that share common functions.
2. *Redundancy.* Most structures of the CAN are bilateral and reciprocally interconnected, and usually a

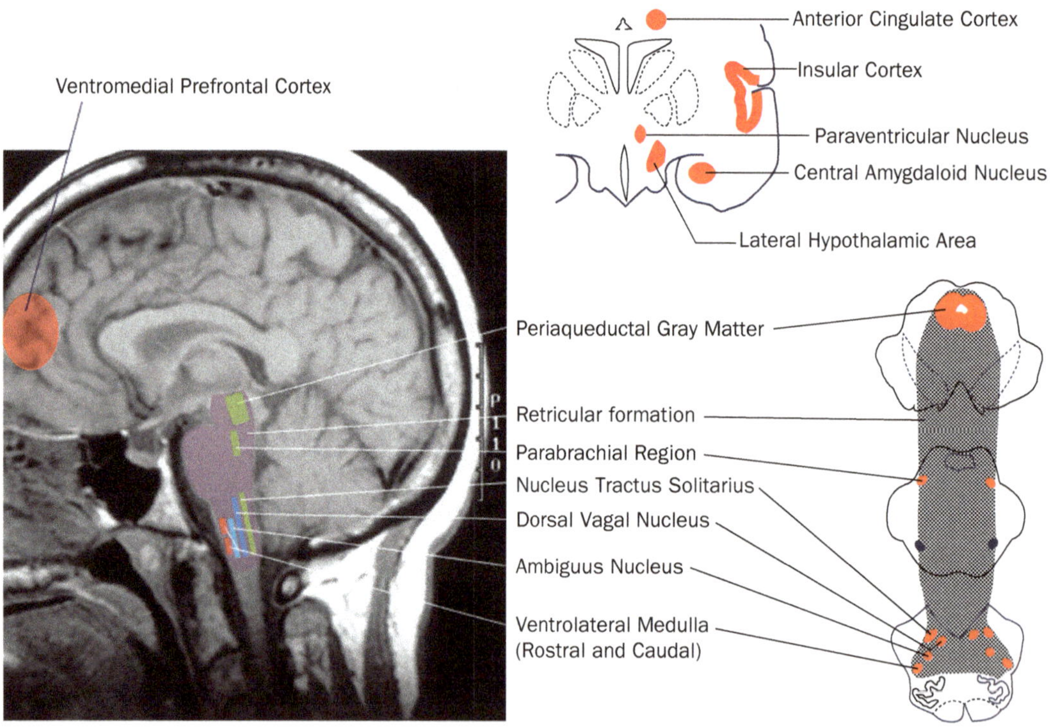

Figure 2.1 Components of the central autonomic network.

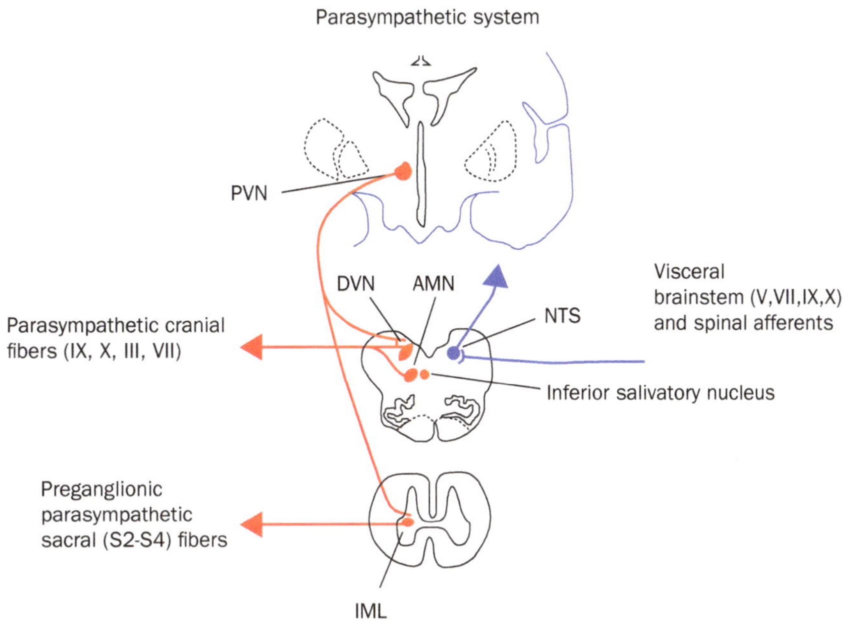

Figure 2.2 Parasympathetic system. DVN, dorsal vagal nucleus; AMN, ambiguus nucleus; IML, intermediolateral column; NTS, nucleus tractus solitarius; PVN, paraventricular nucleus.

bilateral lesion is needed to produce well-defined and lasting effects.

3. *Integration centers.* These are areas where the autonomic and nonautonomic functions are integrated. For example, the periventricular nucleus of the hypothalamus integrates autonomic functions with energy balance.

The CAN forms a network of reciprocally interconnected structures with integration centers at the cortex, hypothalamus, brainstem, medulla, and spinal cord. Thalamus plays an important role in regulating wakefulness and sleep, emotions, and other functions. Cerebellum also appears to influence emotional and affective behavior through the connections to the CAN, brainstem, solitary nucleus, and vagal nerves (Figure 2.3) in addition to postural, balance and coordination control.

PARASYMPATHETIC NERVOUS SYSTEM

The parasympathetic nervous system consists of cranial and sacral portions (Figures 2.2 and 2.3). Cranial preganglionic

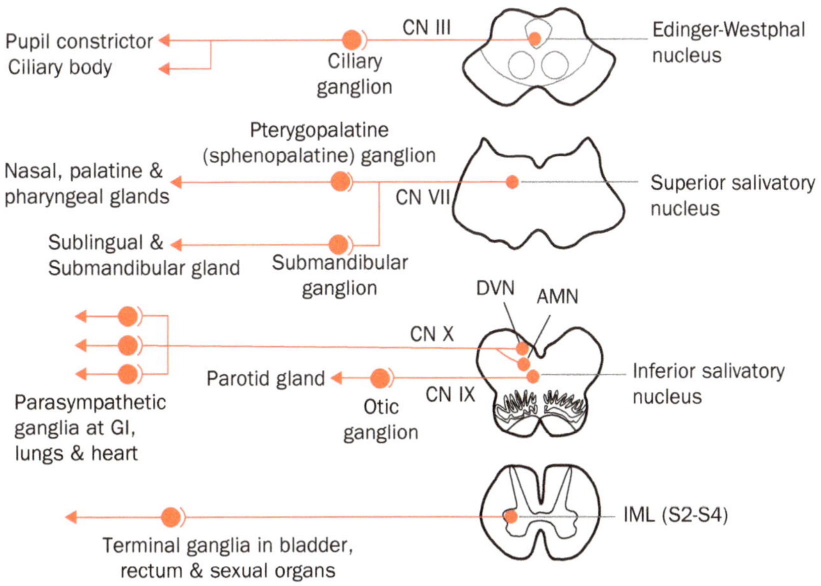

Figure 2.3 Parasympathetic system. DVN, dorsal vagal nucleus; AMN, ambiguus nucleus; IML, intermediolateral column; CN, cranial nerve.

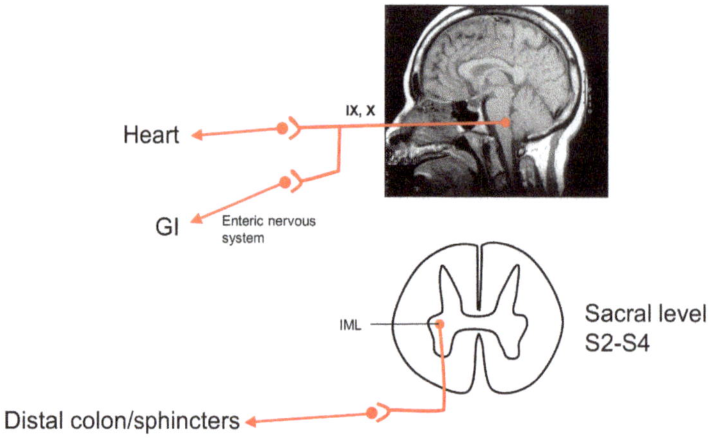

Figure 2.4 Parasympathetic system. IML, intermediolateral column; IX, cranial nerve IX; X, cranial nerve X; GI, gastrointestinal innervation.

fibers originate in the general visceral efferent column in specific nuclei.

The *Edinger-Westphal nucleus* located close to the third nerve nucleus synapses at the ciliary ganglion, which innervates the pupil constrictor and the ciliary body. The superior salivatory nucleus in the pons synapses at the sphenopalatine, pterygopalatine, and submandibular ganglia. The inferior salivatory ganglion in the medulla sends axons via the glossopharyngeal nerve (IX) and synapses at the otic ganglion that innervates the parotid gland.

The dorsal nucleus of the vagus nerve (X) provides the majority of parasympathetic preganglionic fibers. They innervate parasympathetic ganglia cells located at the heart, lung, and enteric ganglia. The nucleus ambiguous also provides preganglionic innervations to the heart.

Postganglionic neurons lie in the gastric, myenteric, or submucosal plexuses. Short postganglionic fibers innervate glands and smooth muscles at target organs. The sacral portion originates in the intermediolateral columns at the S2–S4 level and innervates sphincters and reproductive organs (Figure 2.4). This classic concept has been recently challenged.[3]

SYMPATHETIC NERVOUS SYSTEM

Preganglionic sympathetic neurons originate in the intermediolateral column at the T1–L3 level (Figures 2.5 and 2.6). They synapse at sympathetic ganglionic neurons. There are two types of sympathetic ganglia: paravertebral and prevertebral.

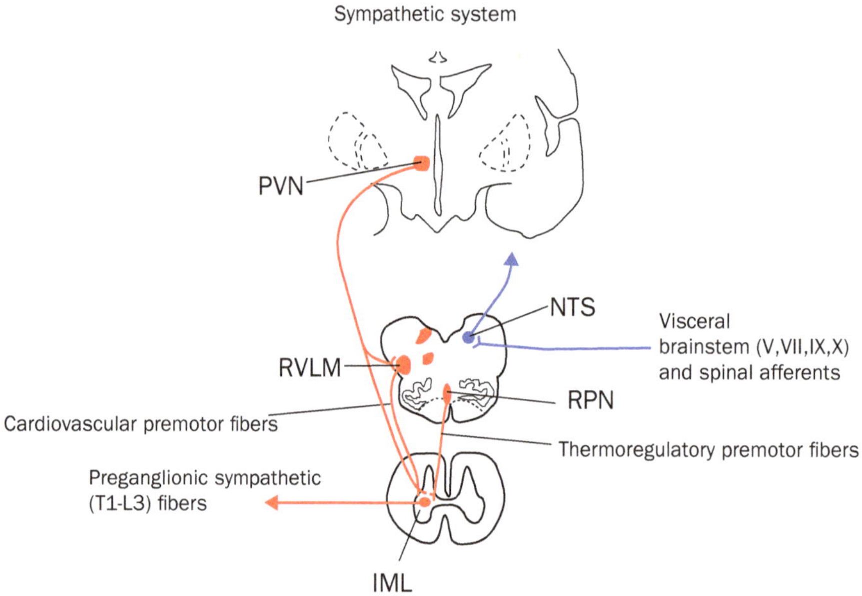

Figure 2.5 Sympathetic system. IML, intermediolateral column; NTS, nucleus of the solitary tract; CVLM, caudal ventrolateral medulla; RVLM, rostral ventrolateral medulla; PVN, paraventricular nucleus; RPN, raphe pontis nucleus.

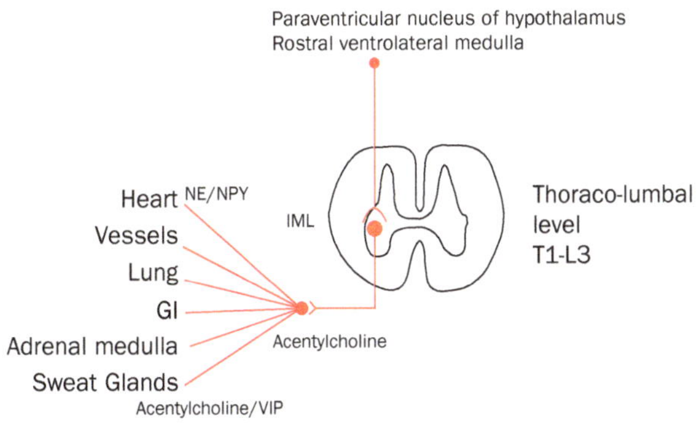

Figure 2.6 Sympathetic system. IML, intermediolateral column; NE, norepinephrine; NPY, neuropeptide Y; VIP, vasoactive intestinal peptide.

Paravertebral ganglia include the cervical, thoracic, lumbar, and chromaffin cells of the adrenal medulla. There are three cervical ganglia: superior, middle, and inferior (stellate). The superior cervical ganglion projects postganglionic fibers to all cranial structures including cerebral vessels, pupils, the pineal, the lacrimal, and the parotid gland. The stellate ganglion sends postganglionic vasomotor and sudomotor fibers to the upper limb. There are 11 thoracic, 4 lumbar, 4 sacral ganglia and 1 coccygeal ganglion. The thoracic and upper two lumber ganglia project to the lower limb.

Prevertebral ganglia include superior mesenteric inferior mesenteric and celiac ganglion.

Postganglionic nerves originating in the sympathetic ganglia innervate organs via splanchnic nerves including the cervical, thoracic, lumbar, and sacral nerves (Figure 2.6).

Skin sympathetic nerves are sudomotor, pilomotor, and vasomotor.

ENTERIC NERVOUS SYSTEM

The enteric nervous system contains about 100 million neurons and innervates the gastrointestinal tract. It is formed by the myenteric and the submucosal plexuses. These plexuses form local integrative circuits mainly controlling peristalsis.

NEURONAL SUBSTRATE OF THE ARTERIAL BARORECEPTOR REFLEX

The baroreceptor reflex (BR) is important in controlling the heart rate and blood pressure. The BR maintains the blood pressure within a narrow range by a feedback loop. An elevation of blood pressure decreases the heart rate and reduces the blood pressure via reduced peripheral resistance.

The baroreflex circuit is shown in Figure 2.7. An increase of arterial pressure activates the baroreceptors in the carotid sinus and aortic arch. Primary afferents from

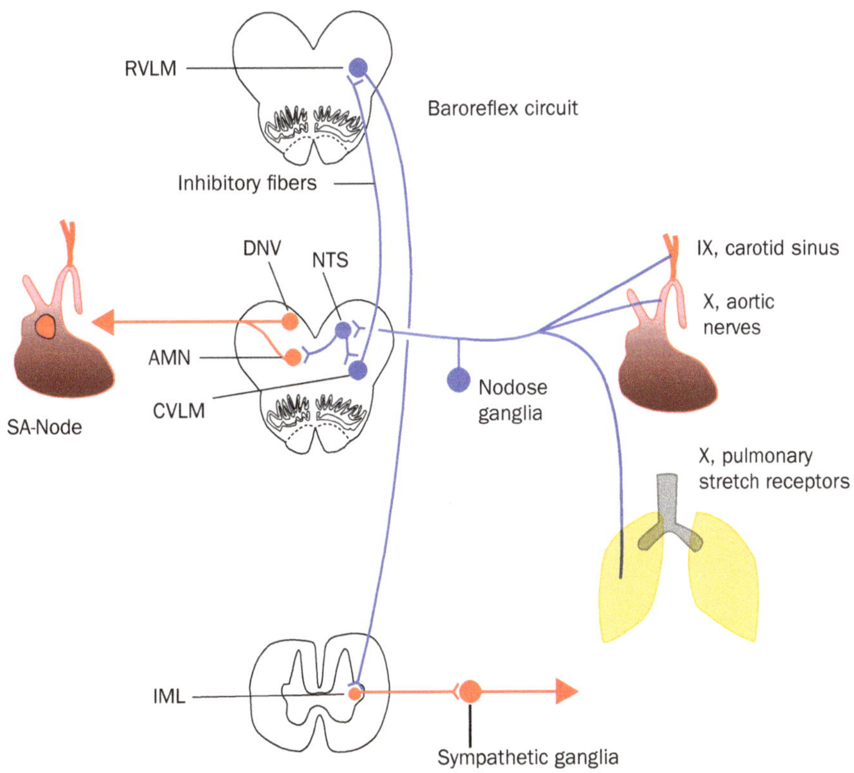

Figure 2.7 Neuronal circuits mediating baroreflex. Stretching of baroreceptors in the carotid body, aortic arc, and lungs activates the NTS, which in turn activates the AMN and the CVLM. The AMN is cardioinhibitory, and its activation results in parasympathetic withdrawal and increasing of the heart rate. The CVLM inhibits the RVLM and IML and causes sympathetic withdrawal. AMN, ambiguus nucleus; NTS, nucleus tractus solitarius; CVLM, caudal ventrolateral medulla; RVLM, rostral ventrolateral medulla; IML, intermediolateral column; DNV, dorsal vagal nucleus.

baroreceptors excite second-order neurons in the nucleus of the solitary tract (NTS) via glutamate. The NTS neurons activate the caudal ventrolateral medulla (CVLM) neurons, then the CVLM GABAergic neurons inhibit the rostral ventrolateral medulla (RVLM) sympathoexcitatory premotor neurons. The net effect is withdrawal of the sympathetic drive and vasodilatation. The NTS also activates the preganglionic parasympathetic cardioinhibitory neurons in the nucleus ambiguus that results in bradycardia.

REFERENCES

1. Shields RW. Functional anatomy of the autonomic nervous system. *J Clin Neurophysiol Off Publ Am Electroencephalogr Soc.* 1993;10(1):2–13.
2. Benarroch EE. The central autonomic network: functional organization, dysfunction, and perspective. *Mayo Clin Proc.* 1993;68(10): 988–1001.
3. Espinosa-Medina I, Saha O, Boismoreau F, et al. The sacral autonomic outflow is sympathetic. *Science.* 2016;354(6314):893–897. doi:10.1126/science.aah5454.

3.

LABORATORY EQUIPMENT

INTRODUCTION

Most autonomic laboratories have a proprietary setting.[1] Typically, various monitors are connected together by a recording system.

MINIMAL REQUIREMENTS

At a bare minimum, the autonomic laboratory should be equipped with the following:

- Respiratory rate monitor
- Electrocardiogram (ECG) monitor
- Continuous noninvasive blood pressure monitor
- System or method for evaluation of the sudomotor functions
- Software and hardware that connects all monitors and records the signals.

All signals should be displayed on monitor simultaneously at various zoom settings. The software should reliably detect the R waves and corresponding systolic and diastolic blood pressure values (Figure 3.1). The software should be able to plot the detected values, including the instantaneous heart rate on-screen or on paper. The software should be able to detect and prompt a user for common abnormalities in ECG that can affect the instantaneous heart rate, such as ectopic beats or runs of tachycardia.

ROOM

The room for autonomic testing should be large enough to accommodate the tilt table and access to tilt table from both sides. The temperature and humidity should be controllable. The room should be shielded from direct sunlight, and the noise level should be low.

TILT TABLE

Several characteristics should be kept in mind when choosing a tilt table. The table should be large enough to accommodate obese patients. For proper measurement of blood pressure, the patient's arms are extended and abducted. The table should be equipped with an electrical motor providing smooth movement. Fast tilt, with a duration of tilt movement of less than 10 seconds, is a preferred option since slow tilt can miss transient oscillations of the heart rate and blood pressure at the onset of tilt. An important safety feature is the presence of a manual override in case of motor failure. Fast tilt down is also an important safety measure that may be necessary in the case of asystole or other potentially serious events. An adjustable armrest is necessary for keeping the arm at heart level during all positions of tilt. This is required for proper calibration when using a finger cuff device or wrist tonometric device for measuring blood pressure. Additional standard features are a footrest and safety belts.

ECG MONITOR

Most available monitors with analog output are suitable. The three-lead system is sufficient. Units with the capability to change filters are preferable. The analog output should be available without averaging. It is advantageous to use standard hospital ECG monitors typically seen in the ICU since these monitors are reliable, and they have standard connectors and cables.

CONTINUOUS NONINVASIVE BLOOD PRESSURE MONITOR

Noninvasive continuous or beat-to-beat pressure is necessary for proper evaluation of sympathetic activity during the Valsalva maneuver, and this also provides dynamic information during the tilt test. Typically, a finger cuff device is used. The blood pressure should be always calibrated using an oscillometric brachial cuff device.[2,3]

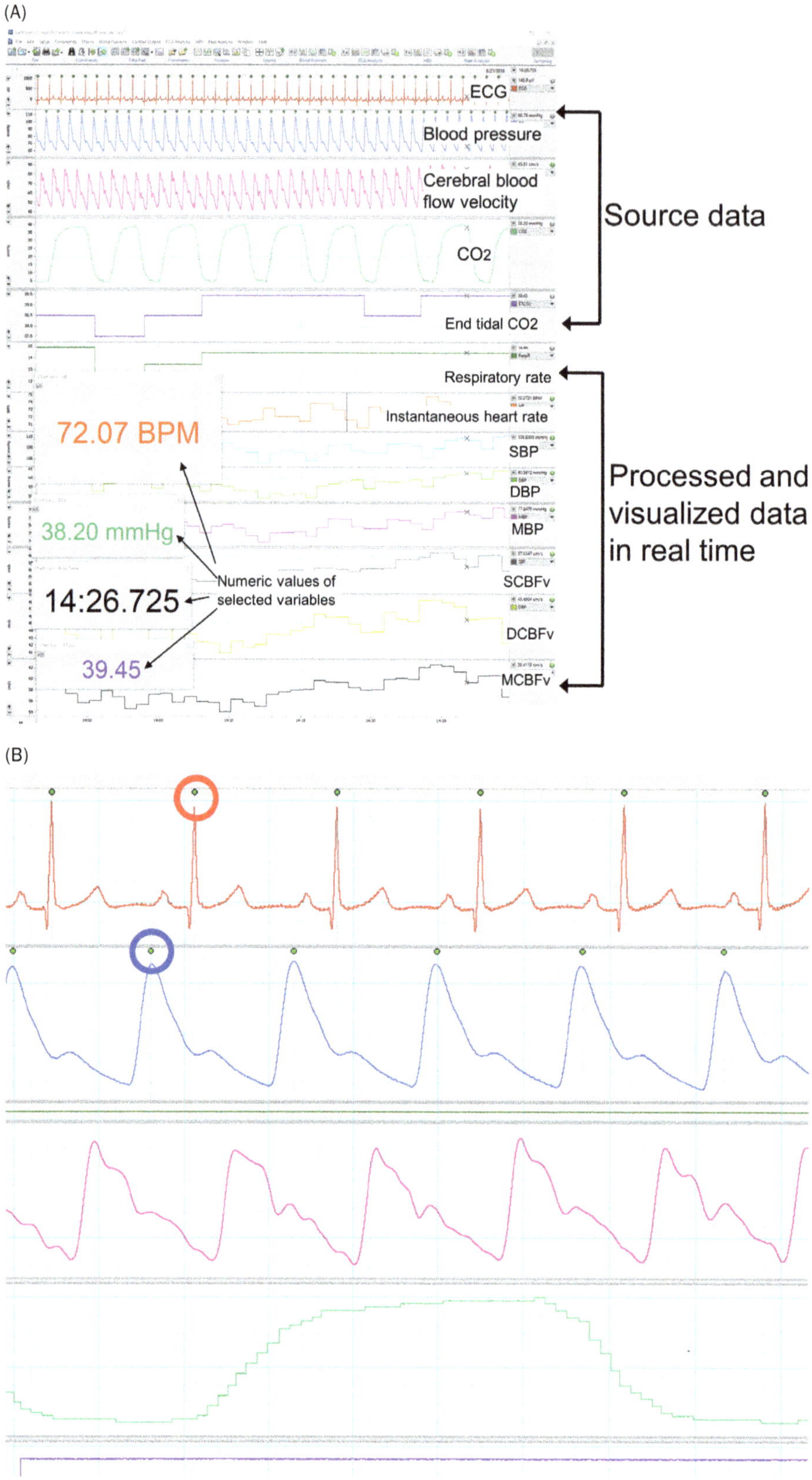

Figure 3.1 Recommended setup of the acquisition and evaluation system. We usually split the screen into upper raw source data and lower processed data (A). Each R wave (red circle) and each systolic blood pressure (blue circle) are detected in real time and the detection is confirmed by a green marker (B). ECG, electrocardiogram; SBP, systolic blood pressure; DBP, diastolic blood pressure; MBP, mean blood pressure; SCBFV, systolic cerebral blood flow velocity; DCBFV, diastolic cerebral blood flow velocity; MCBFV, mean cerebral blood flow velocity.

TRANSCRANIAL DOPPLER MONITOR

A transcranial Doppler (TCD) monitor enables noninvasive blood flow velocity monitoring, usually from the middle cerebral artery although any large cerebral artery can be insonated. Typically, 2 MHz probes are used. The manufacturer should also provide the probe holder that allows the clinician to attach the probe to the patient's head. The holder should have three-dimensional joints for easy probe positioning. TCD monitor should provide blood flow velocity in analog output, preferably with a standardized range (0–1 V). Then, velocity can be recorded and evaluated together with other cardiovascular signals. Newer systems with dual monitoring are preferable since they improve localization of intracranial vessels.

END TIDAL CO_2 MONITOR

End tidal CO_2 monitor is an important part of the equipment. End tidal CO_2 is necessary to correctly interpret the cerebral blood flow velocity, which can be affected either by blood pressure or end tidal CO_2.

RESPIRATORY MOVEMENT MONITOR

Recording of respiratory movements can be done via a nasal thermistor, which provides noncalibrated respiratory frequency, or via a respiratory mask, which enables calibrated data.

AUTONOMIC SOFTWARE

Data acquisition system and software records all signals, plots them on the screen, and enables signal analysis. The software should include a reliable method for R-wave detection and detection of systolic and diastolic pressure that can be also expanded to detect the systolic and diastolic blood flows. The software should allow independent setting adjustments for each channel.

R-WAVE DETECTION

Most cardiovascular signals are related to R-waves. Hence reliable detection of the R-wave is of utmost importance. There are several methods for R-wave detection. It is preferable to use pattern recognition over threshold recognition since the latter method is too sensitive to artifacts. A high-quality ECG recording is necessary because, in the presence of excessive noise, all detection methods can fail.

It is customary to plot successive R-waves in the form of either RR intervals or as the instant heart rate. Usually, the RR intervals are used in the research literature while the instant heart rate is used more often for clinical applications.

It is highly desirable that R-wave detection is done in real-time during recordings. This provides immediate feedback to the technician as long as the quality of the recording is acceptable. In our setting, each detected R-wave is marked by a green ball. We also simultaneously mark the systolic pressure.

HEART RATE PROCESSING

It is important to detect the R-wave correctly. Ectopic beats should be ignored, and compensatory pauses should be ignored as well. It is customary to interpolate for missing values in research studies. If these abnormal beats are not corrected, the deep breathing results can lead to false values. Hence, a practical knowledge of the basic ECG pattern is required.

BLOOD PRESSURE PROCESSING

Typically, systolic and diastolic values are detected and plotted simultaneously with heart rate. It is advantageous to plot mean blood pressure and pulse pressure. A collapse of the pulse pressure is sometimes the only abnormality on the Valsalva maneuver, and it can be easily detected from the pulse pressure waveform.

SUDOMOTOR TESTING

Sudomotor functions can be evaluated by the quantitative sudomotor axon reflex test (QSART) or by electrochemical skin conductance (ESC).

SKIN BIOPSY

Skin biopsy is minimally invasive method that enables direct morphological evaluation of small nerve fibers. Commonly used epidermal nerve fiber density (ENFD) evaluates sensory fibers while sweat gland nerve fiber density (SGNFD) evaluates sudomotor fibers.

DEVICES

For results presented in this book, ECG was obtained using the Octal Bio Amp module and Power Lab data acquisition system (ADInstruments, Inc., Colorado Springs, CO, USA).

Blood pressure was obtained intermittently using an automated oscillometric blood pressure monitor Welch Allyn CVSM 6400 Monitor (Skaneateles Falls, NY, USA) from arm and continuously using Finometer® (Finapress Medical Systems, Amsterdam, Netherlands). End tidal CO_2 was obtained using Nonin Respsense Capnograph (Nonin Medical Inc., Plymouth, MN, USA). A pulse oximeter (part of Welch Allyn monitor) was used to monitor the oxygen saturation. Cerebral blood flow velocity was monitored using a Transacranial Dopper systemMultiDop T (Multigon, New York, USA). Sudomotor testing was done using the Q - Sweat device (measures QSART) made by WR Medical Electronics Co (Stillwater, MN, USA) and Sudoscan device (measures ESC, Impeto Medical, Paris, France). For skin biopsies, we used biopsy kits with 3 mm circular punch blade and fixatives provided by Therapath (New York, USA).

DATA ACQUISITION SYSTEM

The data were recored using PowerLab 16/35 data acquisition system controlled by LabChart 8 software with ECG analysis, heart rate variability and blood pressure modules (ADInstruments, Inc., Colorado Springs, CO, USA). The recorded data were then exported to a proprietary graphic library written in Matlab programming language for generation of artwork. (MathWorks, Natick, MA, USA).

REFERENCES

1. Novak P. Quantitative autonomic testing. *J Vis Exp JoVE*. 2011;(53). doi:10.3791/2502.
2. Novak V, Novak P, Schondorf R. Accuracy of beat-to-beat noninvasive measurement of finger arterial pressure using the Finapres: a spectral analysis approach. *J Clin Monit*. 1994;10(2):118–126.
3. Lakhal K, Martin M, Faiz S, et al. The CNAP™ finger cuff for noninvasive beat-to-beat monitoring of arterial blood pressure: an evaluation in intensive care unit patients and a comparison with 2 intermittent devices. *Anesth Analg*. 2016;123(5):1126–1135. doi:10.1213/ANE.0000000000001324.

4.

AUTONOMIC TESTS

INTRODUCTION

Historically, autonomic tests have been focused on the cardiovascular and sudomotor systems.[1–3] Established cardiovascular reflex function tests are heart rate variability during paced deep breathing, the Valsalva maneuver, and the tilt test. The deep breathing test measures parasympathetic innervation to the heart. The Valsalva maneuver and tilt test measure predominantly sympathetic function and peripheral vasoconstriction in response to straining and orthostatic challenge. Newer tests include skin biopsies for evaluation of sensory and sweat gland fibers and evaluation of cerebral blood flow using transcranial Doppler.[4]

Sudomotor functions can be evaluated by the quantitative sudomotor axon test (QSART) and electrochemical skin conductance (ESC). Direct methods for evaluation of small nerve fiber damage include skin biopsy for evaluation of sensory fibers using epidermal nerve fiber density (ENFD) and for evaluation of sudomotor fibers using sweat gland nerve fiber density (SGNFD).

PREPARATION FOR AUTONOMIC TESTS

Patients should refrain from smoking and eating for at least 3 hours before the testing. They should avoid caffeinated beverages for several hours before testing. Alcoholic beverages should be avoided altogether on the day of testing.

INTERFERENCE OF CONCOMITANT MEDICATION WITH AUTONOMIC TESTING

Commonly used medications with cardiovascular effects or sudomotor effects may interfere with autonomic testing (e.g., antihypertensive medications including beta-blockers, acetylcholinesterase inhibitors, calcium channel blockers, diuretics, and nitrates). These medications should not be used at least 24 hours before the autonomic testing. Furthermore, anticholinergic medication may interfere with sudomotor testing. Typically, anticholinergic drugs (e.g., tricyclic antidepressants) have long half-lives and should be discontinued several days before testing. Pressor medications (pyridostigmine, ProAmatine, and droxidopa) have short half-lives and should not be used the day of testing. Fludrocortisone has long biological half-life, up 36 hours, and therefore should not be used at least 2 days before testing. It is important to review medication side-effects before scheduling autonomic testing.

Discontinuation of many medications can be either impractical or unsafe. Autonomic testing still can be done while patients are taking medications that affect the autonomic nervous system, but it is important to understand the effects of medication and to discount that effect when interpreting results. It is important to realize that commonly used medications are a common cause of autonomic failure in the elderly.

DEEP BREATHING

Deep breathing is a simple yet important test to evaluate cardiac parasympathetic functions mediated mainly by the vagal nerve.[2,5,6] The test is easy to perform, but requires patient cooperation.

PHYSIOLOGY

The deep breathing test is performed at a breathing frequency of 0.1 Hz (6 breaths per minute) to achieve maximal respiratory variation of heart rate (formerly called *respiratory sinus arrhythmia* [RSA]). During the deep breathing test, inhalation increases and exhalation decreases heart rate. The difference between heart rate maximum during inhalation and minimum during exhalation is used as a measure of parasympathetic modulation to the heart.

The neuronal circuits generating RSA include a central RSA generator in the brainstem and peripheral circuits (Figure 4.1). Afferent inputs are primarily from pulmonary stretch receptors and baroreceptors in the aortic arc and in the carotid body. Lung inflation stimulates pulmonary stretch receptors, which activate the nucleus tractus solitarius (NTS) via the vagus nerve. The NTS synapses to the cardioinhibitory nucleus ambiguus that innervates the heart. Increased activity in the NTS activates the

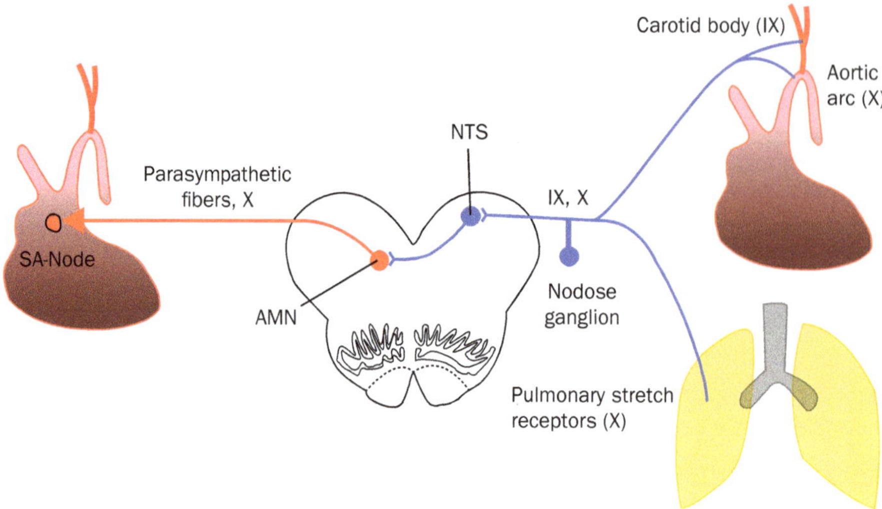

Figure 4.1 Neuronal circuits of deep breathing. Inhalation results in stretching and activation of baroreceptors in the carotid body, aortic arc and lungs. The lungs in turn activate the NTS which also actives the AMN. AMN is cardioinhibitory, its activation results in parasympathetic withdrawal and increasing of the heart rate. Exhalation has opposite effects and the heart rate decreases. AMN, the ambiguous nucleus, NTS, the nucleus tractus solitarius; SA, sinoatrial node.

nucleus ambiguus. The vagal nerve's cardioinhibitory activity decreases during inspiration and increases during exhalation.

TECHNIQUE

The test is performed in the supine position. Deep breathing is usually performed as the first autonomic test, and therefore the subject should be given an adequate time to relax. This will minimize the effect of anxiety or recent physical activity that can interfere with the testing. It is customary to wait at least 3–5 minutes in addition to time spent for the montage of electrodes before starting the deep breathing test. We usually record at least a 1-minute baseline before proceeding with the deep breathing test.

The patient is instructed breathe at 0.1 Hz frequency, with an inhalation and exhalation of 5 seconds each. Six breathing cycles are typically performed. The patient should breathe continuously and regularly through the nose, with the mouth closed. The respiratory movement trace should resemble a wave. Sudden inhalations/exhalations, breath holding, and hyperventilation should be avoided. The end tidal CO_2 should be monitored to rule out hyperventilation. Figure 4.2.A–C shows a normal (A), moderately abnormal (B), and severely reduced (C) heart rate variability responses to deep breathing.

Mean heart rate should be stable and not to trend up and down during the baseline period. If the heart rate is trending in either direction, then wait until the mean heart rate remains stable. The normal end tidal CO_2 range is 35–45 mm Hg. The patient should not hyperventilate. The deep breathing test can be executed even if end tidal CO_2 is abnormal, but the CO_2 levels need to be accounted for during test interpretation. End tidal CO_2 has a profound effect on cerebral blood flow and may influence the results of autonomic testing.

The amplitude of RSA is defined as the difference in heart rate between the end of inspiration and end of expiration. Typically, six respiratory cycles are identified and the respective RSA amplitudes are averaged (Figure 4.3). The normative data of heart rate variation show a decline with age (Table 4.1) but are not affected by gender. RSA amplitude decreases with age by 3–5 beats per minute per decade. RSA also depends on resting heart rate. Hypocapnia due to hyperventilation and increased sympathetic outflow reduces the RSA amplitude and may increase baseline heart rate. Low limits of normal values are shown in Table 4.1.

INTERPRETATION OF DEEP BREATHING TEST

RSA reflects primarily cardiovagal parasympathetic function. The test results are reported as normal or abnormal (Figure 4.2.A–C). Abnormal results are usually divided into mild, moderate, or severe. Grading of abnormalities is described below. An abnormal deep breathing test can be seen with early polyneuropathy when other tests are still normal. However, the deep breathing test is nonspecific and cannot distinguish, for example, diabetic neuropathy from the cardiovagal failure seen in Parkinson disease or multiple system atrophy.

LIMITATION OF THE TEST

Several systemic conditions may affect deep breathing test results. RSA can decrease due to chronic pulmonary,

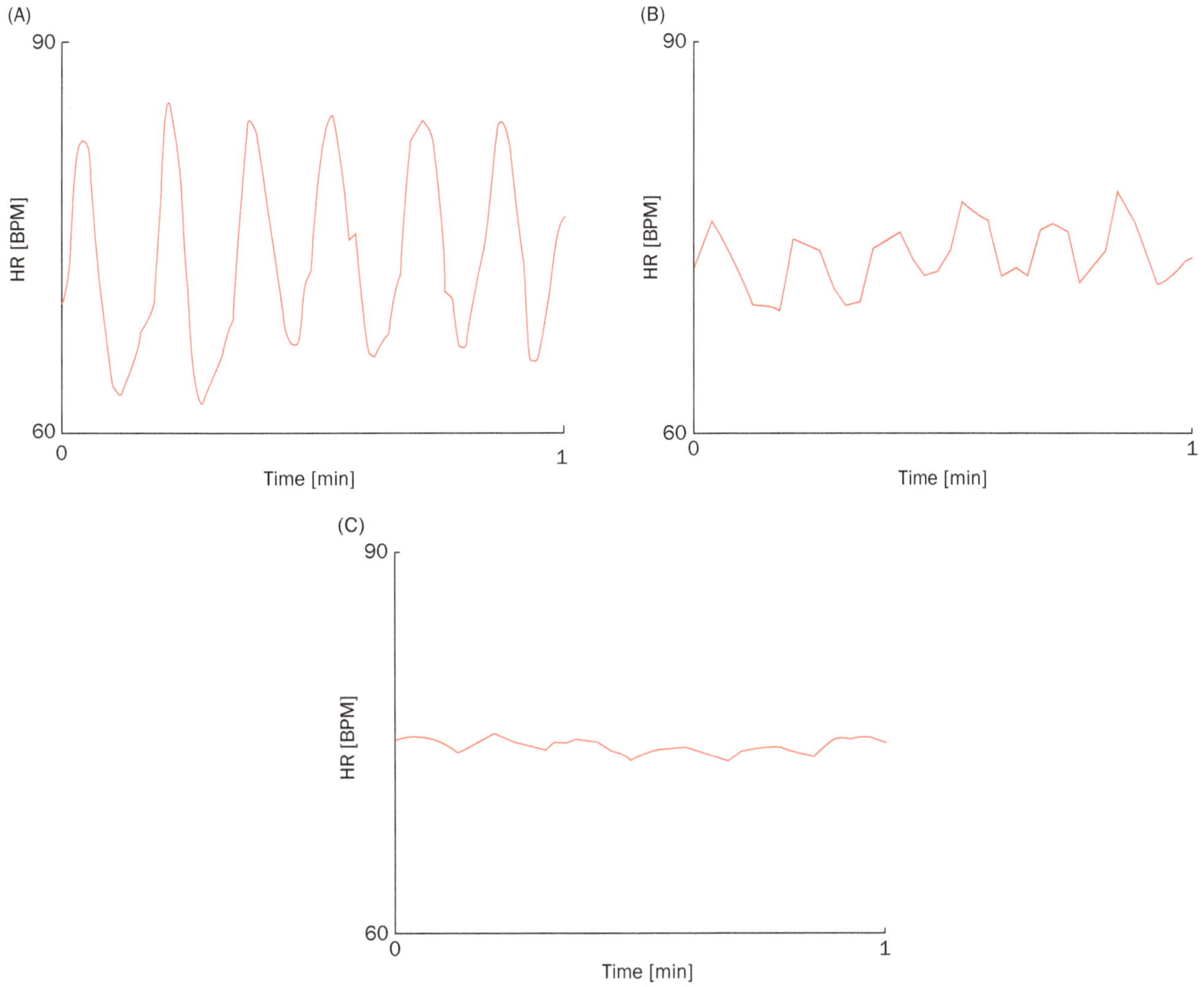

Figure 4.2 Examples of normal deep breathing test results (A, 23 y/o man, RSA= 19.2, normal ≥14 BPM), moderate abnormality (B, 36 y/o woman, RSA=6.3, normal ≥12 BPM) and severe abnormality (C, 76 y/o woman, RSA=1.2, normal ≥7 BPM).

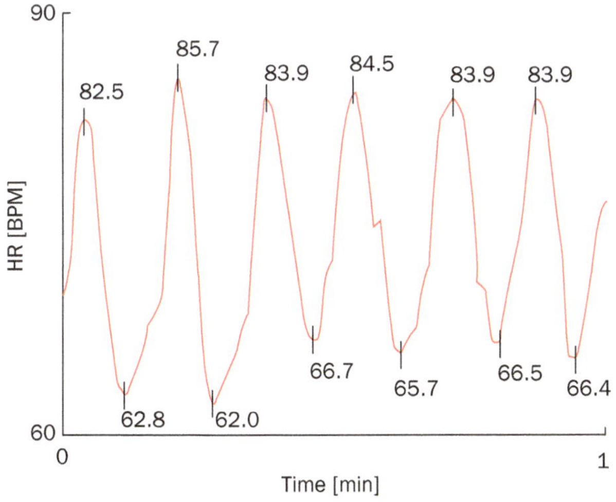

Figure 4.3 Calculation of RSA amplitude. The average RSA amplitude is equal to 19.2 BPM which was obtained by subtracting the minimum from the maximum heart rate for each breathing cycle ((82.5–62.8) + (85.7–62) + (83.9–66.7) + (84.5–65.7) + (83.9–66.5) + (83.9–65.4))/6.

TABLE 4.1 NORMATIVE DATA FOR DEEP BREATHING TEST

Age (years)	Minimum of normal RSA (beats/min)
10–29	14
30–39	12
40–49	10
50–59	9
60–69	7

RSA, average amplitude of the respiratory sinus arrhythmia.

vascular, cardiac, and connective tissue disorders. The deep breathing test requires patient cooperation that might be difficult to achieve in very old or frail patients. Several factors limit interpretation of the deep breathing test. Patients with certain cardiac arrhythmias and pacemaker cannot be evaluated since their heart rate does not accurately reflect vagal function. Medication also may affect the results. Hyperventilation should be avoided. The best technique to exclude hyperventilation is to measure the end tidal CO_2. The test also requires sophisticated software for proper detection of R-waves and proper removal of ectopic beats. A working knowledge of basic ECG patterns is desirable.

VALSALVA MANEUVER

The Valsalva maneuver is a noninvasive test used for evaluations of sympathetic functions.[2,5,7,8] The Valsalva maneuver is perhaps the most sensitive test for detection of sympathetic adrenergic failure.[7]

PHYSIOLOGY

The Valsalva maneuver is defined as forced expiration against a resistance. Neuronal circuits mediating the effects of the Valsalva maneuver are the same as baroreflex circuits (Figure 4.4).[9] In a healthy subject, the Valsalva maneuver evokes a characteristic response in heart rate and blood pressure (Figure 4.5).

The normal Valsalva maneuver has four phases (Figure 4.5–4.6).[10]

Phase 1 is mechanical. Transient elevation of blood pressure during Phase 1 is mainly caused by compression of the aorta with passive transmission of the elevated intrathoracic pressure into the peripheral circulation, an increased stroke volume, and reduced afterload. Phase 1 starts at the onset of the initial deeper breath causing the breathing artifact. Phase 1 duration is about 2–4 seconds.

Phase 2 starts when the expiratory pressure reaches 40 mm Hg and continues for 15 seconds. The blood pressure falls during the early Phase 2. This is caused by reductions in the left atrial and left ventricular dimensions and a decline in stroke volume and cardiac output due to reduced venous return. Blood pressure fall activates sympathetic vasomotor nerves that increase the peripheral resistance. In the late Phase 2, blood pressure then begins to raise, and this response depends on the degree of sympathetic activation. In healthy subjects, blood pressure recovers back to or above the baseline. In sympathetic failure, blood pressure recovery is reduced or absent.

Phase 3 is mechanical. This phase starts with inspiration that releases the strain. Blood pressure falls during Phase 3 due to the release of the expiratory pressure and a related increase in left ventricular afterload and a sudden

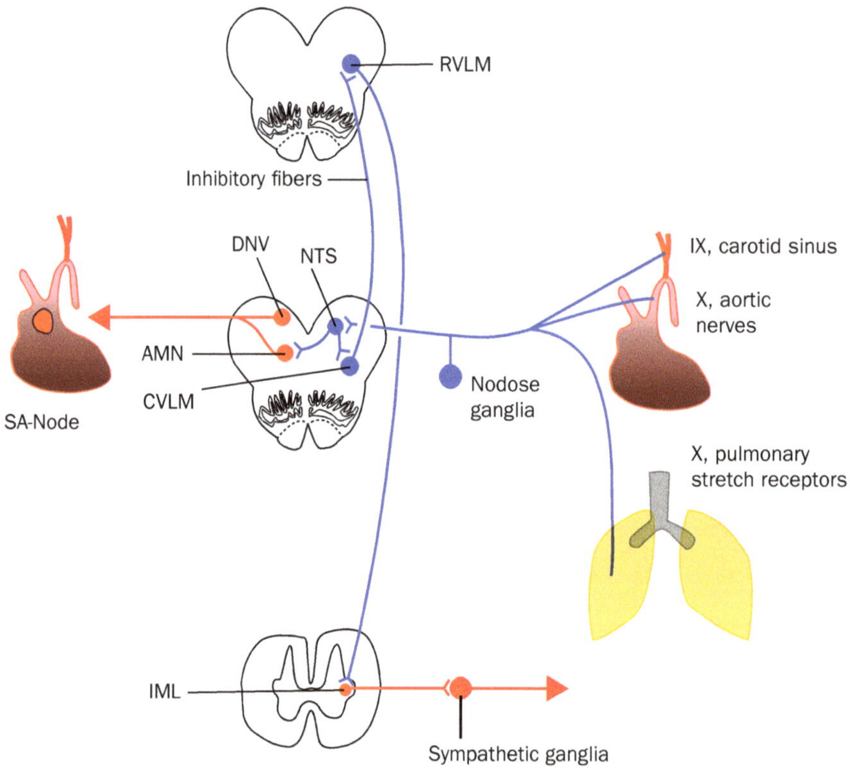

Figure 4.4 Neuronal circuits mediating responses to the Valsalva maneuver are identical to the baroreflex circuits (Fig. 2.7). AMN= the ambiguous nucleus, NTS=the nucleus of the solitary tract, CVLM=the caudal ventrolateral medulla, RVLM= the rostral ventrolateral medulla, IML= the intermediolateral column.

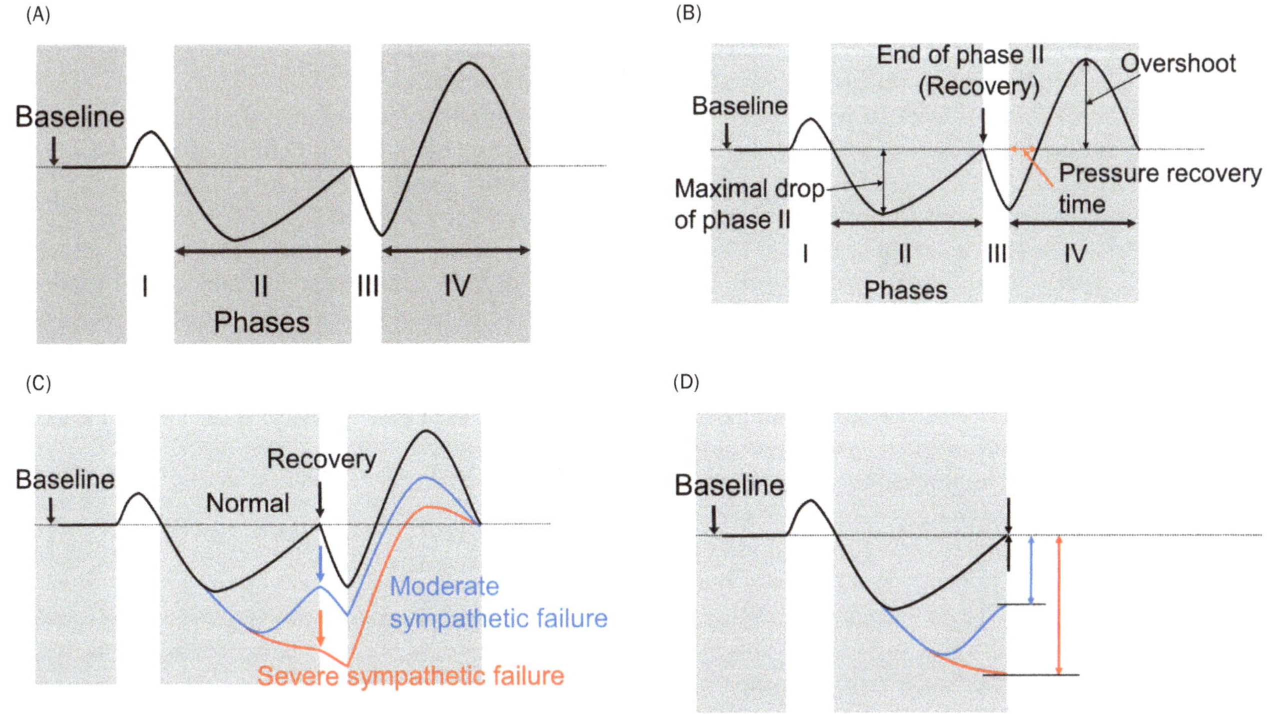

Figure 4.5 The profile of the Valsalva maneuver in mean blood pressure. Valsalva maneuver has four phases (A): Phase I – mechanical, Phase II – straining, Phase III mechanical, Phase IV – recovery. The most important blood pressure response is the recovery at the end of Phase II (B). In healthy subjects, mean blood pressure at the end of Phase II reaches or exceeds the baseline ("recovery"). With graded sympathetic adrenergic failure, there is a progressive reduction of blood pressure recovery (C, D). The recovery of blood pressure is absent in severe sympathetic failure. Panel D shows how to calculate the end of Phase II.

expansion of intrathoracic vessels. The duration of Phase 3 is about 2–3 seconds.

Phase 4 is "the overshoot." Blood pressure rises during Phase 4 is due to persistent vasoconstriction that started during Phase 2. The duration of Phase 4 is about 10–20 seconds.

TECHNIQUE

The Valsalva maneuver is usually performed in the supine position. In our protocol, the target expiratory pressure is 40 mm Hg for 15 seconds. Patients performing the Valsalva maneuver should be given a feedback to

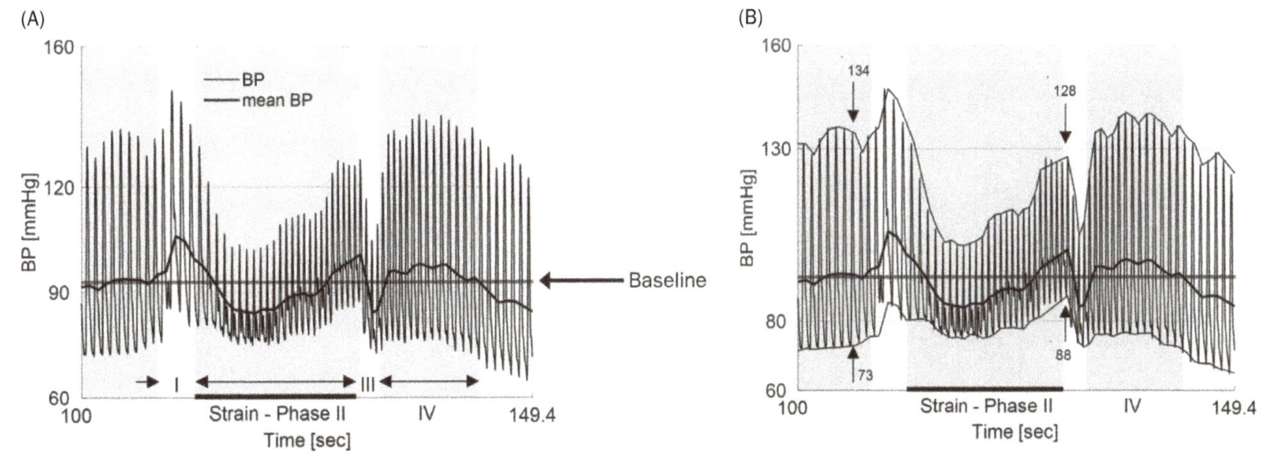

Figure 4.6 Phases of normal Valsalva maneuver in beat-to-beat blood (A) and extraction of values for the analysis (B). The baseline is equal to mean blood pressure just before the Phase I. Phase 2 ends with the end of strain. For analysis we use systolic and diastolic values obtained at the baseline (134/73 mmHg) and at the end of Phase 2 (128/88 mmHg). The systolic/diastolic values are preferable over the mean blood pressure, which is a derived measure. The errors in automatic detection of systolic/diastolic values would be magnified in mean blood pressure calculations. The mean blood pressure is used to grade severity of abnormal results.

assure correct technique. Expiratory pressure should be measured. A convenient way to measure the expiratory pressure is to connect the tonometer to a 5–10 mL plastic syringe and ask the subject to blow into the syringe. A small air leak in the tubing prevents closing of the glottis.

In healthy people, blood pressure decline during Phase 2 is short, about 7 seconds minimum, from the beginning of Phase 2. This local minimum separates early Phase 2 from the late Phase 2. In more advanced sympathetic failure (Figure 4.7–4.8), blood pressure continues to decline, thus shifting the local minimum in blood pressure toward the end of the Phase 2. In severe sympathetic failure, the local minimum in blood pressure is shifted to the end of Phase 2 as blood pressure continues to fall without recovery. In our laboratory, location of minimal blood pressure during Phase 2 is obtained from diastolic blood pressure. Lower peripheral resistance may reduce the recovery at the end of Phase 2. Figure 4.7 shows the Valsalva maneuver in a healthy control (A) and in subjects with mild (B), moderate (C), and severe (D) sympathetic failure. The Valsalva maneuver is performed three times (Figure 4.9), and the most representative tracing is chosen for the final analysis.

A variant of the Valsalva maneuver is a square wave response (Figure 4.10). This is defined as a response where blood pressure remains above the baseline during Phase 2. The square wave response can be seen in healthy subjects and also in subjects with congestive heart failure. Tilting up to 30 degrees may change the square wave variant to the usual four-phase pattern. The Valsalva maneuver in hyperadrenergic state, such as in hyperadrenergic variant of postural tachycardia syndrome, may show markedly elevated Phase 4, the Phase 2 may be below or above the baseline (Figure 4.11).

CEREBRAL BLOOD FLOW MONITORING IN VALSALVA MANEUVER

Cerebral blood flow monitoring using transcranial Doppler ultrasound is a new feature of autonomic testing that enables assessment of cerebral autoregulation

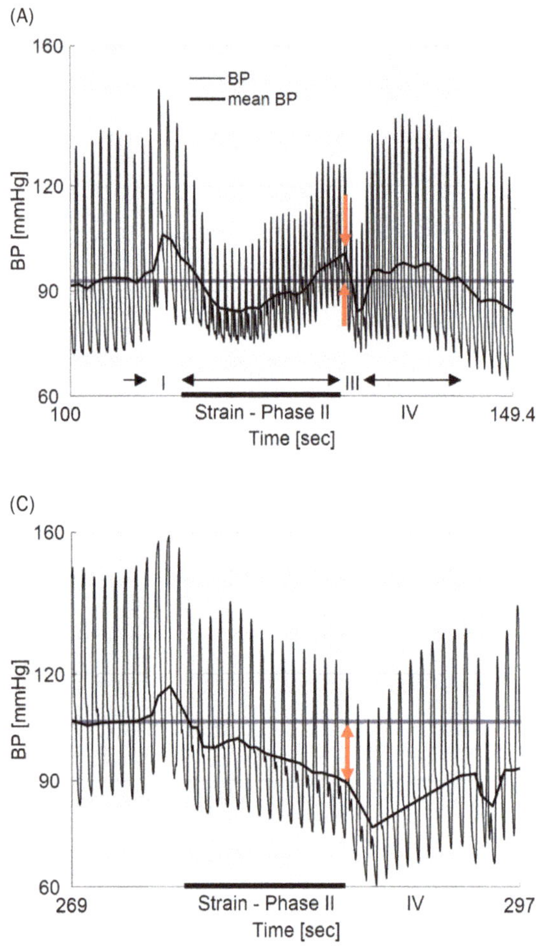

Figure 4.7 Valsalva maneuver in a normal person (A) and in a subject with mild (B), moderate (C) and severe (D) sympathetic failure. Note the y scale in panel D ranges 20–160 mmHg.

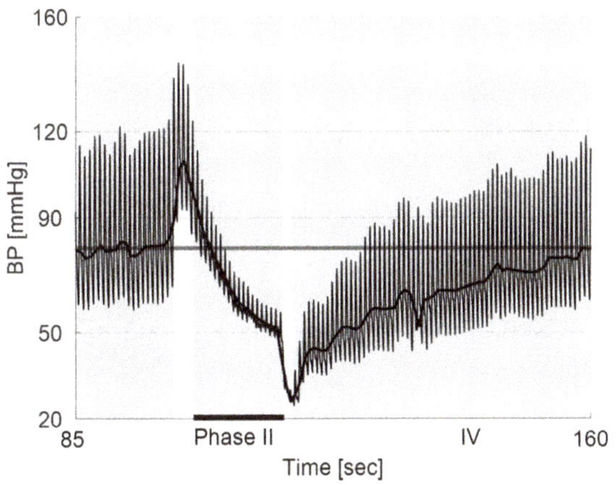

Figure 4.8 The Valsalva maneuver in severe sympathetic adrenergic failure. The recovery at the Phase II is absent. It took 46 seconds till the mean blood pressure returned to baseline.

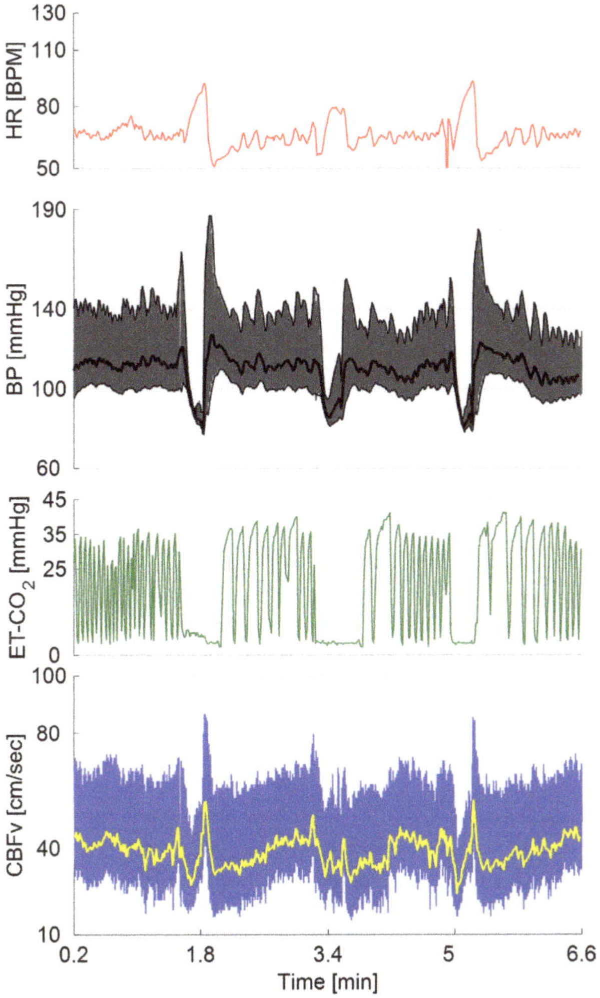

Figure 4.9 Examples of Valsalva maneuvers. Three Valsalva maneuvers are usually done by each patient to assess reproducibility. The first and third maneuvers looks similar, the second maneuver is associated with reduced Phase IV in both blood pressure and cerebral blood flow velocity. The third Valsalva maneuver was chosen for the analysis.

in response to blood pressure variations during the Valsalva maneuver.[4,8] Cerebral blood flow velocity (CBFv) is measured from the middle cerebral artery that is insonated from the temporal window using a 1.6–2 MHz probe at a depth of 35–55 mm. It is important to stabilize the probe using a 3-D holder in order to achieve recordings of good quality. A typical CBFv profile has four phases, similar to a blood pressure profile (Figure 4.12). All three CBFv signals (systolic, mean, and diastolic) are needed for the analysis. Figure 4.13 is an example of normal CBFv response, showing a decline during Phase 2, recovery in the late Phase 2 when CBFv exceeds baseline, and an overshoot during Phase 4 (Table 4.3).

Patterns of CBFv during the Valsalva maneuver can differentiate between normal and abnormal cerebrovascular responses. Figure 4.14 illustrates a mildly abnormal Valsalva maneuver in both blood pressure and normal CBFv response, indicating normal autoregulation. Figure 4.15 is an example of a moderately abnormal Valsalva maneuver where both blood pressure and CBFv failed to return to the baseline at the end of Phase 2. Figure 4.16 is an example of a severely abnormal Valsalva maneuver, where both blood pressure and CBFv are markedly reduced during Phase 2. Figures 4.17–4.19 further illustrate the usefulness of CBFv monitoring during the Valsalva maneuver, as well as the reproducibility of blood flow responses.

INTERPRETATION OF VALSALVA MANEUVER

The Valsalva maneuver provides an index of sympathetic functions. Several indexes have been defined (Table 4.2). The adrenergic sympathetic index that is based on blood pressure changes at the end of Phase 2 was found superior to other indexes.[7] Mean blood pressure at the end of Phase 2 "recovers" in healthy controls and reaches or exceeds the baseline (Figure 4.2). In sympathetic failure, blood pressure does not reach baseline at the end of Phase 2. The grading of sympathetic failure is described below. Severe pulse pressure collapse can be seen in hypovolemia. Pressure recovery time can also be prolonged in sympathetic failure.[11]

Historically, the *Valsalva ratio* was used also as an index of parasympathetic functions. The Valsalva ratio is defined as the ratio between the fastest and shortest heart rate during the Valsalva maneuver. However, the Valsalva ratio is not widely used since it does not take into account the underlying blood pressure response.[12]

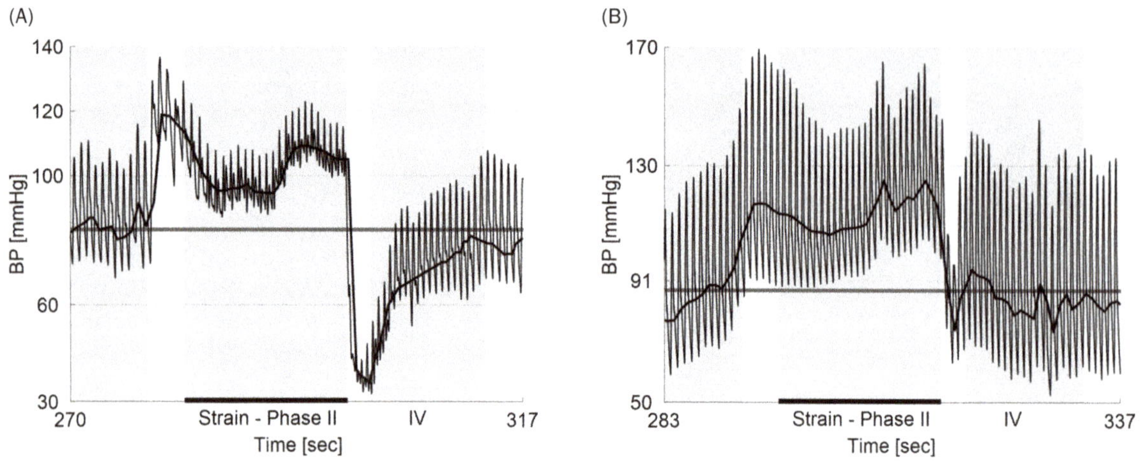

Figure 4.10 The square wave variants of Valsalva maneuver (A–B). Blood pressure during Phase II is above the baseline.

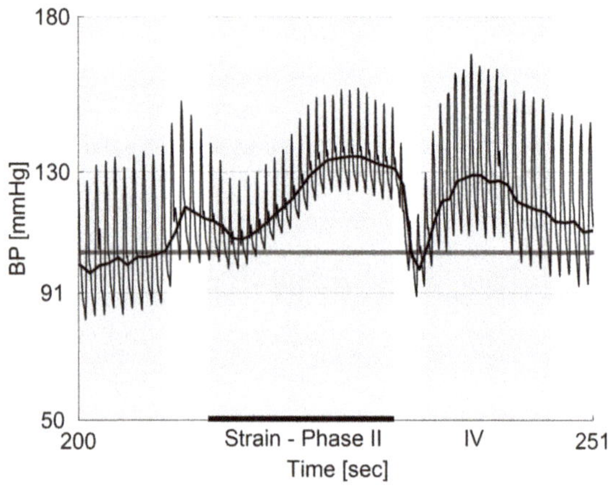

Figure 4.11 Profile of Valsalva maneuver in hyperadrenergic state. Blood pressure is noticeably elevated at the end of Phase II and Phase IV. This patterrn can be seen in hypertension or in postural tachycardia syndrome where particularly phase IV can be markedly elevated.

LIMITATIONS OF VALSALVA MANEUVER

The Valsalva maneuver requires considerable subject cooperation. It also assumes certain level of physical fitness, and many elderly or sicker people and children cannot perform the Valsalva maneuver correctly either because of inability to develop the adequate pressure or hold it for the required time. A square wave variant of the Valsalva maneuver precludes analysis of sympathetic functions. Partial square wave response can mimic normal response in sympathetic failure. At present, there are no criteria on how to differentiate the partial square wave response. The Valsalva ratio, although used as a parasympathetic marker, also depends on sympathetic influences.

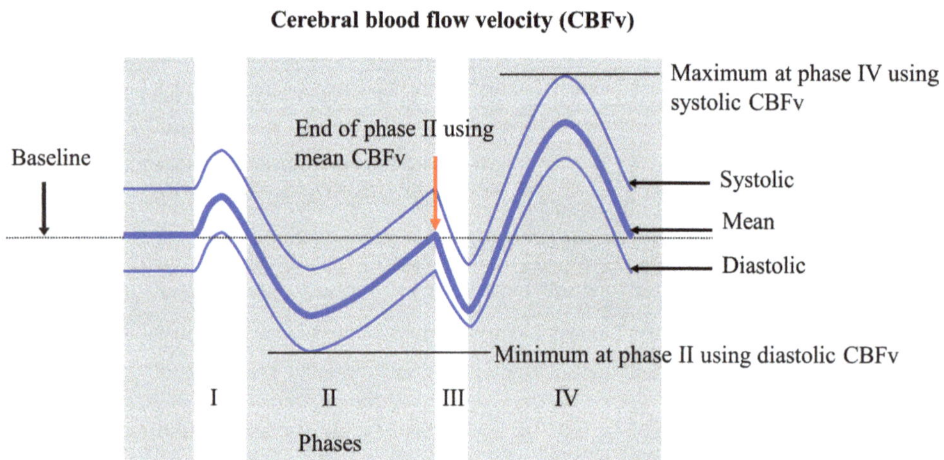

Figure 4.12 Principles of evaluation of the Valsalva maneuver using cerebral blood flow velocity. All three signals (systolic, mean and diastolic) are needed for the analysis.

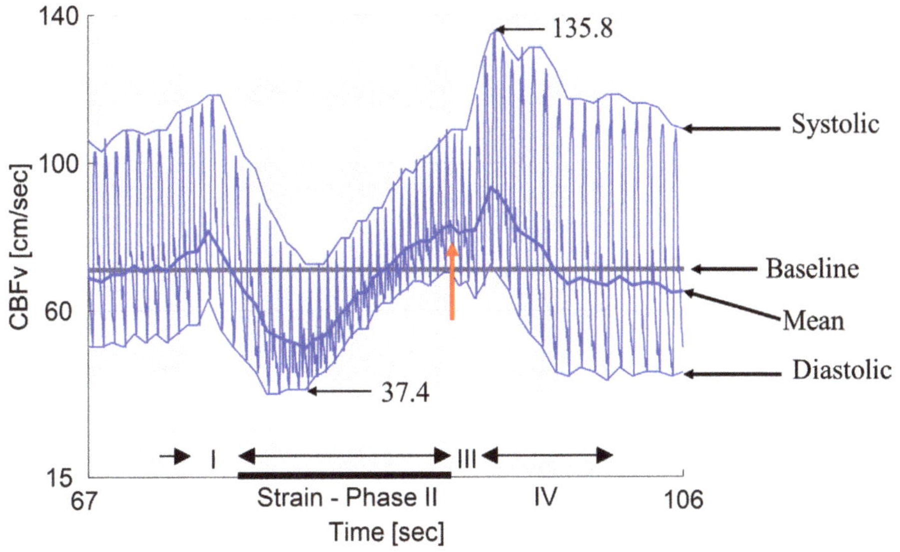

Figure 4.13 An example of normal cerebral blood flow velocity (CBFv) during the Valsalva maneuver. The mean CBFv exceeds the baseline (red arrow).

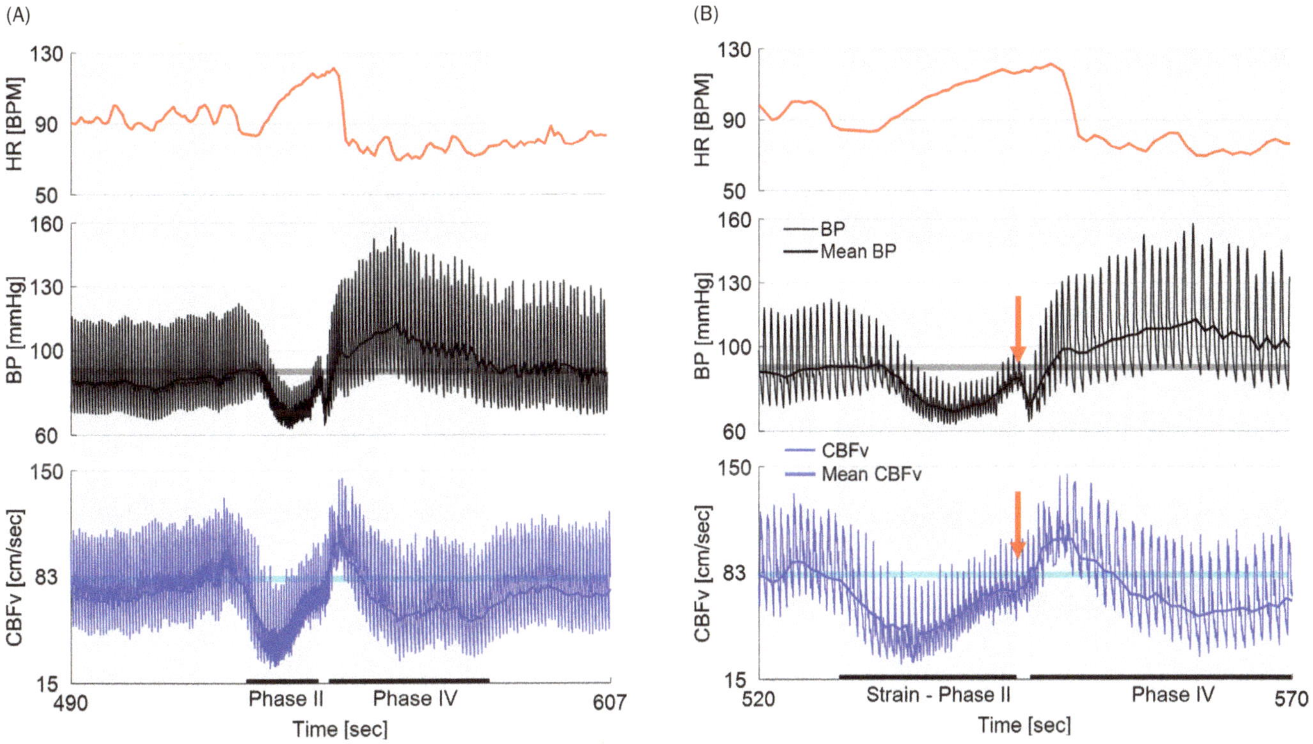

Figure 4.14 An example of mildly abnormal Valsalva maneuver in both blood pressure and cerebral blood flow velocity (CBFv). Magnified Valsalva maneuver (B).

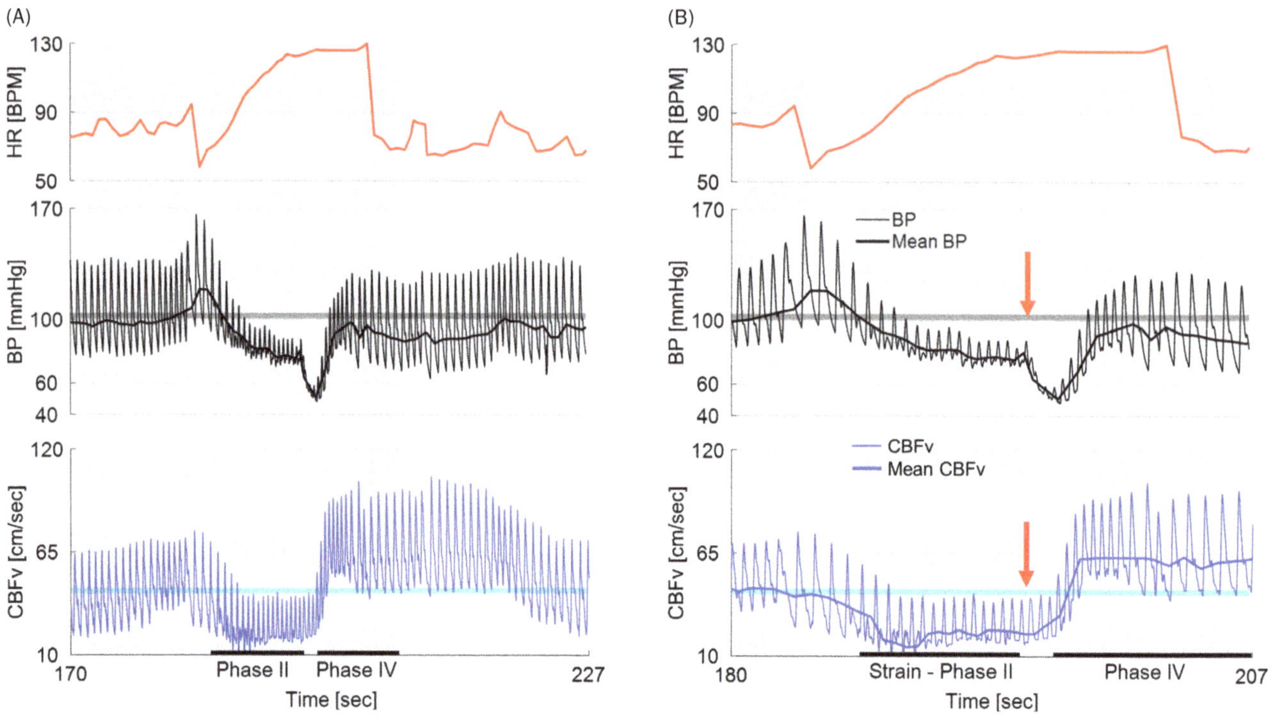

Figure 4.15 An example of moderately abnormal Valsalva maneuver. Both blood pressure and cerebral blood flow velocity failed to return to the baseline at the end of Phase II.

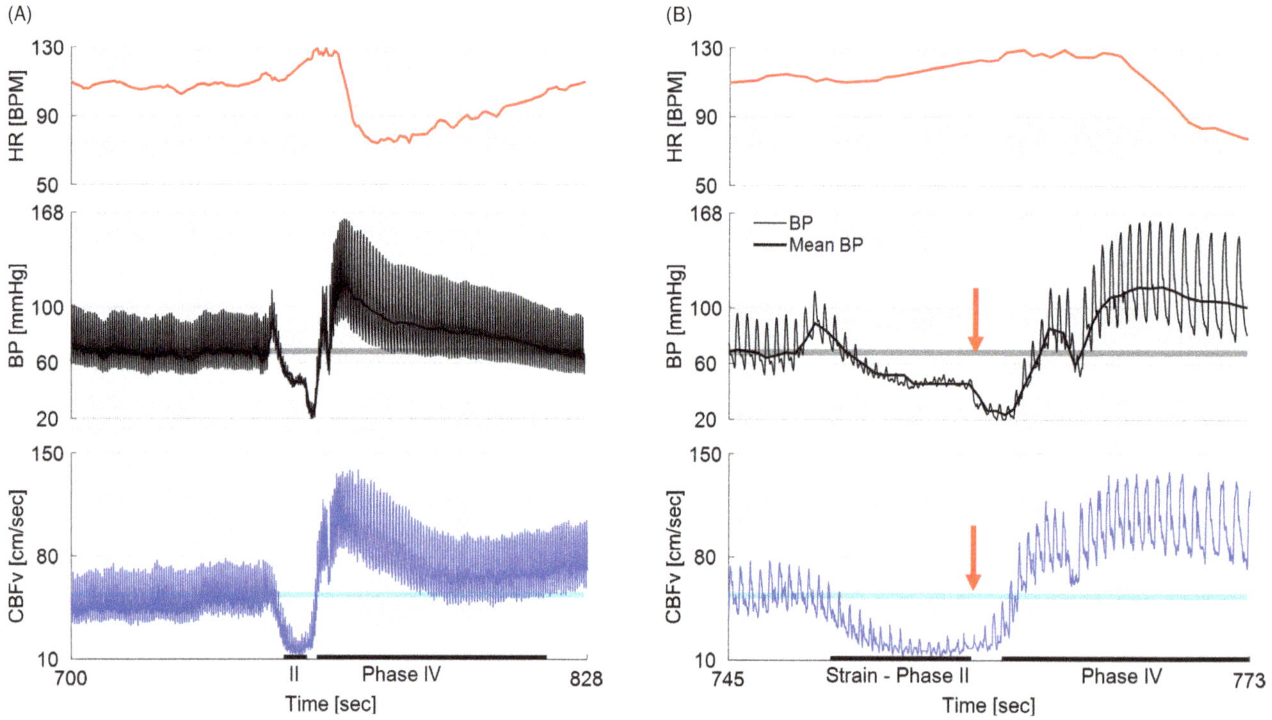

Figure 4.16 An example of severely abnormal Valsalva maneuver. Both blood pressure and cerebral blood flow velocities are markedly reduced during the Phase II.

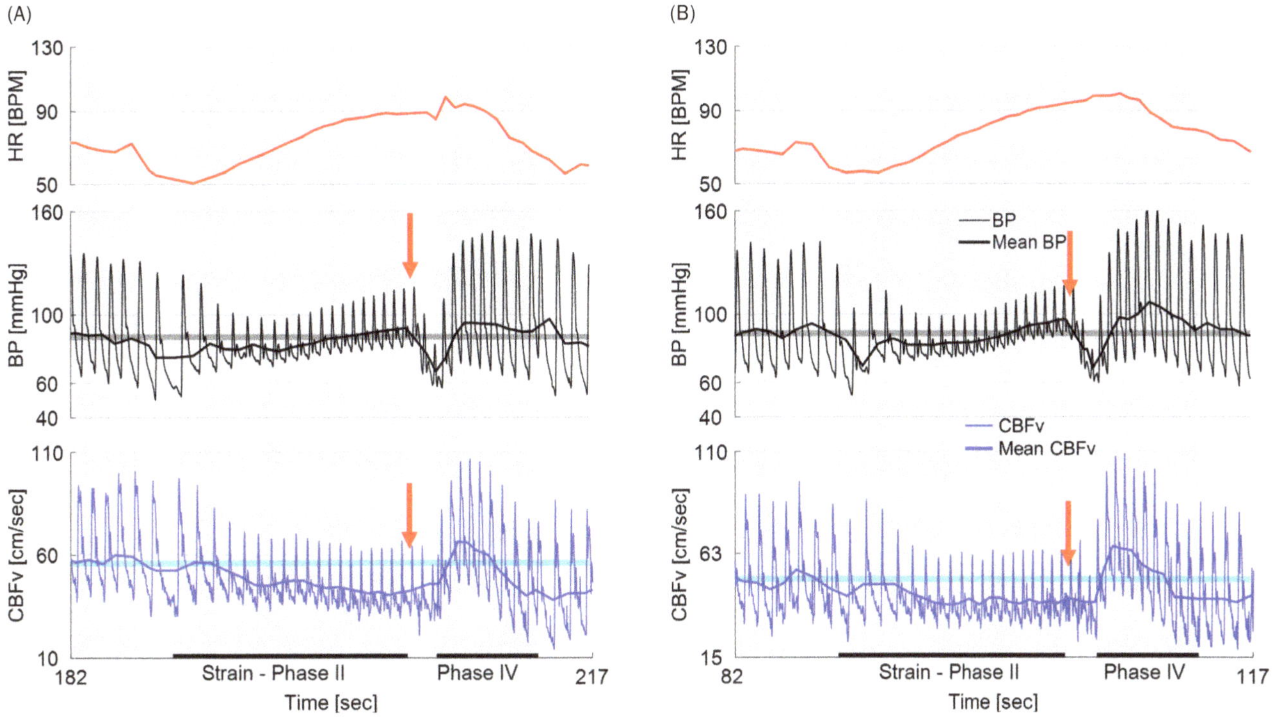

Figure 4.17 Two successive Valsalva maneuvers form the same person. Both maneuvers show normal blood pressure responses (end of Phase II exceeds baseline, red arrow) but abnormal cerebral blood flow velocity responses (end of Phase II is below the baseline). Both maneuvers look very similar which is consistent with high reproducibility of Valsalva maneuvers when done correctly.

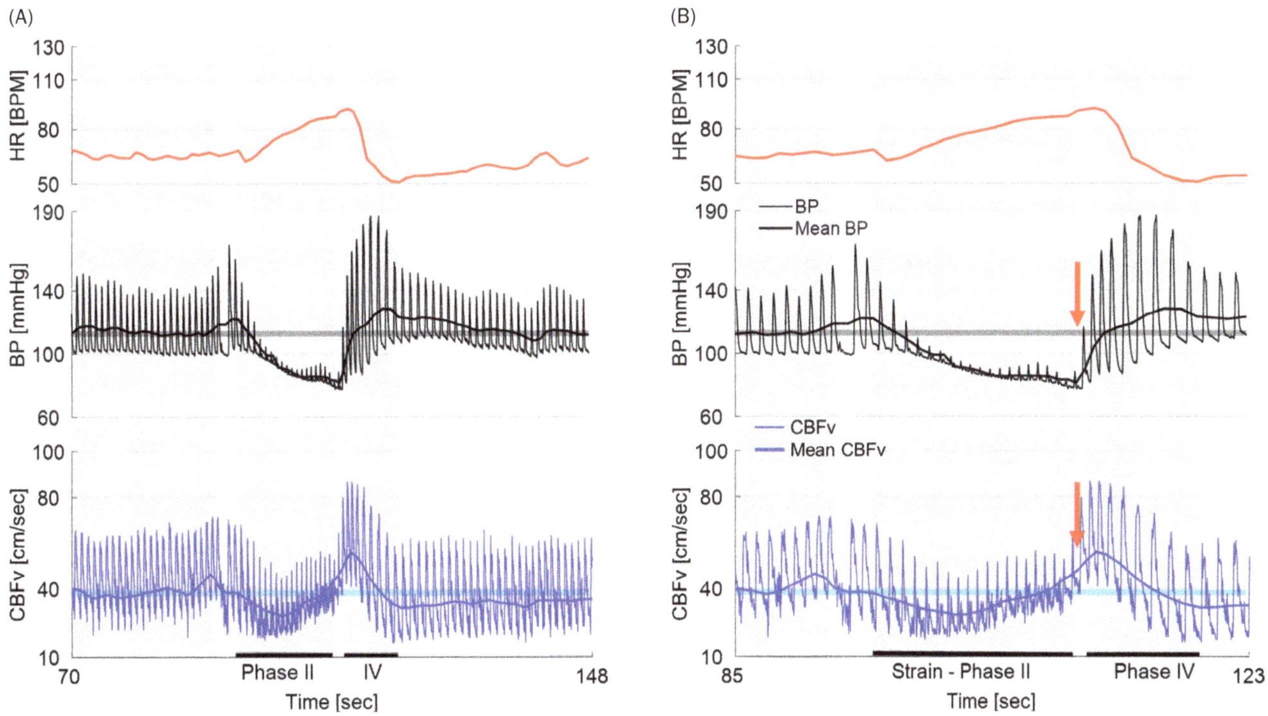

Figure 4.18 Blood pressure responses to Valsalva maneuver are abnormal (end of Phase II is below the baseline, red arrow) but the cerebral blood flow velocity responses are normal (end of Phase II exceeds the baseline, blue arrow).

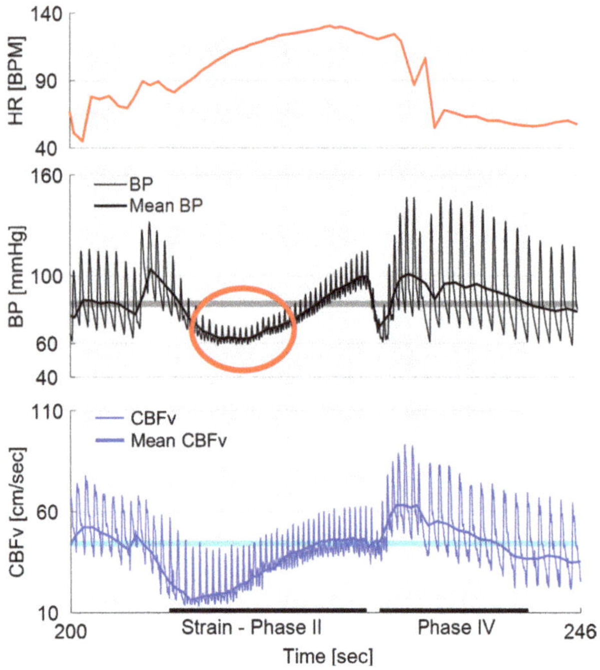

Figure 4.19 This Valsalva maneuver shows pulse pressure collapse (difference between systolic and diastolic blood pressure, red oval) which is consistent with hypovolemia. Blood pressure increase at the end of Phase II exceeds baseline. This is a normal response that indicates normal adrenergic function. Cerebral blood flow velocity (CBFv) was extremely low during the Phase II (diastolic CBFv close to 10 cm/s) that is typically seen in severe cerebral hypoperfusion. Indeed, patient became encephalopathic during the Phase II.

TABLE 4.2 BLOOD PRESSURE PARAMETERS OBTAINED FROM VALSALVA MANEUVER

Parameter	Comments
Mean blood pressure at the end of Phase 2, "recovery"	The end of Phase 2 ≥ the baseline in normal controls
Drop in mean blood pressure during Phase 2	Early Phase 2 drop reduction <40 >25 mm Hg indicate mild sympathetic failure
Pulse pressure reduction during Phase 2	Normal response is ≤50% of baseline
Pressure recovery time (PRT)	PRT is defined as the time for the systolic blood pressure to return to baseline during Phase 4. Normal PRT is <4 seconds.
Phase 4	Absent Phase 4 is seen in severe sympathetic failure

TABLE 4.3 CEREBRAL BLOOD FLOW VELOCITY (CBFV) PARAMETERS OBTAINED FROM VALSALVA MANEUVER

Parameter	Comments
Mean CBFv at the end of Phase 2	The end of Phase 2 ≥ the baseline in normal controls
Minimum in diastolic CBFv during Phase 2	The normal value is >20 cm/s
Maximum in systolic CBFv during Phase 4	Normal response is <190 cm/s

TILT TEST

The head-up tilt is one of the most important tools for evaluation of autonomic functions. It is particularly useful in the diagnosis of orthostatic intolerance. Tilting to upright position provokes blood pooling in the splanchnic and lower extremity circulation, which triggers the neural and humoral compensatory mechanisms aiming to maintain stable blood pressure and cerebral perfusion.[13] The tilt test assesses the integrity of parasympathetic and sympathetic innervation. The tilt test was initially introduced to diagnose vasovagal syncope.[14] Since then, the diagnostic utility of the tilt test has been expanded for diagnosis of orthostatic hypotension, autonomic failure, postural tachycardia syndrome, and other forms of orthostatic intolerance.[15]

The test stimulates the autonomic nervous system with orthostatic stress induced by passive movement from a supine position to an upright tilt in a controlled laboratory setting. Typically, respiratory movement, blood pressure, and heart rate are recorded during the test. Additional variables which can be monitored include end tidal CO_2 and CBFv from the middle or other cerebral arteries. Under special circumstances, simultaneous electroencephalogram recordings may have clinical value. The testing requires special equipment and trained technicians.

PHYSIOLOGICAL BASIS OF TILT TESTING

Passive body movement from the supine to standing position induces pooling of venous blood (300–800 mL) in the splanchnic circulation, pelvis, and lower extremities venous system. Venous pooling decreases venous return to the heart. Compensatory mechanisms regulate cardiovascular and cerebrovascular response to maintain stable blood pressure and cerebral perfusion in the upright position. Compensatory responses are complex and include withdrawal of vagal tone, sympathetic activation, activation of the renin-angiotensin system, activation of the vasopressin system and muscle pumping in the legs, and cerebral autoregulation.

Upright tilt activates low-pressure atrial baroreceptors through the vagus nerve. This neural firing input is transmitted to nucleus tractus solitarius (NTS) that acts as an integration center. The NTS then directly and indirectly inhibits the dorsal motor nucleus of the vagus and excites the ventrolateral medulla that is a preganglionic sympathoexcitatory center. The net effect is parasympathetic (cardiovagal) withdrawal associated with increased heart rate and increased peripheral resistance via sympathetic vasomotor activation. The decrease of parasympathetic tone is followed by sympathetic activation that occurs within 30 seconds of the tilt. Elevated norepinephrine and vasopressin can be detected within a minute of tilt.

TILT TABLE TEST PROTOCOL

The tilt test is usually done after deep breathing and the Valsalva maneuver. Supine rest before the tilt should be at least 3–5 minutes, although 10 minutes of rest is preferable. The supine period serves to establish a baseline heart rate, blood pressure, and other parameters. The patient is tilted upright to an angle of 70 degrees. The duration of tilt table test depends on the question being studied. Five minutes is considered a minimum; our standard protocol uses a 10-minute tilt. The tilting may continue up 40 minutes or more if the tilt test does not provide explanatory results and there is strong clinical suspicion of autonomic impairment or orthostatic intolerance, particularly in younger subjects.

In a healthy subject, a typical response to tilt consists of a mild increase in heart rate, decrease in systolic blood pressure, increase in diastolic blood pressure, decrease in end tidal CO_2, and a decrease or no change in CBFv. Table 4.4 shows criteria for normal tilt response.

INTERPRETATION OF RESULTS

There are several cardiovascular and cerebrovascular patterns that can be detected using the tilt test.[3,15] Table 4.5 provides the criteria and description of common abnormal orthostatic patterns. However, many patterns may overlap. For example, syncope may occur with postural tachycardia syndrome (POTS). However, many patterns may overlap. For example, syncope may occur with POTS or orthostatic hypotension. Figures 4.20–4.26 illustrate typical orthostatic patterns such as a normal response (Figure 4.20), POTS (Figure 4.21), inappropriate sinus tachycardia (IST) (Figure 4.22), orthostatic cerebral hypoperfusion syndrome (OCHOS) (Figure 4.23), transient compensated orthostatic hypotension (Figure 4.24), sustained uncompensated orthostatic hypotension (Figure 4.25), and compensated orthostatic hypotension (Figure 4.26). These patterns are further discussed in subsequent case studies.

The tilt table test is easy to perform, requires minimal subject cooperation, and is very sensitive in revealing autonomic dysfunction, which are its main advantages. However, at the same time, it is the most complex test to interpret. The tilt test can facilitate the diagnosis of syncope, orthostatic hypotension, POTS, and abnormal cerebral autoregulation.

TABLE 4.4 **NORMAL RESPONSE TO TILT TEST**

Variable	Definition
Heart rate	Heart rate increment <30 and ≥10 beats per minute.
Blood pressure	[a]Systolic blood pressure <20 mm Hg or mean blood pressure <10 mm Hg [b]Systolic blood pressure ≤80% or mean blood pressure ≤85% of a supine baseline where the baseline = 100%
Decline in end tidal CO_2	≤3 mm Hg
Cerebral blood flow velocity	Abnormal decline in mean CBFv during tilt test is <90 % (1st minute), <89% (5th minute), and <85% (10th minute) of the supine baseline where the baseline is equal to 100%. For example if supine baseline is 100 cm/s (=100%) and the CBFv is 85 cm/s (=85%) at the first minute of the tilt, this is abnormal decline.

All definitions use supine baseline as a reference.

[a]Classic definition of orthostatic hypotension.

[b]QASAT definition of orthostatic hypotension.

SAFETY ISSUES

Tilt testing has high safety margin. During the tilt, the patients are continuously monitored for presence of shortness of breath, chest pain, and changes of consciousness in addition to changes in ECG or other measured cardiovascular parameters. A physician trained in autonomic testing should be readily available. Patients are attached to the table with a belt to avoid falls. In the case of loss of consciousness, the tilting should be aborted. Every member of the testing team should be familiar with life support procedures.

QUANTITATIVE SUDOMOTOR AXON REFLEX TEST

QSART evaluates the postganglionic sympathetic cholinergic functions.[16]

NEURONAL CIRCUITS

The principle of the QSART is based on the diluted acetylcholine stored in a capsule reservoir and transferred to the cholinergic terminals via iontophoresis to stimulate the sweat glands (Figure 4.27).

There are two types of sweat responses, spontaneous and evoked. The following applies for a Q-Sweat device made by WR Medical Electronics Co (Stillwater, MN). Larger capsules (sampling area 5.06 cm^2, volume 3.614 cm^3) are used for spontaneous responses and smaller capsules (sampling area 0.7871 cm^2, volume 0.1229 cm^3) are used for evoked responses. The typical electrical stimulation uses a 2 mA current for 5 minutes. Spontaneous sweat volume can be detected by other methods.

TECHNIQUE

Four standardized recording sites are typically used. Additional sites can be used if clinically justified, for example when evaluating complex regional pain syndrome.

TABLE 4.5 **TILT TEST PATTERNS**

Pattern	Definitions or description
Postural tachycardia syndrome (POTS)	Symptoms of OI + sustained (>30 seconds) heart rate increment ≥30 BPM during the tilt and heart rate exceeding 120 BPM
Inappropriate sinus tachycardia (IST)	Persistent or recurrent tachycardia (>100 BPM) during supine + heart rate increment (≥30 BPM) during tilt
Paroxysmal sinus tachycardia (PST)	Intermittent (<2 min) tachycardia (heart rate >100 BPM) + heart rate increment (≥30 BPM) during supine or tilt
Hypocapnic cerebral hypoperfusion (HYCH)	Reduced orthostatic CBFv due to reduced end tidal CO_2
Orthostatic cerebral hypoperfusion syndrome (OCHOS)	Reduced orthostatic CBFv with normal heart rate, blood pressure, and end tidal CO_2
Syncope	Systolic blood pressure <60 mm Hg and very low diastolic CBFv
Cardiovagal	Heart rate is <40 BPM during syncope
Vasodepressor	Heart rate is unchanged or increased during syncope
Mixed	Heart rate is decelerating before and/or during syncope but still above 40 BPM
Psychogenic pseudosyncope	Apparent loss of consciousness and normal cerebral blood flow
Orthostatic hypotension	Historical definition: 1. Decrease in systolic blood pressure ≥20 mm Hg or ≥10 mm Hg in diastolic blood pressure 2. QASAT definition (takes baseline into account): A relative drop to 80% and 85% in systolic and mean blood pressure, respectively, where supine baseline is 100% (Example: supine systolic blood pressure = 160 mm Hg, orthostatic blood pressure = 140 mm Hg A relative drop = 87.5% (= 140/160*100) = not OH)
Neurogenic	Associated with abnormal Valsalva maneuver and reduced heart rate response to the tilt
Nonneurogenic	Due volume depletion; typically associated with normal or exaggerated heart rate response to tilt and pulse pressure collapse (reduced difference between systolic and diastolic pressure) during the tilt and/or during Valsalva maneuver. Due medication effect
Transient	Blood pressure recovers during the tilt
Progressive	A progressive decline in blood pressure during the tilt; may result in syncope
Persistent	Constant but not progressing OH
Compensated	CBFv stable in spite of OH
Uncompensated	CBFv reduced during OH
Delayed	OH after the third minute of the tilt
Orthostatic hypertension	Postural increase of systolic blood pressure ≥20mm Hg or an increase in systolic blood pressure during the tilt to 120% and above where supine baseline is equal to 100%
Initial orthostatic hypotension	Transient orthostatic hypotension upon tilt initiation
Primary cerebral autoregulatory failure	Low cerebral blood flow, both at supine and during the tilt, without orthostatic hypotension and hypocapnia Supine normal range of cerebral blood flow velocity: Males lower limits: 72.09–0.38* age(cm/s) Males upper limits: 84.35–0.38* age(cm/s) Females lower limit: 82.2–0.45 * age (cm/s) Females upper limit: 90.8–0.45 * age(cm/s)
Vasomotor oscillations	

OI, orthostatic intolerance; CBFv, cerebral blood flow velocity.

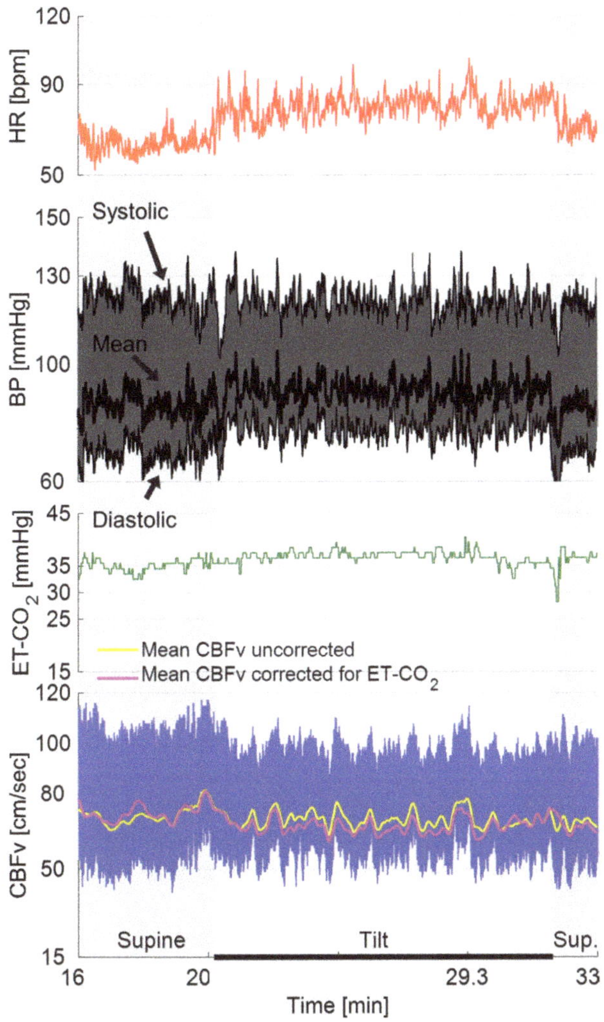

Figure 4.20 Normal response to tilt. The heart rate response consists of mild orthostatic heart rate increment (10–30 BPM). Mean blood pressure is essentially unchanged during the tilt, while there is mild increase in diastolic and decrease in systolic blood pressure. End tidal (ET) CO_2 is also unchanged during the tilt. Orthostatic cerebral blood flow velocity is also stable, normally the mean CBFv is unchanged or there is a mild decline in CBFv during the tilt. Data from 25 year old woman.

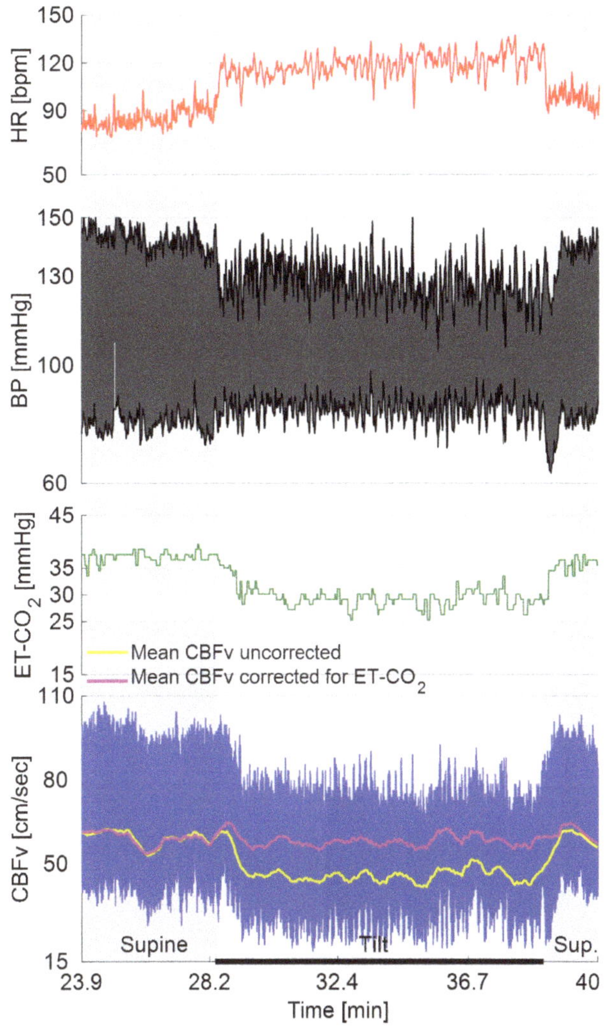

Figure 4.21 Postural tachycardia syndrome (POTS). Data from 25 year old woman.

There are four standardized sites:

1. Medial forearm (75% distance from the ulnar epicondyle to the pisiform bone)
2. Proximal leg (5 cm distal to the fibular head laterally)
3. Distal leg (5 cm proximal to the medial malleolus medially)
4. Proximal foot over the extensor digitorum brevis muscle

An instructional video provides details.[2] The skin should be vigorously cleaned with alcohol at all recording sites. Then the capsules should be attached tightly, but not so tight that they cause significant discomfort to the patient. Once attached, the capsules are filled with 10% acetylcholine diluted in sterile water (not normal saline!).

Then a baseline sweat recording is used to verify that no capsule leak is present. In the case of a leak, the capsule placement should be fixed. The ground electrode for stimulation is placed about 5 cm away from the capsule. It is important to wait until the baseline sweat is flat, below 100 nanoliters per minute, and all channels give similar baseline sweat output (difference <15%). Once the baseline sweat output is stable, the stimulation with 2 mA current for 5 minutes starts. Duration of recording is 10 minutes: 5 minutes with and 5 minutes without stimulation. Normative data adjusted for age and gender are shown in Table 4.6.[2] Men have significantly higher sweat output compared to women, and there is also a small decline of sweating with age.

INTERPRETATION OF RESULTS

Abnormal QSART indicates a postganglionic lesion. The abnormalities vary from mild to severe generalized anhidrosis. Mild abnormalities are associated with reduced food volume only or with a length-dependent pattern. These abnormalities can be seen also in healthy people. Short

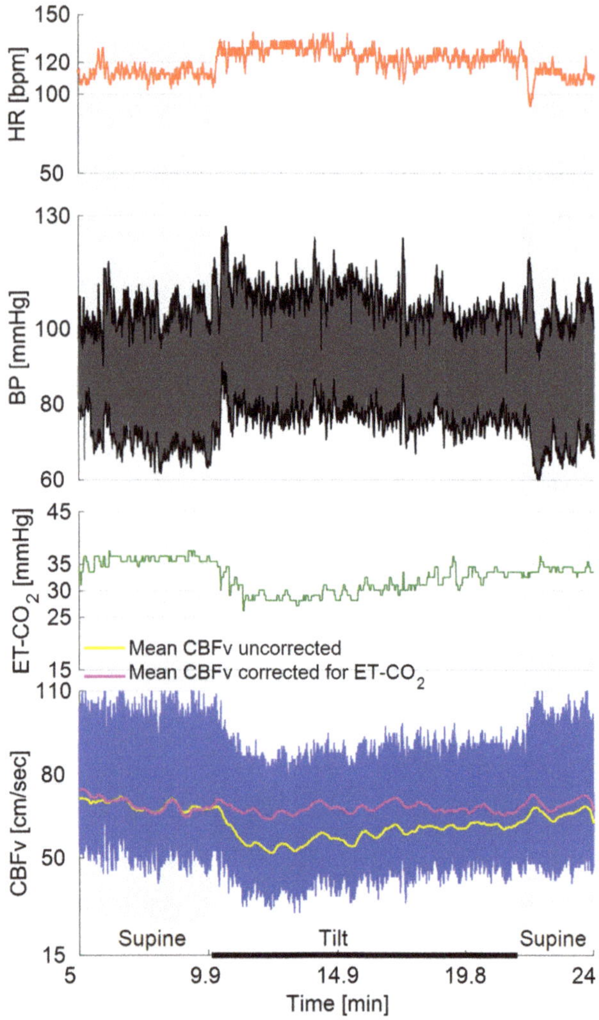

Figure 4.22 Inappropriate sinus tachycardia (IST). Data from 23 year old woman.

latencies can be due to a pain-induced somatosympathetic reflex. More widespread abnormalities, such as reduced volume at two or more sites, are indicative of small fiber neuropathy affecting cholinergic fibers. Below are described details on grading of abnormal results.

LIMITATIONS OF THE TEST

The QSART is time-consuming, can cause significant discomfort to a patient, and requires considerable skills to do correctly. Many commonly used medications have anticholinergic effect and interfere with the results. There are also some concerns about the reproducibility of the test.

ELECTROCHEMICAL SKIN CONDUCTANCE (ESC)

ESC evaluates the function of sweat glands and related sudomotor fibers.[17–20]

PRINCIPLE OF ESC MEASUREMENTS

ESC measures the flow of chloride ions induced by an electrical current (Figure 4.28). According to a theoretical model, electrical current stimulates sudomotor fibers innervating the sweat glands.[18] The activated sweat glands produce sweat with chloride ions. Chloride ions are consumed at the anode, mimicking the corrosion process using principles of reverse electrophoresis (also called *electro-osmotic flow*). In reverse iontophoresis, the molecules are extracted from the medium.[21]

Due to the high capacitance of human skin due to its dense lipid layers, the chloride ions cannot penetrate the stratum corneum at low voltages.[20,22] However, ions driven by electric current can move in an electric field via sweat duct pores. In vitro electrochemical studies[23] showed that the concentration of chloride had a strong influence on the anodic potential. The chloride ion flow produced by sweat glands is then proportional to the level of stimulus and sweat gland function.

Since the stimulus is electrical, it is possible to exactly define the intensity of the stimulation level, which may be a key factor in reproducibility.

During ESC measurement, an incremental, low, direct voltage (<4 V) is applied for several seconds between two electrodes at either the feet or hands. The voltage applied to skin electrodes generates a current between the anode and the cathode. The current is measured by using a Wheatstone bridge. Then, the voltage applied on the anode is increased and a new measurement is performed. Such a progressive step-by-step increase of 0.2 V during 1 second is applied until a maximal voltage of 3.8 V is reached. The same steps of incremental voltage are applied on all four electrodes. The ESC is calculated from the generated current, which is a function of the anodic and cathodic potentials. Results are expressed as a ratio of the current generated and the direct voltage stimulus in microSiemens (μS). Two ESC values are usually provided separately for the average of both hands and the average of both feet.

TECHNIQUE

The testing is typically done in the standing position. The patient places both palms and soles on large stainless-steel electrodes. The whole test takes about 3 minutes to complete.

NORMATIVE VALUES

Our normative data are hands ≥1.03 μS/kg; feet ≥1.14 μS/kg.

INTERPRETATION OF RESULTS

Abnormal ESC indicates abnormal function of sweat glands or a postganglionic sudomotor lesion.

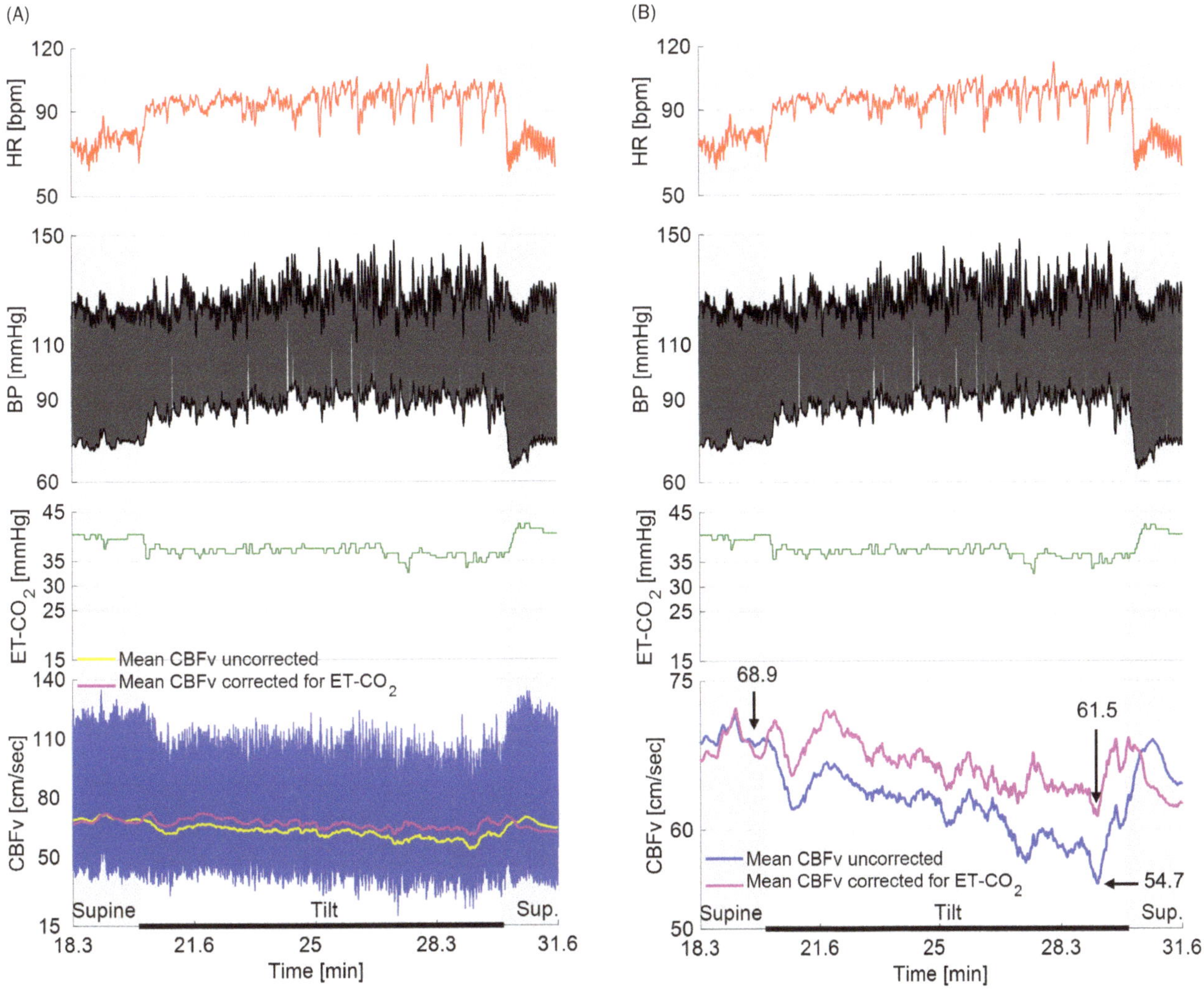

Figure 4.23 Orthostatic cerebral hypoperfusion syndrome (OCHOS). Data from 23 y/o man.

LIMITATIONS OF THE TEST

Although ESC correlates with skin biopsy, the correlation is not high enough to justify replacement of skin biopsies with ESC.

SKIN BIOPSY

Direct small fiber damage can be assessed using skin biopsies, which is a minimally invasive procedure[8]. Available techniques include assessment of sensory fibers using epidermal nerve fiber density (ENFD) and sudomotor fibers using sweat gland nerve fiber density (SGNFD). Skin biopsy samples can be obtained using a 3-mm circular disposable punch tool. Typically, one sample is taken from the proximal thigh 20 cm distal to the iliac spine and the other at the calf (10 cm above the lateral malleolus). Usually the skin samples are immediately transferred to appropriate fixative and processed at the skin pathology laboratory. Samples are commonly immunoperoxidase-stained for the pan-axonal marker PGP 9.5. Then the density of fibers is calculated per length (density/mm). The processing should be done at the certified laboratory. The limits of normality for ENFD at the thigh are 6.2/8.3 (men/women) fibers per millimeter of epidermal length (Therapath, NY, USA). The University of Massachusetts' limits of normal ENFD (fibers per millimeter of epidermal length) at the calf are equal to 9.5–0.075* age for men and 11.1–0.08* age for women). The limits of normality for SGN FD at the thigh and the calf are 37.8 and 36.5 fibers per millimeter (Therapath, NY, USA).

AUXILIARY TESTS

Numerous methods for direct or indirect evaluation of autonomic functions have been designed. Many of these tests require a specialized laboratory, extensive experience, or were not

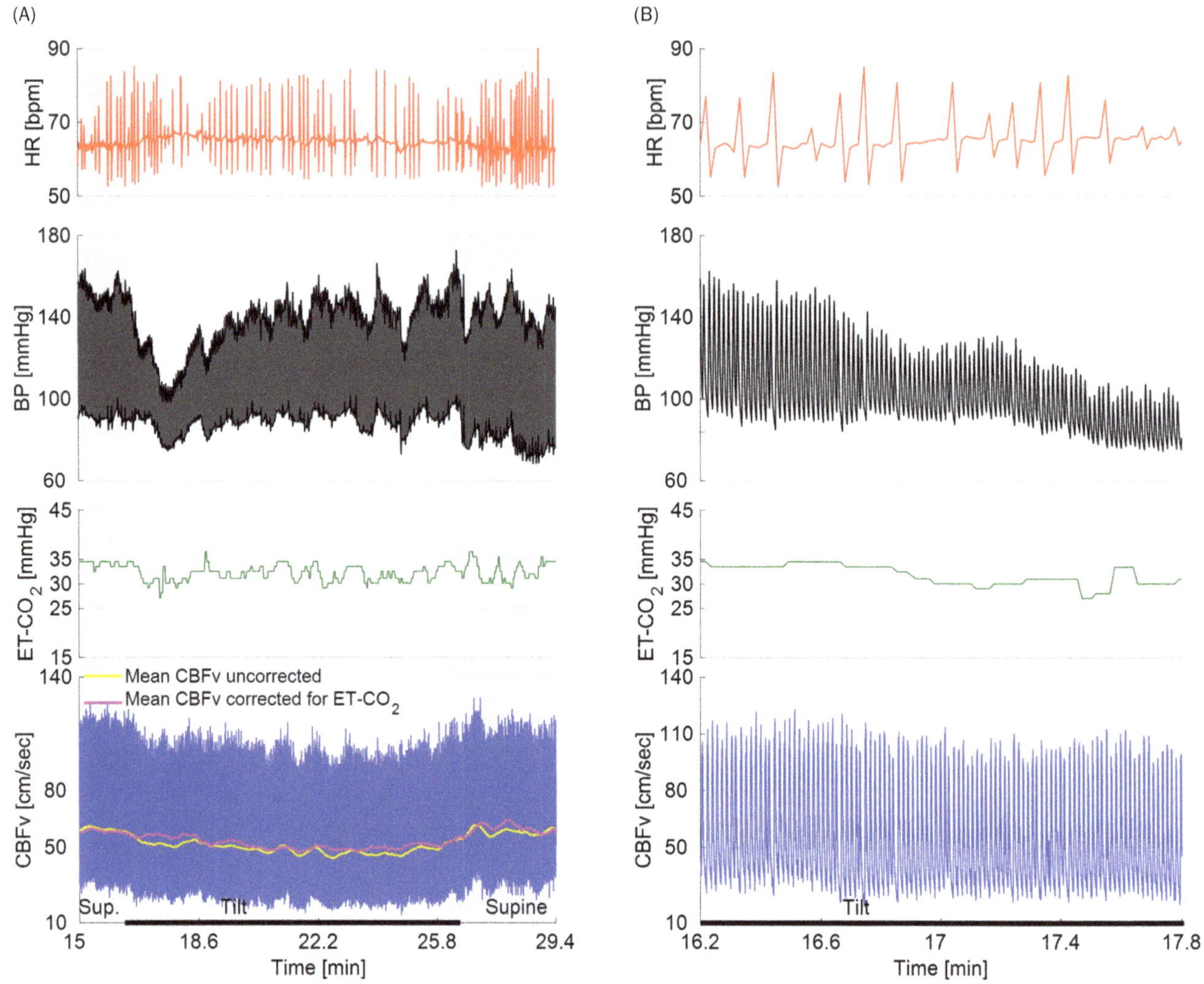

Figure 4.24 Transient orthostatic hypotension, compensated. In spite of transient decline of systolic blood pressure by 52 mmHg at the beginning of the tilt, cerebral blood flow velocity was relatively stable. The stable cerebral blood flow velocity indicate compensatory cerebral vasodilation and cerebral autoregulation. Patient was asymptomatic. Data from 76 y/o man.

validated with adequate clinical studies. Some of these tests are listed here. It is out of the scope of this textbook to describe each testing protocol; for details, consult corresponding texts.[1,6]

- Thermoregulatory sweat test
- Sweat imprint method
- Skin potentials
- Cold pressor test
- Handgrip maneuver
- Venoarterioral reflex
- Flare response
- Microneurography
- Neck suction
- Lower body negative pressure
- Laser Doppler techniques
- Venous plethysmography
- Positron emission tomography (PET)
- Single-proton emission computed tomography (SPECT)

Pharmacological assessment of postganglionic sympathetic outflow
- IV phenylephrine, low-dose (25 mg)
- IV tyramine
- Isoproterenol infusion test

Pupillary function
- Pupillary response to dilute pilocarpine
- Hydroxyamphetamine (1%) or n-methyl hydroxyamphetamine (5%)

Lacrimal/salivary functions
- Schirmer's test

Gastrointestinal motility
- Video-cinefluoroscopy
- Oesophageal manometry
- Small bowel manometry
- Telemetric devices

Bladder function
- Urodynamic studies
- Cystoscopy

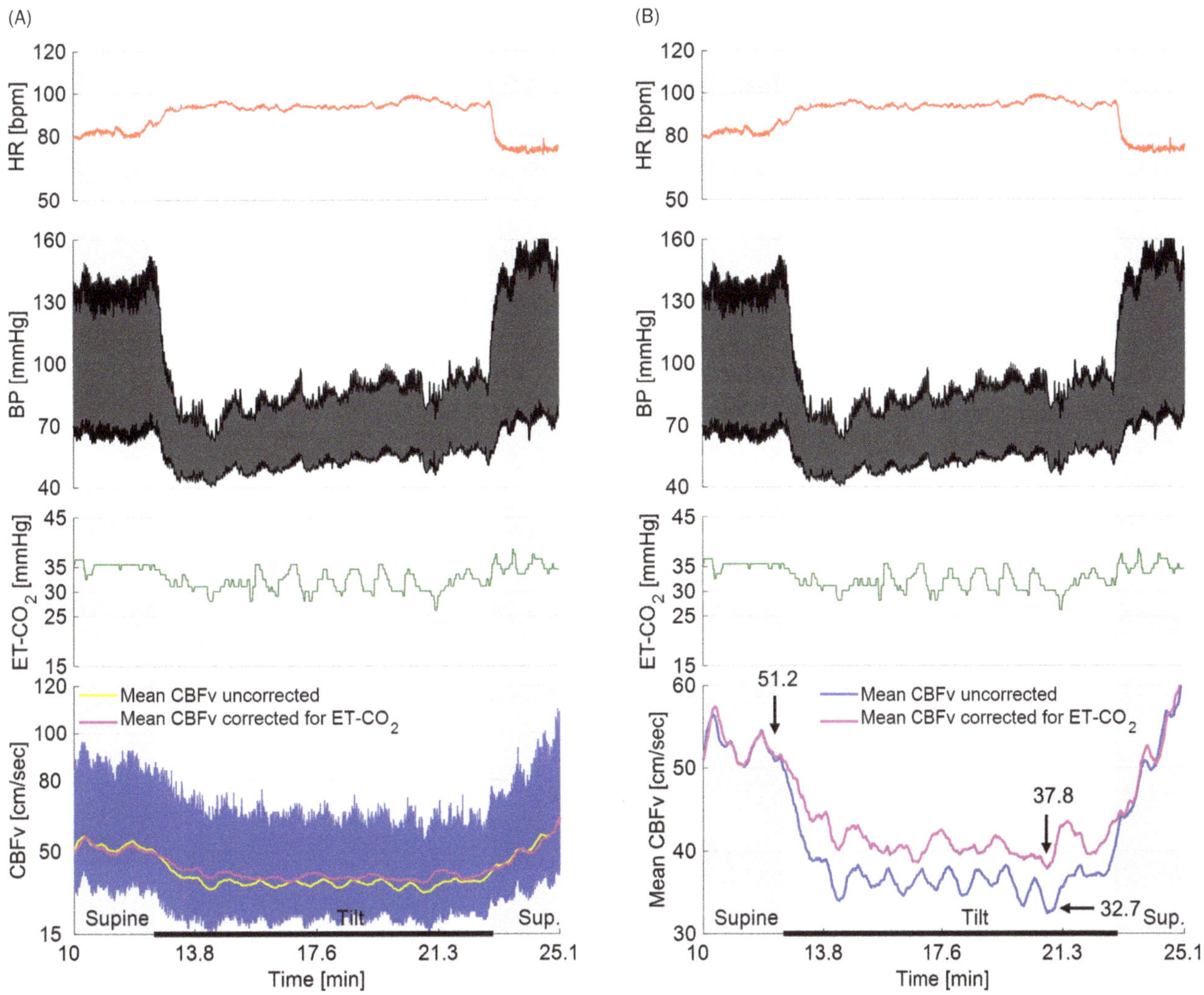

Figure 4.25 Orthostatic hypotension, sustained, uncompensated (A) and detail of mean cerebral blood flow velocity decline with and without end tidal (ET) CO_2 correction (B). Data from 71 y/o man.

Sexual function

Penile plethysmography

Intracavernosal papaverine

EVALUATIONS OF CAUSES OF SMALL FIBER NEUROPATHY

INTRODUCTION

Skin biopsy and/or sudomotor testing are useful for diagnosis of small fiber neuropathy, but the findings are usually nonspecific and do not point to the cause of neuropathy. Therefore, additional testing is commonly recommended to delineate underlying pathology.

The first-tier screening blood work for a typical length-dependent small fiber neuropathy includes cell count with differential, basic metabolic panel including electrolytes, renal and hepatic function tests, hemoglobin A1c, protein electrophoresis with immunofixation in serum and urine, lipid profile, hepatitis panel, erythrocyte sedimentation rate, extractable nuclear antigens (SS-A/Ro, SS-B/La, RNP, and SM), vitamin B_{12} levels, thyroid stimulating hormone, and immunoglobulin A anti-tissue transglutaminase antibody (IgA TTG, for celiac disease).[24]

The second-tier tests are typically used if the first-tier tests are unrevealing, and they depend on the underlying clinical context. Second-tier tests include catecholamines supine and standing, plasma free metanephrine, plasma renin, aldosterone, plasma chromogranin A, urinary 5-HIAA, 24-hour urinary sodium, tryptase, urinary methylhistamine, urinary prostaglandin F, and alpha galactosidase.

Commonly available catecholamines are norepinephrine, epinephrine, dopamine, and plasma free metanephrines. Plasma norepinephrine reflects sympathetic neural activity, and plasma epinephrine measures adrenal medullary activity. Norepinephrine is usually obtained in supine and

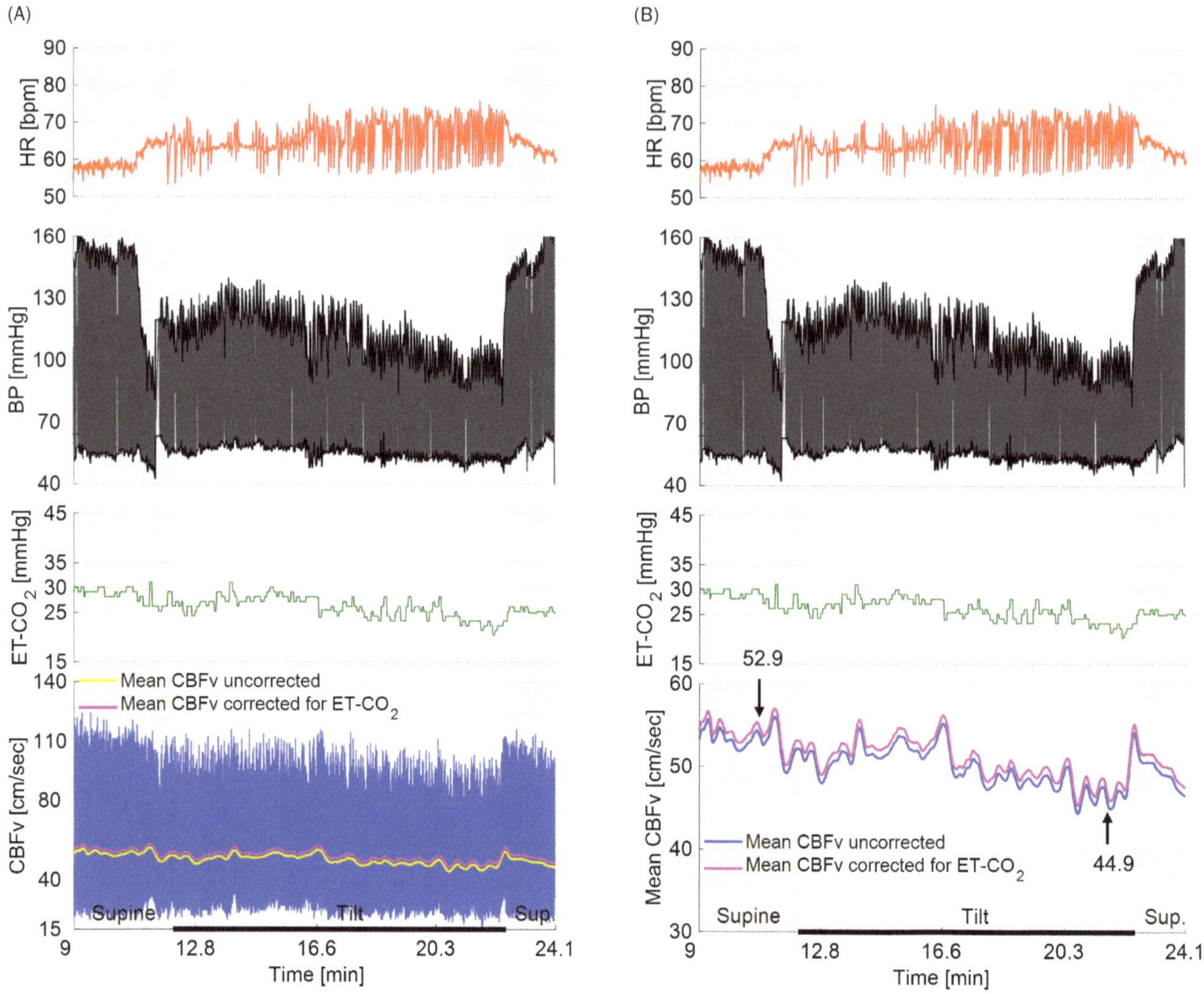

Figure 4.26 Orthostatic hypotension, compensated (A) and detail of stable cerebral blood flow velocity with and without end tidal (ET) CO_2 correction (B). Data from 69 y/o woman.

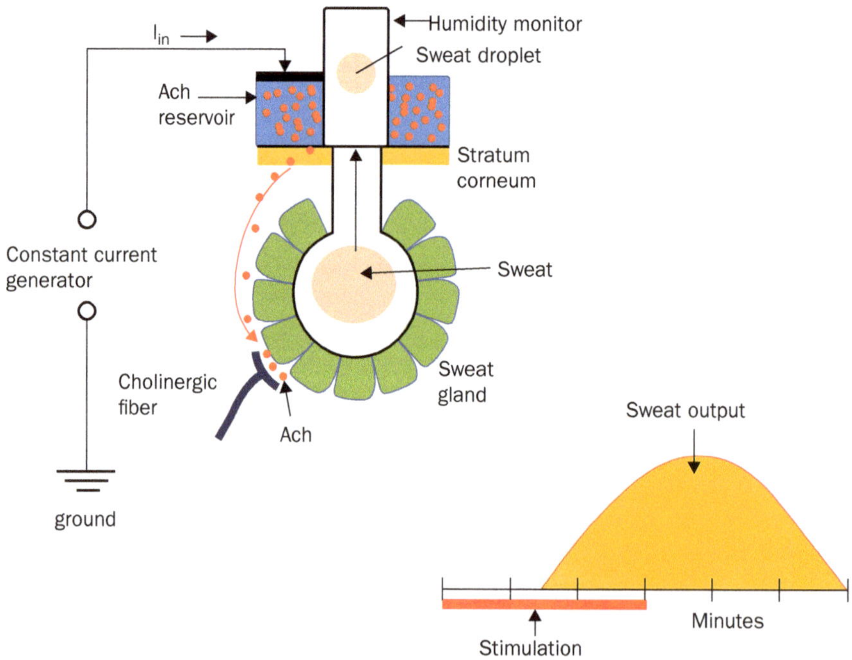

Figure 4.27 Principle of Quantitative Sudomotor Axon Reflex Test (QSART). Diluted acetylcholine stored in a capsule reservoir is transported to the cholinergic terminals via iontophoresis and stimulates sweat glands.

TABLE 4.6 NORMATIVE DATA FOR Q-SWEAT DEVICE. ALL VALUES ARE IN MICROLITERS.

		Age range		
Location	Gender	10–29	30–49	≥50
Forearm	Female	0.1–1.39	0.1–1.39	0.1–1.39
	Male	0.38–2.53	0.38–2.53	0.38–2.53
Proximal leg	Female	0.23–1.99	0.23–1.99	0.23–1.99
	Male	0.80–2.86	0.58–2.64	0.36–2.42
Distal leg	Female	0.32–1.51	0.21–1.21	0.10–0.90
	Male	0.72–2.79	0.52–2.41	0.31–2.02
Foot	Female	0.10–1.38	0.08–1.28	0.05–1.19
	Male	0.39–2.02	0.35–1.83	0.31–1.64

after 3–10 minutes in an upright position while the other catecholamines are obtained only once in the supine position.

Supine and upright norepinephrine can be used for differentiation of central versus peripheral dysautonomia. In peripheral autonomic neuropathies, the supine norepinephrine is reduced, but it can increase during standing. In central dysautonomia, supine norepinephrine is normal, but it fails to rise during standing due to reduced central drive. In general, catecholamines are insensitive as the only tool for detection of dysautonomia, and they correlate poorly with autonomic failure grade. They are useful in the diagnosis of the hyperadrenergic variant of POTS and in the diagnosis of hypoadrenergic state associated with painful small fiber neuropathies and the hyperadrenergic state associated with hypertension.

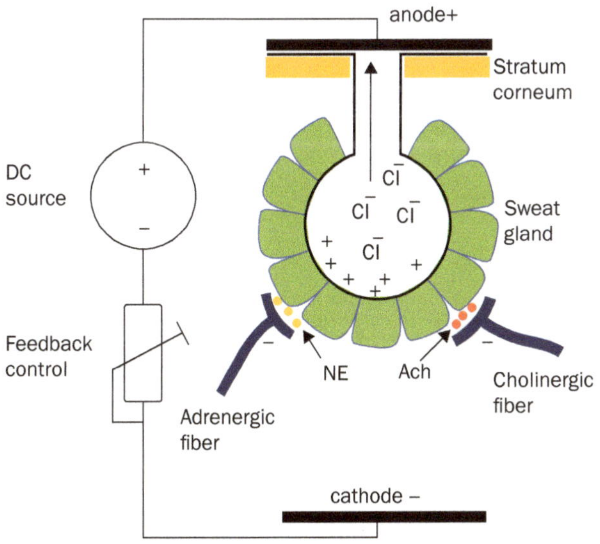

Figure 4.28 Principle of Electrochemical skin conductance (ESC). An electrical current activates sweat glands which induces the flow of chloride ions. The flow of chloride ions results in a changes in skin conductance which is measured.

In a pheochromocytoma, plasma free metanephrines, norepinephrine, and epinephrine are elevated. In dopamine β-hydroxylase deficiency, the dopamine level is high, and both norepinephrine and epinephrine are undetectable.[25] Both plasma renin and aldosterone can be low in diabetic autonomic neuropathy. Renin can be elevated in Addison disease. Plasma chromogranin A or elevated urinary of 5-hydrozyindoleacetic acid (5-HIAA) can be elevated in carcinoid tumors. Twenty-four-hour urinary sodium can be useful in evaluation of hypovolemia. Urinary methylhistamine can be elevated in mast cell activation disorders. Elevated urinary 5-HIAA can indicate carcinoid tumor. α-Galactosidase is reduced in Fabry disease.

Neuronal antibodies may be obtained if autoimmune mechanisms are suspected.[26–28] They can be obtained usually as a panel from either serum or cerebrospinal fluid. Table 4.7 shows common antibodies associated with paraneoplastic or autoimmune small fiber autonomic or sensory neuropathy.[26,33]

Several genes are associated with inherited small fiber neuropathy (Table 4.8).[29–32]

QASAT VERSION 1.1

INTRODUCTION

Quantitative Scale for Grading of Cardiovascular Autonomic Reflex Tests and Small Fibers from Skin Biopsies (QASAT) is a quantitative scale for grading of cardiovascular reflex tests, transcranial Doppler, quantitative sudomotor axon reflex test, and small fiber (epidermal sensory and sweat gland) densities from skin biopsies. It is the validated objective instrument for grading of dysautonomia, related small fiber neuropathy, and cerebral blood flow.[8] The version 1.1 described here defines the ESC and end tidal CO_2 module.

TABLE 4.7 **ANTIBODIES ASSOCIATED WITH SMALL FIBER NEUROPATHY AND DYSAUTONOMIA**

Antibody	Underlying tumor/disease	Autonomic syndromes
NMO/AGP4	Devic disease/Neuromyelitis optica	
Anti-Hu/ANNA-1	Small-cell lung carcinoma	Sensory and autonomic neuropathy, autonomic ganglionopathy, enteric neuropathy
ANNA-2	Bladder and cervical cancer	Unclear
ANNA-3	Small-cell lung carcinoma	Autonomic neuropathy?
AGNA-1		Autonomic neuropathy, pseudoobstruction
CRMP-5/anti-CV2	Small-cell lung carcinoma, thymoma	Autonomic neuropathy, enteric neuropathy
Anti-Yo/PCA-1	Ovarian, breast cancer	Cerebellar degeneration, GI dysmotility
PCA-2	Small-cell lung carcinoma	Autonomic neuropathy
PCA-TR	Hodgkin lymphoma	Unclear
CRMP-5 IgG	Small-cell lung carcinoma	
Anti-amphiphysin	Lung or breast cancer	Stiff person syndrome, various autonomic dysfunction
P/Q-type voltage-gated calcium channel	Small-cell lung carcinoma, Lambert-Eaton myasthenic syndrome	Lambert-Eaton syndrome
N-type voltage-gated calcium channel	Small-cell lung carcinoma	Lambert-Eaton syndrome, sensory and autonomic neuropathy
Ganglionic (α3) acetylcholine receptor	Small-cell lung carcinoma	Postural tachycardia, GI dysmotility, autonomic ganglionopathy
Muscarinic (M3) acetylcholine receptor		Sjögren syndrome
Voltage-gated potassium channel (VGKC)	Thymoma	Limbic encephalitis with autonomic hyperactivity
CASPR2 (contactin-associated protein-2-IgG)		CASPR2 should be assessed if VGKC is positive
LGli (glioma inactivated 1 protein-IgG)		LGli should be assessed if VGKC is positive
TS-HDS		Painful SFN
FGFR3		
Striated muscle antibody	Thymoma, myasthenia, Lambert-Eaton myasthenic syndrome, small-cell lung carcinoma, breast carcinoma	
GAD65	Thymoma, renal cell carcinoma, breast cancer, colon adenocarcinoma	

QASAT DESCRIPTION

QASAT (Table 4.9) is a fully quantitative, modular, and expandable instrument for grading autonomic dysfunction, abnormal cerebral blood flow and small fiber neuropathy. QASAT uses established tests evaluating autonomic functions and damage of small fibers, including deep breathing, the Valsalva maneuver, tilt test, QSART, ENFD, and SGNFD.[2,8,34,35]

QASAT is grouped into three main categories: cardiovascular, cerebral blood flow, and small fibers. The specific QASAT sections are heart rate, blood pressure, cerebral blood flow, sudomotor, and sensory. The heart rate section assesses the presence of supine bradycardia, supine tachycardia, heart responses to tilt, and heart rate variability. Heart rate variation during the breathing test is used as a marker of cardiovagal or parasympathetic functions. The blood pressure section describes blood pressure responses to the Valsalva maneuver and to the tilt. The QASAT index of blood pressure quantifies both reduced (orthostatic hypotension) and increased (orthostatic hypertension) blood pressure during the tilt. The severity of orthostatic hypotension is used as a marker of sympathetic/adrenergic failure. The cerebral blood flow section of the QASAT is based on blood flow velocity from the middle cerebral artery during

TABLE 4.8 GENES ASSOCIATED WITH SMALL FIBER NEUROPATHY

Gene	Disease	Comment
SPTLC1,RAB7A, DNMT1	HSAN type I	
HSN2	HSAN type II	
ELP1 (formerly IKBKAP)	HSAN type III	Familial dysautonomia
NTRK1	HSAN type IV	Congenital insensitivity to pain with anhidrosis
NGFb	HSAN type V	Congenital insensitivity to pain with partial anhidrosis
MTHFR (Methylenetetrahydrofolate reductase)	Cardiac autonomic dysfunction?	
SCN9A	Painful SFN	Encode the voltage-gated sodium channels Na_v 1.7, gain of function mutation
SCN10A	Painful SFN	Encode the voltage-gated sodium channels Na_v 1.8, gain of function mutation
SCN11A		Encode the voltage-gated sodium channels Na_v 1.9
TTR	Hereditary transthyretin amyloidosis	
TRPA1	Episodic painful SFN	
Acid α-1,4-glucosidase	Pompe disease	
α-galactosidase A	Fabry disease	Painful SFN

HSAN, Hereditary sensory and autonomic neuropathy.

TABLE 4.9 DEFINITION OF QASAT

Cardiovascular

Heart rate

Bradycardia: Supine and/or during tilt

Results	Grading	Value	Definition
Normal		0	HR ≥50 BPM
Abnormal		1	HR <50 BPM

HR, Heart rate; BPM, Beats per minute, at least 10 minutes of the rest should be obtained

Tachycardia: Supine

Results	Grading	Value	Definition
Normal		0	HR ≤100 BPM
Abnormal	Mild	1	HR >100 BPM

Increased heart rate response to tilt

Results	Grading	Value	Definition
Normal		0	HR increment ≥10 BPM and <30 BPM and maximal HR ≤110
Abnormal	Mild	1	For HR increment ≥30 BPM but maximal HR <120 BPM throughout the tilt, assign the value 1. For HR increment ≥30 BPM but maximal HR ≥120 BPM assign the value 0 for normal results and 1 for abnormal results at each measurement (each minute) and sum the results.
	Moderate	2,3	
	Severe	4,5,6	
	Marked	>6	

HR should be obtained at baseline and every minute of tilt up 10 minutes of the tilt. For tilt longer than 10 minutes, additional measurements should be obtained every 5 minutes.

(continued)

TABLE 4.9 CONTINUED

Reduced heart rate response to tilt test

Results	Grading	Value	Definition
Normal		0	HR increment ≥10 BPM and <30 BPM during tilt
Abnormal		1	HR increment during tilt <10 BPM

Heart rate variability

Results	Grading	Value	Definition
Normal		0	Heart rate variations to deep breathing test abnormal but ≥50% of normal value* <50% but ≥35% of normal value <35% of normal value
Abnormal	Mild	1	
	Moderate	2	
	Severe	3	

Valsalva ratio

Results	Grading	Value	Definition
Normal		0	Abnormal but ≥50% of normal value* <50% but ≥35% of normal value <35% of normal value
Abnormal	Mild	1	
	Moderate	2	
	Severe	3	

Blood pressure

Supine hypotension

Results	Grading	Value	Definition
Normal		0	SBP ≥90 and DBP ≥60
Abnormal		1	SBP <90 or DBP <60

Orthostatic hypotension during tilt test

Results	Grading	Value	Definition
Normal		0	At each measurement, assign the value 0 for normal results and 1 for abnormal results. Abnormal result is defined as a systolic BP ≤80% of baseline or mean BP ≤85% of baseline. Baseline is defined as the BP in supine position just before the tilt test.
Abnormal	Mild	1,2	
	Moderate	3,4	
	Severe	5,6	
	Marked	>6	

BP should be obtained at baseline and every minute of tilt up 10 minutes of the tilt. For tilt longer than 10 minutes, additional measurements should be obtained every 5 minutes.

Valsalva maneuver: Blood pressure

Results	Grading	Value	Definition
Normal		0	End of Phase 2 returns to or exceeds the baseline

TABLE 4.9 CONTINUED

Abnormal	Mild	1	≥90% and <100% of baseline
	Moderate	2	<90% and ≥60% of baseline
	Severe	3	<60% of baseline

Use mean BP expressed as changes in percent. Baseline is defined as the last mean BP just before Valsalva maneuver. The flat top response defined by minimum of Phase 2 above the baseline is discarded.

Supine hypertension

Results	Grading	Value	Definition
Normal		0	SBP <140 or DBP <90
Abnormal	Mild	1	(SBP ≥140 or DBP ≥90) and (SBP< 160 or DBP< 100)
	Moderate	2	(SBP ≥160 or DBP ≥100) and (SBP <180 or DBP <110)
	Severe	3	SBP ≥180 or DBP ≥110

Orthostatic hypertension during tilt test

Results	Grading	Value	Definition
Normal	Normal	0	SBP ≤120% of baseline
Abnormal	Abnormal	>1	SBP >120% of baseline

Calculate the difference between systolic BP obtained every minute of the tilt and supine baseline. The total score is summation of all scores obtained at each minute.

Cerebral blood flow

Valsalva maneuver: Cerebral blood flow

Results	Grading	Value	Definition
Normal		0	≥85% of baseline*
Abnormal	Mild	1	≥80 and <85% of baseline
	Moderate	2	≥65 and <80% of baseline
	Severe	3	<65% of baseline

Using systolic CBFv. * Systolic CBFv at the end of Phase 2, baseline is defined as the CBFv just before the Valsalva maneuver

Cerebral autoregulation

Results	Grading	Value	Definition
Normal		0	
Abnormal		1	Systolic CBFv >160 cm/s during Phase 4 and (Systolic CBFv–Diastolic CBFv) Phase 4/(Systolic CBFv–Diastolic CBFv) baseline) >140%

Supine cerebral blood flow low

Results	Grading	Value	Definition
Normal		0	
Abnormal		1	<Lower normal limit

Supine cerebral blood flow high

Results	Grading	Value	Definition
Normal		0	
Abnormal		1	>Upper normal limit

(continued)

Cerebral blood flow response to tilt

Results	Grading	Value	Definition*
Normal		0	Using mean CBFv. CBFv should be measured at baseline, and at 1, 5, and 10 minutes of tilt. *At each measurement, assign the value 0 for normal results. Abnormal results are defined as CBFv less than normal limit. Normal limit is defined as follows: At 1 minute: normal drop of CBFv ≥90%. Assign 1 for CBFv 80–89% of baseline, 2 for 70–79% of baseline, and 3 for <70% of baseline. At 5 minutes: Normal drop of CBFv ≥89%. Assign 1 for CBFv 79– 88% of baseline, 2 for 69–78% of baseline, and 3 for <69% of baseline. At 10 minutes: Normal drop of CBFv ≥86%. Assign 1 for CBFv 77–85% of baseline, 2 for 67–76% of baseline, and 3 for <67% of baseline. Total score is obtained by sum of all score.
Abnormal	Mild	1,2	
	Moderate	3,4	
	Severe	>4	

QSART (Quantitative sudomotor axon reflex test)

Results	Grading	Value	Definition
Normal		0	
Abnormal	Mild	1	Single site ≥50% and <100% or Length-dependent pattern* or Persistent sweat activity
	Moderate	2	Single site <50% or two or more sites ≥50% and <100%
	Severe	3	Two or more sites <50%

ESC (Electrochemical skin conductance)

Results	Grading	Value	Definition
Normal		0	
Abnormal	Mild	1	At least one site ≥75% and <100% or asymmetry between left or right side >20%
	Moderate	2	At least 2 sites ≥55%, <75%, or single site <55%
	Severe	3	Two or more sites <55%

One limb counts as one site; average ESC from both legs count as two sites.

Epidermal nerve fiber density (ENFD)

Results	Grading	Value	
Normal		0	
Abnormal	Mild	1	Single site <100% and ≥70%
	Moderate	2	Single site <70% and ≥40% or two sites <100% and ≥70%
	Severe	3	One site <40% or two or more sites <70% and ≥40%
	Marked	4	One site <20% or two or more sites <40%

*100%: normal limit. At least one biopsy should be done at the distal leg (10 cm above the lateral malleolus), with a second site at the thigh (20 cm distal to the iliac spine).

TABLE 4.9 **CONTINUED**

Sweat gland nerve fiber density (SGNFD)

Results	Grading	Value	Definition
Normal		0	
Abnormal	Mild	1	
	Moderate	2	Single site <85% and ≥65% or two sites <100% and ≥85%
	Severe	3	One site <65% or two or more sites <85% and ≥65%
	Marked	4	One site <50% or two or more sites <65%

*100%: normal limit. At least one biopsy should be done at the distal leg (10 cm above the lateral malleolus), with a second site at the thigh (20 cm distal to the iliac spine).

End tidal CO2

Supine end tidal CO_2 low

Results	Grading	Value	Definition
Normal		0	35-45 mmHg
Abnormal		1	< 35 mmHg

Supine end tidal CO_2 high

Results	Grading	Value	Definition
Normal		0	35–45 mm Hg
Abnormal		1	>45 mm Hg

Orthostatic end tidal CO_2 during the tilt

Results	Grading	Value	Definition*
Normal		0	* End tidal (ET) CO_2 should be measured at baseline, and at 1, 5, and 10 minutes of tilt. At each measurement, assign the value 0 for normal results which is defined as ET CO_2 32–45 mm Hg and drop of ET CO_2 ≤3 mm Hg during the tilt test. Abnormal results are defined as follows: At each measurement period (minute 1, 5, and 10), assign the value 1 for ET CO_2 (≥27 mm Hg and <32 mm Hg) OR (≥32 mm Hg and drop of ET CO_2 >3 mm Hg during the tilt test compared to supine); 2 for ET CO_2 ≥22 mm Hg and <27 mm Hg; 3 for ET CO_2 <22 mm Hg. For tilt longer than 10 minutes, additional measurements should be obtained every 5 minutes. Total score is obtained by sum of all scores.
Abnormal	Mild	1-2	
	Moderate	3-4	
	Severe	>4	

the tilt and the Valsalva maneuver and is used to characterize cerebral blood flow, as well as cerebral autoregulation. The end tidal CO_2 module complements the cerebral blood flow section and grades respiratory parameters in the supine position and their changes during tilt. End tidal CO_2 has a powerful effect on cerebral blood flow[36] (inducing both vasoconstriction with low blood flow velocity during hyperventilation with low end tidal CO_2, as well as vasodilatation with an increased blood flow velocity with high end tidal CO_2). Therefore, measurement of end tidal CO_2 is an essential instrument to correctly interpret cerebral blood flow changes during tilt.

The sudomotor section is divided into (1) functional sudomotor tests (QSART and ESC), and (2) the morphological section that grades SGNFD using skin biopsy. The sensory section grades the ENFD abnormalities.

QASAT was developed using genetic algorithms[37] that solve optimization problems mimicking processes of natural selection. The main sections (heart rate, blood pressure, blood flow velocity, sudomotor, and sensory) were determined using physiological and clinical judgment.[8] In general, the initial criteria for the degree of abnormalities (mild, moderate, severe, marked) at each section were generated randomly, and were then adjusted by successive iterations until the best match with a reference test was achieved.

QASAT was written in the Matlab programming language (MathWorks, Natick, MA), and all scores were generated automatically.

TABLE 4.10 **INTERPRETATION OF QASAT**

QASAT—interpretation			
Autonomic failure			
Autonomic domain	QASAT module	Score	Comments
Cardiovagal	Heart rate variability	0–3	
	Tachycardia-supine	0–1	Supine tachycardia can be due to cardiovagal failure or du to adrenergic hyperactivity in addition to other factors
Adrenergic	Valsalva maneuver	0–3	
	Tilt test	0–10	
	Supine hypertension	0–3	
	Total adrenergic score	0–16	= Valsalva maneuver + Tilt test+ supine hypertension
Sudomotor	QSART	0–3	
	ESC	0–3	
Total autonomic failure score		0–23	Uses either QSART or ESC
Autonomic overactivity			
Autonomic domain	QASAT module	Score	Comments
Cardiovagal	Bradycardia supine	0–1	
Adrenergic	Tachycardia supine	0–1	
	Increased heart rate response to tilt	0–10	
	Supine hypertension	0–3	
	Orthostatic hypertension	0–1	
Total adrenergic hyperactivity score		0–15	
Small fiber neuropathy (SFN)			
SFN domain	QASAT module		
Sensory	ENFD	0–3	
Sudomotor	QSART or ESC	0–3	
	SGNFD	0–3	
Total small fiber neuropathy score		0–9	Uses either QSART or ESC
Tachycardia syndromes (POTS, IST, PST)			
Heart rate	Increased heart rate response to tilt	0–10	POTS=postural tachycardia syndrome, IST=inappropriate sinus tachycardia, PST=paroxysmal sinus tachycardia
Cerebral blood flow			
Low supine	Supine blood flow low	0–1	
Reduced orthostatic cerebral blood flow	Blood flow response to tilt	0–9	

TABLE 4.10 CONTINUED

Low cerebral blood flow total score		0–10	
Cerebral autoregulation	Cerebral autoregulation	0–1	Uses Valsalva maneuver
Respiratory system			
Hypocapnia	Orthostatic end tidal CO_2 during the tilt	0–12	

INTERPRETATION OF QASAT

Table 4.10 provides instructions on how to use QASAT. QASAT modules enable quantitative assessment and grading of several syndromes of autonomic dysfunction (e.g., autonomic failure, autonomic overactivity, tachycardia syndromes, small fiber neuropathy, cerebral blood flow, cerebral autoregulation and respiratory abnormalities).

QASAT reflects the functioning of integrative systems, and grading is based on implicit assumptions that certain conditions are met. For example, grading of adrenergic failure using orthostatic hypotension is valid only if nonautonomic causes of orthostatic hypotension are ruled out. Furthermore, is not unusual to have combinations of two or more patterns during autonomic testing. For example, paroxysmal sinus tachycardia or syncope can be superimposed on other patterns.[35] Therefore, it is important that the expert physiologist interprets QASAT scores in the proper context.

AUTONOMIC FAILURE

Autonomic failure assessment includes cardiovagal, adrenergic, and sudomotor systems.

Cardiovagal Failure

QASAT-Heart rate variability is a marker of cardiovagal activity and is compatible with the cardiovagal score as defined in the Composite Autonomic Scoring Scale (CASS).[5] Patients with cardiovagal failure may also have supine tachycardia. Multiple factors affect heart rate variability, including the sensory afferent pathways, parasympathetic and sympathetic modulation, chest mechanics, resting heart rate, and volemic and cardiac status.[35]

Adrenergic Failure

An abnormal Phase 2 in the Valsalva maneuver is the most sensitive marker of adrenergic failure.[7] Orthostatic hypotension is present in more advanced autonomic adrenergic failure. QASAT uses relative changes in blood pressure, which increases sensitivity to detect adrenergic failure in patients with low supine blood pressure and reduces sensitivity to detect adrenergic failure in patients with elevated supine blood pressure. In QASAT, the total adrenergic failure score is calculated as the sum of the Valsalva maneuver—blood pressure, orthostatic hypotension, and supine hypertension scores.

Sudomotor Failure

Grading of sudomotor failure can be obtained from QASAT-QSART, which is same as to the QSART module in CASS[5] or from the QASAT-ESC module.

Total Autonomic Failure

QASAT defines total autonomic failure by a summation of cardiovagal, adrenergic, and sudomotor failure score. QASAT stratifies total autonomic failure as none (total score 0), mild (total score 1–3), moderate (total score 4–6), or severe (total score >7).

Autonomic Overactivity

Cardiovagal parasympathetic overactivity can be obtained from the QASAT-Bradycardia module. Total adrenergic overactivity can be obtained as a sum of QASAT-tachycardia supine, QASAT-increased heart rate response to tilt, QASAT-supine hypertension, and QASAT-orthostatic hypertension scores.

Orthostatic Intolerance Associated with Tachycardia

Tachycardia syndromes, particularly POTS, are common and they can be graded using the QASAT-increased heart rate increment during the tilt.

Small Fiber Neuropathy

The small fiber neuropathy grading uses both direct measures of small fiber damage using skin biopsies (QASAT-ENFD and QASAT-SGNFD) as well as functional sudomotor evaluations using the QASAT-ESC and QASAT-QSART modules. This module can be used to grade severity and type of small fiber neuropathy (sensory, autonomic, mixed) or used in combination with other portions of the QASAT, for example to evaluate neuropathic versus non-neuropathic form of POTS.

Cerebral Blood Flow

Sings of orthostatic intolerance are frequently associated with cerebral hypoperfusion, particularly in POTS patients.[38] The QASAT-cerebral blood flow response to tilt can be used to grade cerebral orthostatic blood flow changes which may reflect cerebral hypoperfusion. Low cerebral orthostatic blood flow can be associated with orthostatic hypotension (which can be assessed by QASAT-orthostatic hypotension during the tilt test module), hypocapnia (which can be assessed by QASAT-orthostatic end tidal CO_2 during tilt test module), or absent orthostatic hypotension/hypocapnia as seen in OCHOS.[39]

MODULARITY OF QASAT

QASAT has a modular design; therefore, not all modules have to be used. An example of a reduced, inexpensive autonomic setup is assessment of cardiovagal score using the heart rate variability module (using a deep breathing test) and assessment of the adrenergic score using orthostatic hypotension during tilt test module by evaluating blood pressure responses to active standing obtained at every minute. The above described limited setting evaluating cardiovagal and adrernergic score can be done in any office with an ECG device and arm blood pressure.

TESTING PROTOCOLS

The testing should be tailored to clinical needs. Several protocols are used in our laboratory. The most common is the Brigham protocol, which includes functional autonomic testing and skin biopsies for assessments of small fibers.[2,8] The grading of abnormalities is evaluated using QASAT.

Another protocol is the syncope protocol, where the skin biopsies are omitted. This protocol is used for younger subjects (age <30 years) when the history or examination is not suggestive of autonomic failure or small fiber dysfunction. However, if the autonomic testing is consistent with autonomic failure or orthostatic intolerance, skin biopsies may be recommended.

The Brigham Protocol

1. Autonomic functional testing: Deep breathing, Valsalva and tilt test with monitoring of heart rate, blood pressure (both continuous from finger and intermittent from arm), end tidal CO_2, respiratory frequency, and CBFv from middle cerebral artery.
2. Skin biopsy for evaluation of ENFD and SGNFD.
3. Sudomotor function evaluation (QSART or ESC).

Syncope Protocol

1. Autonomic functional testing (deep breathing, Valsalva and tilt test) with monitoring of heart rate, blood pressure, end tidal CO_2, respiratory frequency, and CBFv
2. Sudomotor function evaluation (QSART or ESC).

Depending on clinical context, the testing may be expanded using active standing, prolonged tilt, carotid massage, postprandial challenge, exercise, or reverse tilt. Reverse tilt (head-down tilt at 50–60 degrees) is useful to differentiate psychogenic hypocapnic hyperventilation (e.g., due to anxiety) from metabolic/physiologic hypocapnia. The hypocapnia typically persists in the psychogenic hyperventilation syndrome but disappears in the case of metabolic/physiologic hypocapnia during reverse tilt.

REFERENCES

1. Low PA, Tomalia VA, Park K-J. Autonomic function tests: some clinical applications. *J Clin Neurol Seoul Korea*. 2013;9(1):1–8. doi:10.3988/jcn.2013.9.1.1.
2. Novak P. Quantitative autonomic testing. *J Vis Exp JoVE*. 2011;(53). doi:10.3791/2502.
3. Novak P. Cerebral blood flow, heart rate, and blood pressure patterns during the tilt test in common orthostatic syndromes. *Neurosci J*. 2016;2016:6127340. doi:10.1155/2016/6127340.
4. Norcliffe-Kaufmann L, Galindo-Mendez B, Garcia-Guarniz A-L, Villarreal-Vitorica E, Novak V. Transcranial Doppler in autonomic testing: standards and clinical applications. *Clin Auton Res Off J Clin Auton Res Soc*. 2018;28(2):187–202. doi:10.1007/s10286-017-0454-2.
5. Low PA. Composite autonomic scoring scale for laboratory quantification of generalized autonomic failure. *Mayo Clin Proc*. 1993;68(8):748–752.
6. Hilz MJ, Dütsch M. Quantitative studies of autonomic function. *Muscle Nerve*. 2006;33(1):6–20. doi:10.1002/mus.20365.
7. Novak P. Assessment of sympathetic index from the Valsalva maneuver. *Neurology*. 2011;76(23):2010–2016. doi:10.1212/WNL.0b013e31821e5563.
8. Novak P. Quantitative scale for grading of cardiovascular autonomic reflex tests and small fibers from skin biopsies (QASAT). *J Neurol Disord*. April 2015. doi:10.4172/2329-6895.1000226
9. Schreihofer AM, Guyenet PG. The baroreflex and beyond: control of sympathetic vasomotor tone by GABAergic neurons in the ventrolateral medulla. *Clin Exp Pharmacol Physiol*. 2002;29(5-6):514–521.
10. Fritsch-Yelle JM, Convertino VA, Schlegel TT. Acute manipulations of plasma volume alter arterial pressure responses during Valsalva maneuvers. *J Appl Physiol Bethesda Md 1985*. 1999;86(6):1852–1857. doi:10.1152/jappl.1999.86.6.1852.
11. Vogel ER, Sandroni P, Low PA. Blood pressure recovery from Valsalva maneuver in patients with autonomic failure. *Neurology*. 2005;65(10):1533–1537. doi:10.1212/01.wnl.0000184504.13173.ef.
12. Goldstein DS, Cheshire WP. Beat-to-beat blood pressure and heart rate responses to the Valsalva maneuver. *Clin Auton Res Off J Clin Auton Res Soc*. 2017;27(6):361–367. doi:10.1007/s10286-017-0474-y.

13. Smith JJ, Porth CM, Erickson M. Hemodynamic response to the upright posture. *J Clin Pharmacol.* 1994;34(5):375–386.
14. Kenny RA, Ingram A, Bayliss J, Sutton R. Head-up tilt: a useful test for investigating unexplained syncope. *Lancet Lond Engl.* 1986;1(8494):1352–1355.
15. Task Force for the Diagnosis and Management of Syncope, European Society of Cardiology (ESC), European Heart Rhythm Association (EHRA), et al. Guidelines for the diagnosis and management of syncope (version 2009). *Eur Heart J.* 2009;30(21):2631–2671. doi:10.1093/eurheartj/ehp298.
16. Low PA, Caskey PE, Tuck RR, Fealey RD, Dyck PJ. Quantitative sudomotor axon reflex test in normal and neuropathic subjects. *Ann Neurol.* 1983;14(5):573–580. doi:10.1002/ana.410140513.
17. Ayoub H, Calvet JH, Lair V, Griveau S, Bedioui F, Cassir M. Electrochemical basis for EZSCAN/SUDOSCAN: a quick, simple, and non-invasive method to evaluate sudomotor dysfunctions. 2012. doi:10.5772/53965.
18. Ayoub H, Lair V, Griveau S, Brunswick P, Bedioui F, Cassir M. Electrochemical characterization of stainless steel as a new electrode material in a medical device for the diagnosis of sudomotor dysfunction. *Electroanalysis.* 2012;24(6):1324–1333. doi:10.1002/elan.201200058.
19. Vinik AI, Nevoret M-L, Casellini C. The new age of sudomotor function testing: a sensitive and specific biomarker for diagnosis, estimation of severity, monitoring progression, and regression in response to intervention. *Front Endocrinol.* 2015;6:94. doi:10.3389/fendo.2015.00094.
20. Hubert D, Brunswick P, Calvet J-H, Dusser D, Fajac I. Abnormal electrochemical skin conductance in cystic fibrosis. *J Cyst Fibros Off J Eur Cyst Fibros Soc.* 2011;10(1):15–20. doi:10.1016/j.jcf.2010.09.002.
21. Leboulanger B, Guy RH, Delgado-Charro MB. Reverse iontophoresis for non-invasive transdermal monitoring. *Physiol Meas.* 2004;25(3):R35–R50.
22. Chizmadzhev YA, Indenbom AV, Kuzmin PI, Galichenko SV, Weaver JC, Potts RO. Electrical properties of skin at moderate voltages: contribution of appendageal macropores. *Biophys J.* 1998;74(2 Pt 1):843–856. doi:10.1016/S0006-3495(98)74008-1.
23. Brunswick P, Mayaudon H, Albin V, Lair V, Ringuede A, Cassir M. Use of Ni electrodes chronoamperometry for improved diagnostics of diabetes and cardiac diseases. *Conf Proc Annu Int Conf IEEE Eng Med Biol Soc IEEE Eng Med Biol Soc Annu Conf.* 2007;2007:4544–4547. doi:10.1109/IEMBS.2007.4353350.
24. Gorson KC, Herrmann DN, Thiagarajan R, et al. Non-length dependent small fibre neuropathy/ganglionopathy. *J Neurol Neurosurg Psychiatry.* 2008;79(2):163–169. doi:10.1136/jnnp.2007.128801.
25. Robertson D, Haile V, Perry SE, Robertson RM, Phillips JA, Biaggioni I. Dopamine beta-hydroxylase deficiency. A genetic disorder of cardiovascular regulation. *Hypertens Dallas Tex 1979.* 1991;18(1):1–8.
26. Vernino S. Antibody testing as a diagnostic tool in autonomic disorders. *Clin Auton Res Off J Clin Auton Res Soc.* 2009;19(1):13–19. doi:10.1007/s10286-008-0488-6.
27. Dhamija R, Tan KM, Pittock SJ, Foxx-Orenstein A, Benarroch E, Lennon VA. Serological profiles aiding the diagnosis of autoimmune gastrointestinal dysmotility. *Clin Gastroenterol Hepatol Off Clin Pract J Am Gastroenterol Assoc.* 2008;6(9):988–992. doi:10.1016/j.cgh.2008.04.009.
28. McKeon A, Lennon VA, Jacob A, et al. Coexistence of myasthenia gravis and serological markers of neurological autoimmunity in neuromyelitis optica. *Muscle Nerve.* 2009;39(1):87–90. doi:10.1002/mus.21197.
29. Themistocleous AC, Ramirez JD, Serra J, Bennett DLH. The clinical approach to small fibre neuropathy and painful channelopathy. *Pract Neurol.* 2014;14(6):368–379. doi:10.1136/practneurol-2013-000758.
30. Huang J, Han C, Estacion M, et al. Gain-of-function mutations in sodium channel Na(v)1.9 in painful neuropathy. *Brain J Neurol.* 2014;137(Pt 6):1627–1642. doi:10.1093/brain/awu079.
31. Faber CG, Hoeijmakers JGJ, Ahn H-S, et al. Gain of function Nav1.7 mutations in idiopathic small fiber neuropathy. *Ann Neurol.* 2012;71(1):26–39. doi:10.1002/ana.22485.
32. Baccarelli A, Cassano PA, Litonjua A, et al. Cardiac autonomic dysfunction: effects from particulate air pollution and protection by dietary methyl nutrients and metabolic polymorphisms. *Circulation.* 2008;117(14):1802–1809. doi:10.1161/CIRCULATIONAHA.107.726067.
33. Pestronk A, Schmidt RE, Choksi RM, Sommerville RB, Al-Lozi MT. Clinical and laboratory features of neuropathies with serum IgM binding to TS-HDS. *Muscle Nerve.* 2012;45(6):866–872. doi:10.1002/mus.23256.
34. Lauria G, Hsieh ST, Johansson O, et al. European Federation of Neurological Societies/Peripheral Nerve Society Guideline on the use of skin biopsy in the diagnosis of small fiber neuropathy. Report of a joint task force of the European Federation of Neurological Societies and the Peripheral Nerve Society. *Eur J Neurol.* 2010;17(7):903–912, e44–e49. doi:10.1111/j.1468-1331.2010.03023.x.
35. Novak P. Cerebral blood flow, heart rate, and blood pressure patterns during the tilt test in common orthostatic syndromes. *Neurosci J.* 2016;2016:6127340. doi:10.1155/2016/6127340.
36. Van Lieshout JJ, Wieling W, Karemaker JM, Secher NH. Syncope, cerebral perfusion, and oxygenation. *J Appl Physiol Bethesda Md 1985.* 2003;94(3):833–848. doi:10.1152/japplphysiol.00260.2002.
37. Forrest S. Genetic algorithms: principles of natural selection applied to computation. *Science.* 1993;261(5123):872–878.
38. Novak V, Spies JM, Novak P, McPhee BR, Rummans TA, Low PA. Hypocapnia and cerebral hypoperfusion in orthostatic intolerance. *Stroke.* 1998;29(9):1876–1881.
39. Novak P. Orthostatic cerebral hypoperfusion syndrome. *Front Aging Neurosci.* 2016;8:22. doi:10.3389/fnagi.2016.00022.

5.

ARTIFACTS

It is of paramount importance to recognize artifacts since they can mimic various abnormalities. Most artifacts are easily recognized by trained personnel, such as a disconnected electrode or cable leading to either absent or distorted signals. There is, however, another category of artifacts that is more difficult to recognize. These artifacts may change the character of signals in a subtle way. For example a finger cuff device may introduce artificial drift in blood pressure (Figures 5.1 and 5.2).[1] It is advised to measure blood pressure from arm and use it as a calibration reference for the finger cuff device.

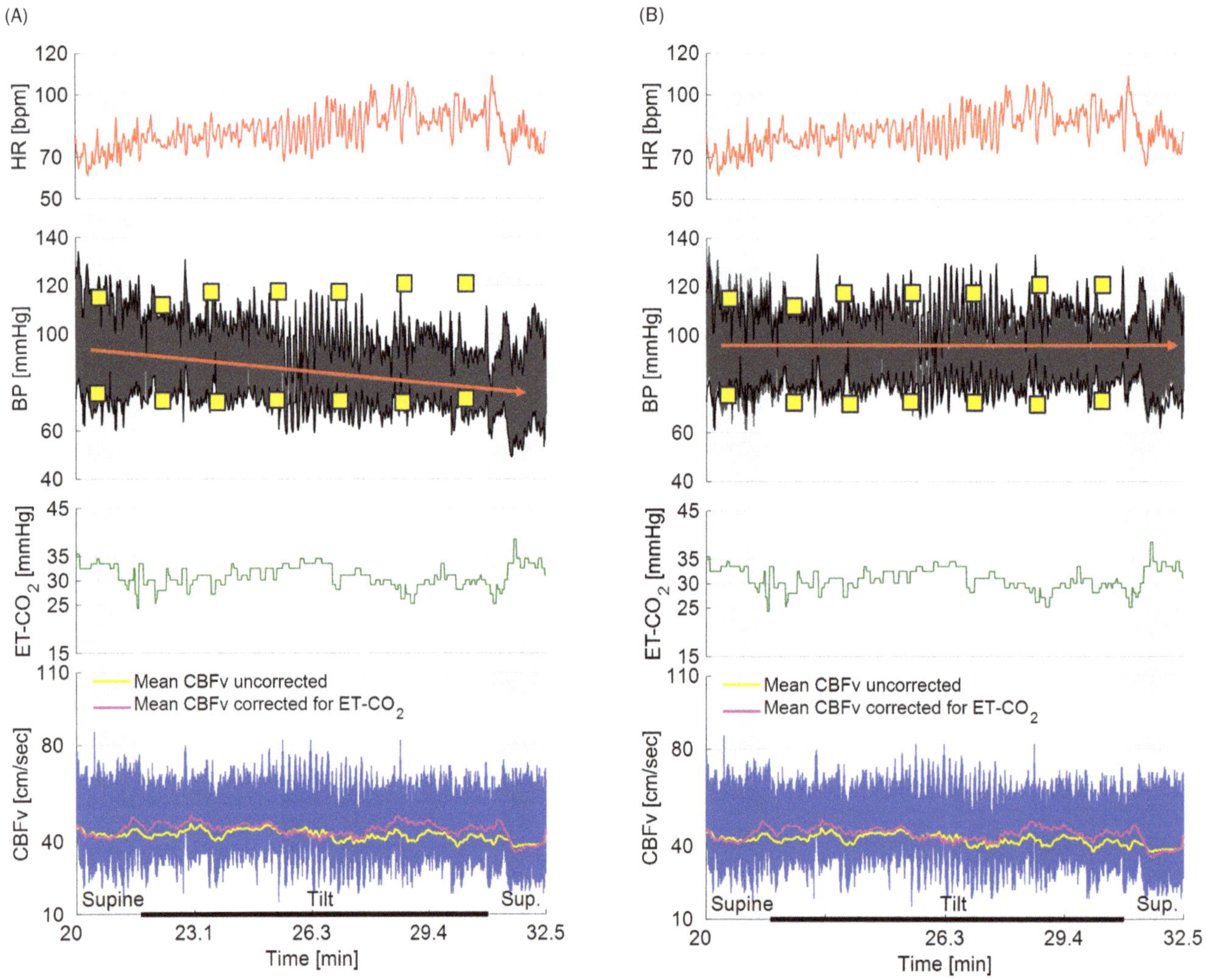

Figure 5.1 Finapres device may generate artificial drifts in blood pressure, as seen in this example (A). Despite the fact that the Finapress calibration was turned on several times during the tilt, there was a progressive decline in blood pressure. If not corrected, the drift would be incorrectly interpreted as orthostatic hypotension. The blood pressure signal corrected for the drift using the arm blood pressure (B) shows no orthostatic hypotension. Yellow boxes show blood pressure obtained from the arm.

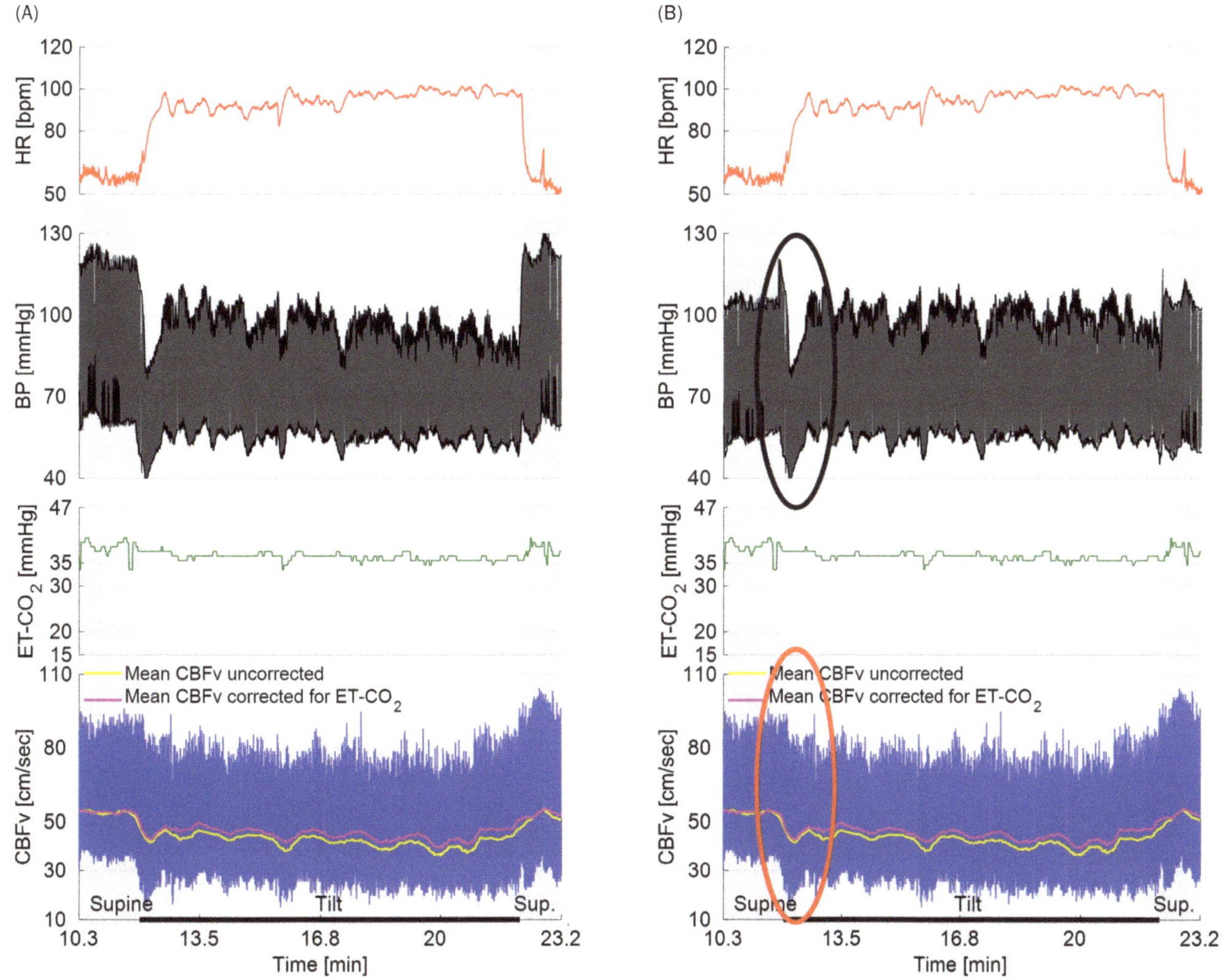

Figure 5.2 A finger cuff device may generate an artificial drift in blood pressure provoked by movement of the tilt table. Uncorrected blood pressure signal showed artificial orthostatic hypotension (A). The corrected blood pressure shows only initial orthostatic hypotension (*black oval*) confirmed by a decline in cerebral blood flow velocity (*red oval*, B). Orthostatic hypotension was absent (B).

Inappropriate placement of a transcranial probe may generate artificially lower cerebral blood flow velocity (CBFv) or a distorted signal. Unusual artifacts may occur when the upright position causes a shifting of the intracranial contents down, causing a sudden decrease in the CBFv (Figure 5.3).

End tidal CO_2 may be artificially low if the patient talks during testing. Therefore it is important to document when the patient was talking, particularly during the tilt test. Correct end tidal CO_2 is necessary for correct interpretation of CBFv changes. For example, end tidal CO_2 differentiates between orthostatic cerebral hypoperfusion syndrome (OCHOS, end tidal CO_2 is normal) and hypocapnic cerebral hypoperfusion (HYCH, end tidal CO_2 is reduced) in patients with reduced CBFv without orthostatic hypotension.

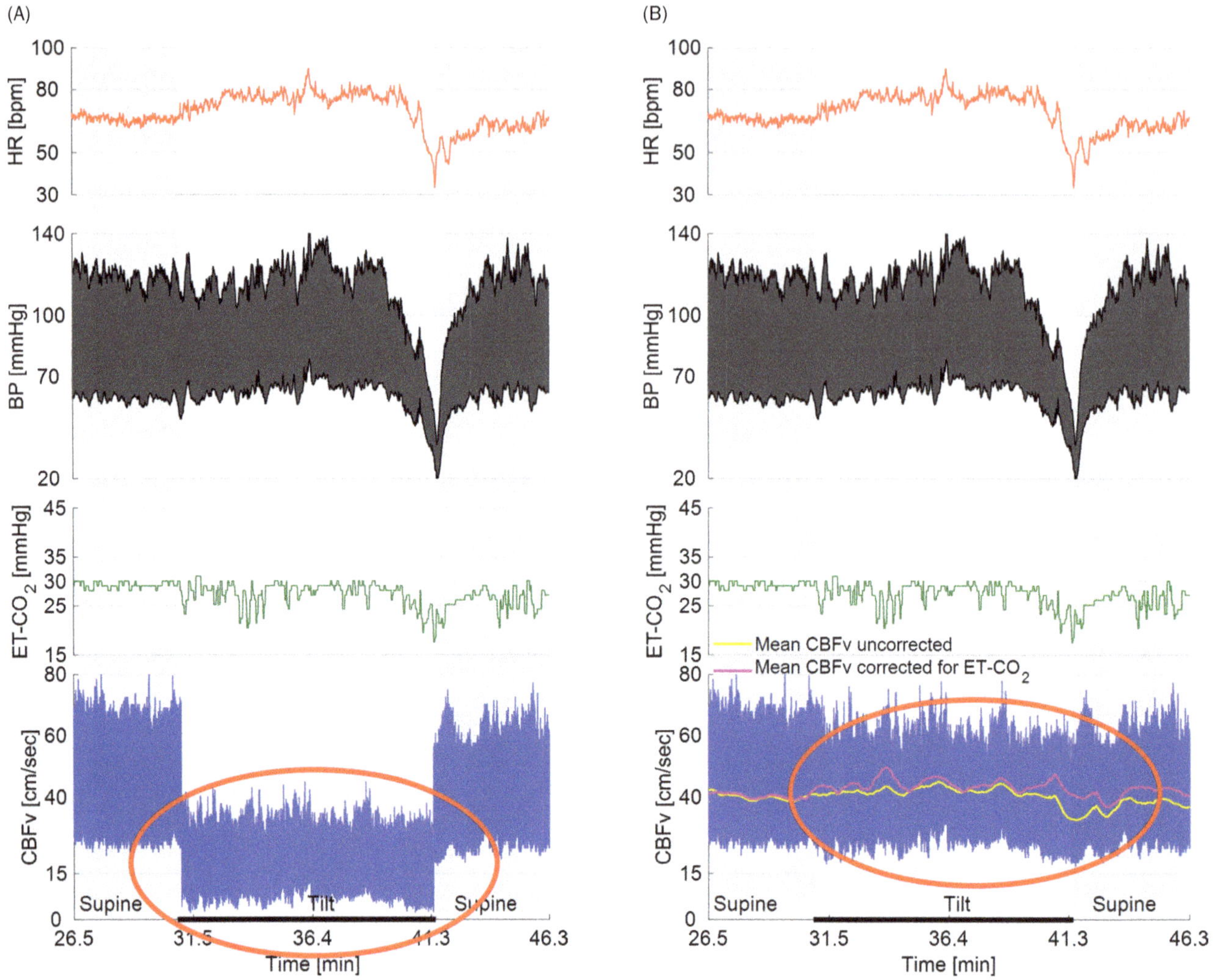

Figure 5.3 Cerebral blood flow velocity (CBFv, A–D) declined suddenly at the tilt onset and increased at the tilt end. Such sudden changes in CBFv are not physiological. In this patient, it was caused by shifting of the probe induced by tilt movement. This patient had a very narrow temporal window and adjustment of the Doppler probe during the tilt did not correct the signal. The patient experienced syncope at the 11th minute of the tilt, and the corrected CBFv showed a vasodilation pattern (increase in systolic and decrease in diastolic CBFv).

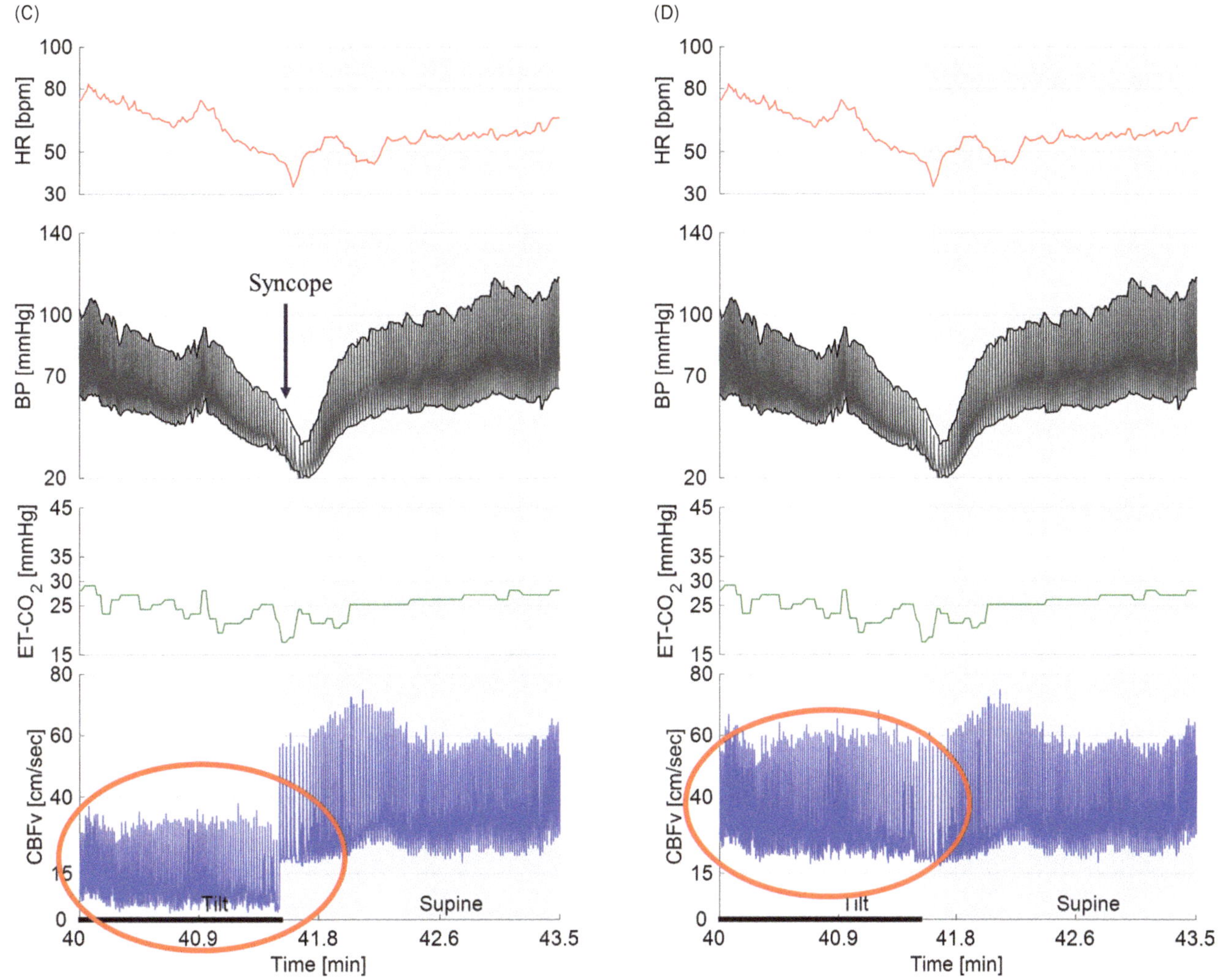

Figure 5.3 Continued

REFERENCE

1. Novak V, Novak P, Schondorf R. Accuracy of beat-to-beat noninvasive measurement of finger arterial pressure using the Finapres: a spectral analysis approach. *J Clin Monit*. 1994;10(2):118–126.

6.

CASE 1: NORMAL EXAMPLE

Chief complaint: None.

Case presentation: A 50-year-old woman presents for autonomic testing as a volunteer.

Past medical history: None.

Current medication: None.

Assessment plan: Functional autonomic tests and skin biopsy

AUTONOMIC TESTING EVALUATION

See Table 6.1.

Heart rate: Supine heart rate was normal. Heart rate responses to deep breathing were normal. Heart rate increment during the tilt (18 BPM) was normal.

Blood pressure:

Valsalva maneuver: Blood pressure responses were normal.

Tilt: Supine blood pressure was normal. Blood pressure responses to tilt were normal.

Sudomotor Evaluation: Sweat output was normal at forearm, normal at proximal leg, normal at distal leg, and normal at foot.

Respiratory system: Respiratory frequency and end tidal CO_2 were normal in supine position and during the tilt.

Cerebral blood flow velocity (CBFv): CBFv in middle cerebral artery was normal in supine position. CBFv in middle cerebral artery was stable during the tilt.

Skin biopsy (sensory-epidermal): Epidermal nerve fiber density was normal at proximal leg and normal at distal leg.

Skin biopsy (sweat glands): Sweat gland nerve fiber density was normal at proximal leg and normal at distal leg.

Patient-reported symptoms during testing: None during the tilt.

Patient-reported symptoms for past 2 weeks:

Lightheadedness or dizziness: None
Dry eyes or mouth: None
Pale feet: None
Cold feet: None
Reduced sweating: None
Reduced sweating after exercise: None
Increased sweating: None
Nausea: None
Diarrhea: None
Constipation: None
Urinary leaks: None
Current pain severity: 0
Aching pain: None
Allodynia: None
Burning pain: None
Lancinating pain: None
Numbness: None
Prickling sensation: None

TABLE 6.1 **RESULTS OF AUTONOMIC TESTING**

Blood pressure evaluation					
Test: Valsalva maneuver					
Pressure [mmHg]	Baseline	Phase 2			Phase 4
		Early	End		
Systolic	113	103	124		
Mean	79.7	74.3	83.3	n/a	
Diastolic	63	60	63	n/a	

Heart rate evaluation	
Test: Deep breathing	
Results	Norm*
20.4	≥9
Test: Valsalva ratio	
2.26	≥1.47
* adjusted for a gender and age	

TABLE 6.1 CONTINUED

Test: Tilt test											
Position		HR [BPM]	Blood pressure [mmHg]		MCA Blood flow velocity [cm/s]				Respiratory frequency [breaths/min]	End tidal CO_2 [mmHg]
			Systolic	Diastolic	Systolic	Mean	Mean drop [%]	Diastolic		
Supine		64	115	77	100	66.7		50	13	38
Tilt [min]	1	67	117	81	111	66.3	0.6	44	14	37
	2	67	118	70						
	3	72	112	76						
	4	72	112	76						
	5	74	115.4	75	108	65.3	2.1	44	15	36
	6	74	113	72						
	7	77	116.7	74						
	8	77	112	79						
	9	82	111	77						
	10	79	118	82	111	67.7	−1.5	46	14	37
	15									
	20									
	30									
	40									

Sudomotor evaluation—functional

Test: Quantitative sudomotor axon reflex test (QSART)				
Location	Site (l/r)	Latency [min]	Volume [μl]	Norm [μl]*
Forearm	l	1.5	0.6	≥0.08
Prox. leg	l	1.7	0.61	≥0.14
Distal leg	l	1.5	0.49	≥0.07
Foot	l	1.8	0.42	≥0.05

* normative data are adjusted for a gender and age of a patient

Test: Electrochemical skin conductance (ESC)				
Location	Left [μS]	Right [μS]	Average [μS/k]	Norm [μS/kg]
Hand				≥1.03
Feet				≥1.14
Forehead				

For grading uses ESC [μS] adjusted for weight [μS/k].

(continued)

TABLE 6.1 **CONTINUED**

Small fiber (sensory + sudomotor) evaluation—morphological					
Test: Skin biopsy					
		Nerve fibers			
		Epidermal*		Sweat glands	
Location	Site (l/r)	Density	Norm	Density	Norm
Proximal leg—thigh	Right	12.4	≥8.3	66.7	≥37.8
Distal leg—calf	Right	7.6	≥7.1	45.5	≥36.5
Foot	Right		≥3.11		≥34.8

* normative data for distal leg are adjusted for a gender and age of a patient

QASAT*											
Heart rate		BP		CBFv		ET-CO2		Sudomotor			Total QASAT score
S. bradycardia	0	Low supine	0	Low supine	0	Low supine	0	QSART	0		
S. tachycardia	0	High supine	0	High supine	0	High supine	0	ESC			
Increase tilt	0	OH	0	Tilt response	0	Tilt low	0				
Decrease tilt	0	OHTN	0	CA	0	Tilt high	0	**Skin biopsy**			0
Deep breathing	0	VM	0	CVR	0			Epidermal	0		
VR	0			VM	0			Sweat gland	0		
Total	0	Total	0	Total	0	Total	0				

*QASAT. See Novak. Quantitative Scale for Grading of Cardiovascular Autonomic Reflex Tests and Small Fibers from Skin Biopsies. *J Neurol Disord* 2015;3:2.

S, supine; Increase tilt, increased response to tilt; Decrease tilt, decreased response to tilt; BP, blood pressure; VM, Valsalva maneuver; CBFv, cerebral blood flow velocity; CA, cerebral autoregulation; MCA, middle cerebral artery; VR, Valsalva ratio; CVR, cerebral vasoreactivity.

AUTONOMIC TESTING INTERPRETATION

- The autonomic testing was normal.[1,2]
- There was no evidence of autonomic failure.
- There was no evidence of small fiber neuropathy on skin biopsy.
- Cerebral blood flow was normal in supine position. Orthostatic cerebral blood flow was stable.
- Respiratory functions were normal; there was no evidence of hyperventilation or hypoventilation.

COMMENT

Parasympathetic functions are evaluated by the deep breathing test. Adrenergic sympathetic functions are evaluated by the Valsalva maneuver and tilt test. Small fiber neuropathy is evaluated by both morphological tests (skin biopsy) and functional tests (quantitative sudomotor reflex axon test [QSART] and/or electrochemical skin conductance [ESC]). Cerebral blood flow is evaluated by transcranial Doppler, which depends on blood pressure and end tidal CO_2.

TREATMENT AND FOLLOW-UP

- None.

CAVEATS

- The report should summarize main findings.

REFERENCES

1. Novak P. Quantitative autonomic testing. *J Vis Exp JoVE*. 2011;(53). doi:10.3791/2502.
2. Novak P. Quantitative Scale for Grading of Cardiovascular Autonomic Reflex Tests and Small Fibers from Skin Biopsies (QASAT). *J Neurol Disord*. April 2015. doi:10.4172/2329-6895.1000226.

PART II

SYNCOPE, NEURALLY MEDIATED

7.

CASE 2: SYNCOPE, NEURALLY MEDIATED, MIXED

Chief complaint: Orthostatic intolerance.

Case presentation: A 19-year-old woman presents with unexplained heat and cold intolerance, dizziness, hearing loss, stomach cramps, shortness of breath, headaches, and chest pain for 1 year. All symptoms were intermittent, duration is minutes, usually orthostatic, and adding considerable anxiety. She passed out several times. Neurological examination was entirely normal. She was suspected to have postural tachycardia syndrome.

Past medical history: Depression, suspected postural tachycardia syndrome, anxiety.

Current medication: None.

Assessment plan: Functional autonomic tests and skin biopsy for evaluation of small fiber neuropathy since patient has history of cold intolerance which can be seen in small fiber neuropathy affecting sudomotor fibers.

AUTONOMIC TESTING EVALUATION

See Table 7.1.

Heart rate: Supine heart rate was normal. Heart rate responses to deep breathing were normal. Heart rate increment during the tilt (23 BPM) was normal.

Blood pressure:

Valsalva maneuver: Blood pressure responses were normal.

Tilt: Supine blood pressure was normal. There was a progressive decline in blood pressure until minute 4 of tilt, when the patient lost consciousness.

Sudomotor evaluation: Electrochemical skin conductance (ESC) was normal at hands and abnormal (reduced to 89.8% of normal limit) at feet.

Respiratory system: Respiratory frequency was normal in supine position and during the tilt. End tidal CO_2 was normal during supine position but was reduced during the tilt.

Cerebral blood flow velocity (CBFv): CBFv in middle cerebral artery was normal in supine position but was severely reduced during the tilt.

Skin biopsy (sensory-epidermal): Epidermal nerve fiber density was normal at proximal leg and normal at distal leg.

Skin biopsy (sweat glands): Sweat gland nerve fiber density was normal at proximal leg and normal at distal leg.

Patient-reported symptoms during testing: Dizziness and loss of consciousness during the tilt test.

TABLE 7.1 **RESULTS OF AUTONOMIC TESTING**

Blood pressure evaluation					
Test: Valsalva maneuver					
Pressure [mmHg]	Baseline	Phase 2			Phase 4
		Early	End		
Systolic	84	68	73		
Mean	58.7	56.7	65	n/a	
Diastolic	46	51	61	n/a	

Heart rate evaluation	
Test: Deep breathing	
Results	Norm*
27.6	≥14
Test: Valsalva ratio	
1.63	≥1.46
* Adjusted for a gender and age	

(continued)

TABLE 7.1 **CONTINUED**

Test: Tilt test										
Position			HR [BPM]	Blood pressure [mmHg]		MCA Blood flow velocity [cm/s]			Respiratory frequency [breaths/min]	End tidal CO_2 [mmHg]
			Systolic	Diastolic	Systolic	Mean	Mean drop [%]	Diastolic		
Supine		57	101	62	114	68		45	15	41
Tilt [min]	1	73	93	63	111	68.3	-0.4	47	16	36
	2	80	86	55						
	3	64	83	55						
	4	48	65	37						
	5									
	6									
	7									
	8									
	9									
	10									
	15									
	20									
	30									
	40									

Sudomotor evaluation - functional

Test: Quantitative sudomotor axon reflex test (QSART)				
Location	Site (l/r)	Latency [min]	Volume [μl]	Norm [μl]*
Forearm				≥0.08
Prox. leg				≥0.14
Distal leg				≥0.24
Foot				≥0.09

* Normative data are adjusted for gender and age of patient.

Test: Electrochemical skin conductance (ESC)				
Location	Left [μS]	Right [μS]	Average [μS/k]	Norm [μS/kg]
Hand	77	73	1.18	≥1.03
Feet	65	65	1.02	≥1.14
Forehead				

For grading uses ESC [μS] adjusted for weight [μS/k].

TABLE 7.1 CONTINUED

Small fiber (sensory + sudomotor) evaluation - morphological					
Test: Skin biopsy					
Location	Site (l/r)	Nerve fibers			
		Epidermal*		Sweat glands	
		Density	Norm	Density	Norm
Proximal leg – thigh	Right	17.34	≥8.3	45	≥37.8
Distal leg – calf	Right	14.9	≥9.58	48.6	≥36.5
Foot	Right		≥3.11		≥34.8

* Normative data for distal leg are adjusted for gender and age of patient.

QASAT*										
Heart rate		**BP**		**CBFv**		**ET-CO2**		**Sudomotor**		**Total QASAT score**
S. bradycardia	0	Low supine	0	Low supine	0	Low supine	0	QSART		
S. tachycardia	0	High supine	0	High supine	0	High supine	0	ESC	1	
Increase tilt		OH		Tilt response		Tilt low				
Decrease tilt		OHTN		CA	0	Tilt high		**Skin biopsy**		1
Deep breathing	0	VM	0	CVR	0			Epidermal	0	
VR	0			VM	0			Sweat gland	0	
Total	0	Total	0	Total	0	Total	0			

*QASAT. See Novak. Quantitative Scale for Grading of Cardiovascular Autonomic Reflex Tests and Small Fibers from Skin Biopsies. *J Neurol Disord* 2015;3:2. Orthostatic (tilt) responses were not graded since QASAT requires the duration of the tilt at least 10 minutes.

S, supine; Increase tilt, increased response to tilt; Decrease tilt, decreased response to tilt; BP, blood pressure; VM, Valsalva maneuver; CBFv, cerebral blood flow velocity; CA, cerebral autoregulation; MCA, middle cerebral artery; VR, Valsalva ratio; CVR, cerebral vasoreactivity.

Patient reported symptoms for past 2 weeks:

Lightheadedness or dizziness: Occasionally
Dry eyes or mouth: Occasionally
Pale feet: Occasionally
Cold feet: Often
Reduced sweating: None
Reduced sweating after exercise: None
Increased sweating: Occasionally
Nausea: Occasionally
Diarrhea: Occasionally
Constipation: Occasionally
Urinary leaks: None
Current pain severity: 4
Aching pain: Often, moderate
Allodynia: None
Burning pain: Occasionally, moderate
Lancinating pain: None
Numbness: Often, severe
Prickling sensation: Often, severe

AUTONOMIC TESTING INTERPRETATION

- Syncope, neurally mediated, mixed.
- Mild sudomotor dysfunction, which can be seen in early small fiber neuropathy.
- No evidence of significant autonomic failure, orthostatic hypotension, or postural tachycardia syndrome.

COMMENT

Initial response to the tilt was normal (Figure 7.1). The patient became dizzy, complained of shortness of breath, and started to hyperventilate at minute 2 of the tilt. Subsequently she became dizzier, anxious, and her vision became blurred. The latter symptoms were accompanied by a progressive decline in blood pressure and in end tidal CO_2 until she passed out at the minute 5. ECG showed bradycardia and sinus rhythm. Decline in blood pressure during syncope was accompanied by characteristic widening of Doppler signal (reduction of diastolic and an increase in systolic flow velocity) that indicates compensatory cerebral arteriolar vasodilation and normal cerebral autoregulation.[1] Simultaneous decline in blood pressure and heart rate is consistent with mixed syncope.

TREATMENT AND FOLLOW-UP

- Reassurance is important in the case of neurally mediated syncope. Patient's anxiety was greatly relieved after it was explained that neurally mediated syncope has a good prognosis.
- Patient was educated on how to avoid trigger events, how to recognize the symptoms, and how to perform maneuvres to abort syncope. She was also recommended exercise training and a high-volume fluid and salt diet.

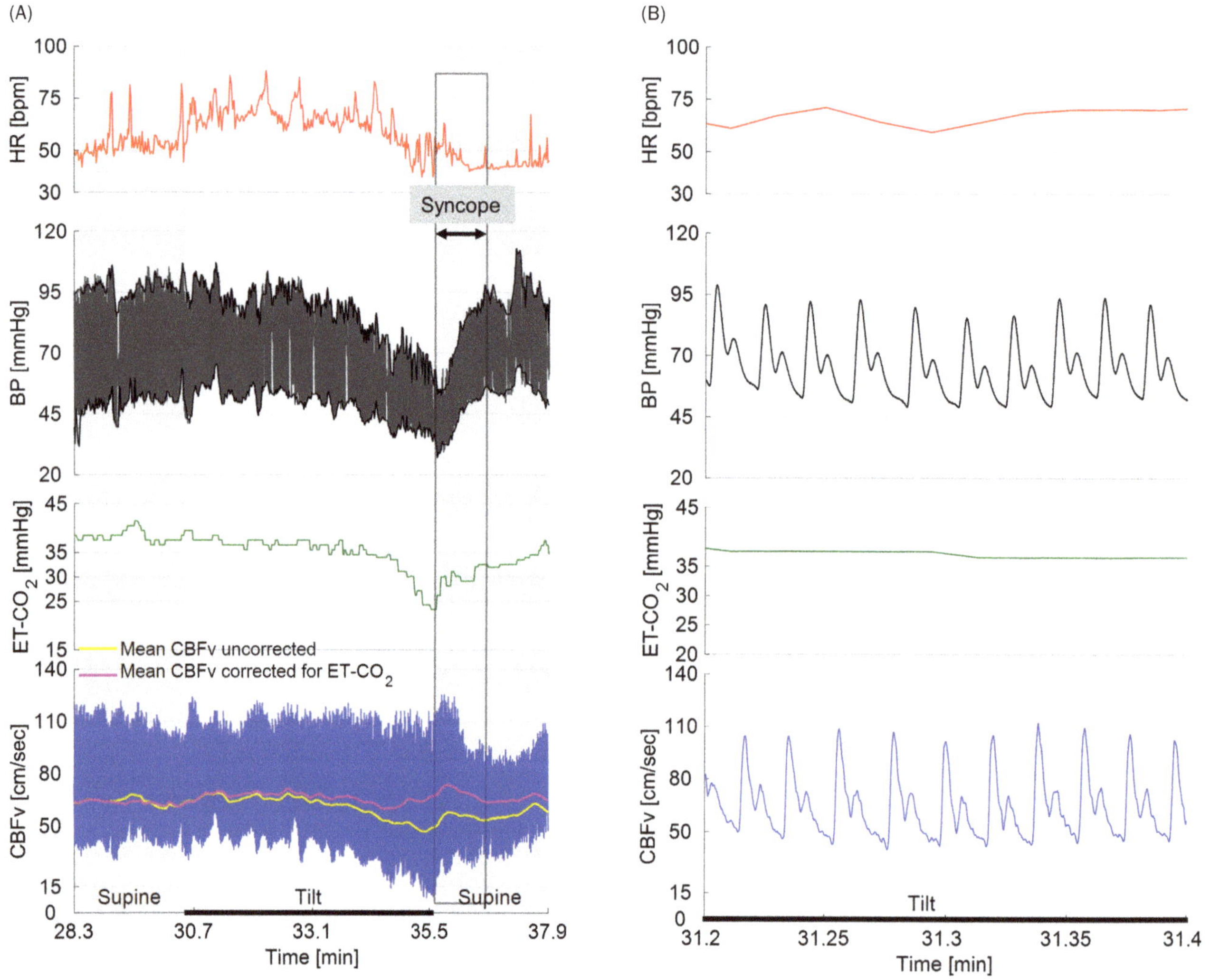

Figure 7.1 The tilt test provoked syncope of mixed type (A–C). The initial responses to tilting were normal. Then, starting at minute 5 of the tilt, there was a progressive decline in heart rate, blood pressure, end tidal CO_2, and diastolic cerebral blood flow velocity (CBFv) until the patient lost consciousness. Details of signals just before (B) and during the syncope (C) show characteristic patterns typical of syncope of mixed type. Cerebral vasodilation pattern (reduced diastolic more than systolic CBFv) was present during syncope despite severe hyperventilation (end tidal CO_2 ~22 mm Hg during syncope, normal range 35–45 mm Hg) which causes cerebral vasoconstriction and reduction in systolic CBFv.

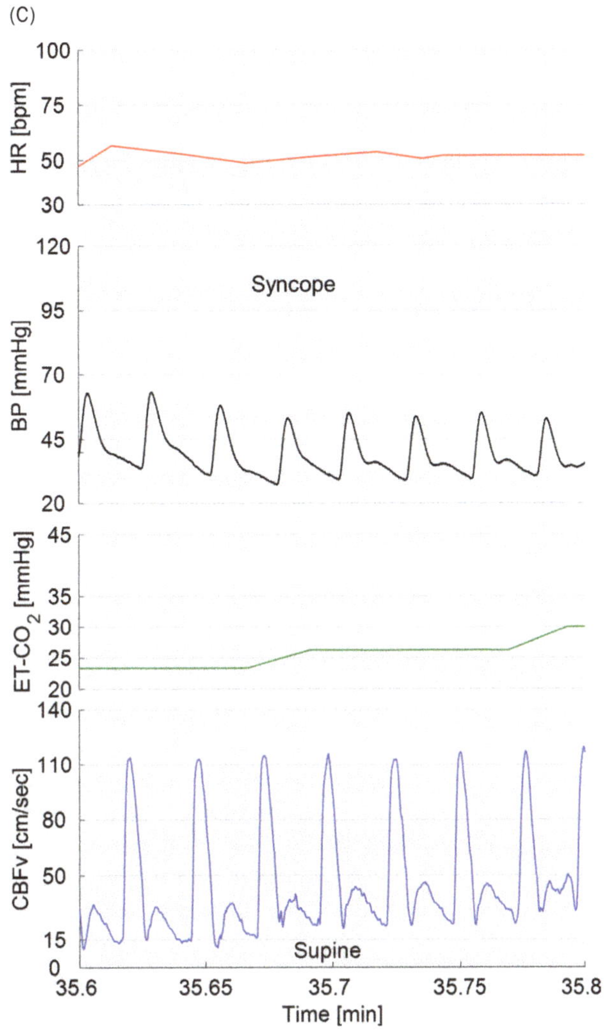

Figure 7.1 Continued

CAVEATS

- Neurally mediated syncope has a characteristic pattern on the tilt test.[1]
- Neurally mediated syncope is a benign syndrome with favorable prognosis.[2]

REFERENCES

1. Novak P. Cerebral blood flow, heart rate, and blood pressure patterns during the tilt test in common orthostatic syndromes. *Neurosci J*. 2016;2016:6127340. doi:10.1155/2016/6127340.
2. Soteriades ES, Evans JC, Larson MG, et al. Incidence and prognosis of syncope. *N Engl J Med*. 2002;347(12):878–885. doi:10.1056/NEJMoa012407.

8.

CASE 3: SYNCOPE WITHOUT HYPERVENTILATION

Chief complaint: Dizziness.

Case presentation: A 20-year-old woman presents with orthostatic dizziness, hot flashes, and memory problems for 2 years. For the past weeks, she experienced burning sensation in the distal legs and occasional widespread deeper pain. She was diagnosed with Lyme disease and tried multiple antibiotics. Neurological examination was entirely normal.

Past medical history: Lyme disease.

Current medication: Vancomycin.

Assessment plan: Functional autonomic tests and skin biopsy.

AUTONOMIC TESTING EVALUATION

See Table 8.1.

Heart rate: Supine heart rate was normal. Heart rate responses to deep breathing were normal. Heart rate increment during the tilt (40 BPM) was exaggerated.

Blood pressure:

Valsalva maneuver: Blood pressure responses were normal.

Tilt: Supine blood pressure was within normal range. Blood pressure responses to tilt were normal within the initial 12 minutes of the tilt. Then at minute 13 of the tilt, there was a rapid and progressive decline in blood pressure until the patient developed syncope and the tilt was aborted.

Sudomotor evaluation: Sweat output was normal at forearm, normal at proximal leg, normal at distal leg, and normal at foot. Quantitative sudomotor axon reflex tests (QSART) showed length dependent pattern with a decrease of sweat output distally at least 33%.

Respiratory system: Respiratory frequency was normal in supine position and during the tilt. End tidal CO_2 was mildly reduced in supine position and during the tilt.

Cerebral blood flow velocity (CBFv): CBFv in middle cerebral artery was normal in supine position. CBFv in middle cerebral artery was reduced during the tilt test.

Skin biopsy (sensory-epidermal): Epidermal nerve fiber density was normal at proximal leg and abnormal (reduced to 96.3% of normal limit) at distal leg.

Skin biopsy (sweat glands): Sweat gland nerve fiber density was normal at distal leg.

Patient-reported symptoms during testing: Dizziness, loss of consciousness during the tilt.

Patient-reported symptoms for past 2 weeks:

Lightheadedness or dizziness: Occasionally
Dry eyes or mouth: Occasionally
Pale feet: Occasionally
Cold feet: Occasionally

TABLE 8.1 **RESULTS OF AUTONOMIC TESTING**

Blood pressure evaluation					
Test: Valsalva maneuver					
Pressure [mmHg]	Baseline	Phase 2			Phase 4
		Early	End		
Systolic	127	119	139		
Mean	87	84.3	99.7	n/a	
Diastolic	67	67	80	n/a	

Heart rate evaluation	
Test: Deep breathing	
Results	Norm*
28.67	≥14
Test: Valsalva ratio	
1.69	≥1.46
* adjusted for a gender and age	

TABLE 8.1 CONTINUED

Test: Tilt test										
Position		HR [BPM]	Blood pressure [mmHg]		MCA Blood flow velocity [cm/s]				Respiratory frequency [breaths/min]	End tidal CO2 [mmHg]
			Systolic	Diastolic	Systolic	Mean	Mean drop [%]	Diastolic		
Supine		80	116	72	118	72.7		50	13	34
Tilt [min]	1	79	123	76	110	65.3	10.2	43	9	32
	2	74	117	81						
	3	84	112	79						
	4	82	116	80						
	5	90	115	79	101	59	18.8	38	9	30
	6	92	113	80						
	7	90	110	79						
	8	107	118	82						
	9	115	117	83						
	10	120	112	78	114	71.3	1.9	50	19	30
	15									
	20									
	30									
	40									

Sudomotor evaluation – functional

Test: Quantitative sudomotor axon reflex test (QSART)				
Location	Site (l/r)	Latency [min]	Volume [µl]	Norm [µl]*
Forearm	l	1.39	0.573	≥0.08
Prox. leg	l	0.18	0.471	≥0.14
Distal leg	l	0.06	0.914	≥0.24
Foot	l	1.57	0.151	≥0.09

* Normative data are adjusted for gender and age of patient.

Test: Electrochemical skin conductance (ESC)				
Location	Left [µS]	Right [µS]	Average [µS/k]	Norm [µS/kg]
Hand				≥1.03
Feet				≥1.14
Forehead				

For grading uses ESC [µS] adjusted for weight [µS/k].

(continued)

TABLE 8.1 **CONTINUED**

Small fiber (sensory + sudomotor) evaluation – morphological					
Test: Skin biopsy					
Location	Site (l/r)	Nerve fibers			
		Epidermal*		Sweat glands	
		Density	Norm	Density	Norm
Proximal leg – thigh	Right	9.32	≥8.3		≥37.8
Distal leg - calf	Right	9.15	≥9.5	39.7	≥36.5
Foot	Right		≥3.11		≥34.8

* Normative data for distal leg are adjusted for gender and age of patient.

QASAT*											
Heart rate		**BP**		**CBFv**		**ET CO2**		**Sudomotor**			**Total QASAT score**
S. bradycardia	0	Low sup.	0	Low sup.	0	Low sup.	1	QSART	1		
S. tachycardia	0	High sup.	0	High sup.	0	High sup.	0	ESC			
Increase. tilt	1	OH	0	Tilt resp.	2	Tilt low	1				
Decreas. tilt	0	OHTN	0	CA	0	Tilt high	0	**Skin biopsy**			7
Deep breath	0	VM	0	CVR	0			Epidermal	1		
VR	0			VM	0			Sweat gland	0		
Total	1	Total	0	Total	2	Total	2				

*QASAT. See Novak. Quantitative Scale for Grading of Cardiovascular Autonomic Reflex Tests and Small Fibers from Skin Biopsies. *J Neurol Disord* 2015;3:2.

S, supine; Increase tilt, increased response to tilt; Decrease tilt, decreased response to tilt; BP, blood pressure; VM, Valsalva maneuver; CBFv, cerebral blood flow velocity; CA, cerebral autoregulation; MCA, middle cerebral artery; VR, Valsalva ratio; CVR, cerebral vasoreactivity.

Reduced sweating: Occasionally
Reduced sweating after exercise: Occasionally
Increased sweating: Occasionally
Nausea: Occasionally
Diarrhea: Occasionally
Constipation: Occasionally
Urinary leaks: Yes, minor annoyance
Current pain severity: 0
Aching pain: Often, moderate
Allodynia: Occasionally, mild
Burning pain: Occasionally, mild
Lancinating pain: Often, moderate
Numbness: Often, mild
Prickling sensation: Occasionally, mild

Cardiovascular and cerebrovascular recordings before and during syncope (B-C) show characteristic changes seen in syncope of mixed type including the cerebral vasodilation pattern (reduced diastolic signal more than systolic cerebral blood flow velocity).

AUTONOMIC TESTING INTERPRETATION

- Syncope, neurally mediated, mixed.[1–3]
- Postural orthostatic intolerance syndrome (POTS), mild.
- Small fiber neuropathy, mixed, length dependent.

COMMENT

Two main findings were detected through autonomic testing: POTS/syncope and sensory small fiber neuropathy (Figure 8.1). The findings are relevant to the patient symptoms as the testing explains the reason for orthostatic intolerance (POTS/syncope) and pain (small fiber neuropathy). Furthermore, syncope is usually accompanied by hyperventilation, but, as illustrated by this case, syncope can occur without hyperventilation.

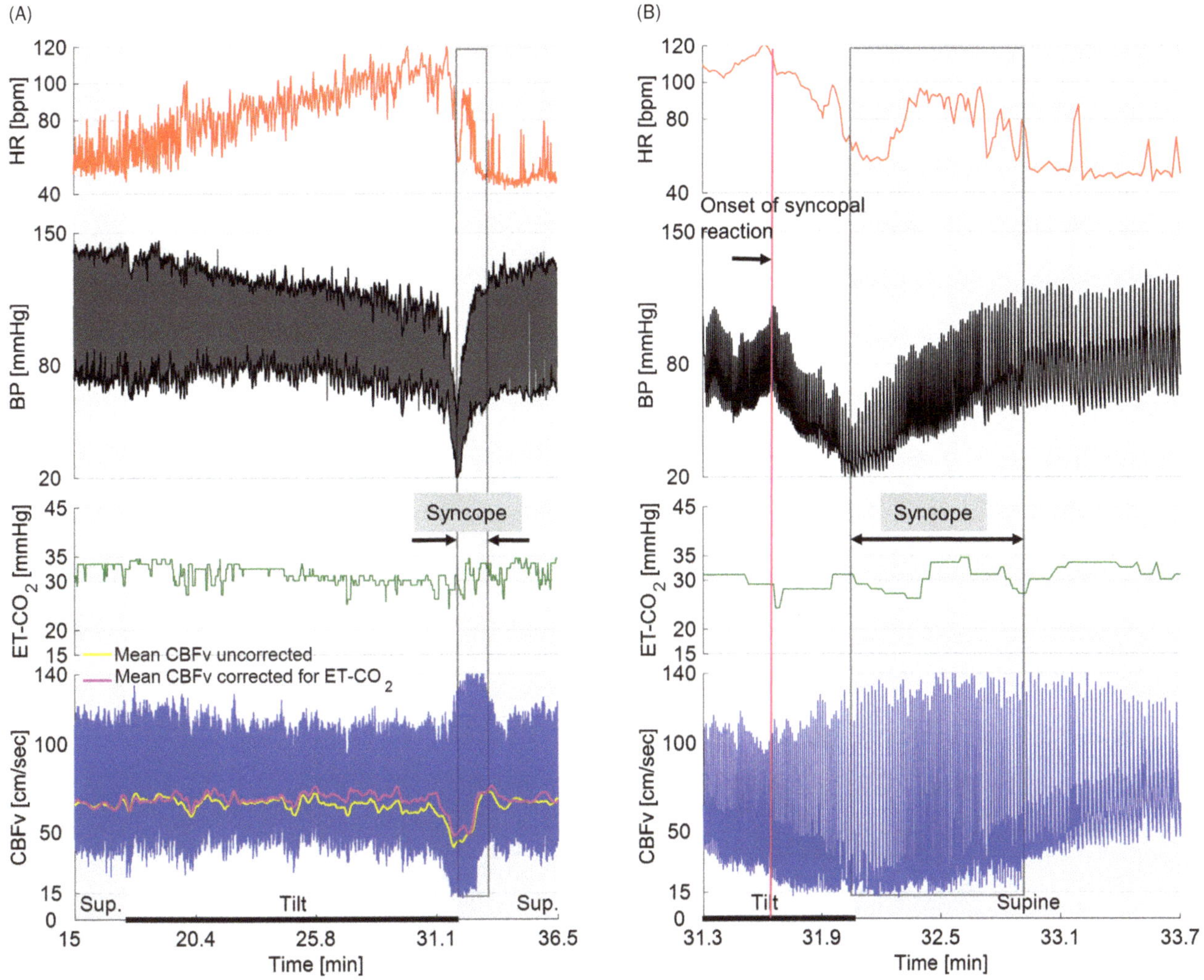

Figure 8.1 The tilt test provoked syncope (A–C). The responses to tilting were normal during the first 10 minutes of the tilt. Then, suddenly at minute 13 of the tilt, there was a fast (within 20 seconds) decline in heart rate, blood pressure, and diastolic cerebral blood flow velocity until the patient lost consciousness. At baseline, there was a mild hypocapnia (32–34 mm Hg, normal range 35–45 mm Hg of end tidal CO_2). However, the typical hyperventilatory response with decline of end tidal CO_2 just before syncope was absent.

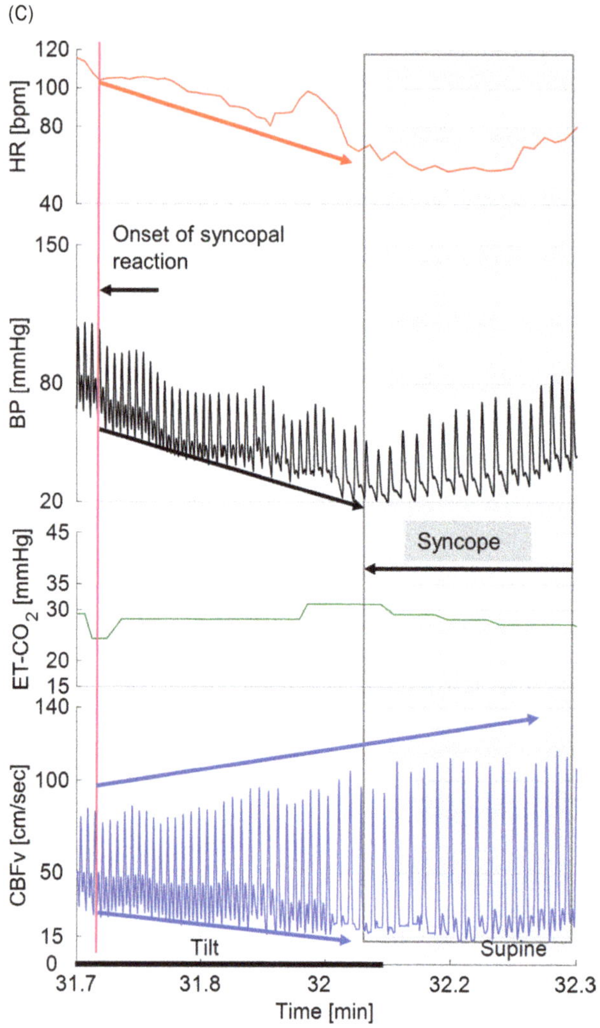

Figure 8.1 Continued

TREATMENT AND FOLLOW-UP

- Clinical workup for neuropathy.
- Volume expansion through high fluid and high salt intake.

CAVEATS

- Syncope may occur without hyperventilation.
- The tilt test that is longer than 10 minute may be necessary to provoke syncope.
- Syncope may be independent from small fiber sensory neuropathy.

REFERENCES

1. Novak P. Cerebral blood flow, heart rate, and blood pressure patterns during the tilt test in common orthostatic syndromes. *Neurosci J.* 2016;2016:6127340. doi:10.1155/2016/6127340.
2. Brignole M. Neurally-mediated syncope. *Ital Heart J Off J Ital Fed Cardiol.* 2005;6(3):249–255.
3. Can I, Cytron J, Jhanjee R, Nguyen J, Benditt DG. Neurally-mediated syncope. *Minerva Med.* 2009;100(4):275–292.

9.

CASE 4: SYNCOPE, VASODEPRESSOR

Chief complaint: Dizziness.

Case presentation: A 22-year-old woman presents with orthostatic intolerance. She used to be very active, and was even active in rock climbing, until she was diagnosed with mononucleosis 3 years ago. Subsequently, she noticed dizziness during prolonged standing with intermittent tingling and numbness in her legs. Even mild exercise induced fatigue and leg weakness. Dizziness became the most disabling symptom. She has good and bad days; bad days are related to menstrual periods. She was evaluated by several neurologists and cardiologists, but examinations were unrevealing. MRI of the brain and EEG was normal. Patient was referred for evaluation of orthostatic intolerance.

Past medical history: Low vitamin D and B_{12}.

Current medication: Sertraline, gabapentin, vitamins D and B_{12}.

Assessment plan: Functional autonomic tests and skin biopsy.

AUTONOMIC TESTING EVALUATION

See Table 9.1.

Heart rate: Supine heart rate was normal. Heart rate responses to deep breathing were normal. Heart rate increment during the tilt (39 BPM) was exaggerated.

Blood pressure:

Valsalva maneuver: Blood pressure responses were normal.

Tilt: Supine blood pressure was within normal range. There was a progressive decline in blood pressure until the patient developed a syncope at minute 3 of tilt, then the tilt was aborted.

Sudomotor evaluation: Sweat output was normal at forearm, normal at proximal leg, normal at distal leg, and normal at foot. Quantitative sudomotor axon reflex test (QSART) showed length-dependent pattern with a decrease of sweat output distally of at least 33%.

Respiratory system: Respiratory frequency was normal during supine and during the tilt. End tidal CO_2 was reduced during supine position and further declined during the tilt.

Cerebral blood flow velocity (CBFv): CBFv in middle cerebral artery was normal in supine position. CBFv in middle cerebral artery was mildly reduced during the tilt test.

Skin biopsy (sensory-epidermal): Epidermal nerve fiber density was normal at proximal leg and normal at distal leg.

Skin biopsy (sweat glands): Sweat gland nerve fiber density was normal at proximal leg and normal at distal leg.

Patient-reported symptoms during testing: Dizziness during the tilt.

TABLE 9.1 RESULTS OF AUTONOMIC TESTING

Blood pressure evaluation					
Test: Valsalva maneuver					
Pressure [mmHg]	Baseline	Phase 2			Phase 4
		Early	End		
Systolic	128	108	138		
Mean	90.7	81.3	113.3	n/a	
Diastolic	72	68	101	n/a	

Heart rate evaluation	
Test: Deep breathing	
Results	Norm*
18.43	≥14
Test: Valsalva ratio	
1.68	≥1.46
* Adjusted for a gender and age	

(continued)

TABLE 9.1 **CONTINUED**

Test: Tilt test											
Position		HR [BPM]	Blood pressure [mmHg]		MCA Blood flow velocity [cm/s]				Respiratory frequency [breaths/min]	End tidal CO_2 [mmHg]
			Systolic	Diastolic	Systolic	Mean	Mean drop [%]	Diastolic		
Supine		66	94	60	110	66.7		45	11	27
Tilt [min]	1	93	111	72	112	68.7	–3	47	17	26
	2	105	98	63						
	3	83	80	50						
	4									
	5									
	6									
	7									
	8									
	9									
	10									
	15									
	20									
	30									
	40									

Sudomotor evaluation - functional

Test: Quantitative sudomotor axon reflex test (QSART)				
Location	Site (l/r)	Latency [min]	Volume [μl]	Norm [μl]*
Forearm	l	2.45	0.106	≥0.08
Prox. leg	l	2.23	0.656	≥0.14
Distal leg	l	3.37	0.449	≥0.24
Foot	l	2.47	0.298	≥0.09

* Normative data are adjusted for gender and age of patient.

Test: Electrochemical skin conductance (ESC)				
Location	Left [μS]	Right [μS]	Average [μS/k]	Norm [μS/kg]
Hand				≥1.03
Feet				≥1.14
Forehead				

For grading, use ESC [μS] adjusted for weight [μS/k].

TABLE 9.1 **CONTINUED**

Small fiber (sensory + sudomotor) evaluation - morphological					
Test: Skin biopsy					
Location	Site (l/r)	Nerve fibers			
		Epidermal*		Sweat glands	
		Density	Norm	Density	Norm
Proximal leg – thigh	Right	11.18	≥8.3	53.1	≥37.8
Distal leg - calf	Right	13.62	≥9.34	55.3	≥36.5
Foot	Right		≥3.11		≥34.8

* Normative data for distal leg are adjusted for gender and age of patient.

QASAT*										
Heart rate		**BP**		**CBFv**		**ET-CO2**		**Sudomotor**		**Total QASAT score**
S. bradycardia	0	Low supine	0	Low supine	0	Low supine	1	QSART	1	
S. tachycardia	0	High supine	0	High supine	0	High supine	0	ESC		
Increase tilt		OH		Tilt response		Tilt low				
Decrease tilt		OHTN		CA	0	Tilt high		**Skin biopsy**		2
Deep breathing	0	VM	0	CVR	0			Epidermal	0	
VR	0			VM	0			Sweat gland	0	
Total	0	Total	0	Total	0	Total	1			

*QASAT. See Novak. Quantitative Scale for Grading of Cardiovascular Autonomic Reflex Tests and Small Fibers from Skin Biopsies. *J Neurol Disord* 2015;3:2. Orthostatic (tilt) responses were not graded since QASAT requires the duration of the tilt at least 10 minutes.

S, supine; Increase tilt, increased response to tilt; Decrease tilt, decreased response to tilt; BP, blood pressure; VM, Valsalva maneuver; CBFv, cerebral blood flow velocity; CA, cerebral autoregulation; MCA, middle cerebral artery; VR, Valsalva ratio; CVR, cerebral vasoreactivity.

Patient-reported symptoms for past 2 weeks:

Lightheadedness or dizziness: Occasionally
Dry eyes or mouth: None
Pale feet: Yes, minor annoyance
Cold feet: Occasionally
Reduced sweating: None
Reduced sweating after exercise: Occasionally
Increased sweating: Occasionally
Nausea: Occasionally
Diarrhea: None
Constipation: Yes, minor annoyance
Urinary leaks: Yes, minor annoyance
Aching pain: Continuous, severe
Allodynia: Occasionally, moderate
Burning pain: Occasionally, mild
Lancinating pain: Often, moderate
Numbness: Occasionally, mild
Prickling sensation: Continuous, moderate

AUTONOMIC TESTING INTERPRETATION

- Syncope, neurally mediated, vasodepressor.
- Mild sudomotor dysfunction can be seen in early small fiber neuropathy.
- There was no evidence of autonomic failure.

COMMENT

The autonomic testing revealed vasodepressor syncope (Figure 9.1). The decline in blood pressure while the heart rate remains unchanged, is characteristic for vasodepressor syncope.[1,2] This is a rare type of syncope. It is important to differentiate among various types of syncope because the therapy differs by syncope type.

In spite of several sensory complaints, the skin biopsy did not reveal small fiber neuropathy. Mild sudomotor dysfunction detected in the testing may indicate early damage of small fibers.[3]

Patient was doing temporarily well on diet and exercise adjustment. Two years after initial autonomic evaluations, she experienced worsening sensory symptoms and developed autonomic failure. Subsequently, she was unable to work.

TREATMENT AND FOLLOW-UP

- Volume expansion by high fluid and high salt intake, strenuous exercise.

CAVEATS

- Syncope can be the first manifestation of small fiber neuropathy and autonomic failure.

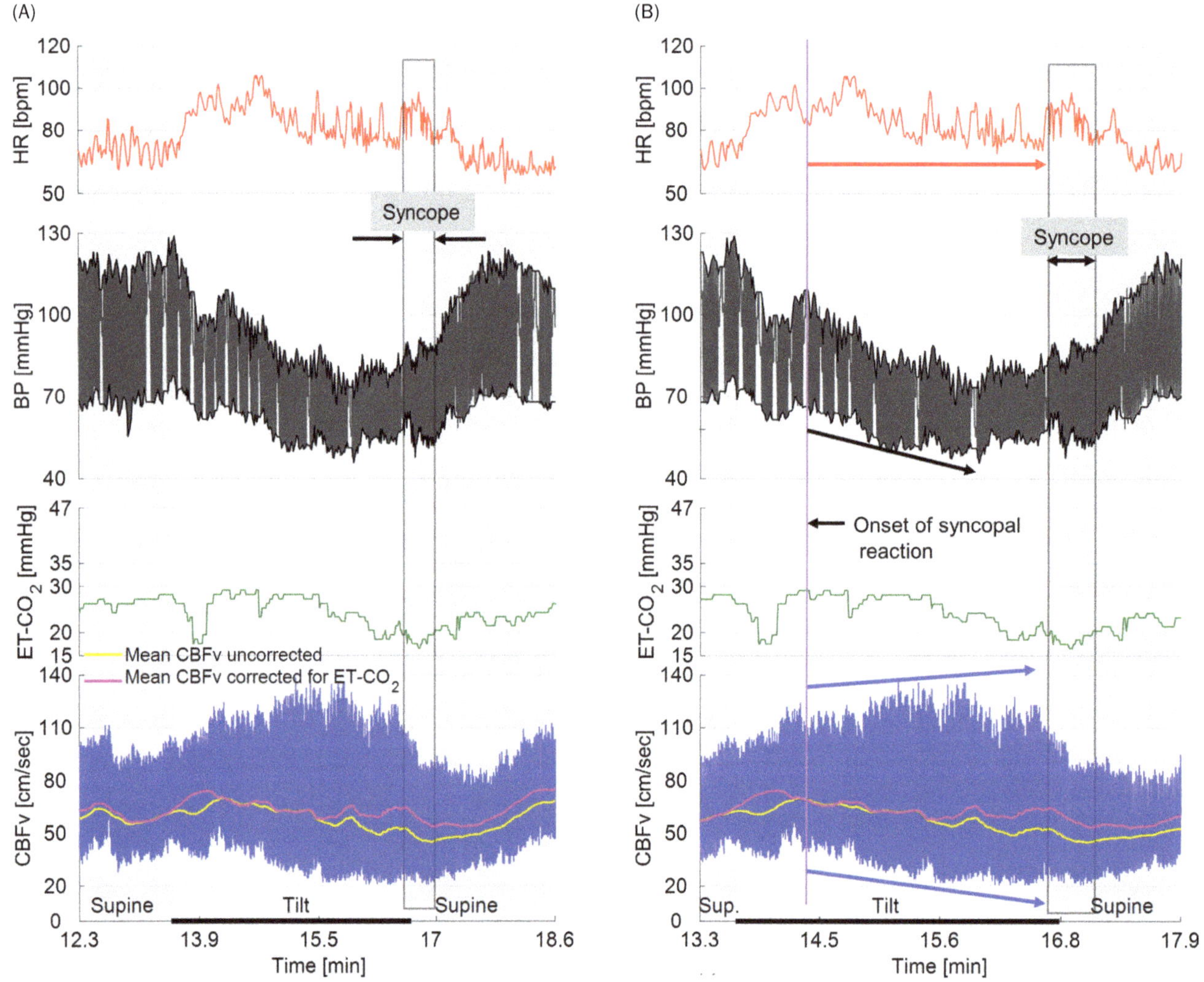

Figure 9.1 The tilt test provoked syncope early after tilt onset (A–D). The progressive decline in blood pressure (*black descending arrows*, B) started after the first minute of the tilt. Heart rate did not change significantly (*horizontal red arrow*). Patient was hyperventilating, as indicated by hypocapnia (end tidal CO_2 <35 mm Hg). Cerebral blood flow velocity showed a vasodilation pattern with a widening of the velocity signal, reduction of the diastolic (*descending blue arrow*), and increase in systolic (*ascending blue arrow*) cerebral blood flow velocities.

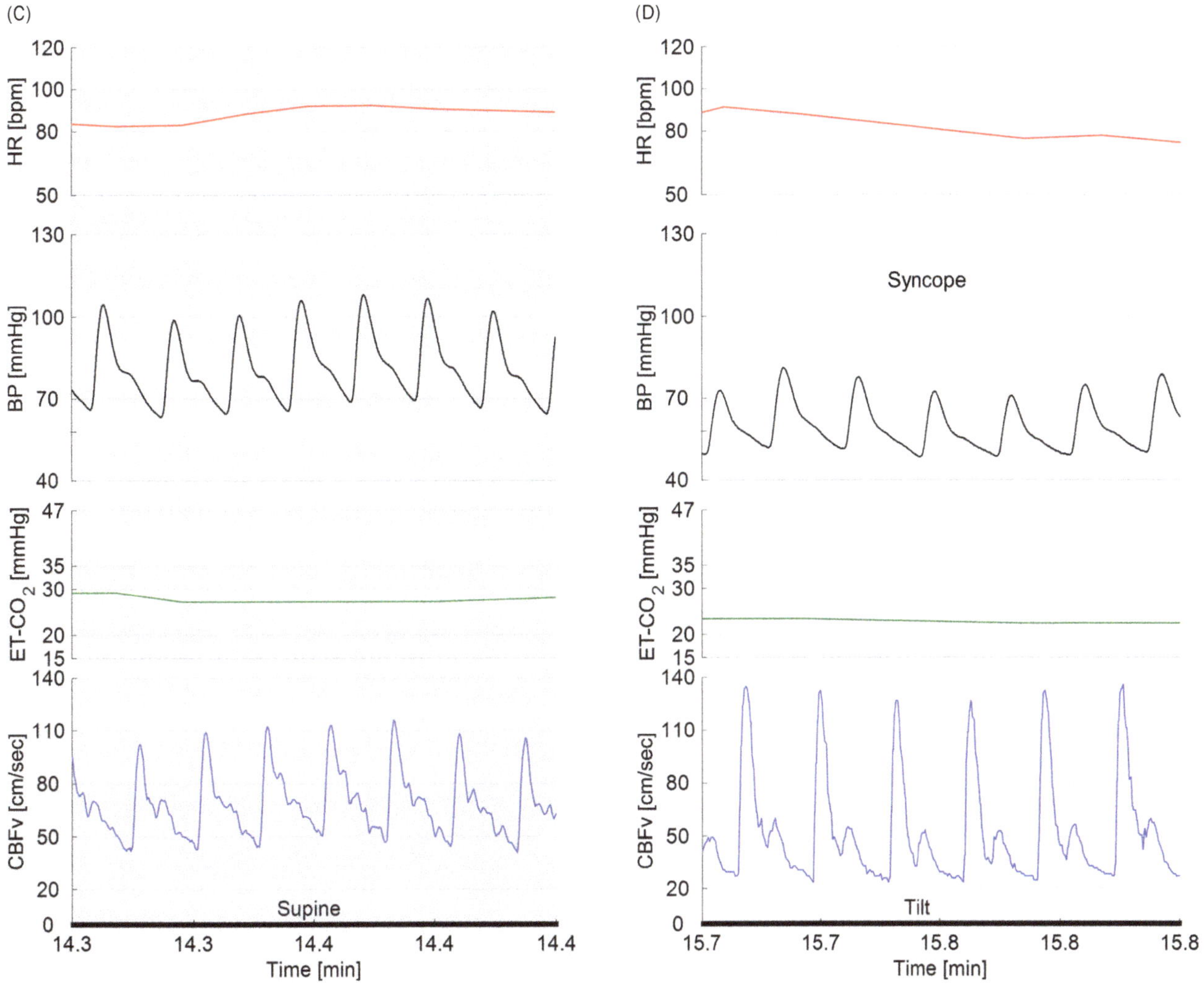

Figure 9.1 Continued

REFERENCES

1. Weissler AM, Warren JV, Estes EH, Mcintosh HD, Leonard JJ. Vasodepressor syncope: factors influencing cardiac output. *Circulation*. 1957;15(6):875–882.
2. Novak P. Cerebral blood flow, heart rate, and blood pressure patterns during the tilt test in common orthostatic syndromes. *Neurosci J*. 2016;2016:6127340. doi:10.1155/2016/6127340.
3. Low VA, Sandroni P, Fealey RD, Low PA. Detection of small-fiber neuropathy by sudomotor testing. *Muscle Nerve*. 2006;34(1):57–61. doi:10.1002/mus.20551.

10.

CASE 5: SYNCOPE, NEURALLY MEDIATED VASODEPRESSOR WITH CEREBRAL AUTOREGULATORY FAILURE

Chief complaint: Loss of consciousness.

Case presentation: A 76-year-old woman presents with episodic loss of consciousness. As a child she had several episodes of passing out which resolved. She had hip replacement surgery 4 years ago, and since then she has been passing out once per year. Her warning symptom is usually dizziness, but not always. At times she can stop the spell by lying down. She also passed out at her trip to Asia during hot weather after having a beer. She also passed out in the street; at that time her blood pressure was around 80/60 mm Hg. Neurological evaluation was unrevealing; she was not orthostatic at the office. Cardiac evaluation was unrevealing as well, and Holter monitoring did not record any spells. Patient was referred for autonomic testing for evaluation of suspected syncope.

Past medical history: Dyslipidemia, vitamin D deficiency, hypertension.

Current medication: Aspirin, atorvastatin, lisinopril, gabapentin.

Assessment plan: Functional autonomic tests and skin biopsy.

AUTONOMIC TESTING EVALUATION

See Table 10.1.

Heart rate: Supine heart rate was normal. Heart rate responses to deep breathing were reduced to 35.7% of normal value. Heart rate increment during the tilt (16 BPM) was normal.

Blood pressure:

Valsalva maneuver: Mean blood pressure failed to return to baseline at the end of Phase 2 by 37.3 mm Hg; that is 65.6% of baseline.

Tilt: Supine blood pressure was normal. Blood pressure was stable for the first 6 minutes. Afterward, there was a progressive decline in blood pressure until patient lost consciousness, which was consistent with syncope. Heart rate did not change during the syncope.

Sudomotor evaluation: Electrochemical skin conductance was abnormal (reduced to 66.9% of normal limit) at hands and abnormal (reduced to 55.1% of normal limit) at feet.

Respiratory system: Respiratory frequency was normal in supine position and during the tilt. End tidal CO_2 was reduced during in supine position and was further reduced during the tilt test.

Cerebral blood flow velocity (CBFv): CBFv in middle cerebral artery was reduced in supine position. CBFv in middle cerebral artery was severely reduced during the tilt test.

Skin biopsy (sensory-epidermal): N/A

Skin biopsy (sweat glands): N/A

Patient-reported symptoms during testing: Dizziness during the tilt test.

TABLE 10.1 RESULTS OF AUTONOMIC TESTING

Blood pressure evaluation					
Test: Valsalva maneuver					
Pressure [mmHg]	Baseline	Phase 2			Phase 4
		Early	End		
Systolic	157	74	77		
Mean	108.3	67.3	71	n/a	
Diastolic	84	64	68	n/a	

Heart rate evaluation	
Test: Deep breathing	
Results	Norm*
2.5	≥7
Test: Valsalva ratio	
1.769	≥1.39
* adjusted for a gender and age	

TABLE 10.1 **CONTINUED**

Test: Tilt test										
Position		HR [BPM]	Blood pressure [mmHg]		MCA Blood flow velocity [cm/s]				Respiratory frequency [breaths/min]	End tidal CO_2 [mmHg]
			Systolic	Diastolic	Systolic	Mean	Mean drop [%]	Diastolic		
Supine		60	135	79	72	38		21	13	32
Tilt [min]	1	70	124	79	68	35.3	7.1	19	10	33
	2	68	124	80						
	3	76	115	68						
	4	69	115	74						
	5	66	105	69	59	31.7	16.6	18	10	33
	6	68	98	65						
	7	69	80	83						
	8									
	9									
	10									
	15									
	20									
	30									
	40									

Sudomotor evaluation - functional

Test: Quantitative sudomotor axon reflex test (QSART)				
Location	Site (l/r)	Latency [min]	Volume [µl]	Norm [µl]*
Forearm				≥0.08
Prox. leg				≥0.14
Distal leg				≥0.07
Foot				≥0.05

* Normative data are adjusted for gender and age of patient.

Test: Electrochemical skin conductance (ESC)				
Location	Left [µS]	Right [µS]	Average [µS/k]	Norm [µS/kg]
Hand	46	45	0.69	≥1.03
Feet	39	44	0.67	≥1.14
Forehead				

For grading uses ESC [µS] adjusted for weight [µS/k].

(continued)

Small fiber (sensory + sudomotor) evaluation - morphological					
Test: Skin biopsy					
Location	Site (l/r)	Nerve fibers			
		Epidermal*		Sweat glands	
		Density	Norm	Density	Norm
Proximal leg – thigh	Right		≥8.3		≥37.8
Distal leg - calf	Right		≥5.02		≥36.5
Foot	Right		≥3.11		≥34.8

* Normative data for distal leg are adjusted for gender and age of patient.

QASAT*											
Heart rate		BP		CBFv		ET-CO2		Sudomotor			Total QASAT score
S. bradycardia	0	Low supine	0	Low supine	1	Low supine	1	QSART			
S. tachycardia	0	High supine	0	High supine	0	High supine	0	ESC	3		
Increase tilt		OH		Tilt response		Tilt low	0				
Decrease tilt		OHTN		CA	0	Tilt high	0	**Skin biopsy**			9
Deep breathing	2	VM	2	CVR	0			Epidermal			
VR	0			VM	0			Sweat gland			
Total	2	Total	2	Total	1	Total	1				

*QASAT. See Novak. Quantitative Scale for Grading of Cardiovascular Autonomic Reflex Tests and Small Fibers from Skin Biopsies. *J Neurol Disord* 2015;3:2. Orthostatic (tilt) responses were not graded since QASAT requires the duration of the tilt at least 10 minutes.

S, supine; Increase tilt, increased response to tilt; Decrease tilt, decreased response to tilt; BP, blood pressure; VM, Valsalva maneuver; CBFv, cerebral blood flow velocity; CA, cerebral autoregulation; MCA, middle cerebral artery; VR, Valsalva ratio; CVR, cerebral vasoreactivity.

Patient-reported symptoms for past 2 weeks:

Lightheadedness or dizziness: Occasionally
Dry eyes or mouth: None
Pale feet: None
Cold feet: None
Reduced sweating: None
Reduced sweating after exercise: None
Increased sweating: None
Nausea: None
Diarrhea: None
Constipation: None
Urinary leaks: None
Current pain severity: 0
Aching pain: Occasionally, mild
Allodynia: None
Burning pain: None
Lancinating pain: None
Numbness: Occasionally, mild
Prickling sensation: Occasionally, mild

AUTONOMIC TESTING INTERPRETATION

- Syncope, neurally mediated, vasodepressor.
- Cerebral autoregulatory failure associated with abnormal vasoconstriction since the compensatory vasodilation during syncope was absent and supine CBFv was reduced despite of normal supine blood pressure.
- Generalized autonomic failure, mild, affecting all major branches of autonomic nervous system (parasympathetic, adrenergic, and sudomotor).
- Hypocapnic hyperventilation during the supine position and during tilt.

COMMENT

The tilt test revealed vasodepressor syncope with characteristic decline in blood pressure with stable heart rate

(Figure 10.1).[1,2] The patient had minimal prodromal signs, which is atypical for syncope. She denied having dizziness whatsoever, but she felt "unusual" a few second before the syncope.

A second abnormality detected in the autonomic testing was the presence of cerebral autoregulatory failure as evidenced by (1) low supine CBFv in the context of normal supine blood pressure and (2) lack of compensatory cerebral vasodilation during syncope. Cerebral autoregulatory failure may worsen clinical outcome of syncope.

A third abnormality detected on the testing was generalized but mild autonomic failure, likely not contributing significantly to orthostatic intolerance.

TREATMENT AND FOLLOW-UP

- Volume expansion through high fluid and high salt intake, strenuous exercise.
- Consider cerebral perfusion study to assess cerebral autoregulation.

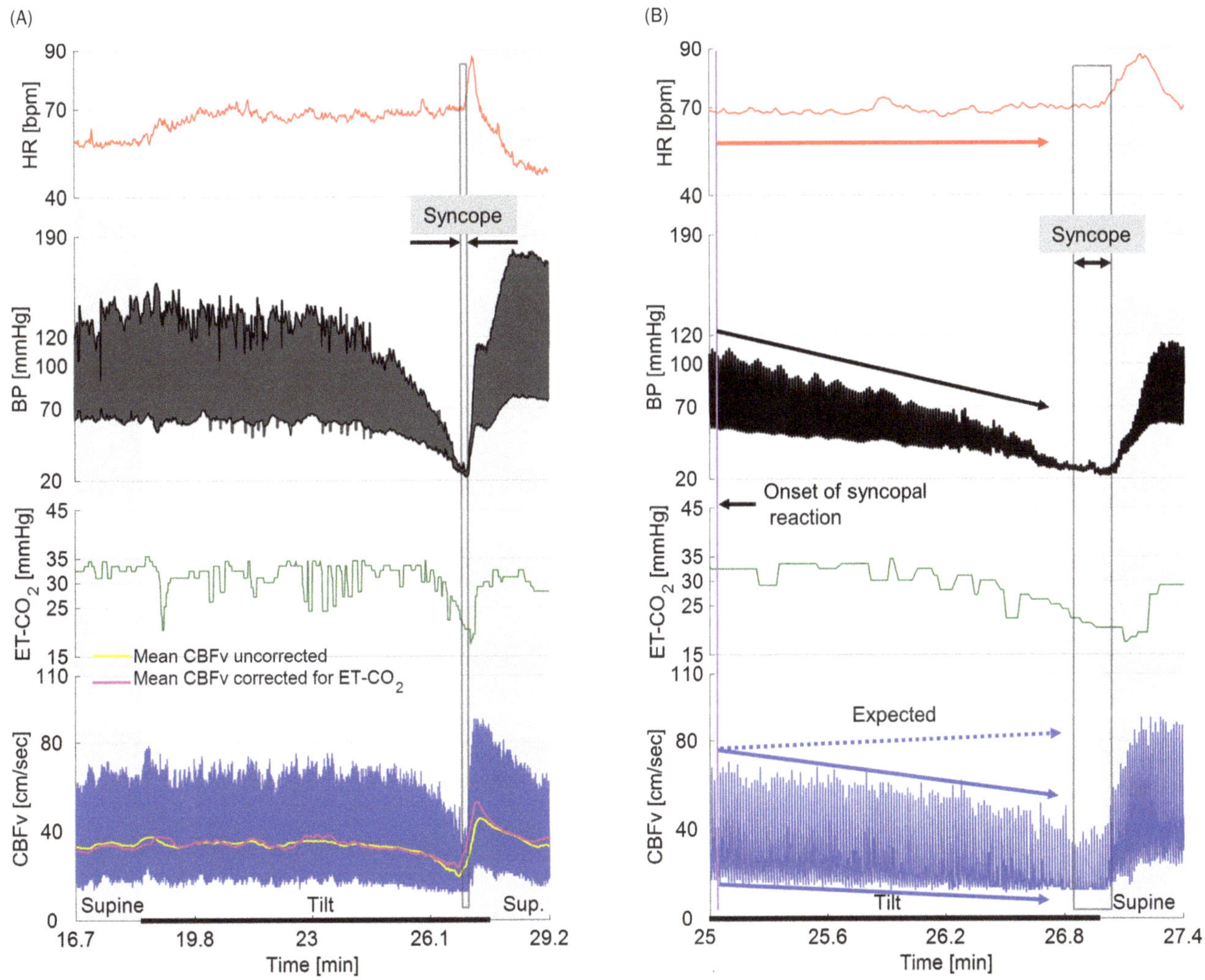

Figure 10.1 The tilt test provoked syncope (A–D). The blood pressure was stable for the initial 6 minutes of the tilt. Then, suddenly, there was a progressive decline in blood pressure (*black descending arrows*) (B) that started after minute 7 of the tilt. Heart rate did not change significantly (*horizontal red arrow*). Patient was hyperventilating, as indicated by hypocapnia (end tidal CO_2 <35 mm Hg). Cerebral blood flow velocity (CBFv) declined as blood pressure declined. Both systolic and diastolic CBFv declined, and the vasodilation pattern (widening of the velocity signal, reduction of the diastolic, and increase in systolic CBFv) was absent. Patient had minimal prodromes; in fact, she denied dizziness until seconds before passing out, when she felt "unusual."

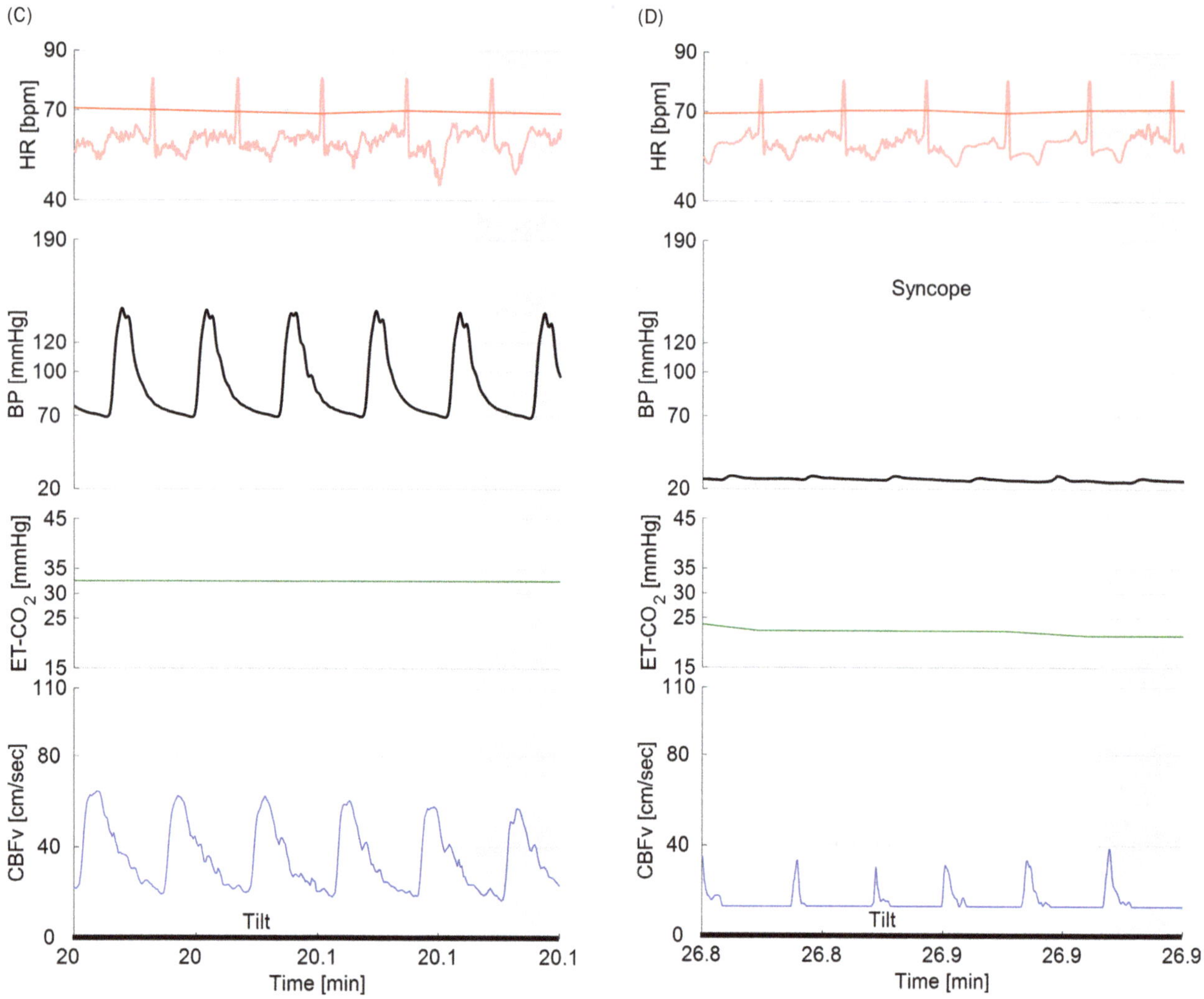

Figure 10.1 Continued

CAVEATS

- Syncope may have minimal prodromes.
- Vasodepressor syncope can be associated with loss of cerebral autoregulation.

REFERENCES

1. Weissler AM, Warren JV, Estes EH, Mcintosh HD, Leonard JJ. Vasodepressor syncope; factors influencing cardiac output. *Circulation*. 1957;15(6):875–882.
2. Novak P. Cerebral blood flow, heart rate, and blood pressure patterns during the tilt test in common orthostatic syndromes. *Neurosci J*. 2016;2016:6127340. doi:10.1155/2016/6127340.

11.

CASE 6: SYNCOPE, NEURALLY MEDIATED WITH PROLONGED ASYSTOLE

Chief complaint: Dizziness.

Case presentation: A 25-year-old woman presents with episodic loss of consciousness. She had multiple witnessed spells since age 15. The usual spells occur while standing or sitting and sometimes are associated with prodromes including dizziness, but not always. She is typically unconscious for about 1 minute during the spell. The witnesses observed the whole body stiffening, a gargling sound, and foam at mouth. She is then tired for about a day, until she returns to her baseline. She has the stereotypical spells every 3 months. MRI of the brain was normal. Several electroencephalograms and Holter monitors were normal, but no spell has been recorded. Patient was treated with seizure medication for suspected epilepsy, but medication was discontinued since it was ineffective.

Past medical history: Anxiety.

Current medication: Lorazepam.

Assessment plan: Functional autonomic tests.

AUTONOMIC TESTING EVALUATION

See Table 11.1.

Heart rate: Supine heart rate was normal. Heart rate responses to deep breathing were normal. Heart rate increment during the tilt (11 BPM) was normal.

Blood pressure:

Valsalva maneuver: Blood pressure responses were normal.

Tilt: Supine blood pressure was within normal range. Blood pressure responses to tilt were normal for the initial 10 minutes of the tilt. Then there was a progressive decline in blood pressure until the patient developed syncope; the tilt was aborted, but the asystole lasted 73 seconds.

Sudomotor evaluation: After the syncope, the patient was unable to tolerate sudomotor evaluation.

Respiratory system: Supine respiratory frequency was normal. The respiratory frequency during the tilt was normal. The end tidal CO_2 was normal in supine position. The end tidal CO_2 was normal during the tilt test.

Cerebral blood flow velocity (CBFv): CBFv in middle cerebral artery was normal in supine position. CBFv in middle cerebral artery was stable during the first 9 minutes of the tilt test, then declined during the syncope.

Skin biopsy (sensory-epidermal): N/A

Skin biopsy (sweat glands): N/A

Patient-reported symptoms during testing: Dizziness during the tilt test. The patient experienced stiffening of the whole body, eyes rolling up, gargling sound, and foam at her mouth. Her airways were kept protected. Once the stiffening resolved, the heart restarted, and she regained consciousness within a minute. She complained of headache

TABLE 11.1 **RESULTS OF AUTONOMIC TESTING**

Blood pressure evaluation					
Test: Valsalva maneuver					
Pressure [mmHg]	Baseline	Phase 2			Phase 4
		Early	End		
Systolic	89	66	122		
Mean	59.7	60.7	98.7	n/a	
Diastolic	45	58	87	n/a	

Heart rate evaluation	
Test: Deep breathing	
Results	Norm*
14.14	≥14
Test: Valsalva ratio	
1.6	≥1.46
* adjusted for a gender and age	

(continued)

Test: Tilt test										
Position		HR [BPM]	Blood pressure [mmHg]		MCA Blood flow velocity [cm/s]				Respiratory frequency [breaths/min]	End tidal CO_2 [mmHg]
			Systolic	Diastolic	Systolic	Mean	Mean drop [%]	Diastolic		
Supine		59	116	74	102	66		48	13	39
Tilt [min]	1	61	118	74	101	62.3	5.6	43	8	36
	2	63	122	80						
	3	59	119	77						
	4	61	117	73						
	5	63	113	75	96	60	9.1	42	15	35
	6	64	113	76						
	7	66	116	74						
	8	68	118	75						
	9	67	110	68						
	10	70	123	79	93	57.7	12.6	40	8	36
	15									
	20									
	30									
	40									

Sudomotor evaluation - functional

Test: Quantitative sudomotor axon reflex test (QSART)				
Location	Site (l/r)	Latency [min]	Volume [μl]	Norm [μl]*
Forearm				≥0.08
Prox. leg				≥0.14
Distal leg				≥0.24
Foot				≥0.09

* Normative data are adjusted for gender and age of patient

Test: Electrochemical skin conductance (ESC)				
Location	Left [μS]	Right [μS]	Average [μS/k]	Norm [μS/kg]
Hand				≥1.03
Feet				≥1.14
Forehead				

For grading uses ESC [μS] adjusted for weight [μS/k].

Small fiber (sensory + sudomotor) evaluation - morphological					
Test: Skin biopsy					
Location	Site (l/r)	Nerve fibers			
		Epidermal*		Sweat glands	
		Density	Norm	Density	Norm
Proximal leg – thigh	Right		≥8.3		≥37.8
Distal leg - calf	Right		≥9.1		≥36.5
Foot	Right		≥3.11		≥34.8

* Normative data for distal leg are adjusted for gender and age of patient

QASAT*											
Heart rate		BP		CBFv		ET-CO2		Sudomotor			Total QASAT score
S. bradycardia	0	Low supine	0	Low supine	0	Low supine	0	QSART			
S. tachycardia	0	High supine	0	High supine	0	High supine	0	ESC			
Increase tilt	0	OH	0	Tilt response	0	Tilt low	0				
Decrease tilt	0	OHTN	0	CA	0	Tilt high	0	Skin biopsy			0
Deep breathing	0	VM	0	CVR	0			Epidermal			
VR	0			VM	0			Sweat gland			
Total	0	Total	0	Total	0	Total	0				

*QASAT. See Novak. Quantitative Scale for Grading of Cardiovascular Autonomic Reflex Tests and Small Fibers from Skin Biopsies. *J Neurol Disord* 2015;3:2.

S, supine; Increase tilt, increased response to tilt; Decrease tilt, decreased response to tilt; BP, blood pressure; VM, Valsalva maneuver; CBFv, cerebral blood flow velocity; CA, cerebral autoregulation; MCA, middle cerebral artery; VR, Valsalva ratio; CVR, cerebral vasoreactivity.

and fatigue. According to her mother who witnessed the testing, this was her typical spell.

Patient-reported symptoms for past 2 weeks:

Lightheadedness or dizziness: Occasionally
Dry eyes or mouth: Occasionally
Pale feet: None
Cold feet: None
Reduced sweating: None
Reduced sweating after exercise: None
Increased sweating: Often
Nausea: None
Diarrhea: None
Constipation: None
Urinary leaks: None
Current pain severity: 3
Aching pain: None
Allodynia: None
Burning pain: None
Lancinating pain: None
Numbness: Occasionally, mild
Prickling sensation: Occasionally, mild

AUTONOMIC TESTING INTERPRETATION

- Syncope, neurally mediated, mixed (since both blood pressure and heart rate declined at the onset of syncopal reaction) with strong cardioinhibitory component.
- No evidence of autonomic adrenergic failure.

COMMENT

The tilt provoked syncope and reproduced the patient's typical spell (Figure 11.1). The syncope was unusual in several respects. First, the presyncopal reaction was extremely short: the asystole occurred within 6–8 seconds after the onset of bradycardia, hypotension, and cerebral vasodilation. Second, the duration of asystole was very long.

Syncope was associated with bradycardia and hyperventilation. CBFv showed a characteristic vasodilation pattern (signal widening due to reduction of diastolic and increase in systolic velocities) indicating active compensatory autoregulation (Figure 11.1).

TREATMENT AND FOLLOW-UP

- Patient was reassured that she does not have psychiatric illness or epilepsy.
- Urgent referral to cardiology for cardiac pacemaker placement.

CAVEATS

- An asystolic tilt response is consistent with neurally mediated syncope with strong cardioinhibitory reflex.[1]
- For older patients (age ≥40 years), cardiac pacing for cardioinhibitory syncope may be beneficial as shown by randomized blinded studies.[2,3] Although

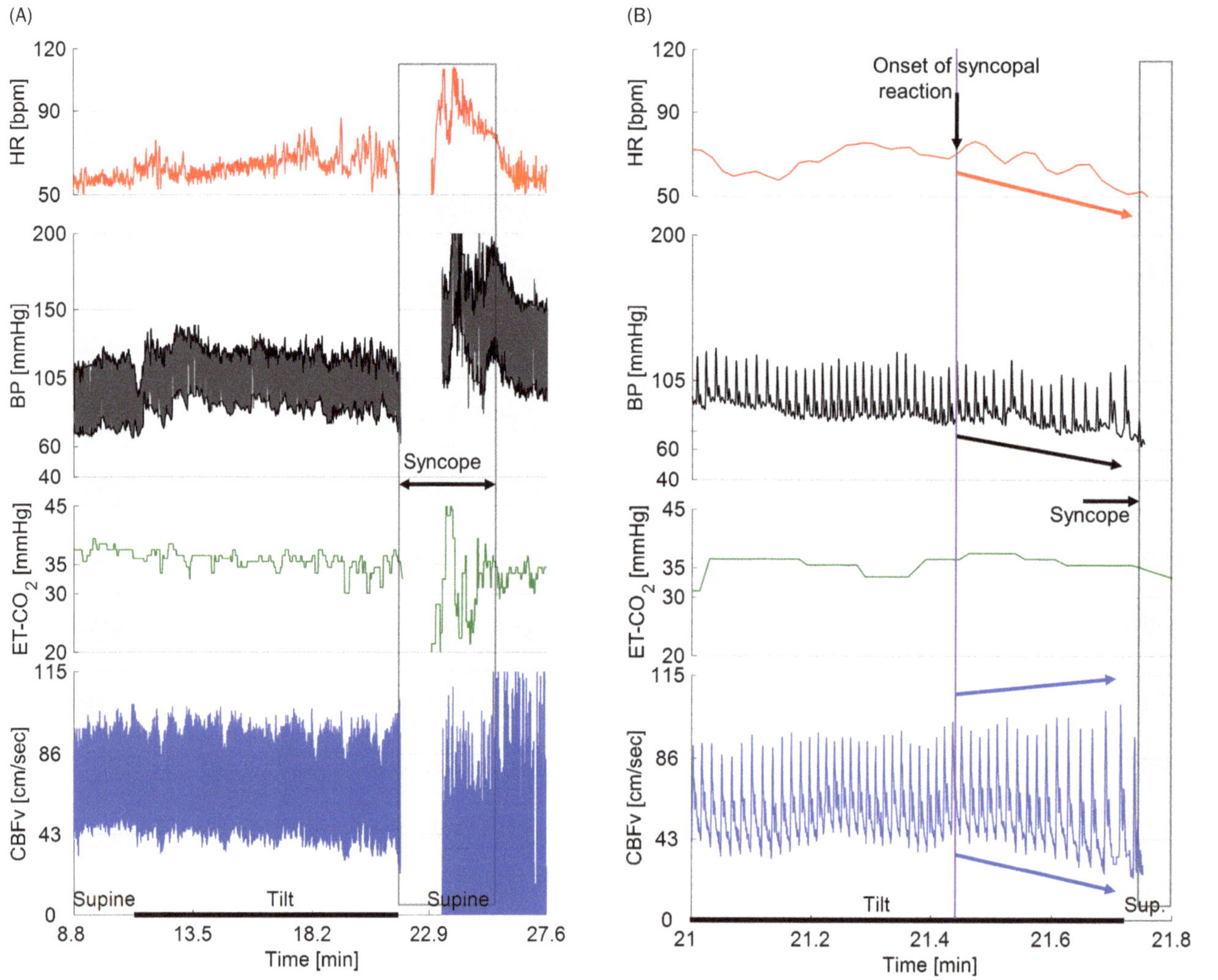

Figure 11.1 The tilt test provoked syncope at minute 10 (A). The onset of syncopal reaction was associated with simultaneous decline in heart rate (*red arrow*), blood pressure (*black arrow*), and cerebral vasodilation (*blue arrows*). The tilt was terminated immediately when the patient lost consciousness. Nevertheless, asystole continued in supine position for total duration of 73 seconds. Details of asystole are shown in C and D.

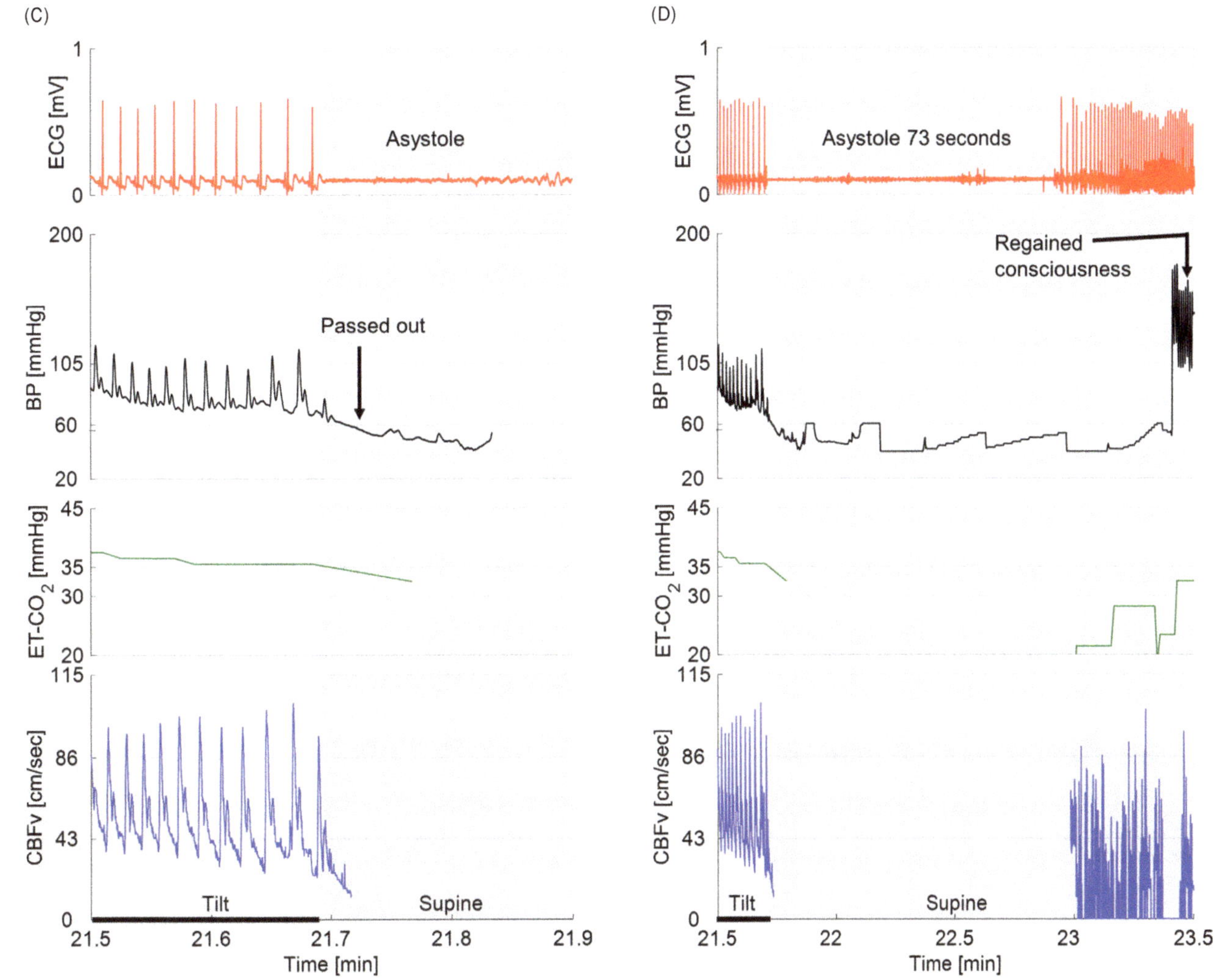

Figure 11.1 Continued

evidence is somewhat limited, even younger patients with cardioinhibitory response may benefit from cardiac pacing.[4]

REFERENCES

1. Brignole M, Tomaino M, Gargaro A. Vasovagal syncope with asystole: the role of cardiac pacing. *Clin Auton Res Off J Clin Auton Res Soc*. 2017;27(4):245–251. doi:10.1007/s10286-017-0441-7.
2. Baron-Esquivias G, Morillo CA, Moya-Mitjans A, et al. Dual-chamber pacing with closed loop stimulation in recurrent reflex vasovagal syncope: the SPAIN study. *J Am Coll Cardiol*. 2017;70(14):1720–1728. doi:10.1016/j.jacc.2017.08.026.
3. Palmisano P, Dell'Era G, Russo V, et al. Effects of closed-loop stimulation vs. DDD pacing on haemodynamic variations and occurrence of syncope induced by head-up tilt test in older patients with refractory cardioinhibitory vasovagal syncope: the Tilt test-Induced REsponse in Closed-loop Stimulation multicentre, prospective, single blind, randomized study. *Eur Pacing Arrhythm Card Electrophysiol J Work Groups Card Pacing Arrhythm Card Cell Electrophysiol Eur Soc Cardiol*. April 2017. doi:10.1093/europace/eux015.
4. Olshansky B. Vasovagal syncope: to pace or not to pace. *J Am Coll Cardiol*. 2017;70(14):1729–1731. doi:10.1016/j.jacc.2017.08.025.

12.

CASE 7: SYNCOPE, DOUBLE

Chief complaint: Syncope.

Case presentation: A 36-year-old woman presents with frequent spells of passing out. The spells usually occur in an upright posture, but not always, and are associated with feeling hot and lightheaded. Neurological examination, MRI of the brain, and EEG were normal.

Past medical history: Migraine with aura, syncope.

Current medication: Topiramate, duloxetine, ranitidine, rizatriptan.

Assessment plan: Functional autonomic tests.

AUTONOMIC TESTING EVALUATION

See Table 12.1.

Heart rate: Supine heart rate was normal. Heart rate responses to deep breathing were normal. Heart rate increment during the tilt (17 BPM) was normal.

Blood pressure:

Valsalva maneuver: Mean blood pressure failed to return to baseline at the end of Phase 2 by 1 mm Hg (i.e., 98.8% of baseline).

Tilt: Supine blood pressure was within normal range. There was a progressive decline of blood pressure until minute 3 of tilt, when patient developed syncope and the tilt was aborted. The patient developed a second syncope in supine position.

Sudomotor evaluation: Electrochemical skin conductance was abnormal (reduced to 55.6% of normal limit) at hands and abnormal (reduced to 71.6% of normal limit) at feet.

Respiratory system: Respiratory frequency was normal in supine position and during the tilt. End tidal CO_2 was normal in supine position but was severely reduced during the tilt test.

Cerebral blood flow velocity (CBFv): CBFv in middle cerebral artery was normal in supine position. CBFv in middle cerebral artery was severely reduced during the tilt test.

Skin biopsy (sensory-epidermal): N/A

Skin biopsy (sweat glands): N/A

Patient-reported symptoms during testing: Loss of consciousness and dizziness during the tilt.

Patient-reported symptoms for past 2 weeks:

Lightheadedness or dizziness: Occasionally
Dry eyes or mouth: Occasionally
Pale feet: Occasionally
Cold feet: Occasionally
Reduced sweating: Yes, minor annoyance
Reduced sweating after exercise: None
Increased sweating: None
Nausea: Occasionally
Diarrhea: None
Constipation: None
Urinary leaks: None
Current pain severity: 0
Aching pain: Occasionally, mild
Allodynia: None

TABLE 12.1 **RESULTS OF AUTONOMIC TESTING**

Blood pressure evaluation					
Test: Valsalva maneuver					
Pressure [mmHg]	Baseline	Phase 2			Phase 4
		Early	End		
Systolic	115	108	112		
Mean	83.7	78	82.7	n/a	
Diastolic	68	63	68	n/a	

Heart rate evaluation	
Test: Deep breathing	
Results	Norm*
15.5	≥12
Test: Valsalva ratio	
1.24	≥1.5

* adjusted for a gender and age

TABLE 12.1 CONTINUED

Test: Tilt test										
Position		HR [BPM]	Blood pressure [mmHg]		MCA Blood flow velocity [cm/s]				Respiratory frequency [breaths/min]	End tidal CO_2 [mmHg]
			Systolic	Diastolic	Systolic	Mean	Mean drop [%]	Diastolic		
Supine		65	119	80	108	73.3		56	13	35
Tilt [min]	1	77	124	87	83	49	33.2	32	17	31
	2	82	130	91						
	3	40	60	40						
	4									
	5									
	6									
	7									
	8									
	9									
	10									
	15									
	20									
	30									
	40									

Sudomotor evaluation - functional

Test: Quantitative sudomotor axon reflex test (QSART)				
Location	Site (l/r)	Latency [min]	Volume [µl]	Norm [µl]*
Forearm				≥0.08
Prox. leg				≥0.14
Distal leg				≥0.15
Foot				≥0.07

* Normative data are adjusted for gender and age of patient.

Test: Electrochemical skin conductance (ESC)				
Location	Left [µS]	Right [µS]	Average [µS/k]	Norm [µS/kg]
Hand	62	56	0.57	≥1.03
Feet	84	85	0.83	≥1.14
Forehead				

For grading uses ESC [µS] adjusted for weight [µS/k].

(continued)

Small fiber (sensory + sudomotor) evaluation - morphological					
Test: Skin biopsy					
Location	Site (l/r)	Nerve fibers			
		Epidermal*		Sweat glands	
		Density	Norm	Density	Norm
Proximal leg – thigh	Right		≥8.3		≥37.8
Distal leg - calf	Right		≥8.22		≥36.5
Foot	Right		≥3.11		≥34.8

* Normative data for distal leg are adjusted for gender and age of patient.

QASAT*											
Heart rate		**BP**		**CBFv**		**ET-CO2**		**Sudomotor**			**Total QASAT score**
S. bradycardia	0	Low supine	0	Low supine	0	Low supine	0	QSART			
S. tachycardia	0	High supine	0	High supine	0	High supine	0	ESC	2		
Increase tilt		OH		Tilt response		Tilt low					
Decrease tilt		OHTN		CA	0	Tilt high		**Skin biopsy**			4
Deep breathing	0	VM	1	CVR	0			Epidermal			
VR	1			VM	0			Sweat gland			
Total	1	Total	1	Total	0	Total	0				

*QASAT. See Novak. Quantitative Scale for Grading of Cardiovascular Autonomic Reflex Tests and Small Fibers from Skin Biopsies. *J Neurol Disord* 2015;3:2. Orthostatic (tilt) responses were not graded since QASAT requires the duration of the tilt at least 10 minutes.

S, supine; Increase tilt, increased response to tilt; Decrease tilt, decreased response to tilt; BP, blood pressure; VM, Valsalva maneuver; CBFv, cerebral blood flow velocity; CA, cerebral autoregulation; MCA, middle cerebral artery; VR, Valsalva ratio; CVR, cerebral vasoreactivity.

Burning pain: None
Lancinating pain: None
Numbness: Often, mild
Prickling sensation: Often, moderate

AUTONOMIC TESTING INTERPRETATION

- Syncope, neurally mediated, mixed.
- Mild autonomic failure.

COMMENT

The tilt test provoked two neurally mediated syncope, mixed type (Figure 12.1).[1] The first syncope occurred during the tilt, and the second syncope occurred in the supine position a second later.

TREATMENT AND FOLLOW-UP

- Volume expansion through high fluid and high salt intake.

CAVEATS

- Although rare, neutrally mediated syncope can occur in the supine position.[2]
- Another syncope can follow the previous syncope almost immediately.

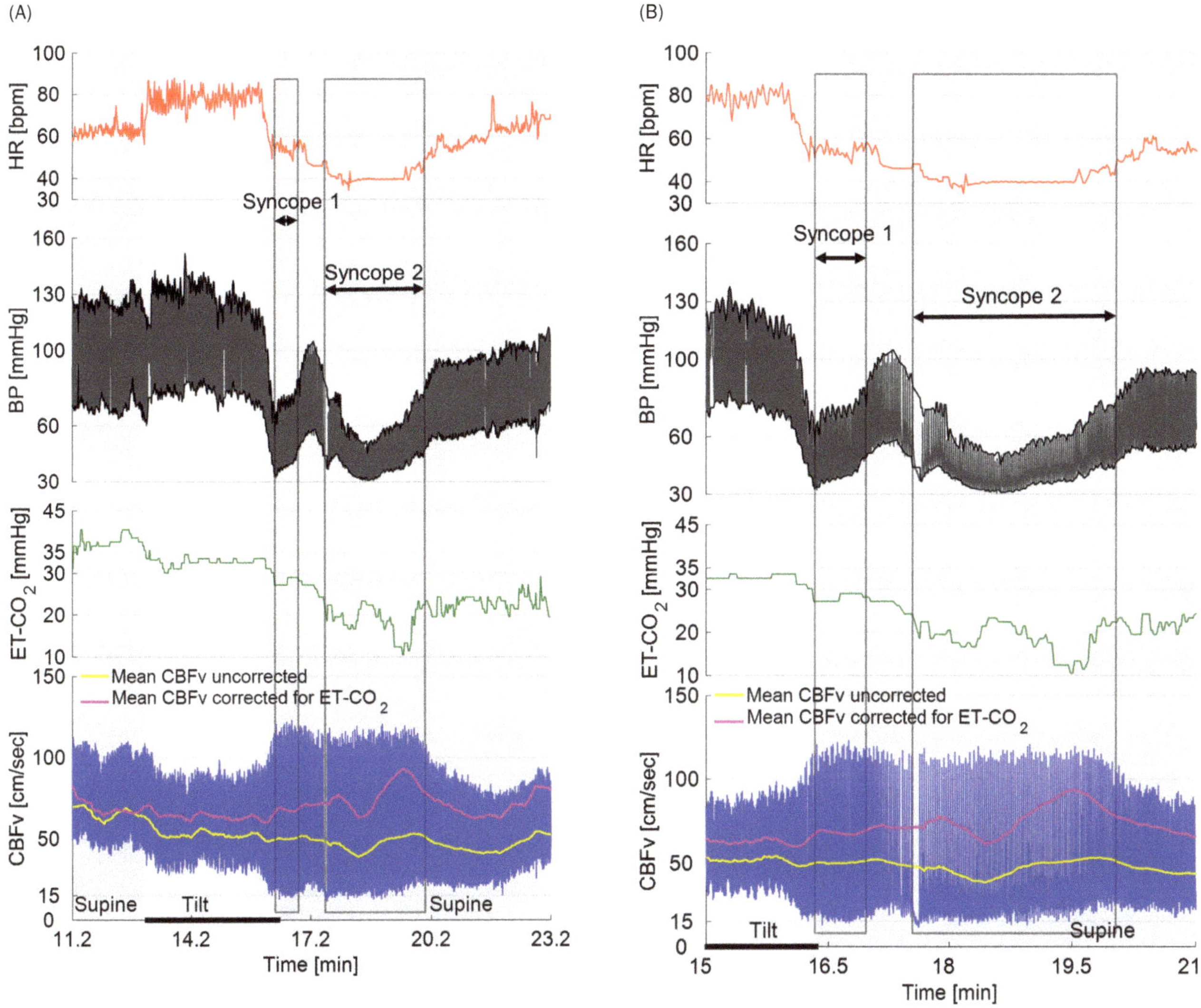

Figure 12.1 The tilt test provoked two neurally mediated syncopes, mixed type (A, B). The first syncopal reaction was associated with a characteristic decline in heart rate and blood pressure and widening of the Doppler signal. The tilt was aborted immediately after the patient lost consciousness. The second syncope occurred in supine position. Details for the first syncope during the tilt (C) and second syncope that occurred in supine position (D). The patient regained consciousness a few seconds after being positioned in supine, which was associated with an increase in blood pressure and diastolic cerebral blood flow velocity (CBFv). However, a few seconds later patient passed out again in the supine position, which was accompanied by another decline in blood pressure and diastolic blood flow velocity. The second syncope was longer compared to the first syncope. The second syncopal reaction was associated with bradycardia, decline of blood pressure, low end tidal CO_2, and decline in diastolic CBFv.

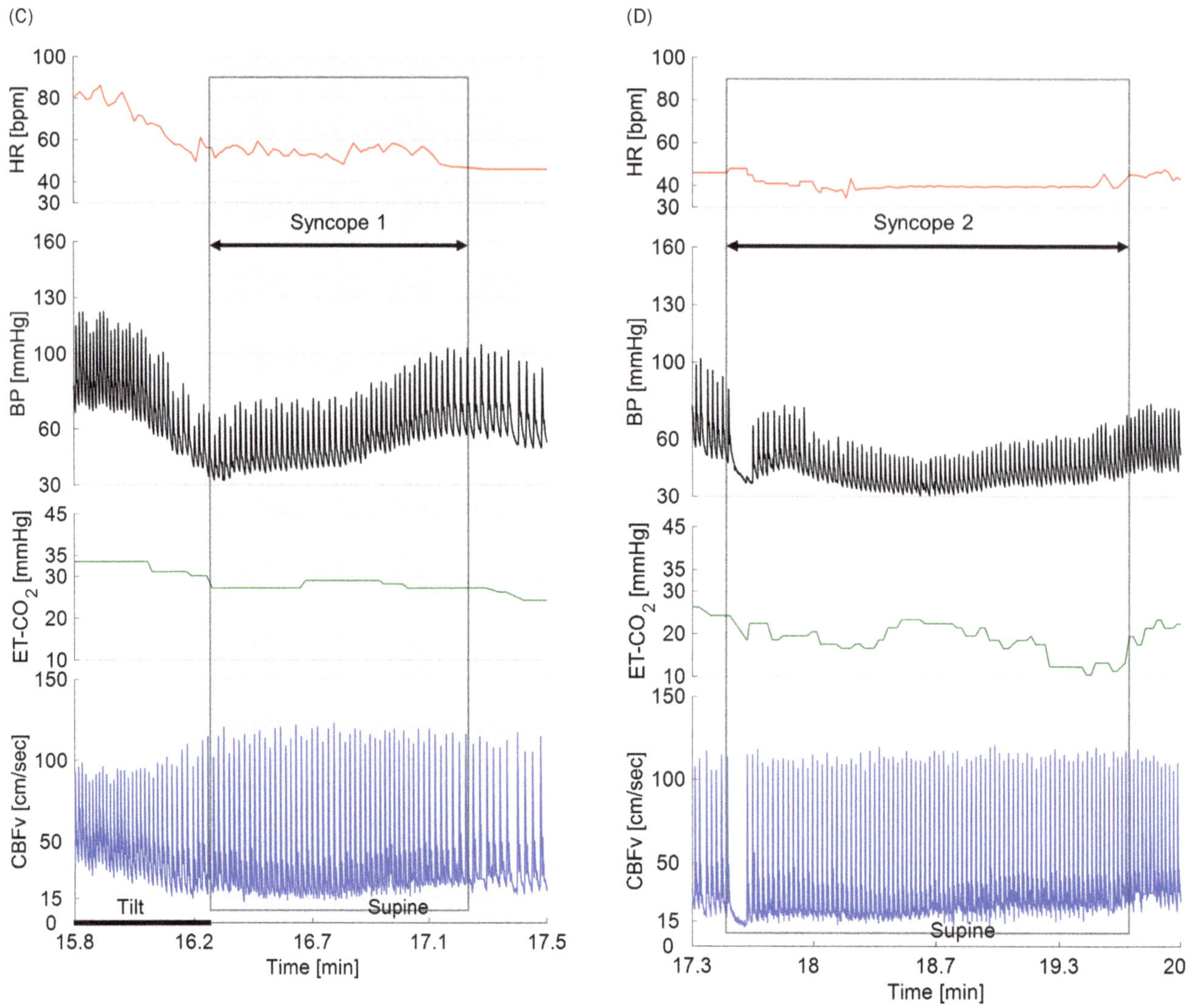

Figure 12.1 Continued

REFERENCES

1. Novak P. Cerebral blood flow, heart rate, and blood pressure patterns during the tilt test in common orthostatic syndromes. *Neurosci J.* 2016;2016:6127340. doi:10.1155/2016/6127340.
2. Khadilkar SV, Yadav RS, Jagiasi KA. Are syncopes in sitting and supine positions different? Body positions and syncope: a study of 111 patients. *Neurol India.* 2013;61(3):239–243. doi:10.4103/0028-3886.115060.

13.

CASE 8: SYNCOPE DUE TO AUTONOMIC FAILURE

Chief complaint: Dizziness.

Case presentation: A 45-year-old woman with past medical history of severe alcohol abuse and recurrent thromboembolic events presented with postural dizziness. She also reports episodes of heart racing that occur while she is at rest. She states her heart rate rises rather abruptly and is associated with shortness of breath and chest pain. She has history of a sinus tachycardia but could not tolerate β-blockers because they induced hypotension. In addition, she became inactive for months. She gets dizzy within seconds of standing. The dizziness is associated with blurred vision and hearing loss. She was referred for evaluation of suspected autonomic failure.

Past medical history: Thromboembolism, alcohol abuse, anxiety, anemia (now corrected).

Current medication: Duloxetine, clonazepam, omeprazole, trazodone, inferior vena cava filter.

Assessment plan: Functional autonomic tests and skin biopsy.

AUTONOMIC TESTING EVALUATION

See Table 13.1.

Heart rate: Supine heart rate was normal. Heart rate responses to deep breathing were reduced to 10% of normal value. Heart rate increment during the tilt (1 BPM) was reduced.

Blood pressure:

Valsalva maneuver: Mean blood pressure failed to return to baseline at the end of Phase 2 by 28.6 mm Hg (i.e., 74.8% of baseline).

Tilt: Supine blood pressure was elevated. There was a progressive decline in blood pressure until the patient developed a syncope at minute 5 of tilt, then the tilt was aborted.

Sudomotor evaluation: Electrochemical skin conductance was abnormal (reduced to 45.4% of normal limit) at hands and abnormal (reduced to 70.3% of normal limit) at feet.

Respiratory system: The respiratory frequency was normal during supine and during the tilt. The end tidal CO_2 was normal during supine position, but it mildly declined during the tilt.

Cerebral blood flow velocity (CBFv): CBFv in middle cerebral artery was normal in supine position, but it was severely reduced during the tilt.

Skin biopsy (sensory-epidermal): Epidermal nerve fiber density was normal at proximal leg and normal at distal leg.

Skin biopsy (sweat glands): N/A

Patient-reported symptoms during testing: Dizziness during the tilt test.

Patient-reported symptoms for past 2 weeks:

Lightheadedness or dizziness: Often
Dry eyes or mouth: Occasionally

TABLE 13.1 **RESULTS OF AUTONOMIC TESTING**

Blood pressure evaluation					
Test: Valsalva maneuver					
Pressure [mmHg]	Baseline	Phase 2			Phase 4
		Early	End		
Systolic	152	80	96		
Mean	113.3	72.7	84.7	n/a	
Diastolic	94	69	79	n/a	

Heart rate evaluation	
Test: Deep breathing	
Results	Norm*
1	≥10
Test: Valsalva ratio	
1.25	≥1.51
* adjusted for a gender and age	

(continued)

Test: Tilt test										
Position		HR [BPM]	Blood pressure [mmHg]		MCA Blood flow velocity [cm/s]				Respiratory frequency [breaths/min]	End tidal CO_2 [mmHg]
			Systolic	Diastolic	Systolic	Mean	Mean drop [%]	Diastolic		
Supine		80	149.6	93.4	84	57.3		44	14	35
Tilt [min]	1	81	105.6	81.6	70	50	12.7	40	13	32
	2	80	93.6	61						
	3	80.3	78.5	56.6						
	4	79.3	70.2	52.1						
	5	78.4	67.8	42.7	58	30	47.6	16	17	29
	6									
	7									
	8									
	9									
	10									
	15									
	20									
	30									
	40									

Sudomotor evaluation - functional

Test: Quantitative sudomotor axon reflex test (QSART)				
Location	Site (l/r)	Latency [min]	Volume [µl]	Norm [µl]*
Forearm				≥0.08
Prox. leg				≥0.14
Distal leg				≥0.15
Foot				≥0.07

* Normative data are adjusted for gender and age of patient.

Test: Electrochemical skin conductance (ESC)				
Location	Left [µS]	Right [µS]	Average [µS/k]	Norm [µS/kg]
Hand	36	34	0.47	≥1.03
Feet	63	58	0.77	≥1.14
Forehead				

For grading uses ESC [µS] adjusted for weight [µS/k].

TABLE 13.1 CONTINUED

Small fiber (sensory + sudomotor) evaluation - morphological					
Test: Skin biopsy					
Location	Site (l/r)	Nerve fibers			
		Epidermal*		Sweat glands	
		Density	Norm	Density	Norm
Proximal leg – thigh	Right	14.73	≥8.3		≥37.8
Distal leg - calf	Right	9.7	≥7.5		≥36.5
Foot	Right		≥3.11		≥34.8

* Normative data for distal leg are adjusted for gender and age of patient.

QASAT*											
Heart rate		BP		CBFv		ET-CO2		Sudomotor			Total QASAT score
S. bradycardia	0	Low supine	0	Low supine	0	Low supine	0	QSART			
S. tachycardia	0	High supine	1	High supine	0	High supine	0	ESC	2		
Increase tilt		OH		Tilt response		Tilt low					
Decrease tilt		OHTN		CA	0	Tilt high		**Skin biopsy**			9
Deep breathing	3	VM	2	CVR	0			Epidermal	0		
VR	1			VM	0			Sweat gland			
Total	4	Total	3	Total	0	Total	0				

*QASAT. See Novak. Quantitative Scale for Grading of Cardiovascular Autonomic Reflex Tests and Small Fibers from Skin Biopsies. *J Neurol Disord* 2015;3:2. Orthostatic (tilt) responses were not graded since QASAT requires the duration of the tilt at least 10 minutes.

S, supine; Increase tilt, increased response to tilt; Decrease tilt, decreased response to tilt; BP, blood pressure; VM, Valsalva maneuver; CBFv, cerebral blood flow velocity; CA, cerebral autoregulation; MCA, middle cerebral artery; VR, Valsalva ratio; CVR, cerebral vasoreactivity.

Pale feet: None
Cold feet: None
Reduced sweating: None
Reduced sweating after exercise: None
Increased sweating: None
Nausea: None
Diarrhea: None
Constipation: None
Urinary leaks: None
Current pain severity: 0
Aching pain: None
Allodynia: None
Burning pain: None
Lancinating pain: None
Numbness: Occasionally, mild
Prickling sensation: Occasionally, mild

AUTONOMIC TESTING INTERPRETATION

- Syncope, neurally mediated, due to sympathetic adrenergic failure.
- Generalized autonomic failure.

COMMENT

Autonomic testing showed severe generalized autonomic failure with a progressive orthostatic hypotension until the patient lost consciousness (Figure 13.1). This pattern is characteristic for a syncope associated with autonomic failure.[1,2]

During the tilt, the patient experienced her typical prodromes—dizziness, blurred vision, and hearing loss—indicative of cerebral hypoperfusion. Subsequent thorough

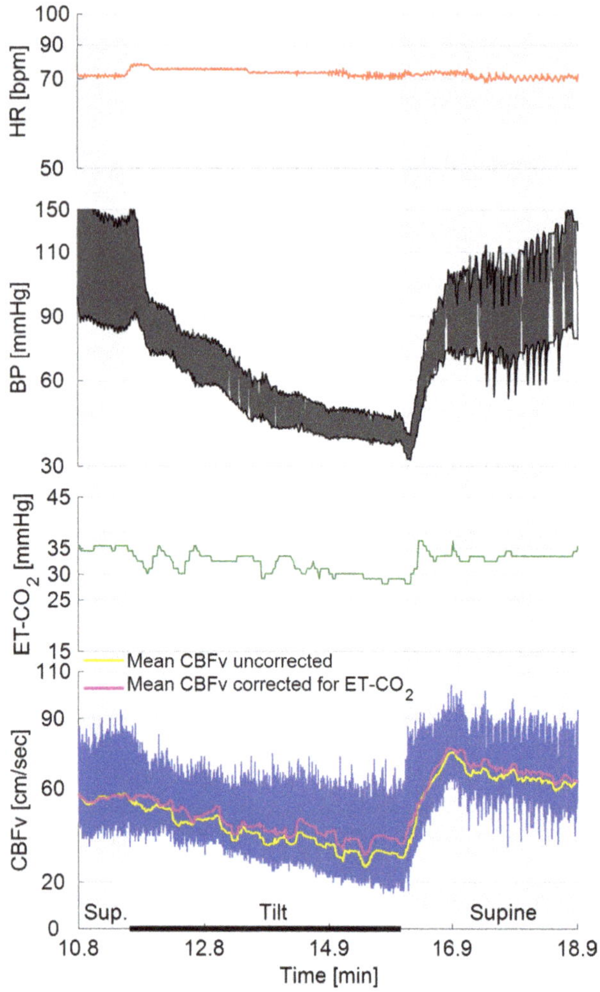

Figure 13.1 The tilt test induced gradual decline in blood pressure and cerebral blood flow velocity (CBFv). The compensatory heart rate increment to tilt was absent. Patient lost consciousness at minute 5 of the tilt.

evaluations for causes of autonomic failure including infectious, systemic, neurodegenerative, paraneoplastic, autoimmune, genetic, and nutritional were all unrevealing except for a history of alcohol abuse. Therefore, toxic effect of alcohol has been implicated as a cause of autonomic failure in this patient. In most alcoholics, the dysautonomia is milder than in this patient and affects predominantly parasympathetic cardiovagal fibers.[3]

TREATMENT AND FOLLOW-UP

- Abstinence of alcohol.
- Volume expansion through high fluid and high salt intake, pressor medications.

CAVEATS

- Syncope associated with autonomic failure has a distinct profile.
- Alcohol abuse can be associated with severe generalized autonomic failure.

REFERENCES

1. Brignole M. Neurally-mediated syncope. *Ital Heart J Off J Ital Fed Cardiol.* 2005;6(3):249–255.
2. Sheldon RS, Grubb BP, Olshansky B, et al. 2015 heart rhythm society expert consensus statement on the diagnosis and treatment of postural tachycardia syndrome, inappropriate sinus tachycardia, and vasovagal syncope. *Heart Rhythm.* 2015;12(6):e41–e63. doi:10.1016/j.hrthm.2015.03.029.
3. Novak DJ, Victor M. The vagus and sympathetic nerves in alcoholic polyneuropathy. *Arch Neurol.* 1974;30(4):273–284.

PART III

POSTURAL TACHYCARDIA SYNDROMES

CASE 9: POSTURAL TACHYCARDIA SYNDROME, NEUROPATHIC TYPE

Chief complaint: Dizziness.

Case presentation: A 25-year-old woman presents with anxiety and intermittent palpitations. She also has chronic aching pain and numbness affecting the limbs. Palpitations are responding to propranolol, and pain is relieved by duloxetine. The referring physician suspects the postural tachycardia syndrome (POTS) and/or small fiber neuropathy.

Past medical history: Anxiety, POTS.

Current medication: Duloxetine, buspirone.

Assessment plan: Functional autonomic tests and skin biopsy because of sensory complaints.

AUTONOMIC TESTING EVALUATION

See Table 14.1.

Heart rate: Supine heart rate was normal. Heart rate responses to deep breathing were normal. Heart rate increment during the tilt (53 BPM) was exaggerated and exceeded 120 BPM.

Blood pressure:

Valsalva maneuver: Mean blood pressure failed to return to baseline at the end of Phase 2 by 42 mm Hg (i.e., 56.7% of baseline).

Tilt: Supine blood pressure was within normal range. Blood pressure responses to tilt were normal.

Sudomotor evaluation: Electrochemical skin conductance was abnormal (reduced to 91% of normal limit) at hands and abnormal (reduced to 89% of normal limit) at feet.

Respiratory system: Respiratory frequency was normal during supine, but increased transiently during the tilt. The end tidal CO_2 was normal during supine position but decreased during the tilt.

Cerebral blood flow velocity (CBFv): CBFv in the middle cerebral artery was normal in supine position. CBFv was severely reduced during the tilt test.

Skin biopsy (sensory-epidermal): Epidermal nerve fiber density was normal at proximal leg and abnormal (reduced to 78.4% of normal limit) at distal leg.

Skin biopsy (sweat glands): Sweat gland nerve fiber density was abnormal (reduced to 31.8% of normal limit) at distal leg.

Patient-reported symptoms during testing: Dizziness, shortness of breath, palpitations during the tilt test.

Patient-reported symptoms for past 2 weeks:

Lightheadedness or dizziness: Often
Dry eyes or mouth: Often

TABLE 14.1 RESULTS OF AUTONOMIC TESTING

Blood pressure evaluation					
Test: Valsalva maneuver					
Pressure [mmHg]	Baseline	Phase 2			Phase 4
		Early	End		
Systolic	129	60	63		
Mean	97	52	55	n/a	
Diastolic	81	48	51	n/a	

Heart rate evaluation	
Test: Deep breathing	
Results	Norm*
33.6	≥14
Test: Valsalva ratio	
2.17	≥1.46
* adjusted for a gender and age	

(continued)

TABLE 14.1 **CONTINUED**

Test: Tilt test										
Position		HR [BPM]	Blood pressure [mmHg]		MCA Blood flow velocity [cm/s]				Respiratory frequency [breaths/min]	End tidal CO_2 [mmHg]
			Systolic	Diastolic	Systolic	Mean	Mean drop [%]	Diastolic		
Supine		88	127	84	96	62.7		46	16	36
Tilt [min]	1	137	124	86	77	48.3	23	34	16	27
	2	138	121	89						
	3	131	125	90						
	4	138	126	88						
	5	131	121	87	84	53.3	15	38	21	36
	6	136	128	91						
	7	136	123	89						
	8	141	132	90						
	9	134	128	87						
	10	140	128	88	75	47.7	23.9	34	18	30
	15									
	20									
	30									
	40									

Sudomotor evaluation - functional

Test: Quantitative sudomotor axon reflex test (QSART)				
Location	Site (l/r)	Latency [min]	Volume [µl]	Norm [µl]*
Forearm				≥0.08
Prox. leg				≥0.14
Distal leg				≥0.24
Foot				≥0.09

* Normative data are adjusted for gender and age of patient.

Test: Electrochemical skin conductance (ESC)				
Location	Left [µS]	Right [µS]	Average [µS/k]	Norm [µS/kg]
Hand	85	86	0.94	≥1.03
Feet	92	92	1.01	≥1.14
Forehead				

For grading uses ESC [µS] adjusted for weight [µS/k].

TABLE 14.1 CONTINUED

Small fiber (sensory + sudomotor) evaluation - morphological					
Test: Skin biopsy					
Location	Site (l/r)	Nerve fibers			
		Epidermal*		Sweat glands	
		Density	Norm	Density	Norm
Proximal leg – thigh	Right	10.55	≥8.3		≥37.8
Distal leg - calf	Right	7.13	≥9.1	11.6	≥36.5
Foot	Right		≥3.11		≥34.8

* Normative data for distal leg are adjusted for gender and age of patient.

QASAT*										
Heart rate		**BP**		**CBFv**		**ET-CO2**		**Sudomotor**		**Total QASAT score**
S. bradycardia	0	Low supine	0	Low supine	0	Low supine	0	QSART		
S. tachycardia	0	High supine	0	High supine	0	High supine	0	ESC	1	
Increase tilt	10	OH	0	Tilt response	5	Tilt low	2			
Decrease tilt	0	OHTN	0	CA	0	Tilt high	0	**Skin biopsy**		26
Deep breathing	0	VM	3	CVR	0			Epidermal	1	
VR	0			VM	0			Sweat gland	4	
Total	10	Total	3	Total	5	Total	2			

*QASAT. See Novak. Quantitative Scale for Grading of Cardiovascular Autonomic Reflex Tests and Small Fibers from Skin Biopsies. *J Neurol Disord* 2015;3:2.

S, supine; Increase tilt, increased response to tilt; Decrease tilt, decreased response to tilt; BP, blood pressure; VM, Valsalva maneuver; CBFv, cerebral blood flow velocity; CA, cerebral autoregulation; MCA, middle cerebral artery; VR, Valsalva ratio; CVR, cerebral vasoreactivity.

Pale feet: None
Cold feet: None
Reduced sweating: Occasionally
Reduced sweating after exercise: None
Increased sweating: Occasionally
Nausea: Often
Diarrhea: None
Constipation: None
Urinary leaks: None
Current pain severity: 5
Aching pain: Often, moderate
Allodynia: Occasionally, moderate
Burning pain: None
Lancinating pain: Occasionally, moderate
Numbness: Often, mild
Prickling sensation: Often, moderate

AUTONOMIC TESTING INTERPRETATION

- Postural tachycardia syndrome (POTS), neuropathic form.
- Small fiber neuropathy (SFN), mixed, length-dependent.
- Low orthostatic cerebral blood flow velocity.
- Hypocapnic hyperventilation.

COMMENT

Autonomic testing showed characteristic neuropathic POTS.[1,2] The tilt showed orthostatic tachycardia without orthostatic hypotension and reduced CBFv due to hypocapnia (Figure 14.1). The skin biopsy showed damage to both

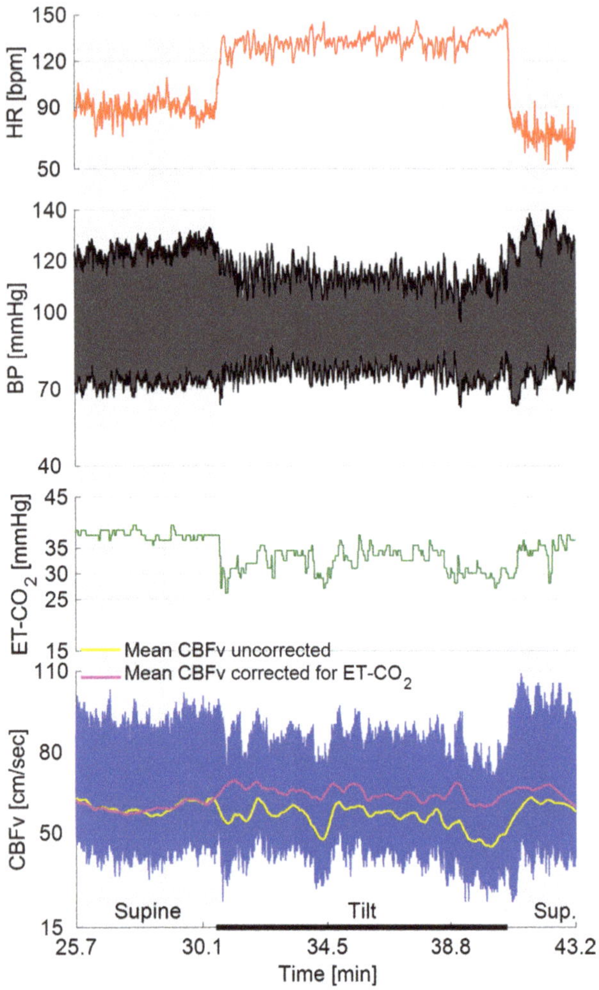

Figure 14.1 The tilt test showed excessive tachycardia with heart rate increment above 30 BPM and exceeding the 120 threshold, while the blood pressure was stable. The end tidal CO_2 declined at the onset of the tilt, then fluctuated and declined again at tilt end. Cerebral blood flow velocity (CBFv) was reduced during the tilt. CBFv adjusted for the effect of end tidal CO2 was stable. Patient was dizzy, short of breath, and experienced palpitations during the tilt.

sensory and sudomotor fibers, which is consistent with mixed small fiber neuropathy. The Valsalva maneuver showed an adrenergic vasoconstrictive deficit. Sudomotor testing showed sympathetic dysfunction. These abnormalities are consistent with the neuropathic form of POTS. Patient's typical orthostatic symptoms were reproduced. In addition, abnormal skin biopsy also explains patient's chronic pain syndrome, which can be related to the damage of epidermal sensory fibers.

TREATMENT AND FOLLOW-UP

- Clinical workup for neuropathy.
- Volume expansion through high fluid and high salt intake.

CAVEATS

POTS can be associated with mixed small fiber neuropathy, in which both epidermal and autonomic fibers are affected. Damage of sensory fibers leads to sensory symptoms (pain, numbness) while dysfunction of autonomic fibers (in this case with adrenergic dysfunctions as detected by the Valsalva maneuver and sudomotor deficit as detected by sudomotor testing and confirmed by abnormal sweat gland nerve fibers on the skin biopsy) leads to POTS. Hypocapnia is common in POTS and reduces CBFv due to its vasoconstrictive effect.

REFERENCES

1. Low PA, Sandroni P, Joyner M, Shen W-K. Postural tachycardia syndrome (POTS). *J Cardiovasc Electrophysiol.* 2009;20(3):352–358. doi:10.1111/j.1540-8167.2008.01407.x.
2. Novak P. Cerebral blood flow, heart rate, and blood pressure patterns during the tilt test in common orthostatic syndromes. *Neurosci J.* 2016;2016:6127340. doi:10.1155/2016/6127340.

15.

CASE 10: POSTURAL TACHYCARDIA SYNDROME WITH HYPERVENTILATION

Chief complaint: Dizziness.

Case presentation: A 23-year-old woman presents with orthostatic dizziness associated with dyspnea and palpitations for 2 years. Neurologic and cardiac examination was unrevealing. She was referred for evaluation of suspected postural tachycardia syndrome (POTS).

Past medical history: Migraine.

Current medication: Rizatriptan.

Assessment plan: Functional autonomic tests and skin biopsy.

AUTONOMIC TESTING EVALUATION

See Table 15.1.

Heart rate: Supine heart rate was normal. Heart rate responses to deep breathing were reduced to 87.1% of normal value. Heart rate increment during the tilt (64 BPM) was exaggerated and exceeded 120 BPM.

Blood pressure:

Valsalva maneuver: Blood pressure responses were normal.

Tilt: Supine blood pressure was within normal range. Blood pressure responses to tilt were normal.

Sudomotor evaluation: Electrochemical skin conductance was normal at hands and normal at feet.

Respiratory system: Respiratory frequency was normal during supine and during the tilt. The end tidal CO_2 was reduced during supine position and was further severely reduced during the tilt.

Cerebral blood flow velocity (CBFv): CBFv in the middle cerebral artery was normal in supine position but was severely reduced during the tilt test.

Skin biopsy (sensory-epidermal): Epidermal nerve fiber density was normal at proximal leg and normal at distal leg.

Skin biopsy (sweat glands): Sweat gland nerve fiber density was normal at proximal leg and normal at distal leg.

Patient-reported symptoms during testing: Dizziness, shortness of breath during the tilt test.

Patient-reported symptoms for past 2 weeks:

Lightheadedness or dizziness: Often
Dry eyes or mouth: Occasionally
Pale feet: Occasionally
Cold feet: Often
Reduced sweating: None
Reduced sweating after exercise: None
Increased sweating: None
Nausea: Occasionally
Diarrhea: Occasionally
Constipation: Occasionally
Urinary leaks: None

TABLE 15.1 RESULTS OF AUTONOMIC TESTING

Blood pressure evaluation					
Test: Valsalva maneuver					
Pressure [mmHg]	Baseline	Phase 2			Phase 4
		Early	End		
Systolic	102	82	123		
Mean	78.7	72	107	n/a	
Diastolic	67	67	99	n/a	

Heart rate evaluation	
Test: Deep breathing	
Results	Norm*
12.2	≥14
Test: Valsalva ratio	
1.96	≥1.46
* adjusted for a gender and age	

(continued)

TABLE 15.1 **CONTINUED**

Test: Tilt test										
Position		HR [BPM]	Blood pressure [mmHg]		MCA Blood flow velocity [cm/s]				Respiratory frequency [breaths/min]	End tidal CO_2 [mmHg]
			Systolic	Diastolic	Systolic	Mean	Mean drop [%]	Diastolic		
Supine		80	111	71	102	60.7		40	11	32
Tilt [min]	1	121	132	89	71	41	32.5	26	20	25
	2	121	127	84						
	3	133	114	81						
	4	138	120	82						
	5	131	132	95	73	41.7	31.3	26	8	24
	6	122	127	82						
	7	129	122	85						
	8	142	119	72						
	9	137	119	72						
	10	144	115	81	70	46	24.2	34	17	19
	15									
	20									
	30									
	40									

Sudomotor evaluation - functional

Test: Quantitative sudomotor axon reflex test (QSART)				
Location	Site (l/r)	Latency [min]	Volume [μl]	Norm [μl]*
Forearm				≥0.08
Prox. leg				≥0.14
Distal leg				≥0.24
Foot				≥0.09

* Normative data are adjusted for gender and age of patient.

Test: Electrochemical skin conductance (ESC)				
Location	Left [μS]	Right [μS]	Average [μS/k]	Norm [μS/kg]
Hand	86	86	1.35	≥1.03
Feet	93	93	1.46	≥1.14
Forehead				

For grading uses ESC [μS] adjusted for weight [μS/k].

TABLE 15.1 **CONTINUED**

Small fiber (sensory + sudomotor) evaluation - morphological					
Test: Skin biopsy					
Location	Site (l/r)	Nerve fibers			
		Epidermal*		Sweat glands	
		Density	Norm	Density	Norm
Proximal leg – thigh	Right	12.87	≥8.3	59.7	≥37.8
Distal leg - calf	Right	10.86	≥9.26	40.2	≥36.5
Foot	Right		≥3.11		≥34.8

*Normative data for distal leg are adjusted for gender and age of patient.

QASAT*										
Heart rate		BP		CBFv		ET-CO2		Sudomotor		Total QASAT score
S. bradycardia	0	Low supine	0	Low supine	0	Low supine	1	QSART		
S. tachycardia	0	High supine	0	High supine	0	High supine	0	ESC	0	
Increase tilt	10	OH	0	Tilt response	8	Tilt low	7			
Decrease tilt	0	OHTN	0	CA	0	Tilt high	0	**Skin biopsy**		27
Deep breathing	1	VM	0	CVR	0			Epidermal	0	
VR	0			VM	0			Sweat gland	0	
Total	11	Total	0	Total	8	Total	8			

*QASAT. See Novak. Quantitative Scale for Grading of Cardiovascular Autonomic Reflex Tests and Small Fibers from Skin Biopsies. *J Neurol Disord* 2015;3:2.

S, supine; Increase tilt, increased response to tilt; Decrease tilt, decreased response to tilt; BP, blood pressure; VM, Valsalva maneuver; CBFv, cerebral blood flow velocity; CA, cerebral autoregulation; MCA, middle cerebral artery; VR, Valsalva ratio; CVR, cerebral vasoreactivity.

Current pain severity: 3
Aching pain: Continuous, severe
Allodynia: Often, mild
Burning pain: None
Lancinating pain: Occasionally, moderate
Numbness: Occasionally, mild
Prickling sensation: None

AUTONOMIC TESTING INTERPRETATION

- POTS, mild. There was also evidence of mild parasympathetic cardiovagal dysfunction.
- Reduced postural cerebral blood flow velocity due to the vasoconstrictive effect of hypocapnia.
- Hypocapnic hyperventilation during the tilt.

COMMENT

Tilt test provoked the characteristic POTS response and reproduced the patient's symptoms including postural dizziness, shortness of breath, flushing of the face, blurred vision, and headache (Figure 15.1).

In POTS, signs of orthostatic intolerance are due to cerebral hypoperfusion associated with reduced CBFv. In POTS, the entire decline in CBFv is driven by the changes in end tidal CO_2 since CBFv adjusted for the effect of end tidal CO_2 does not decline during the tilt (Figure 15.1 A, B).

TREATMENT AND FOLLOW-UP

- Volume expansion through high fluid and high salt intake; endurance training.

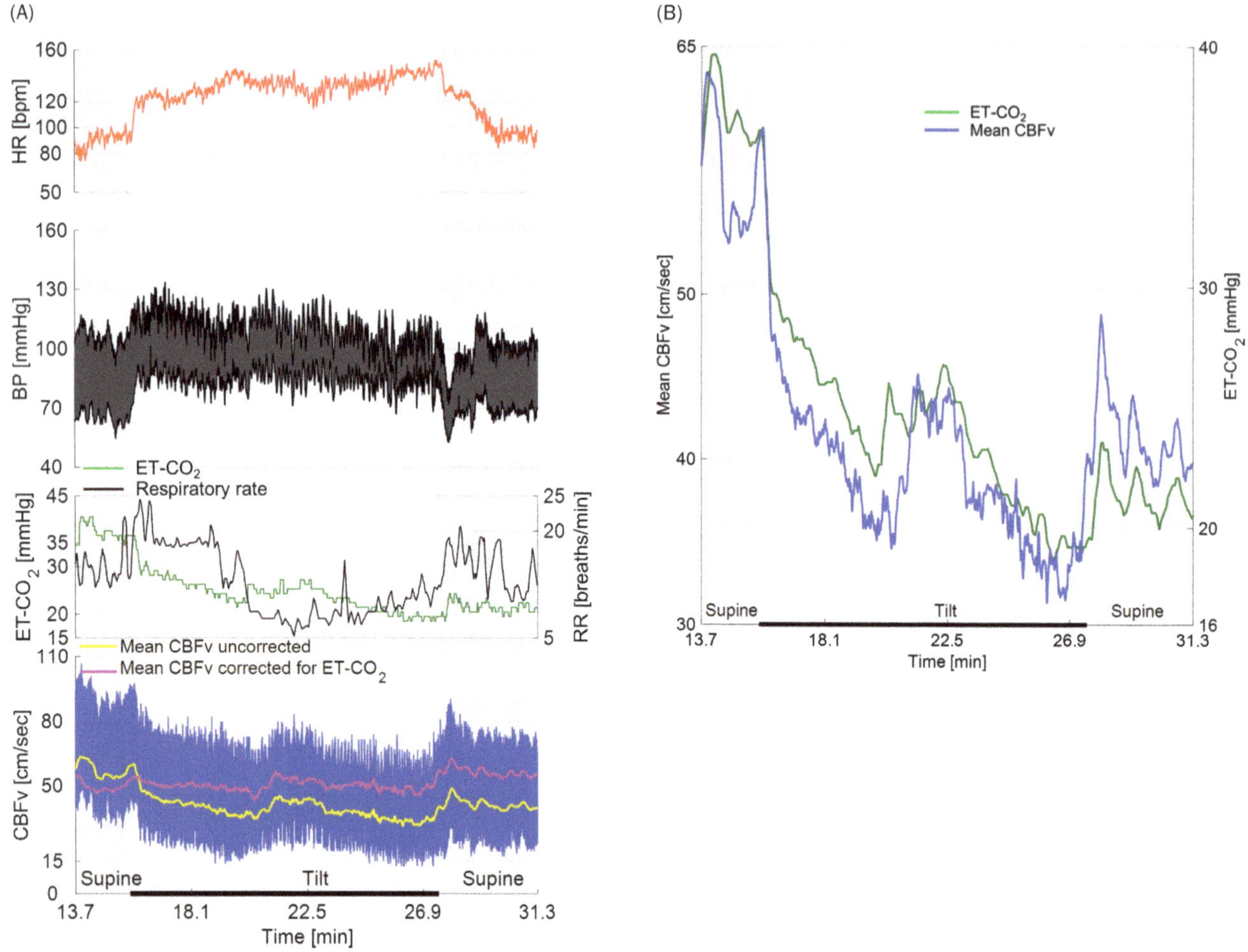

Figure 15.1 The tilt provoked excessive tachycardia, but blood pressure remained stable, which is typical for postural tachycardia syndrome (POTS) (A). End tidal CO_2 was markedly reduced during the tilt (minimum <20 mm Hg), which is consistent with hypocapnic hyperventilation. Cerebral blood flow velocity (CBFv) was also reduced during the tilt. An overlay of mean CBFv and end tidal CO_2 shows that both signals are correlated (B), indicating cerebral vasoconstriction. RR, respiratory rate.

CAVEATS

- POTS patients exhibit signs of cerebral hypoperfusion, which is related to a decline in CBFv.
- End tidal CO_2 has a profound effect on CBFv. Decline in CBFv in POTS is mainly due to hypocapnia. This is a common finding in POTS.[1]

REFERENCE

1. Novak V, Spies JM, Novak P, McPhee BR, Rummans TA, Low PA. Hypocapnia and cerebral hypoperfusion in orthostatic intolerance. *Stroke*. 1998;29(9):1876–1881.

16.

CASE 11: POSTURAL TACHYCARDIA SYNDROME WITH POSITIVE ANTIBODIES AGAINST THE P/Q-TYPE OF CALCIUM CHANNEL

Chief complaint: Dizziness.

Case presentation: A 38-year-old woman presents with unexplained orthostatic dizziness, fatigue, and tachycardia and diffuse, disabling pain at distal legs, including burning sensation, for 6 years. Neurological examination showed normal reflexes, muscle strength, and large fibers examination (soft touch, vibration and proprioception sensation) but abnormal small fiber examination (pin-prick and temperature sensation at distal legs).

Past medical history: Chronic fatigue syndrome.

Current medication: None.

Assessment plan: Functional autonomic tests and skin biopsy.

AUTONOMIC TESTING EVALUATION

See Table 16.1.

Heart rate: Supine heart rate was normal. Heart rate responses to deep breathing were normal. Heart rate increment during the tilt (50 BPM) was exaggerated and exceeded 140 BPM.

Blood pressure:

Valsalva maneuver: Mean blood pressure failed to return to baseline at the end of Phase 2 by 10.5 mm Hg (i.e., 89% of baseline).

Tilt: Supine blood pressure was normal but was elevated during the tilt.

Sudomotor evaluation: Sweat output was normal at forearm, normal at proximal leg, normal at distal leg, and normal at foot.

Respiratory system: Respiratory frequency was normal in supine position and during the tilt. End tidal CO_2 was normal in supine position but was moderately reduced during the tilt.

Cerebral blood flow velocity (CBFv): CBFv in middle cerebral artery was normal in supine position but was severely reduced during the tilt.

Skin biopsy (sensory-epidermal): Epidermal nerve fiber density was abnormal (reduced to 69.2% of normal limit) at proximal leg and abnormal (reduced to 14.4% of normal limit) at distal leg.

Skin biopsy (sweat glands): Sweat gland nerve fiber density was normal at proximal leg and normal at distal leg.

Patient-reported symptoms during testing: Dizziness and shortness of breath during the tilt.

Patient-reported symptoms for past 2 weeks:

Lightheadedness or dizziness: Often
Dry eyes or mouth: Occasionally
Pale feet: None
Cold feet: Often

TABLE 16.1 **RESULTS OF AUTONOMIC TESTING**

Blood pressure evaluation					
Test: Valsalva maneuver					
Pressure [mmHg]	Baseline	Phase 2			Phase 4
		Early	End		
Systolic	128.5	111.6	105.4		
Mean	95.1	88.2	84.6	n/a	
Diastolic	78.4	76.5	74.2	n/a	

Heart rate evaluation	
Test: Deep breathing	
Results	Norm*
17.4	≥12
Test: Valsalva ratio	
1.95	≥1.5
* adjusted for a gender and age	

(continued)

TABLE 16.1 **CONTINUED**

Test: Tilt test										
Position		HR [BPM]	Blood pressure [mmHg]		MCA Blood flow velocity [cm/s]				Respiratory frequency [breaths/min]	End tidal CO_2 [mmHg]
			Systolic	Diastolic	Systolic	Mean	Mean drop [%]	Diastolic		
Supine		98	111	74	98	62.7		45	17	41
Tilt [min]	1	121	122	80	95	57.7	8	39	16	26
	2	125	128	87						
	3	129	123	83						
	4	130	145	92						
	5	134	126	90	78	47.3	24.6	32	14	26
	6	148	130	90						
	7	140	132	96						
	8	137	127	93						
	9	135	120	73						
	10	131	133	91	76	44	29.8	28	13	36
	15									
	20									
	30									
	40									

Sudomotor evaluation - functional

Test: Quantitative sudomotor axon reflex test (QSART)				
Location	Site (l/r)	Latency [min]	Volume [µl]	Norm [µl]*
Forearm	l	1.32	0.666	≥0.08
Prox. leg	l	0.56	0.633	≥0.14
Distal leg	l	1.37	0.42	≥0.15
Foot	l	1.49	0.404	≥0.07

* Normative data are adjusted for gender and age of patient.

Test: Electrochemical skin conductance (ESC)				
Location	Left [µS]	Right [µS]	Average [µS/k]	Norm [µS/kg]
Hand				≥
Feet				≥
Forehead				

For grading uses ESC [µS] adjusted for weight [µS/k].

TABLE 16.1 **CONTINUED**

Small fiber (sensory + sudomotor) evaluation - morphological					
Test: Skin biopsy					
Location	Site (l/r)	Nerve fibers			
		Epidermal*		Sweat glands	
		Density	Norm	Density	Norm
Proximal leg – thigh	Right	5.74	≥8.3	57.8	≥37.8
Distal leg - calf	Right	1.16	≥8.06	48.9	≥36.5
Foot	Right		≥3.11		≥34.8

* Normative data for distal leg are adjusted for gender and age of patient.

QASAT*										
Heart rate		**BP**		**CBFv**		**ET-CO2**		**Sudomotor**		**Total QASAT score**
S. bradycardia	0	Low supine	0	Low supine	0	Low supine	0	QSART	1	
S. tachycardia	0	High supine	0	High supine	0	High supine	0	ESC		
Increase tilt	8	OH	0	Tilt response	4	Tilt low	4			
Decrease tilt	0	OHTN	3	CA	0	Tilt high	0	**Skin biopsy**		26
Deep breathing	0	VM	2	CVR	0			Epidermal	4	
VR	1			VM	0			Sweat gland	0	
Total	8	Total	5	Total	4	Total	4			

*QASAT. See Novak. Quantitative Scale for Grading of Cardiovascular Autonomic Reflex Tests and Small Fibers from Skin Biopsies. *J Neurol Disord* 2015;3:2.

S, supine; Increase tilt, increased response to tilt; Decrease tilt, decreased response to tilt; BP, blood pressure; VM, Valsalva maneuver; CBFv, cerebral blood flow velocity; CA, cerebral autoregulation; MCA, middle cerebral artery; VR, Valsalva ratio; CVR, cerebral vasoreactivity.

Reduced sweating: Often
Reduced sweating after exercise: Often
Increased sweating: None
Nausea: Occasionally
Diarrhea: Occasionally
Constipation: Yes, minor annoyance
Urinary leaks: Occasionally
Current pain severity: 6
Aching pain: Continuous, severe
Allodynia: Often, moderate
Burning pain: Continuous, moderate
Lancinating pain: Often, moderate
Numbness: Continuous, moderate
Prickling sensation: Continuous, moderate

AUTONOMIC TESTING INTERPRETATION

- Postural tachycardia syndrome (POTS), moderate, neuropathic form.
- Small fiber neuropathy, severe, length-dependent.

COMMENT

Patient had both symptoms of autonomic dysfunction (dizziness and tachycardia) and small fibers dysfunction (burning sensation/abnormal sensory examination). Dizziness was present from the beginning of the tilt (Figure 16.1A, B) and was associated with excessive heart rate increment, reduced CBFv, and hypocapnia. This pattern is characteristic for POTS. CBFv was reduced due to hypocapnia-induced cerebral vasoconstriction. Skin biopsy revealed a marked reduction of sensory epidermal fibers, indicating the presence of length-dependent small fiber neuropathy.

Further evaluations showed positive antibodies against the P/Q-type calcium (0.10 nmol/L, normal ≤ 0.02 nmol/L). Antibodies against the P/Q-type calcium channel are detectable in 85% of patients with Lambert-Eaton myasthenic syndrome (LEMS).[1–3] The antibodies are detected on presynaptic cholinergic nerve terminals at the neuromuscular junction and in the autonomic nervous system. Characteristic symptoms of LEMS are an ascending muscle weakness starting

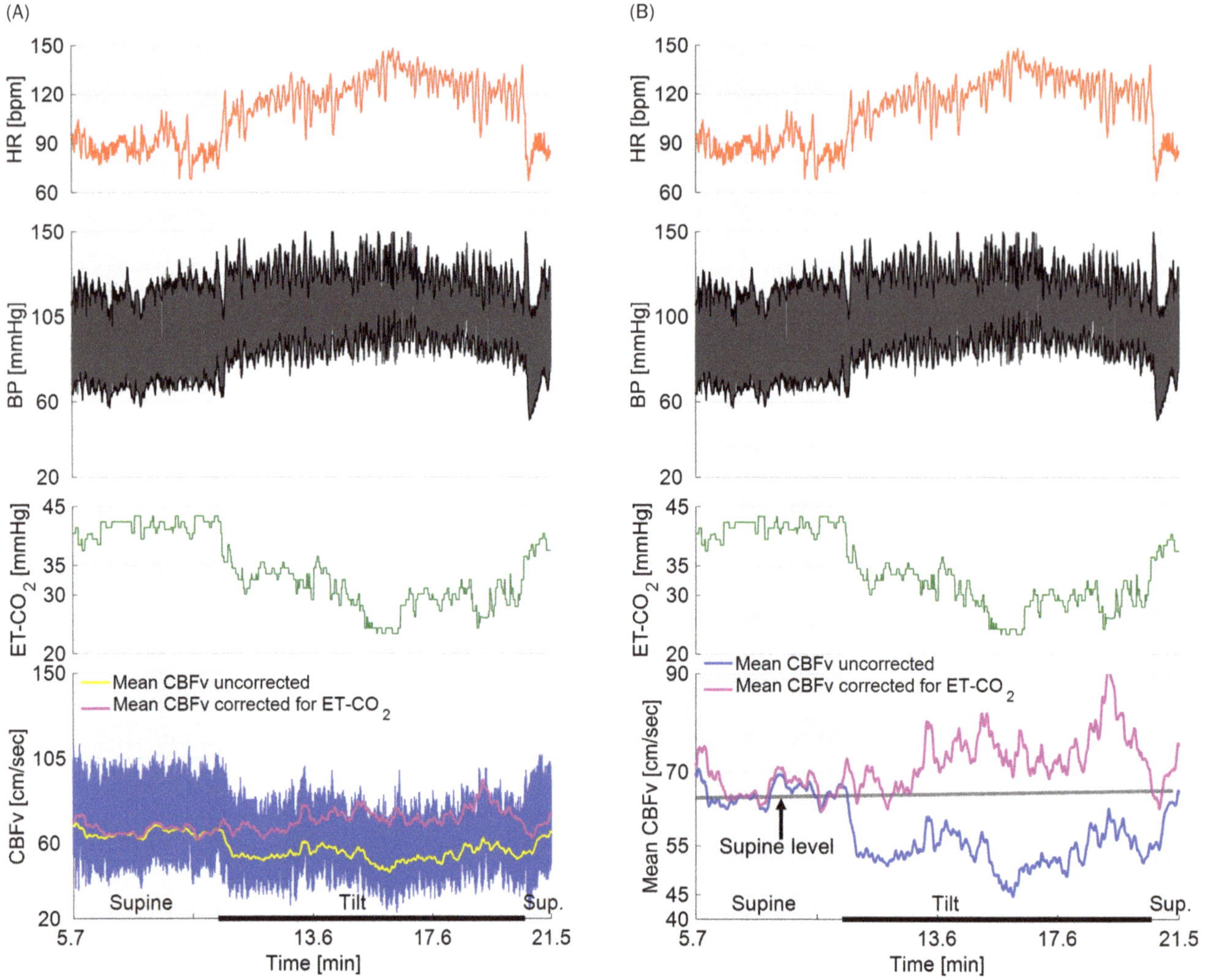

Figure 16.1 The tilt test shows a characteristic POTS pattern with excessive postural tachycardia (an increment in heart rate by >30 and exceeding 120 BPM), decline in cerebral blood flow velocity (CBFv), and low end tidal CO_2 (<25 mm Hg, normal range 35–45 mm Hg) without orthostatic hypotension (A, B). The patient became short of breath at the beginning of the tilt and complained of dizziness. Blood pressure was elevated during the tilt. CBFv declined during the tilt. CBFv corrected for the level of end-tidal CO_2 was not reduced, indicating that the entire drop in CBFv was induced by hypocapnic hyperventilation.

with the lower proximal limb muscles and autonomic dysfunction.

This patient was treated with using immune globulins (2 g/kg, monthly). After approximately 8 months, the chronic fatigue and disabling burning improved. Repeat concentration of the P/Q-type calcium channel after 1 year of immunomodulatory therapy was 0.04 nmol/L.

TREATMENT AND FOLLOW-UP

- Therapy with β-blockers.
- Trial of immunomodulatory therapy using immune globulins.

CAVEATS

- Combination of autonomic testing with skin biopsies may increase diagnostic accuracy of the testing.
- Orthostatic symptoms in POTS (shortness of breath, lightheadedness, fatigue, and others) are due to cerebral hypoperfusion associated with reduced CBFv,[4] which is induced by hypocapnia. Orthostatic hypotension, by definition was absent.
- Elevated orthostatic blood pressure is frequently seen in the hyperadrenergic form of POTS. In this case hyperadrenergic state was later confirmed by findings of elevated norepinephrine on standing. Hyperadrenergic state usually responds to β-blockers.

Neuropathic POTS can be associated with elevated norepinephrine.

- Immunomodulatory therapy using immune globulins may be effective in small fiber neuropathy with positive antibody against the P/Q-type calcium channel.

REFERENCES

1. Motomura M, Lang B, Johnston I, Palace J, Vincent A, Newsom-Davis J. Incidence of serum anti-P/Q-type and anti-N-type calcium channel autoantibodies in the Lambert-Eaton myasthenic syndrome. *J Neurol Sci.* 1997;147(1):35–42. doi:10.1016/S0022-510X(96)05303-8.
2. Lennon VA, Kryzer TJ, Griesmann GE, et al. Calcium-channel antibodies in the Lambert-Eaton syndrome and other paraneoplastic syndromes. *N Engl J Med.* 1995;332(22):1467–1474. doi:10.1056/NEJM199506013322203.
3. Mahadeva B, Phillips LH, Juel VC. Autoimmune disorders of neuromuscular transmission. *Semin Neurol.* 2008;28(2):212–227. doi:10.1055/s-2008-1062260.
4. Low PA, Novak V, Spies JM, Novak P, Petty GW. Cerebrovascular regulation in the postural orthostatic tachycardia syndrome (POTS). *Am J Med Sci.* 1999;317(2):124–133.

17.

CASE 12: POSTURAL TACHYCARDIA SYNDROME WITH PRESYNCOPE AND SYNCOPE

Chief complaint: Dizziness.

Case presentation: A 34-year-old woman presents with unexplained, usually orthostatic, dizziness for several months. She also has a history of cold and heat intolerance, fatigue, insomnia, and anxiety for at least 13 years. Previous neurological and cardiology evaluations were normal. Patient was referred for evaluation of suspected autonomic failure.

Past medical history: Anxiety, anemia.

Current medication: None.

Assessment plan: Functional autonomic tests and skin biopsy.

AUTONOMIC TESTING EVALUATION

See Table 17.1.

Heart rate: Heart rate was within normal range in supine position. Heart rate responses to deep breathing were reduced to 61.4% of normal value. Heart rate increment during the tilt was exaggerated (45 BPM) and exceeded 120 BPM.

Blood pressure:

Valsalva maneuver: Mean blood pressure failed to return to baseline at the end of Phase 2 by 14.3 mm Hg (i.e., 81.3% of baseline).

Tilt: Supine blood pressure was within normal range. Blood pressure responses to tilt were abnormal, consistent with neurally mediated syncope.

Sudomotor evaluation: Electrochemical skin conductance was abnormal (reduced to 67.2% of normal limit) at hands and abnormal (reduced to 85.4% of normal limit) at feet.

Respiratory system: Respiratory frequency was normal during supine. Respiratory frequency was normal during the tilt. The end tidal CO_2 was normal during the supine position. The end tidal CO_2 was normal during the tilt test.

Cerebral blood flow velocity (CBFv): CBFv in middle cerebral artery was normal in supine position. CBFv in middle cerebral artery was moderately reduced during the tilt test and rapidly declined during syncope.

Skin biopsy (sensory-epidermal): Epidermal nerve fiber density was normal at proximal leg and abnormal (reduced to 97.7% of normal limit) at distal leg.

Skin biopsy (sweat glands): Sweat gland nerve fiber density was normal at proximal leg and normal at distal leg.

Patient-reported symptoms during testing: Loss of consciousness, dizziness, and nausea during the tilt.

Patient-reported symptoms for past 2 weeks:

Lightheadedness or dizziness: Occasionally
Dry eyes or mouth: Yes, minor annoyance
Pale feet: Occasionally

TABLE 17.1 **RESULTS OF AUTONOMIC TESTING**

Blood pressure evaluation					
Test: Valsalva maneuver					
Pressure [mmHg]	Baseline	Phase 2			Phase 4
		Early	End		
Systolic	111	69	72		
Mean	76.3	58.3	62	n/a	
Diastolic	59	53	57	n/a	

Heart rate evaluation	
Test: Deep breathing	
Results	Norm*
6.14	≥10
Test: Valsalva ratio	
1.78	≥1.51
* adjusted for a gender and age	

TABLE 17.1 CONTINUED

Test: Tilt test										
Position		HR [BPM]	Blood pressure [mmHg]		MCA Blood flow velocity [cm/s]				Respiratory frequency [breaths/min]	End tidal CO_2 [mmHg]
			Systolic	Diastolic	Systolic	Mean	Mean drop [%]	Diastolic		
Supine		85	119	75	96	62.7		46	14	40
Tilt [min]	1	116	115	81	77	53	15.5	41	12	36
	2	124	115	81						
	3	109	114	81						
	4	107	120	82						
	5	107	118	82	81	54.3	13.4	41	13	37
	6	122	114	82						
	7	118	115	82						
	8	120	111	81						
	9	130	113	79						
	10	82	64	34	78	50	20.3	36	10	36
	15									
	20									
	30									
	40									

Sudomotor evaluation - functional

Test: Quantitative sudomotor axon reflex test (QSART)				
Location	Site (l/r)	Latency [min]	Volume [μl]	Norm [μl]*
Forearm				≥0.08
Prox. leg				≥0.14
Distal leg				≥0.15
Foot				≥0.07

* Normative data are adjusted for gender and age of patient.

Test: Electrochemical skin conductance (ESC)				
Location	Left [μS]	Right [μS]	Average [μS/k]	Norm [μS/kg]
Hand	49	60	0.69	≥1.03
Feet	78	74	0.95	≥1.14
Forehead				

For grading uses ESC [μS] adjusted for weight [μS/k].

(continued)

TABLE 17.1 CONTINUED

Small fiber (sensory + sudomotor) evaluation - morphological					
Test: Skin biopsy					
Location	Site (l/r)	Nerve fibers			
		Epidermal*		Sweat glands	
		Density	Norm	Density	Norm
Proximal leg – thigh	Right	15.1	≥8.3	53.4	≥37.8
Distal leg - calf	Right	7.48	≥7.66	42.4	≥36.5
Foot	Right		≥3.11		≥34.8

* Normative data for distal leg are adjusted for gender and age of patient.

QASAT*												
Heart rate		**BP**		**CBFv**		**ET-CO2**		**Sudomotor**			**Total QASAT score**
S. bradycardia	0	Low supine	0	Low supine	0	Low supine	0	QSART			
S. tachycardia	0	High supine	0	High supine	0	High supine	0	ESC	2		
Increase tilt	5	OH		Tilt response	3	Tilt low	0				
Decrease tilt	0	OHTN	0	CA	0	Tilt high	0	**Skin biopsy**			15
Deep breathing	1	VM	2	CVR	0			Epidermal	1		
VR	0			VM	0			Sweat gland	0		
Total	6	Total	2	Total	3	Total	0				

*QASAT. See Novak. Quantitative Scale for Grading of Cardiovascular Autonomic Reflex Tests and Small Fibers from Skin Biopsies. *J Neurol Disord* 2015;3:2. Only the tilt responses before syncope are graded. Syncope occurred at minute 10. Non syncopal missing values at minute 10 were replaced from minute 9 since QASAT requires 10 minutes of the tilt and cannot grade syncope.

S, supine; Increase tilt, increased response to tilt; Decrease tilt, decreased response to tilt; BP, blood pressure; VM, Valsalva maneuver; CBFv, cerebral blood flow velocity; CA, cerebral autoregulation; MCA, middle cerebral artery; VR, Valsalva ratio; CVR, cerebral vasoreactivity.

Cold feet: Often
Reduced sweating: Often
Reduced sweating after exercise: Often
Increased sweating: None
Nausea: None
Diarrhea: None
Constipation: Often
Urinary leaks: None
Current pain severity: 0
Aching pain: None
Allodynia: None
Burning pain: None
Lancinating pain: None
Numbness: Often, severe
Prickling sensation: Often, severe

AUTONOMIC TESTING INTERPRETATION

- Postural tachycardia syndrome (POTS), neuropathic form.
- Syncope, neurally mediated, mixed.
- Small fiber neuropathy, mixed, length-dependent.

COMMENT

Patient complained of dizziness from the beginning of the tilt (Figure 17.1). This was associated with excessive heart rate increment, reduced CBFv, and hyperventilation. This pattern is typical for POTS. The tilt also provoked presyncope and syncope. Syncope was associated with bradycardia and hyperventilation. CBFv showed a characteristic vasodilation pattern (signal widening due to reduction of diastolic and increase in systolic velocities), indicating active compensatory autoregulation (Figure 17.1B).

TREATMENT AND FOLLOW-UP

- Clinical workup for neuropathy.

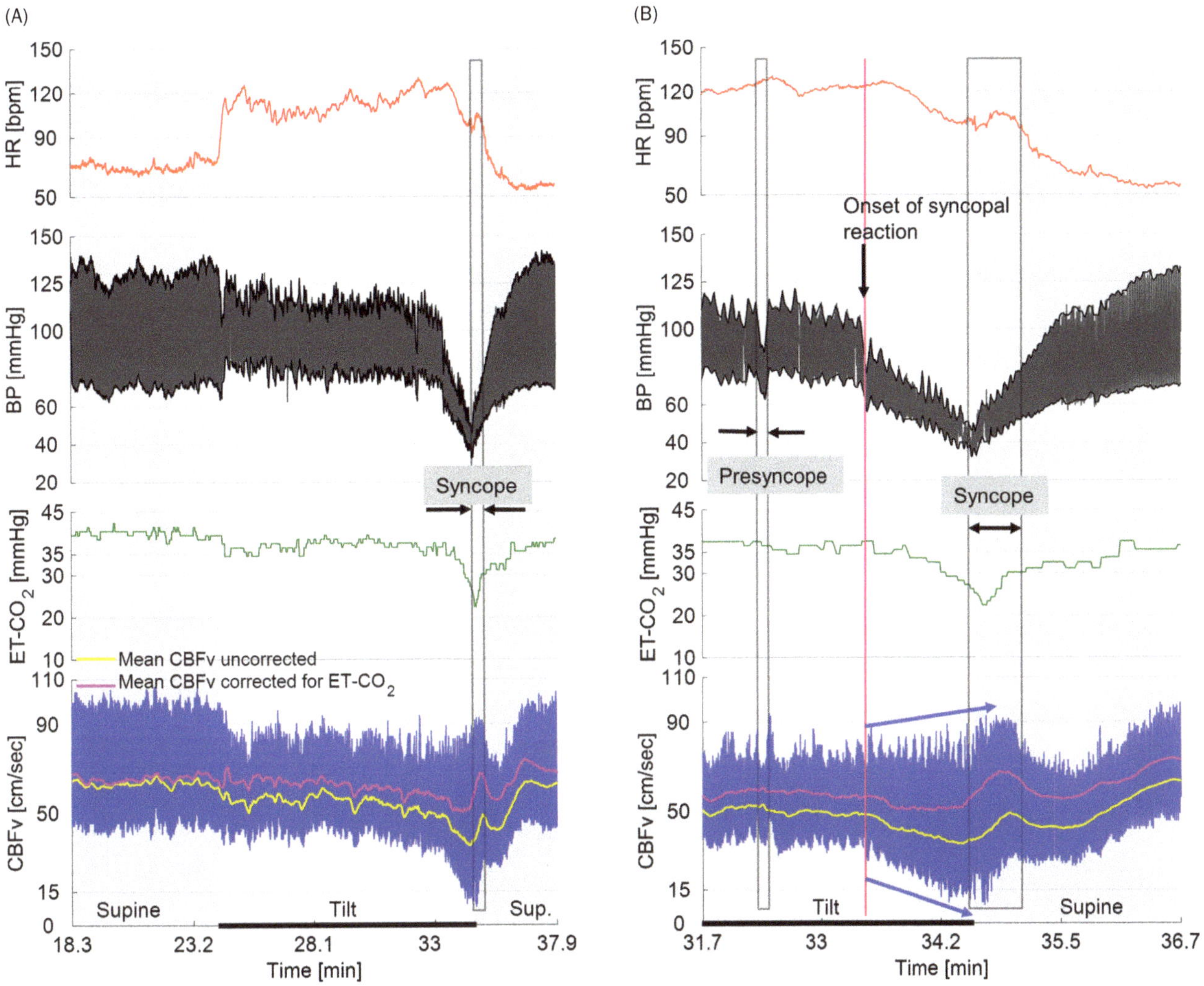

Figure 17.1 The patient became dizzy at the beginning of the tilt and continued to be dizzy and anxious (A). She had a presyncopal reaction that preceded syncope at minute 10 of tilt (A, B, C). The presyncope (B) was associated with a decline in blood pressure and cerebral blood flow velocity (CBFv; C, point 2). Blood pressure recovered (point 3), which was associated with cerebral vasodilation (reduction in diastolic CBFv (C, point 4). The onset of syncopal reaction (C, point 1) was similar, but blood pressure never fully recovered to baseline (C, point 3), which was followed by gradual decrease of blood pressure until the patient lost consciousness. The syncope (A, B) was of mixed type, associated with blood pressure drop and slowing of heart rate. Bradycardia occurred after the syncope in supine position. CBFv showed characteristic vasodilation pattern (reduction of diastolic and increase of systolic velocities, *blue arrows* [B]), which is compensatory and indicates effective cerebral autoregulation.

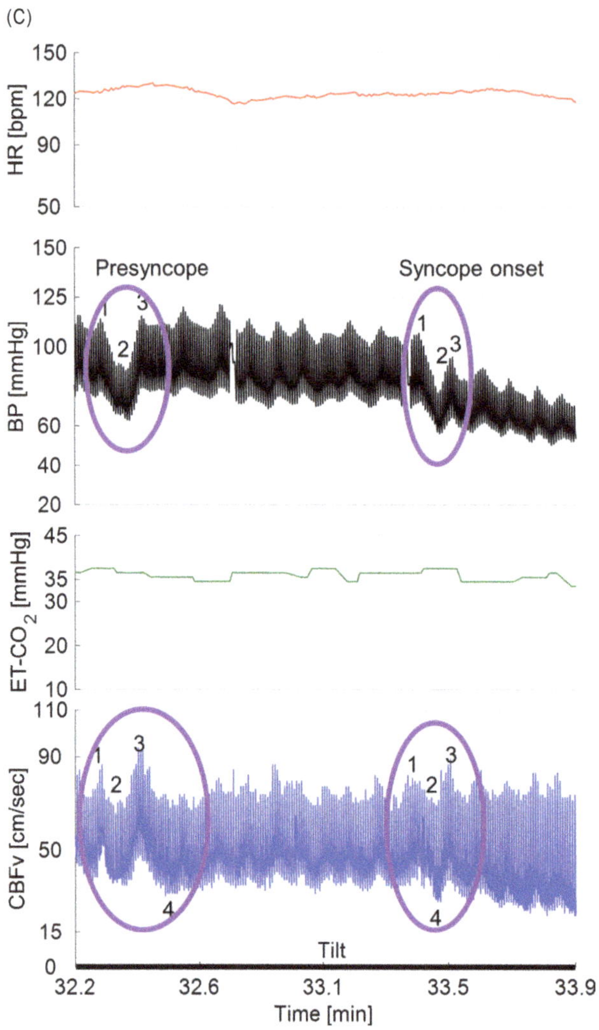

Figure 17.1 Continued

- Volume expansion through high fluid and high salt intake.
- Trial of pyridostigmine[1] since it also may help with gastrointestinal symptoms.

CAVEATS

- Syncope can occur with POTS.[2,3]
- Presyncope may precede syncope during the tilt.

REFERENCES

1. Moon J, Kim D-Y, Lee W-J, et al. Efficacy of propranolol, bisoprolol, and pyridostigmine for postural tachycardia syndrome: a randomized clinical trial. *Neurother J Am Soc Exp Neurother*. March 2018. doi:10.1007/s13311-018-0612-9.
2. Garland EM, Celedonio JE, Raj SR. Postural tachycardia syndrome: beyond orthostatic intolerance. *Curr Neurol Neurosci Rep*. 2015;15(9):60. doi:10.1007/s11910-015-0583-8.
3. Novak P. Cerebral blood flow, heart rate, and blood pressure patterns during the tilt test in common orthostatic syndromes. *Neurosci J*. 2016;2016:6127340. doi:10.1155/2016/6127340.

18.

CASE 13: POSTURAL TACHYCARDIA SYNDROME WITH SYNCOPE

Chief complaint: Dizziness.

Case presentation: A 21-year-old woman presents with unexplained loss of consciousness. As a child, she always became exhausted early in sports. She had scoliosis surgery 6 years ago, and her health has been deteriorating since the surgery. She experienced ringing in the right ear, then she developed fatigue, nausea, abdominal distention, constipation, and bloating. However, she was doing relatively well until 9 months ago, when she noted severe postural dizziness and she started to pass out. She also became more exercise- and temperature-intolerant. She had to stop working at the office. Her 14-year-old cousin was diagnosed with orthostatic intolerance. Extensive evaluation has been unrevealing. Neurologic examination at the office was entirely normal. She had normal MRI of the brain and two normal electroencephalograms. She tried fludrocortisone without any improvement. Somatoform disorder has been suspected. Patient was referred for suspected orthostatic intolerance.

Past medical history: Tachycardia.

Current medication: Pantoprazole.

Assessment plan: Functional autonomic tests and skin biopsy.

AUTONOMIC TESTING EVALUATION

See Table 18.1.

Heart rate: Supine heart rate was normal. Heart rate responses to deep breathing were normal. Heart rate increment during the tilt (66 BPM) was exaggerated and exceeded 150 BPM.

Blood pressure:

Valsalva maneuver: Blood pressure responses were normal.

Tilt: Supine blood pressure was normal. Patient experienced syncope at minute 6 of tilt, then the tilt was aborted.

Sudomotor evaluation: Electrochemical skin conductance was normal at hands and normal at feet.

Respiratory system: Respiratory frequency was normal in supine position and during the tilt. End tidal CO_2 was normal in supine position but was reduced during the tilt.

Cerebral blood flow velocity (CBFv): CBFv in middle cerebral artery was normal in supine position but was severely reduced during the tilt.

Skin biopsy (sensory-epidermal): Epidermal nerve fiber density was normal at proximal leg and normal at distal leg.

Skin biopsy (sweat glands): Sweat gland nerve fiber density was normal at proximal leg.

Patient-reported symptoms during testing: Loss of consciousness, dizziness, nausea during the tilt.

Patient-reported symptoms for past 2 weeks:

Lightheadedness or dizziness: Occasionally
Dry eyes or mouth: Occasionally
Pale feet: Occasionally
Cold feet: Occasionally
Reduced sweating: Yes, minor annoyance

TABLE 18.1 RESULTS OF AUTONOMIC TESTING

Blood pressure evaluation					
Test: Valsalva maneuver					
Pressure [mmHg]	Baseline	Phase 2			Phase 4
		Early	End		
Systolic	130	102	122		
Mean	98	80.7	98.7	n/a	
Diastolic	82	70	87	n/a	

Heart rate evaluation	
Test: Deep breathing	
Results	Norm*
38.7	≥14
Test: Valsalva ratio	
1.3	≥1.46
* adjusted for a gender and age	

(continued)

Test: Tilt test										
Position		HR [BPM]	Blood pressure [mmHg]		MCA Blood flow velocity [cm/s]				Respiratory frequency [breaths/min]	End tidal CO_2 [mmHg]
			Systolic	Diastolic	Systolic	Mean	Mean drop [%]	Diastolic		
Supine		88	115	74	106	66		46	18	41
Tilt [min]	1	142	132	81	88	62.7	5	50	19	35
	2	152	122	89						
	3	152	111	81						
	4	152	111	81						
	5	154	99	70	85	51.7	21.7	35	17	38
	6	70	83	50						
	7									
	8									
	9									
	10									
	15									
	20									
	30									
	40									

Sudomotor evaluation - functional

Test: Quantitative sudomotor axon reflex test (QSART)				
Location	Site (l/r)	Latency [min]	Volume [µl]	Norm [µl]*
Forearm				≥0.08
Prox. leg				≥0.14
Distal leg				≥0.24
Foot				≥0.09

* Normative data are adjusted for gender and age of patient.

Test: Electrochemical skin conductance (ESC)				
Location	Left [µS]	Right [µS]	Average [µS/k]	Norm [µS/kg]
Hand	82	81	1.28	≥1.03
Feet	83	82	1.29	≥1.14
Forehead				

For grading uses ESC [µS] adjusted for weight [µS/k].

TABLE 18.1 CONTINUED

Small fiber (sensory + sudomotor) evaluation - morphological					
Test: Skin biopsy					
Location	Site (l/r)	Nerve fibers			
		Epidermal*		Sweat glands	
		Density	Norm	Density	Norm
Proximal leg – thigh	Right	14.01	≥8.3	61.2	≥37.8
Distal leg - calf	Right	13.03	≥9.42		≥36.5
Foot	Right		≥3.11		≥34.8

* Normative data for distal leg are adjusted for gender and age of patient.

QASAT*											
Heart rate		**BP**		**CBFv**		**ET-CO2**		**Sudomotor**			**Total QASAT score**
S. bradycardia	0	Low supine	0	Low supine	0	Low supine	0	QSART			
S. tachycardia	0	High supine	0	High supine	0	High supine	0	ESC	0		
Increase tilt		OH		Tilt response		Tilt low					
Decrease tilt		OHTN		CA	0	Tilt high		**Skin biopsy**			1
Deep breathing	0	VM	0	CVR	0			Epidermal	0		
VR	1			VM	0			Sweat gland	0		
Total	1	Total	0	Total	0	Total	0				

*QASAT. See Novak. Quantitative Scale for Grading of Cardiovascular Autonomic Reflex Tests and Small Fibers from Skin Biopsies. *J Neurol Disord* 2015;3:2. Orthostatic (tilt) responses were not graded since QASAT requires the duration of the tilt at least 10 minutes.

S, supine; Increase tilt, increased response to tilt; Decrease tilt, decreased response to tilt; BP, blood pressure; VM, Valsalva maneuver; CBFv, cerebral blood flow velocity; CA, cerebral autoregulation; MCA, middle cerebral artery; VR, Valsalva ratio; CVR, cerebral vasoreactivity.

Reduced sweating after exercise: Yes, minor
Increased sweating: Yes, minor annoyance
Nausea: Occasionally
Diarrhea: None
Constipation: Occasionally
Urinary leaks: None
Current pain severity: 5
Aching pain: None
Allodynia: None
Burning pain: Often, severe
Lancinating pain: Occasionally, severe
Numbness: Often, mild
Prickling sensation: Often, moderate

AUTONOMIC TESTING INTERPRETATION

- Postural tachycardia syndrome (POTS) (Figure 18.1).
- Syncope, neurally mediated, mixed.

COMMENT

The tilt provoked most of the patient's symptoms, including dizziness, nausea, and loss of consciousness, which was consistent with postural tachycardia syndrome and neurally mediated mixed syncope (Figure 18.1).[1,2]

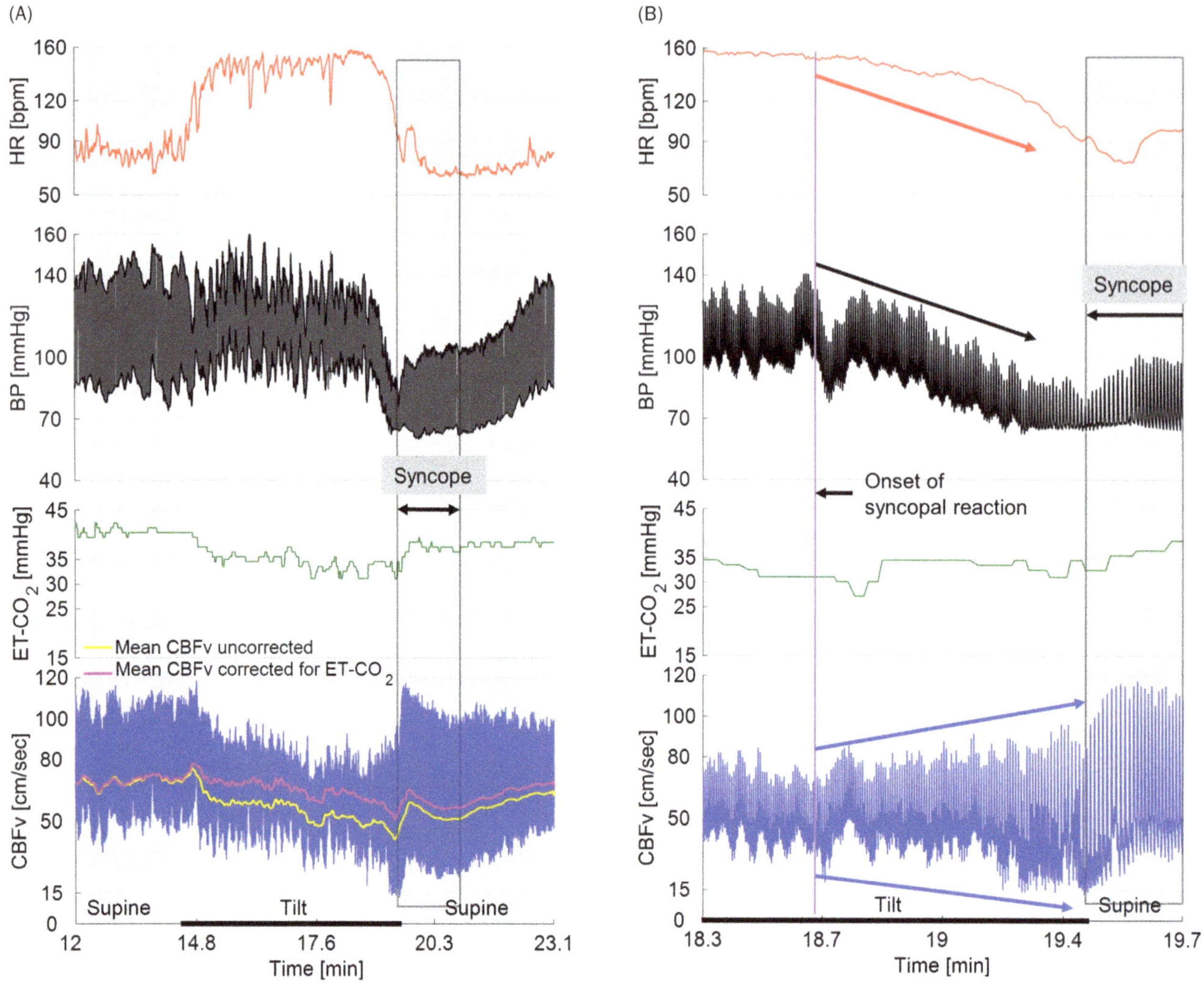

Figure 18.1 The tilt test provoked syncope of mixed type (A, B). The initial response to tilting was tachycardia >150 BPM with stable blood pressure. Starting from the onset of the syncopal reaction (B), there was a progressive decline in heart rate, blood pressure, end tidal CO_2, and diastolic cerebral blood flow velocity (CBFv) until the patient lost consciousness. Cerebral vasodilation pattern (reduced diastolic with increase of systolic CBFv) was present during syncope.

TREATMENT AND FOLLOW-UP

- Volume expansion through high fluid and high salt intake.
- Reconditioning program.

CAVEATS

- Syncope, neutrally mediated, may occur with the POTS.

REFERENCES

1. Garland EM, Celedonio JE, Raj SR. Postural tachycardia syndrome: beyond orthostatic intolerance. *Curr Neurol Neurosci Rep.* 2015;15(9):60. doi:10.1007/s11910-015-0583-8.
2. Novak P. Cerebral blood flow, heart rate, and blood pressure patterns during the tilt test in common orthostatic syndromes. *Neurosci J.* 2016;2016:6127340. doi:10.1155/2016/6127340.

19.

CASE 14: POSTURAL TACHYCARDIA SYNDROME WITH HYPERMOBILE EHLERS-DANLOS SYNDROME

Chief complaint: Dizziness.

Case presentation: A 33-year-old woman has a history of hypermobile Ehlers-Danlos syndrome associated with musculoskeletal problems, chronic pain, and recurrent syncope since childhood. The patient reports joint hypermobility dislocated hips and ribs. Syncope occurs upon standing up from lying or standing up too quickly. The pulse is sometimes too slow or too fast (>130 BPM). Over the past 5 years, her joint pain become worse in her hands and feet but also in spine, hips, and elbow. She has a history of a car accident and a blow to the head, but MRI was normal. She is no longer able to work as a photographer because she is tired, has hand pain, her eyes are not focusing, she sees double, her hands are shaky. These symptoms get worse in summer heat.

Past medical history: Ehlers-Danlos syndrome hypermobility type, posttraumatic stress disorder, gastroparesis, hypokalemia.

Current medication: None.

Assessment plan: Functional autonomic tests and skin biopsy for evaluation of small fiber neuropathy.

AUTONOMIC TESTING EVALUATION

See Table 19.1.

Heart rate: Supine heart rate was normal. Heart rate responses to deep breathing were reduced to 72.6% of normal value. Heart rate increment during the tilt (53 BPM) was exaggerated.

Blood pressure:

Valsalva maneuver: Mean blood pressure failed to return to baseline at the end of Phase 2 by 37.7 mm Hg (i.e., 46.9% of baseline).

Tilt: Supine blood pressure was normal. During the tilt, blood pressure remained stable until the onset of syncope at minute 5.

Sudomotor evaluation: Electrochemical skin conductance was abnormal (reduced to 26.2% of normal limit) at hands and abnormal (reduced to 48.3% of normal limit) at feet.

Respiratory system: Respiratory frequency was normal in supine position but was increased during the tilt. End tidal CO_2 was normal in supine position but was severely reduced during the tilt.

Cerebral blood flow velocity (CBFv): CBFv in middle cerebral artery was normal in supine position. CBFv in middle cerebral artery was moderately reduced during the tilt.

Skin biopsy (sensory-epidermal): Epidermal nerve fiber density was normal at proximal leg and abnormal (reduced to 39% of normal limit) at distal leg.

Skin biopsy (sweat glands): Sweat gland nerve fiber density was normal at distal leg.

TABLE 19.1 **RESULTS OF AUTONOMIC TESTING**

Blood pressure evaluation					
Test: Valsalva maneuver					
Pressure [mmHg]	Baseline	Phase 2			Phase 4
		Early	End		
Systolic	97	40	40		
Mean	71	33.3	33.3	n/a	
Diastolic	58	30	30	n/a	

Heart rate evaluation	
Test: Deep breathing	
Results	Norm*
8.71	≥12
Test: Valsalva ratio	
1.8	≥1.5
* adjusted for a gender and age	

(continued)

TABLE 19.1 **CONTINUED**

Test: Tilt test											
Position		HR [BPM]	Blood pressure [mmHg]		MCA Blood flow velocity [cm/s]				Respiratory frequency [breaths/min]	End tidal CO_2 [mmHg]
			Systolic	Diastolic	Systolic	Mean	Mean drop [%]	Diastolic		
Supine		87	107	78	98	67.3		52	13	39
Tilt [min]	1	120	120	90	89	62.3	7.4	49	23	35
	2	123	120	90						
	3	140	118	90						
	4	140	70	50	94	66.7	0.9	53	24	23
	5									
	6									
	7									
	8									
	9									
	10									
	15									
	20									
	30									
	40									

Sudomotor evaluation - functional

Test: Quantitative sudomotor axon reflex test (QSART)				
Location	Site (l/r)	Latency [min]	Volume [µl]	Norm [µl]*
Forearm				≥0.08
Prox. leg				≥0.14
Distal leg				≥0.15
Foot				≥0.07

* Normative data are adjusted for gender and age of patient.

Test: Electrochemical skin conductance (ESC)				
Location	Left [µS]	Right [µS]	Average [µS/k]	Norm [µS/kg]
Hand	20	25	0.27	≥1.03
Feet	47	44	0.54	≥1.14
Forehead				

For grading uses ESC [µS] adjusted for weight [µS/k].

TABLE 19.1 CONTINUED

Small fiber (sensory + sudomotor) evaluation - morphological					
Test: Skin biopsy					
Location	Site (l/r)	Nerve fibers			
		Epidermal*		Sweat glands	
		Density	Norm	Density	Norm
Proximal leg – thigh	Right	9.22	≥8.3		≥37.8
Distal leg - calf	Right	3.24	≥8.3	38	≥36.5
Foot	Right		≥3.11		≥34.8

* Normative data for distal leg are adjusted for gender and age of patient.

QASAT*										
Heart rate		**BP**		**CBFv**		**ET-CO2**		**Sudomotor**		**Total QASAT score**
S. bradycardia	0	Low supine	0	Low supine	0	Low supine	0	QSART		
S. tachycardia	0	High supine	0	High supine	0	High supine	0	ESC	3	
Increase tilt		OH		Tilt response		Tilt low				
Decrease tilt		OHTN		CA	0	Tilt high		**Skin biopsy**		10
Deep breathing	1	VM	3	CVR	0			Epidermal	3	
VR	0			VM	0			Sweat gland	0	
Total	1	Total	3	Total	0	Total	0			

*QASAT. See Novak. Quantitative Scale for Grading of Cardiovascular Autonomic Reflex Tests and Small Fibers from Skin Biopsies. *J Neurol Disord* 2015;3:2. Orthostatic (tilt) responses were not graded since QASAT requires the duration of the tilt at least 10 minutes.

S, supine; Increase tilt, increased response to tilt; Decrease tilt, decreased response to tilt; BP, blood pressure; VM, Valsalva maneuver; CBFv, cerebral blood flow velocity; CA, cerebral autoregulation; MCA, middle cerebral artery; VR, Valsalva ratio; CVR, cerebral vasoreactivity.

Patient-reported symptoms during testing: Dizziness during the tilt.

Patient-reported symptoms for past 2 weeks:

Lightheadedness or dizziness: Occasionally
Dry eyes or mouth: Often
Pale feet: Occasionally
Cold feet: Occasionally
Reduced sweating: None
Reduced sweating after exercise: None
Increased sweating: None
Nausea: Occasionally
Diarrhea: None
Constipation: None
Urinary leaks: Occasionally, minor
Current pain severity: 0
Aching pain: Often, moderate
Allodynia: Occasionally, mild
Burning pain: Often, severe
Lancinating pain: Occasionally, moderate
Numbness: Occasionally, moderate
Prickling sensation: Occasionally, moderate

AUTONOMIC TESTING INTERPRETATION

- Postural tachycardia syndrome (POTS), neuropathic form (Figure 19.1).
- Syncope, neurally mediated, vasodepressor.
- Small fiber neuropathy, length-dependent, affecting predominantly sensory fibers.
- Generalized autonomic failure, mild, affecting all major branches of autonomic nervous system (parasympathetic, adrenergic, and sudomotor).
- Orthostatic CBFv was reduced at the time of syncope. The compensatory cerebral vasodilation and vasoconstriction has been preserved.

COMMENT

The patient's symptoms were reproduced during the tilt test (Figure 19.1). Her autonomic testing revealed generalized autonomic failure, with small fiber neuropathy that is likely

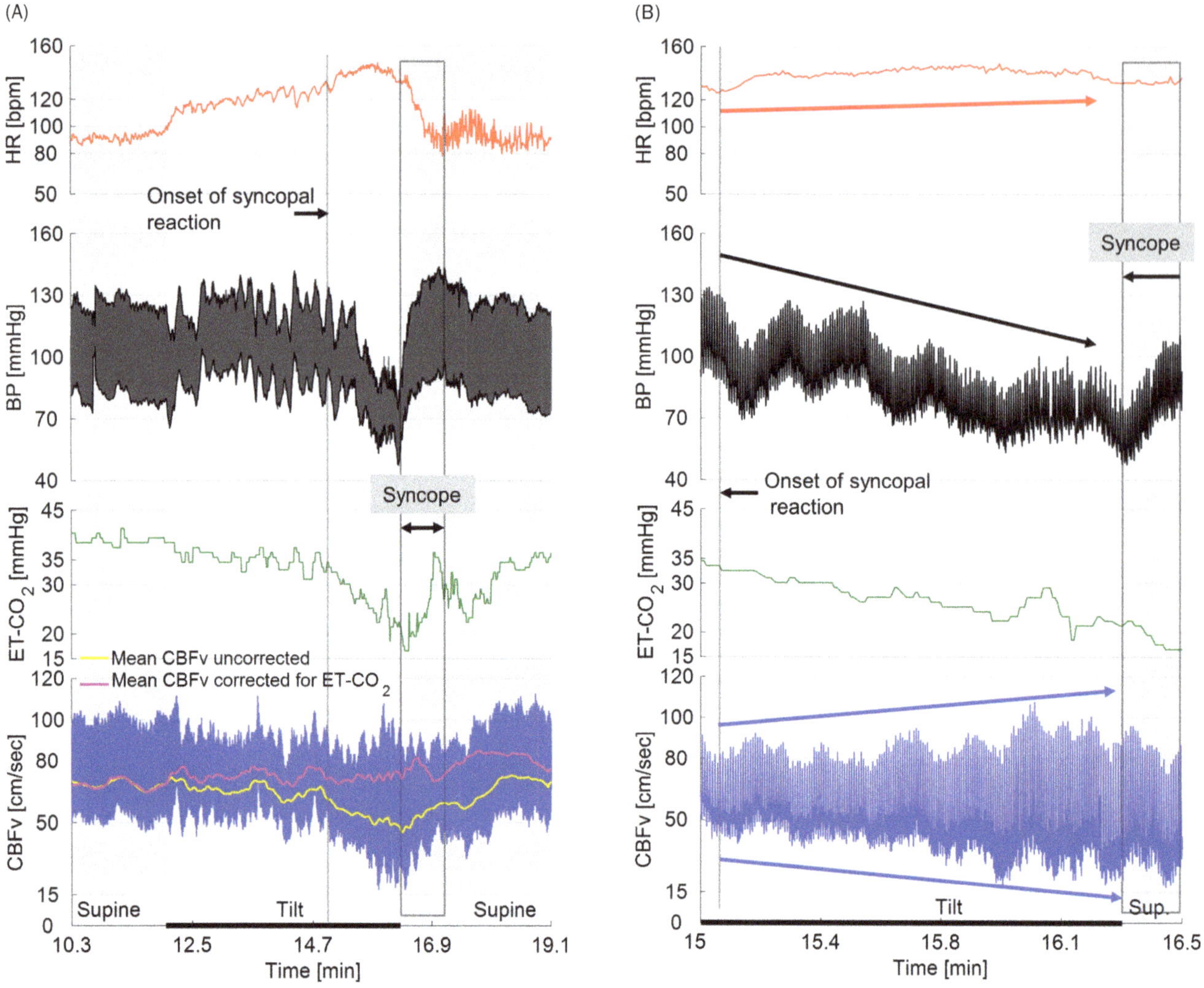

Figure 19.1 The tilt test provoked dizziness, tachycardia, and vasodepressor syncope (A, B). Heart rate progressively increased from the beginning of tilt until >120 BPM at the onset of syncope. With the onset of syncopal reaction (B), there was a progressive decline in heart rate, blood pressure, end tidal CO_2, and diastolic cerebral blood flow velocity (CBFv) until the patient lost consciousness. Cerebral vasodilation pattern (reduced diastolic signal with increase of systolic CBFv) was present during vasodepressor syncope.

to be the underlying mechanisms of orthostatic intolerance and syncope.

Hypermobile Ehlers-Danlos syndrome is relatively common hereditary disorder affecting connective tissue. It is associated with musculoskeletal complaints including joint hypermobility and joint subluxations/dislocations, as well as skin and soft tissue manifestations. Dysautonomia is common in hypermobile Ehlers-Danlos syndrome and includes tachycardia, syncope, dizziness, sudomotor, and gastrointestinal dysfunction as a well as more generalized manifestations including chronic fatigue, sleep disorders, and anxiety.[1–3]

TREATMENT AND FOLLOW-UP

- Volume expansion through high fluid and high salt intake, trial of β-blockers.
- Physical therapy.

CAVEATS

- POTS, syncope, and small fiber neuropathy are associated with hypermobile Ehlers-Danlos syndrome.

REFERENCES

1. Mathias CJ, Low DA, Iodice V, Owens AP, Kirbis M, Grahame R. Postural tachycardia syndrome--current experience and concepts. *Nat Rev Neurol*. 2011;8(1):22–34. doi:10.1038/nrneurol.2011.187.
2. Grigoriou E, Boris JR, Dormans JP. Postural orthostatic tachycardia syndrome (POTS): association with Ehlers-Danlos syndrome and orthopaedic considerations. *Clin Orthop*. 2015;473(2):722–728. doi:10.1007/s11999-014-3898-x.
3. Tinkle B, Castori M, Berglund B, et al. Hypermobile Ehlers-Danlos syndrome (a.k.a. Ehlers-Danlos syndrome Type III and Ehlers-Danlos syndrome hypermobility type): Clinical description and natural history. *Am J Med Genet C Semin Med Genet*. 2017;175(1):48–69. doi:10.1002/ajmg.c.31538.

20.

CASE 15: POSTURAL TACHYCARDIA SYNDROME WITH HYPERVENTILATION AND PRESYNCOPE

Chief complaint: Dizziness.

Case presentation: A 36-year-old woman presents with numerous symptoms since high school (e.g., intermittent chest pain, inner tremor, visual changes [seeing colors when standing up quickly], cramps, pelvic and leg pain, shortness of breath, and fatigue). She has fallen or passed out several times. Extensive neurologic, psychiatric, and cardiologic evaluation was unrevealing. Holter monitoring recorded several periods of sinus tachycardia, but no events were triggered. Neurologic examination was normal except for orthostatic intolerance on active standing. Patient was referred for evaluation of suspected postural tachycardia syndrome (POTS).

Past medical history: Anxiety, migraine.

Current medication: Ibuprofen.

Assessment plan: Functional autonomic tests and skin biopsy.

AUTONOMIC TESTING EVALUATION

See Table 20.1.

Heart rate: Supine heart rate was normal. Heart rate responses to deep breathing were normal. Heart rate increment during the tilt (63 BPM) was exaggerated and exceeded 150 BPM.

Blood pressure:

Valsalva maneuver: Blood pressure responses were normal.

Tilt: Supine blood pressure was normal. Blood pressure was stable during the first 3 minutes of the tilt. Then a progressive decline in blood pressure started and continued until the patient became anxious, disoriented, and asked to terminate the tilt test.

Sudomotor evaluation: Sweat output was normal at forearm, normal at proximal leg, normal at distal leg, and normal at foot. QSART showed length-dependent pattern with a decrease of sweat output distally of at least 33%.

Respiratory system: Respiratory frequency was normal in supine position and during the tilt. End tidal CO_2 was normal in supine position but was severely reduced during the tilt.

Cerebral blood flow velocity (CBFv): CBFv in middle cerebral artery was normal in supine position but was severely reduced during the tilt.

Skin biopsy (sensory-epidermal): Epidermal nerve fiber density was normal at proximal leg and normal at distal leg.

Skin biopsy (sweat glands): Sweat gland nerve fiber density was normal at distal leg.

TABLE 20.1 RESULTS OF AUTONOMIC TESTING

Blood pressure evaluation					
Test: Valsalva maneuver					
Pressure [mmHg]	Baseline	Phase 2			Phase 4
		Early	End		
Systolic	119	97	121		
Mean	89	83	103.7	n/a	
Diastolic	74	76	95	n/a	

Heart rate evaluation	
Test: Deep breathing	
Results	Norm*
12.1	≥12
Test: Valsalva ratio	
1.63	≥1.5
* adjusted for a gender and age	

(continued)

TABLE 20.1 **CONTINUED**

Test: Tilt test										
Position		HR [BPM]	Blood pressure [mmHg]		MCA Blood flow velocity [cm/s]				Respiratory frequency [breaths/min]	End tidal CO_2 [mmHg]
			Systolic	Diastolic	Systolic	Mean	Mean drop [%]	Diastolic		
Supine		93	106	73	95	58.3		40	9	35
Tilt [min]	1	150	112	67	94	56.7	2.7	38	14	22
	2	150	105	61						
	3	154	106	66						
	4	156	62	49	97	42.3	27.4	15	14	21
	5									
	6									
	7									
	8									
	9									
	10									
	15									
	20									
	30									
	40									

Sudomotor evaluation - functional

Test: Quantitative sudomotor axon reflex test (QSART)				
Location	Site (l/r)	Latency [min]	Volume [µl]	Norm [µl]*
Forearm	l	1.34	0.405	≥0.08
Prox. leg	l	0.18	0.617	≥0.14
Distal leg	l	0.47	0.617	≥0.15
Foot	l	1.22	0.159	≥0.07

* Normative data are adjusted for gender and age of patient.

Location	Left [µS]	Right [µS]	Average [µS/k]	Norm [µS/kg]
Hand				≥1.03
Feet				≥1.14
Forehead				

For grading uses ESC [µS] adjusted for weight [µS/k].

TABLE 20.1 CONTINUED

Small fiber (sensory + sudomotor) evaluation - morphological					
Test: Skin biopsy					
Location	Site (l/r)	Nerve fibers			
		Epidermal*		Sweat glands	
		Density	Norm	Density	Norm
Proximal leg – thigh	Right	14.64	≥8.3		≥37.8
Distal leg - calf	Right	12.36	≥8.22	38.3	≥36.5
Foot	Right		≥3.11		≥34.8

* Normative data for distal leg are adjusted for gender and age of patient.

QASAT*												
Heart rate		**BP**		**CBFv**		**ET-CO2**		**Sudomotor**			**Total QASAT score**
S. bradycardia	0	Low supine	0	Low supine	0	Low supine	0	QSART	1		
S. tachycardia	0	High supine	0	High supine	0	High supine	0	ESC			
Increase tilt		OH		Tilt response		Tilt low					
Decrease tilt		OHTN		CA	0	Tilt high		**Skin biopsy**			1
Deep breathing	0	VM	0	CVR	0			Epidermal	0		
VR	0			VM	0			Sweat gland	0		
Total	0	Total	0	Total	0	Total	0				

*QASAT. See Novak. Quantitative Scale for Grading of Cardiovascular Autonomic Reflex Tests and Small Fibers from Skin Biopsies. *J Neurol Disord* 2015;3:2. Orthostatic (tilt) responses were not graded since QASAT requires the duration of the tilt at least 10 minutes.

S, supine; Increase tilt, increased response to tilt; Decrease tilt, decreased response to tilt; BP, blood pressure; VM, Valsalva maneuver; CBFv, cerebral blood flow velocity; CA, cerebral autoregulation; MCA, middle cerebral artery; VR, Valsalva ratio; CVR, cerebral vasoreactivity.

Patient-reported symptoms during testing: Syncope, dizziness, nausea during the tilt.

Patient-reported symptoms for past 2 weeks:

Lightheadedness or dizziness: Occasionally
Dry eyes or mouth: None
Pale feet: None
Cold feet: often
Reduced sweating: None
Reduced sweating after exercise: None
Increased sweating: None
Nausea: None
Diarrhea: None
Constipation: None
Urinary leaks: None
Current pain severity: 0
Aching pain: None
Allodynia: None
Burning pain: None
Lancinating pain: None
Numbness: None
Prickling sensation: Occasionally, mild

AUTONOMIC TESTING INTERPRETATION

- POTS, severe.
- Presyncope, neurally mediated, mixed.
- Severe hypocapnic hyperventilation.

COMMENT

Tilt test showed POTS associated with hypocapnic hyperventilation and low cerebral blood flow velocity which culminated in presyncope (Figure 20.1). Hypocapnia, which is commonly seen in POTS, induces cerebral vasoconstriction and reduces CBFv.[1] Hypocapnia can reduce peripheral resistance, but it is unlikely to be the sole cause of presyncope or syncope. The progressive decline in blood pressure was likely due to decreased cardiac output due hypovolemia potentiated by hypocapnia.

TREATMENT AND FOLLOW-UP

- Further evaluation was directed to assess the type of POTS. A neuropathic form has been ruled out by skin biopsy for assessment of small fibers, which was normal although it can be argued that the length dependent pattern as shown by QSART can be seen in early or minimal small fiber neuropathy (Table 20.1). The autoimmune form of POTS is unlikely since neuronal antibodies, including ganglionic acetylcholine receptor antibodies, were absent. Supine serum norepinephrine level was slightly elevated (820 pg/mL; normal range 70–720 pg/mL), but an increase in standing norepinephrine was normal (1,081 pg/mL; normal range 200–1,700 pg/mL).
- Patient was treated with a combination of volume expansion through high fluid and high salt intake, strenuous exercise, and a combination of pyridostigmine and low-dose metoprolol. Within a year, her functioning improved to the point that she only had mild and intermittent symptoms.

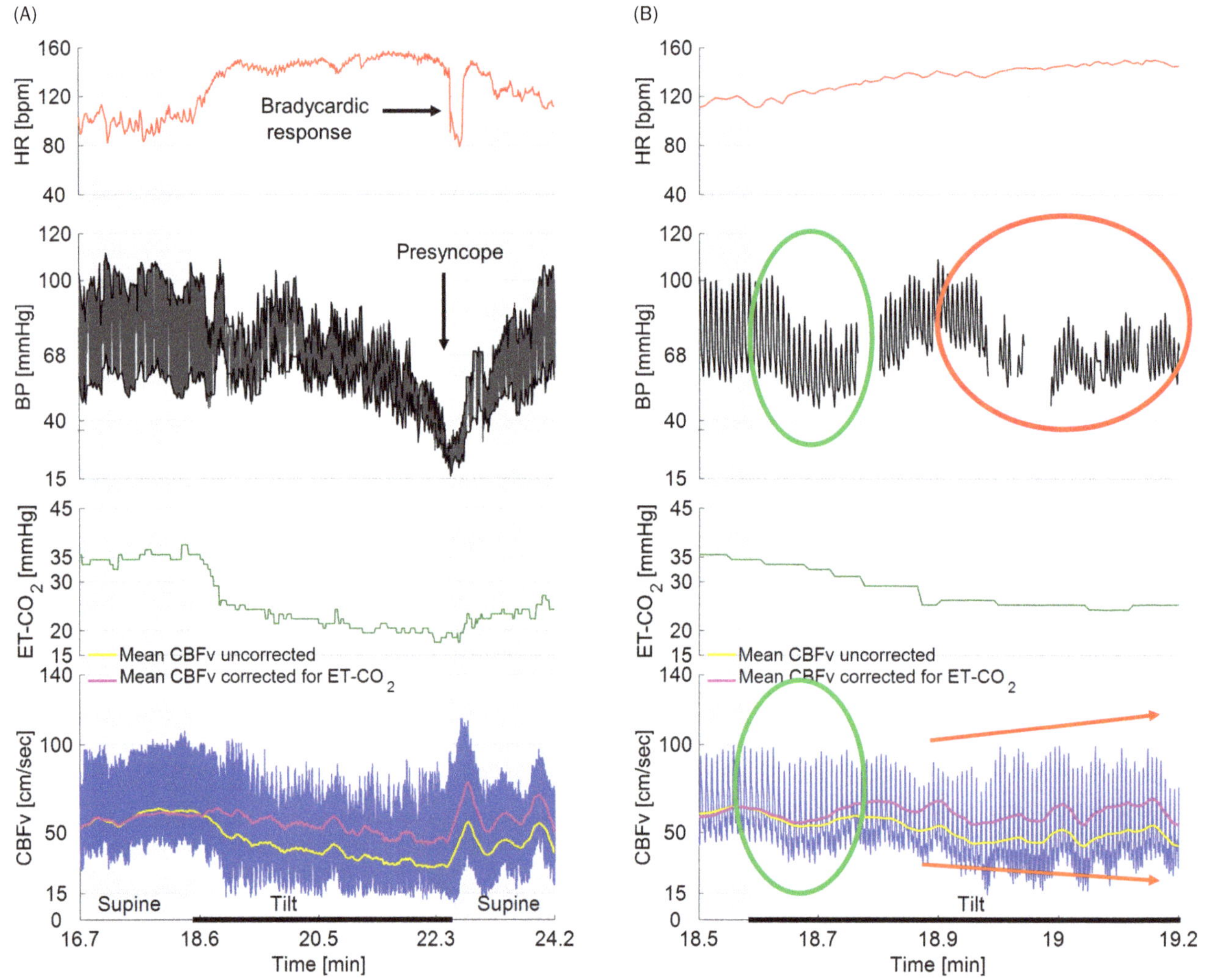

Figure 20.1 The patient became dizzy and anxious at the beginning of the tilt, which was associated with severe tachycardia (heart rate >150 BPM) and hypocapnic hyperventilation (end tidal CO_2. <26 mm Hg) (A, B). The initial decline in blood pressure (*green oval*) recovered (B). However, the second decline in blood pressure (*red oval*) recovered only partially (C). Patient became progressively dizzier, anxious, nauseated, and experienced chest pain and became confused and agitated at minute 3 of the tilt. These symptoms were associated with a progressive decline in blood pressure, end tidal CO_2, and mean cerebral blood flow velocity (CBFv). The widening of the Doppler signal (*red arrows*) indicates compensatory cerebral vasodilation. There was a sudden bradycardic response at minute 3 of the tilt (decline in heart rate from 144 to 82 BPM). The tilt was terminated at minute 4 per patient's request when she became restless and short of breath. Patient never completely lost consciousness. Recordings of blood pressure were interrupted by a calibration signal which has been deleted (C).

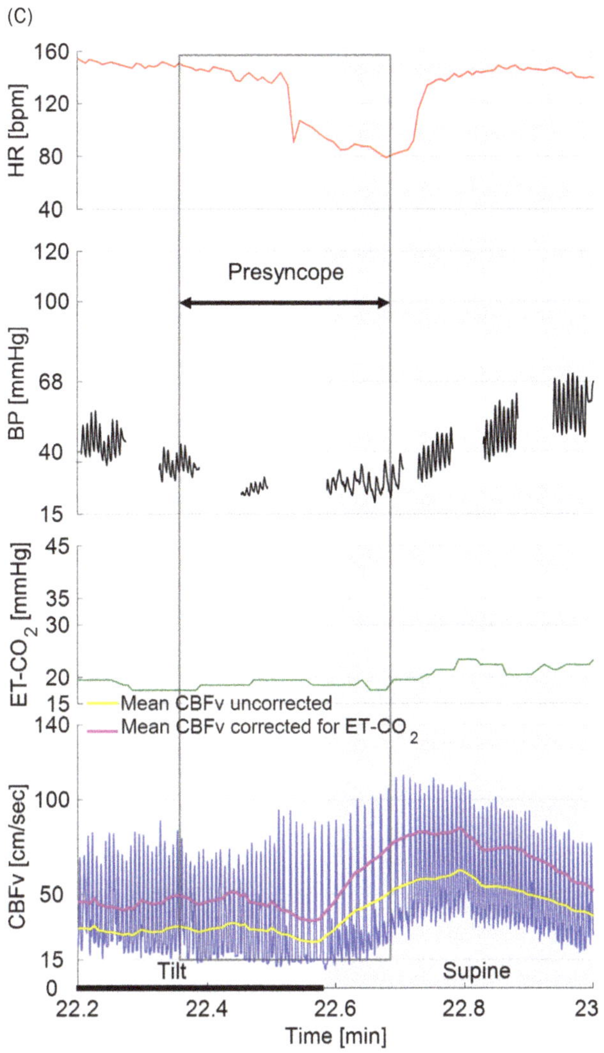

Figure 20.1 Continued

CAVEATS

- POTS without evidence of autoimmunity or neuropathy has good prognosis.
- Early blood pressure decline at the beginning of tilt may provide early warning of impending syncope or other abnormalities during the tilt.[2]
- The finger cuff device overestimated the decline in blood pressure here since this patient never lost consciousness and CBFv was maintained with active autoregulation; thus, the decline did not trigger loss of consciousness.
- Hypocapnic hyperventilation is a common occurrence in POTS.

REFERENCES

1. Novak V, Spies JM, Novak P, McPhee BR, Rummans TA, Low PA. Hypocapnia and cerebral hypoperfusion in orthostatic intolerance. *Stroke*. 1998;29(9):1876–1881.
2. Novak V, Novak P, Opfer-Gehrking TL, O'Brien PC, Low PA. Clinical and laboratory indices that enhance the diagnosis of postural tachycardia syndrome. *Mayo Clin Proc*. 1998;73(12):1141–1150. doi:10.4065/73.12.1141.

21.

CASE 16: AUTONOMIC FAILURE OR POSTURAL TACHYCARDIA SYNDROME?

Chief complaint: Palpitations and dizziness.

Case presentation: A 45-year-old woman presents with orthostatic dizziness, flushing, and palpitations for 7 years. She was treated with β-blockers without improvement. Patient was referred for differential diagnosis of postural tachycardia syndrome (POTS) versus autonomic failure.

Past medical history: Anxiety, mitral valve prolapse, POTS.

Current medication: None.

Plan of testing: Autonomic testing and skin biopsy to evaluate for neuropathic form of POTS.

AUTONOMIC TESTING EVALUATION

See Table 21.1.

Heart rate: Supine heart rate was normal. Heart rate responses to deep breathing were normal. Heart rate increment during the tilt (40 BPM) was exaggerated and exceeded 120 BPM.

Blood pressure:

Valsalva maneuver: Mean blood pressure failed to return to baseline at the end of Phase 2 by 3 mm Hg (i.e., 96.1% of baseline).

Tilt: Supine blood pressure was normal. Blood pressure responses to tilt were abnormal and consistent with mild orthostatic hypotension.

Sudomotor evaluation: Electrochemical skin conductance was normal at hands and abnormal (reduced to 99.1% of normal limit) at feet.

Respiratory system: Respiratory frequency was normal in supine position and during the tilt. End tidal CO_2 was reduced in supine position and during the tilt.

Cerebral blood flow velocity (CBFv): CBFv in middle cerebral artery was normal in supine position but was mildly reduced during the tilt.

Skin biopsy (sensory-epidermal): Epidermal nerve fiber density was abnormal (reduced to 59.8% of normal limit) at proximal leg and abnormal (reduced to 20.1% of normal limit) at distal leg.

Skin biopsy (sweat glands): Sweat gland nerve fiber density was abnormal (reduced to 14.8% of normal limit) at distal leg.

Patient-reported symptoms during testing: Dizziness during the tilt.

Patient-reported symptoms for past 2 weeks:

Lightheadedness or dizziness: Often
Dry eyes or mouth: Often
Pale feet: Occasionally
Cold feet: Often
Reduced sweating: None
Reduced sweating after exercise: None
Increased sweating: Occasionally
Nausea: Often

TABLE 21.1 RESULTS OF AUTONOMIC TESTING

Blood pressure evaluation					
Test: Valsalva maneuver					
Pressure [mmHg]	Baseline	Phase 2			Phase 4
		Early	End		
Systolic	108	97	97		
Mean	77.3	74.3	74.3	n/a	
Diastolic	62	63	63	n/a	

Heart rate evaluation	
Test: Deep breathing	
Results	Norm*
15.6	≥14
Test: Valsalva ratio	
1.7	≥1.46
* adjusted for a gender and age	

TABLE 21.1 CONTINUED

Test: Tilt test										
Position		HR [BPM]	Blood pressure [mmHg]		MCA Blood flow velocity [cm/s]				Respiratory frequency [breaths/min]	End tidal CO_2 [mmHg]
			Systolic	Diastolic	Systolic	Mean	Mean drop [%]	Diastolic		
Supine		87	119	78	91	61.7		47	11	34
Tilt [min]	1	121	108	74	83	56.3	8.8	43	12	32
	2	122	133	89						
	3	125	133	89						
	4	120	104	72						
	5	127	106	75	77	49	20.6	35	12	33
	6	125	128	83						
	7	125	107	70						
	8	123	101	67						
	9	121	110	74						
	10	120	95	64	74	48.7	21.1	36	15	31
	15									
	20									
	30									
	40									

Sudomotor evaluation - functional

Test: Quantitative sudomotor axon reflex test (QSART)				
Location	Site (l/r)	Latency [min]	Volume [µl]	Norm [µl]*
Forearm				≥0.08
Prox. leg				≥0.14
Distal leg				≥0.24
Foot				≥0.09

* Normative data are adjusted for gender and age of patient.

Test: Electrochemical skin conductance (ESC)				
Location	Left [µS]	Right [µS]	Average [µS/k]	Norm [µS/kg]
Hand	81	83	1.14	≥1.03
Feet	86	76	1.06	≥1.14
Forehead				

For grading uses ESC [µS] adjusted for weight [µS/k].

(continued)

TABLE 21.1 **CONTINUED**

Small fiber (sensory + sudomotor) evaluation - morphological					
Test: Skin biopsy					
Location	Site (l/r)	Nerve fibers			
		Epidermal*		Sweat glands	
		Density	Norm	Density	Norm
Proximal leg – thigh	Right	4.96	≥8.3		≥37.8
Distal leg - calf	Right	1.8	≥8.94	5.4	≥36.5
Foot	Right		≥3.11		≥34.8

* Normative data for distal leg are adjusted for gender and age of patient.

Heart rate		**BP**		**CBFv**		**ET-CO2**		**Sudomotor**			**Total QASAT score**
S. bradycardia	0	Low supine	0	Low supine	0	Low supine	1	QSART			
S. tachycardia	0	High supine	0	High supine	0	High supine	0	ESC	1		
Increase tilt	10	OH	1	Tilt response	2	Tilt low	1				
Decrease tilt	0	OHTN	0	CA	0	Tilt high	0	**Skin biopsy**			24
Deep breathing	0	VM	1	CVR	0			Epidermal	3		
VR	0			VM	0			Sweat gland	4		
Total	10	Total	2	Total	2	Total	2				

QASAT*

*QASAT. See Novak. Quantitative Scale for Grading of Cardiovascular Autonomic Reflex Tests and Small Fibers from Skin Biopsies. *J Neurol Disord* 2015;3:2.

S, supine; Increase tilt, increased response to tilt; Decrease tilt, decreased response to tilt; BP, blood pressure; VM, Valsalva maneuver; CBFv, cerebral blood flow velocity; CA, cerebral autoregulation; MCA, middle cerebral artery; VR, Valsalva ratio; CVR, cerebral vasoreactivity.

Diarrhea: Occasionally
Constipation: Often
Urinary leaks: None
Current pain severity: 4
Aching pain: Often, moderate
Allodynia: None
Burning pain: Occasionally, mild
Lancinating pain: Occasionally, moderate
Numbness: None
Prickling sensation: Occasionally, moderate

AUTONOMIC TESTING INTERPRETATION

- Small fiber neuropathy (SFN), severe, mixed, length-dependent, affecting sensory and autonomic fibers, biopsy proven.
- Sympathetic adrenergic failure due to SFN.
- Anxiety.
- Mildly reduced mean orthostatic CBFv due to hypocapnia-induced vasoconstriction.
- Cerebral autoregulatory failure.

COMMENT

Patient was anxious during the testing. During supine baseline, there was a characteristic anxiety reaction[1] consisting of transient elevation of heart rate, blood pressure, and CBFv (Figure 21.1B, green circles). Patient complained of dizziness twice during the tilt—at the onset and at the end. In both cases, the CBFv was reduced (dark gray circles). The first drop was due to a transient drop of CBFv.

The second drop was due combination of hypocapnia and orthostatic hypotension. It can be argued that this patient has POTS since the heart rate response to tilt was excessive. However, the abnormal Valsalva maneuver and orthostatic hypotension during the tilt indicate adrenergic failure. The excessive heart rate response to tilt is probably a compensatory response. The correct interpretation is adrenergic autonomic failure and not POTS. The entire drop in CBFv was due to hypocapnia and not due orthostatic hypotension, as the CBFv adjusted for the effect of end tidal CO_2 was stable during the tilt. Marked oscillations of blood pressure can be seen in adrenergic failure. Marked oscillations of CBFv (Figure 21.1D) can be seen in cerebral autoregulatory failure.

TREATMENT AND FOLLOW-UP

- Clinical workup for small fiber neuropathy.

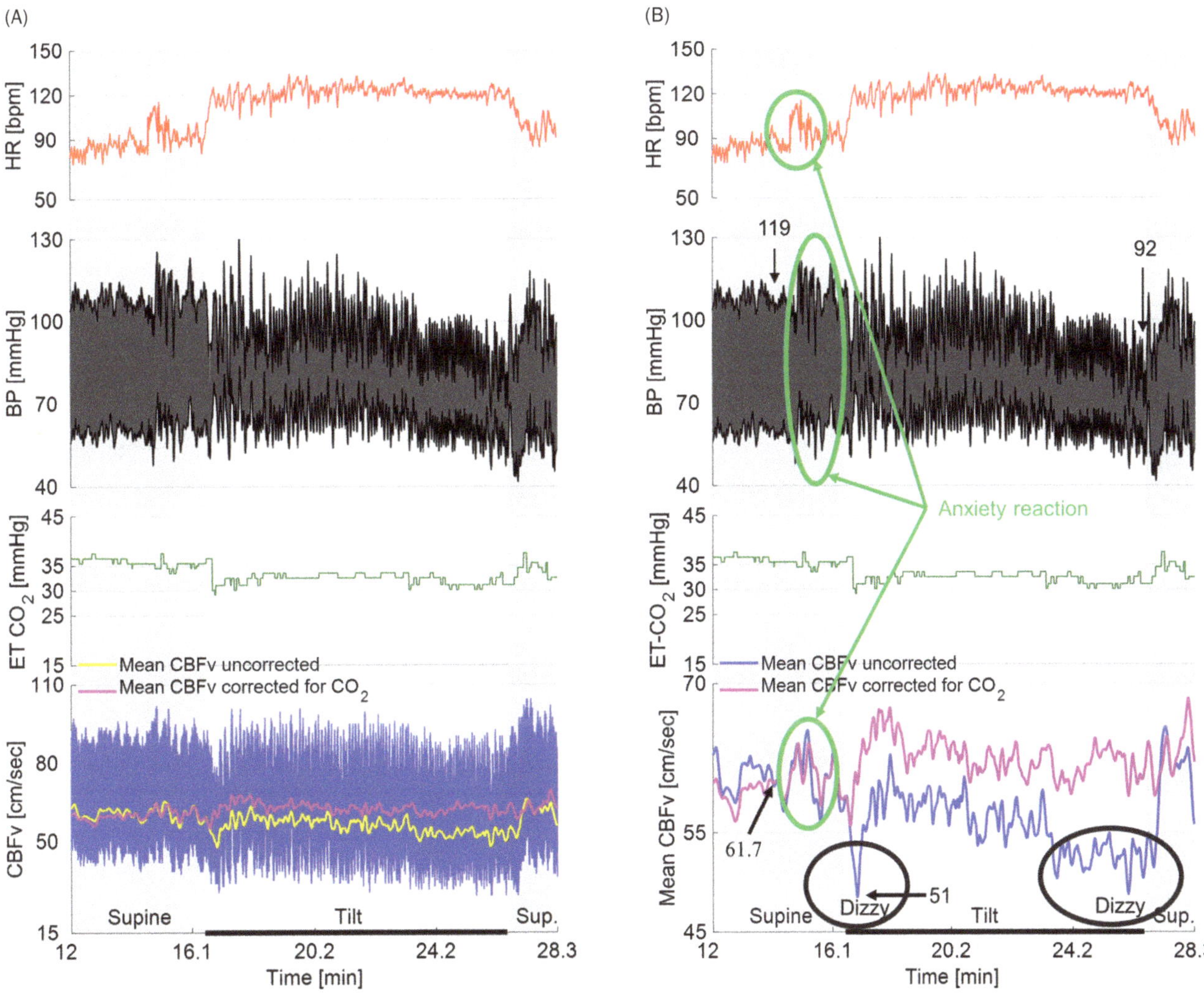

Figure 21.1 Heart rate increment to tilt was exaggerated. Supine systolic blood pressure (119 mm Hg) was normal but declined to 92 mm Hg at the end of the tilt, which is consistent with orthostatic hypotension. Patient felt anxious in supine position, and data (heart rate and blood pressure increase) were consistent with anxiety reaction (*green oval*, B). She became dizzy at the onset of the tilt, which was associated with decline in cerebral blood flow velocity (CBFv) by 17% (from 61.7 to 51 cm/s) and then at the second half of the tilt (B). There were prominent blood pressure and CBFv oscillations (C, D).

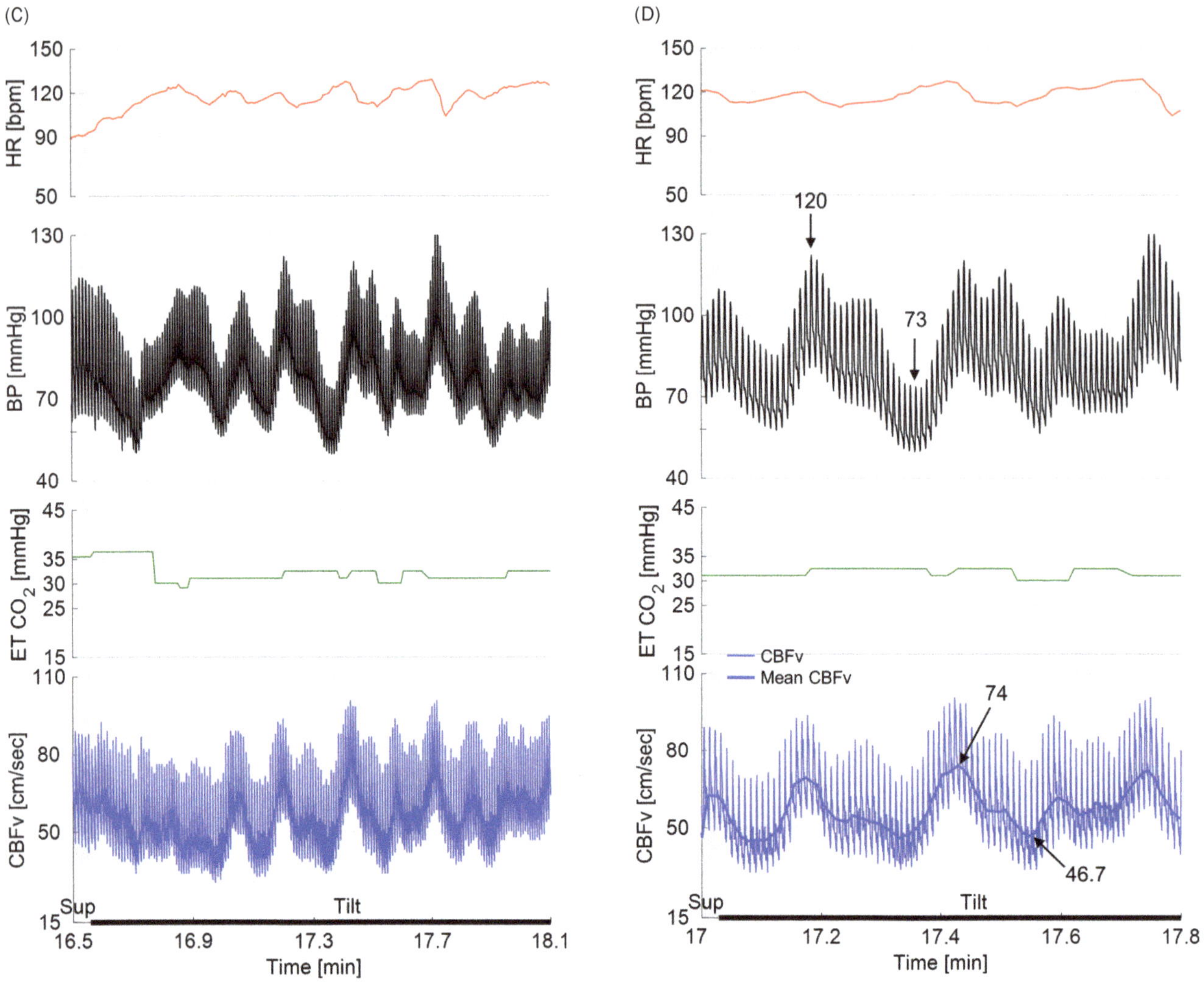

Figure 21.1 Continued

- Volume expansion through high fluid and high salt intake. Patient would also benefit from using the pressor medication.
- Anxiety is common and occasionally can be identified as transient elevation of heart rate, blood pressure, and CBFv.

CAVEATS

- Small fiber neuropathy is associated with adrenergic failure.[1]

REFERENCE

1. Novak P. Cerebral blood flow, heart rate, and blood pressure patterns during the tilt test in common orthostatic syndromes. *Neurosci J.* 2016;2016:6127340. doi:10.1155/2016/6127340.

22.

CASE 17: PAROXYSMAL DIZZINESS IN POSTURAL TACHYCARDIA SYNDROME

Chief complaint: Paroxysmal dizziness.

Case presentation: A 25-year-old woman presents with unexplained, intermittent, usually short (seconds to minutes) orthostatic dizziness for 4 years. She was diagnosed with postural tachycardia syndrome (POTS) but responded poorly to propranolol. She was also suspected of having seizure disorder. She was referred for confirmation of the POTS diagnosis.

Past medical history: POTS, Lyme disease, depression, question of seizure disorder.

Current medication: Lamotrigine, oxcarbazepine.

Assessment plan: Functional autonomic tests and skin biopsy.

AUTONOMIC TESTING EVALUATION

See Table 22.1.

Heart rate: Supine heart rate was normal. Heart rate responses to deep breathing were normal. Heart rate increment during the tilt (40 BPM) was exaggerated.

Blood pressure:

Valsalva maneuver: Mean blood pressure failed to return to baseline at the end of Phase 2 by 13.3 mm Hg (i.e., 83.4% of baseline).

Tilt: Supine blood pressure was normal. Blood pressure responses to tilt were normal.

Sudomotor evaluation: Electrochemical skin conductance was normal at hands and normal at feet.

Respiratory system: Respiratory frequency was normal in supine position but was increased during the tilt. End tidal CO_2 was reduced in supine position and intermittently during the tilt.

Cerebral blood flow velocity (CBFv): CBFv in middle cerebral artery was normal in supine position and was intermittently reduced during the tilt.

Skin biopsy (sensory-epidermal): Epidermal nerve fiber density was normal at proximal leg and normal at distal leg.

Skin biopsy (sweat glands): Sweat gland nerve fiber density was normal at distal leg.

Patient-reported symptoms during testing: Dizziness during the tilt.

Patient-reported symptoms for past 2 weeks:

Lightheadedness or dizziness: Occasionally
Dry eyes or mouth: Occasionally
Pale feet: None
Cold feet: Occasionally
Reduced sweating: Occasionally
Reduced sweating after exercise: Occasionally
Increased sweating: None
Nausea: Occasionally
Diarrhea: Occasionally

TABLE 22.1 **RESULTS OF AUTONOMIC TESTING**

Blood pressure evaluation					
Test: Valsalva maneuver					
Pressure [mmHg]	Baseline	Phase 2			Phase 4
		Early	End		
Systolic	112	80	80		
Mean	80	66.7	66.7	n/a	
Diastolic	64	60	60	n/a	

Heart rate evaluation	
Test: Deep breathing	
Results	Norm*
31.6	≥14
Test: Valsalva ratio	
1.97	≥1.46
* adjusted for a gender and age	

(continued)

TABLE 22.1 **CONTINUED**

Test: Tilt test										
Position		HR [BPM]	Blood pressure [mmHg]		MCA Blood flow velocity [cm/s]				Respiratory frequency [breaths/min]	End tidal CO_2 [mmHg]
			Systolic	Diastolic	Systolic	Mean	Mean drop [%]	Diastolic		
Supine		89	102	68	109	67.7		47	20	32
Tilt [min]	1	115	107	65	103	66.3	2.1	48	21	31
	2	113	106	71						
	3	111	101	71						
	4	121	103	72						
	5	126	110	76	95	63	6.9	47	23	32
	6	123	106	73						
	7	122	106	74						
	8	121	101	71						
	9	129	104	73						
	10	125	108	76	96	60.7	10.3	43	23	31
	15									
	20									
	30									
	40									

Sudomotor evaluation - functional

Test: Quantitative sudomotor axon reflex test (QSART)				
Location	Site (l/r)	Latency [min]	Volume [µl]	Norm [µl]*
Forearm				≥0.08
Prox. leg				≥0.14
Distal leg				≥0.24
Foot				≥0.09

* Normative data are adjusted for gender and age of patient.

Test: Electrochemical skin conductance (ESC)				
Location	Left [µS]	Right [µS]	Average [µS/k]	Norm [µS/kg]
Hand	76	75	1.57	≥1.03
Feet	76	74	1.55	≥1.14
Forehead				

For grading uses ESC [µS] adjusted for weight [µS/k].

TABLE 22.1 **CONTINUED**

Small fiber (sensory + sudomotor) evaluation - morphological					
Test: Skin biopsy					
Location	Site (l/r)	Nerve fibers			
		Epidermal*		Sweat glands	
		Density	Norm	Density	Norm
Proximal leg – thigh	Right	14.25	≥8.3		≥37.8
Distal leg - calf	Right	10.97	≥9.1	40.6	≥36.5
Foot	Right		≥3.11		≥34.8

* Normative data for distal leg are adjusted for gender and age of patient.

QASAT*										
Heart rate		**BP**		**CBFv**		**ET-CO2**		**Sudomotor**		**Total QASAT score**
S. bradycardia	0	Low supine	0	Low supine	0	Low supine	1	QSART		
S. tachycardia	0	High supine	0	High supine	0	High supine	0	ESC	0	
Increase tilt	7	OH	0	Tilt response	0	Tilt low	2			
Decrease tilt	0	OHTN	0	CA	0	Tilt high	0	**Skin biopsy**		12
Deep breathing	0	VM	2	CVR	0			Epidermal	0	
VR	0			VM	0			Sweat gland	0	
Total	7	Total	2	Total	0	Total	3			

*QASAT. See Novak. Quantitative Scale for Grading of Cardiovascular Autonomic Reflex Tests and Small Fibers from Skin Biopsies. *J Neurol Disord* 2015;3:2.

S, supine; Increase tilt, increased response to tilt; Decrease tilt, decreased response to tilt; BP, blood pressure; VM, Valsalva maneuver; CBFv, cerebral blood flow velocity; CA, cerebral autoregulation; MCA, middle cerebral artery; VR, Valsalva ratio; CVR, cerebral vasoreactivity.

Constipation: Occasionally
Urinary leaks: None
Current pain severity: 7
Aching pain: Often, moderate
Allodynia: Often, moderate
Burning pain: Often, moderate
Lancinating pain: Often, moderate
Numbness: Occasionally, mild
Prickling sensation: Occasionally, mild

AUTONOMIC TESTING INTERPRETATION

- POTS

COMMENT

Patient complained of dizziness from the beginning of the tilt (Figure 22.1). This was associated with excessive heart rate increment, reduced CBFv, and hyperventilation. This pattern is typical for POTS.[1] The tilt reproduced a short lasting dizziness, but no syncope or presyncope. Sudden decrease of sympathetic tone with gasping may trigger transient decline in CBFv and dizziness.

TREATMENT AND FOLLOW-UP

- Volume expansion through high fluid and high salt intake

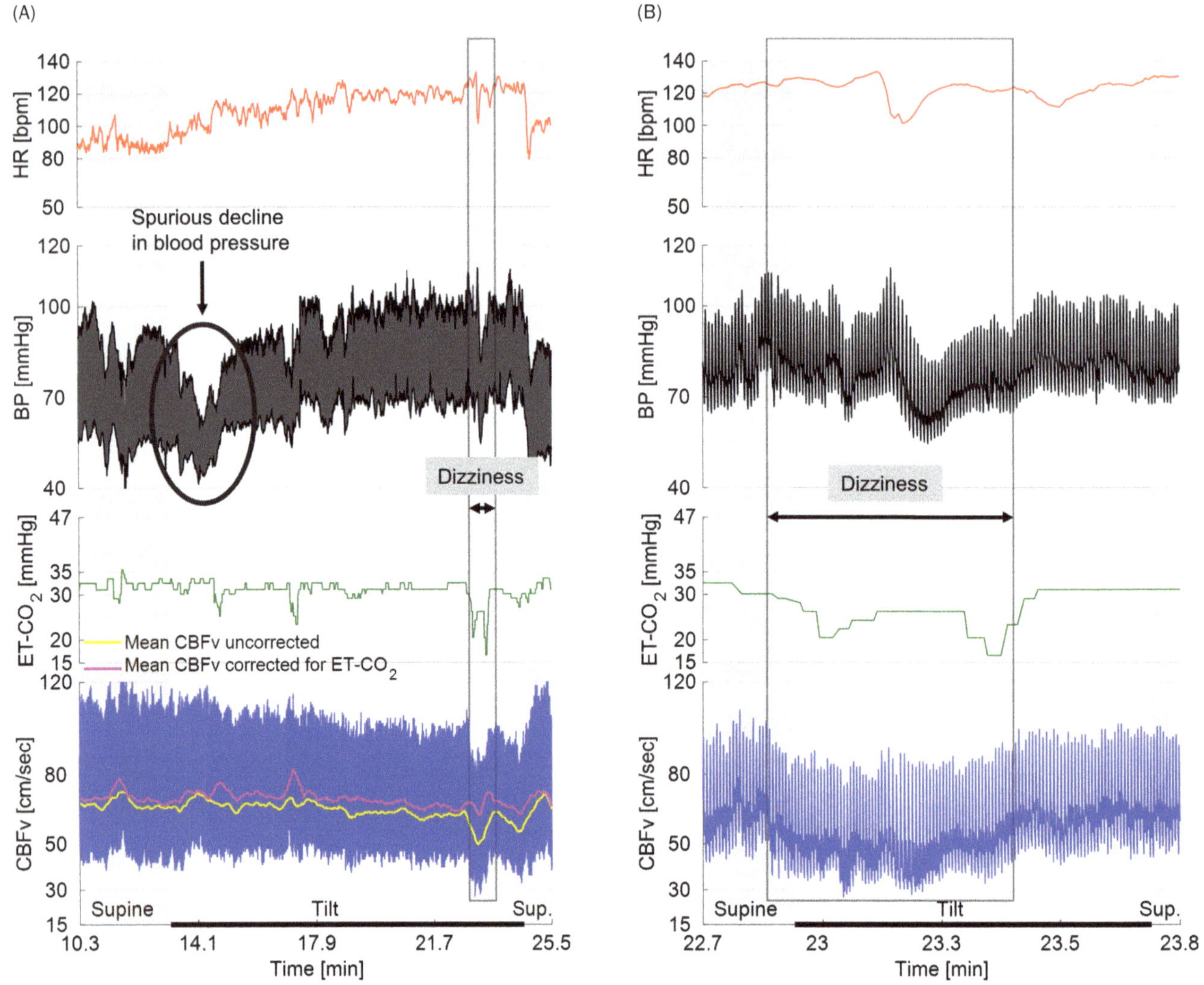

Figure 22.1 Heart rate increment to tilt exceeded 120 BPM. An initial blood pressure decline was an artifact of the finger cuff device. Cerebral blood flow velocity (CBFv) and CO_2 remained stable for most of the tilt. There was an acute onset of dizziness at the end of tilt (A, B) with concomitant decline of heart rate, blood pressure, CO_2, and CBFv, consistent with deep breaths.

CAVEATS

Paroxysmal dysautonomia can be responsible for transient dizziness and POTS.

REFERENCE

1. Low PA, Sandroni P, Joyner M, Shen W-K. Postural tachycardia syndrome (POTS). *J Cardiovasc Electrophysiol.* 2009;20(3):352–358. doi:10.1111/j.1540-8167.2008.01407.x.

CASE 18: POSTURAL TACHYCARDIA SYNDROME AND SMALL FIBER NEUROPATHY IN POLYCYSTIC OVARY SYNDROME

Chief complaint: Dizziness.

Case presentation: A 30-year-old woman has history of dizziness on standing since age 10 years. She had at least two episodes of syncope at the age of 13 and multiple presyncopal episodes associated with loss of vision and severe postural dizziness. A year ago, she began to experience diffuse pain and tingling in the feet that was attributed to fibromyalgia. She had a nerve conduction study that was normal.

Past medical history: Obesity, polycystic ovary syndrome (PCOS), hirsutism, alopecia.

Current medication: Topiramate, venlafaxine, linaclotide, spironolactone, metformin, liraglutide.

Assessment plan: Functional autonomic tests and skin biopsy.

AUTONOMIC TESTING EVALUATION

See Table 23.1.

Heart rate: Supine heart rate was normal. Heart rate responses to deep breathing were normal. Heart rate increment during the tilt (49 BPM) was exaggerated and exceeded 120 BPM (Figure 23.1).

Blood pressure:

Valsalva maneuver: Blood pressure responses were normal.

Tilt: Supine blood pressure was normal. Blood pressure responses to tilt were normal.

Sudomotor evaluation: Electrochemical skin conductance was abnormal (reduced to 64.1% of normal limit) at hands and abnormal (reduced to 63.6% of normal limit) at feet.

Respiratory system: Respiratory frequency was normal in supine position and during the tilt. End tidal CO_2 was reduced in supine position and during the tilt.

Cerebral blood flow velocity (CBFv): CBFv in middle cerebral artery was normal in supine position but was intermittently reduced during the tilt.

Skin biopsy (sensory-epidermal): Epidermal nerve fiber density was normal at proximal leg and abnormal (reduced to 18.4% of normal limit) at distal leg.

Skin biopsy (sweat glands): Sweat gland nerve fiber density was abnormal (reduced to 16.4% of normal limit) at distal leg.

Patient-reported symptoms during testing: Dizziness, shortness of breath, weakness, nausea, and tingling at feet during the tilt.

Patient-reported symptoms for past 2 weeks:

Lightheadedness or dizziness: Occasionally
Dry eyes or mouth: Often
Pale feet: Often

TABLE 23.1 **RESULTS OF AUTONOMIC TESTING**

Blood pressure evaluation					
Test: Valsalva maneuver					
Pressure [mmHg]	Baseline	Phase 2			Phase 4
		Early	End		
Systolic	102	69	104		
Mean	76	63	88.7	n/a	
Diastolic	63	60	81	n/a	

Heart rate evaluation	
Test: Deep breathing	
Results	Norm*
14.33	≥12
Test: Valsalva ratio	
1.55	≥1.5
* adjusted for a gender and age	

(continued)

TABLE 23.1 CONTINUED

Test: Tilt test											
Position		HR [BPM]	Blood pressure [mmHg]		MCA Blood flow velocity [cm/s]				Respiratory frequency [breaths/min]	End tidal CO_2 [mmHg]
			Systolic	Diastolic	Systolic	Mean	Mean drop [%]	Diastolic		
Supine		73	119	79	97	59		40	18	32
Tilt [min]	1	85	131	90	88	51.3	13.1	33	19	28
	2	109	125	93						
	3	109	124	94						
	4	102	122	90						
	5	111	126	93	80	53.3	9.7	40	9	29
	6	107	111	82						
	7	109	127	88						
	8	114	131	92						
	9	122	131	92						
	10	121	127	88	79	52.3	11.4	39	19	29
	15									
	20									
	30									
	40									

Sudomotor evaluation - functional

Test: Quantitative sudomotor axon reflex test (QSART)				
Location	Site (l/r)	Latency [min]	Volume [µl]	Norm [µl]*
Forearm				≥0.08
Prox. leg				≥0.14
Distal leg				≥0.15
Foot				≥0.07

* Normative data are adjusted for gender and age of patient.

Test: Electrochemical skin conductance (ESC)				
Location	Left [µS]	Right [µS]	Average [µS/k]	Norm [µS/kg]
Hand	73	70	0.66	≥1.03
Feet	80	77	0.72	≥1.14
Forehead				

For grading uses ESC [µS] adjusted for weight [µS/k].

TABLE 23.1 CONTINUED

Small fiber (sensory + sudomotor) evaluation - morphological					
Test: Skin biopsy					
Location	Site (l/r)	Nerve fibers			
		Epidermal*		Sweat glands	
		Density	Norm	Density	Norm
Proximal leg – thigh	Right	9.8	≥8.3		≥37.8
Distal leg - calf	Right	1.6	≥8.7	6	≥36.5
Foot	Right		≥3.11		≥34.8

* Normative data for distal leg are adjusted for gender and age of patient.

QASAT*											
Heart rate		**BP**		**CBFv**		**ET-CO2**		**Sudomotor**			**Total QASAT score**
S. bradycardia	0	Low supine	0	Low supine	0	Low supine	1	QSART			
S. tachycardia	0	High supine	0	High supine	0	High supine	0	ESC	3		
Increase tilt	2	OH	0	Tilt response	1	Tilt low	2				
Decrease tilt	0	OHTN	0	CA	0	Tilt high	0	**Skin biopsy**			17
Deep breathing	0	VM	0	CVR	0			Epidermal	4		
VR	0			VM	0			Sweat gland	4		
Total	2	Total	0	Total	1	Total	3				

*QASAT. See Novak. Quantitative Scale for Grading of Cardiovascular Autonomic Reflex Tests and Small Fibers from Skin Biopsies. *J Neurol Disord* 2015;3:2.

S, supine; Increase tilt, increased response to tilt; Decrease tilt, decreased response to tilt; BP, blood pressure; VM, Valsalva maneuver; CBFv, cerebral blood flow velocity; CA, cerebral autoregulation; MCA, middle cerebral artery; VR, Valsalva ratio; CVR, cerebral vasoreactivity.

Cold feet: Often
Reduced sweating: None
Reduced sweating after exercise: None
Increased sweating: None
Nausea: Occasionally
Diarrhea: Occasionally
Constipation: Occasionally
Urinary leaks: None
Current pain severity: 0
Aching pain: Continuous, severe
Allodynia: Often, mild
Burning pain: Often, moderate
Lancinating pain: None
Numbness: Often, mild
Prickling sensation: Continuous, mild

AUTONOMIC TESTING INTERPRETATION

- Small fiber neuropathy, severe, mixed, length-dependent.
- Postural tachycardia syndrome (POTS), mild, neuropathic form.

COMMENT

The testing revealed mild POTS (Figure 23.1) but severe small fiber neuropathy, which can be responsible for fibromyalgia-related complains.[1] She is using metformin for anovulatory infertility due to polycystic ovary syndrome (PCOS).[2] Metformin interferes with vitamin B_{12} metabolism.[3,4] Low vitamin B_{12} can cause small fiber neuropathy[5] as well as POTS.[6] Alternatively, PCOS itself can be associated with dysautonomia.[7]

TREATMENT AND FOLLOW-UP

- Check vitamin B_{12} levels; replace metformin with alternative therapy for PCOS.
- Volume expansion through high fluid and high salt intake for POTS.

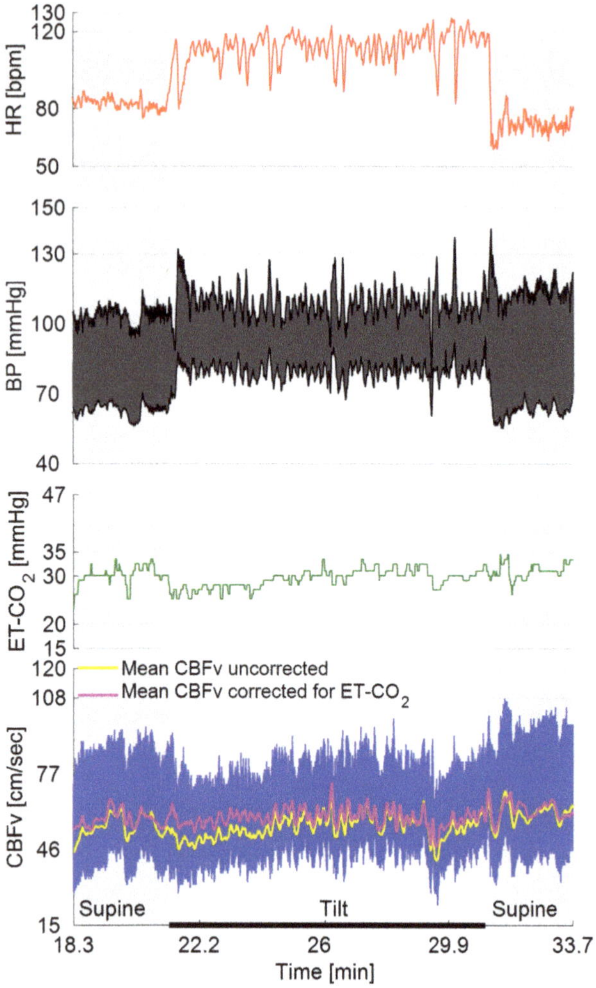

Figure 23.1 Heart rate increment to tilt was exacerbated. Blood pressure responses were normal. End tidal CO_2 and cerebral blood flow velocity were intermittently reduced during the tilt.

CAVEATS

- Postural tachycardia syndrome and small fiber neuropathy can be associated with PCOS or with the use of metformin.
- Small fiber neuropathy can be responsible for fibromyalgia-related complaints.

REFERENCES

1. Caro XJ, Winter EF. The role and importance of small fiber neuropathy in fibromyalgia pain. *Curr Pain Headache Rep*. 2015;19(12):55. doi:10.1007/s11916-015-0527-7.
2. Badawy A, Elnashar A. Treatment options for polycystic ovary syndrome. *Int J Womens Health*. 2011;3:25–35. doi:10.2147/IJWH.S11304.
3. Liu Q, Li S, Quan H, Li J. Vitamin B12 status in metformin treated patients: systematic review. *PloS One*. 2014;9(6):e100379. doi:10.1371/journal.pone.0100379.
4. Chapman LE, Darling AL, Brown JE. Association between metformin and vitamin B12 deficiency in patients with type 2 diabetes: a systematic review and meta-analysis. *Diabetes Metab*. 2016;42(5):316–327. doi:10.1016/j.diabet.2016.03.008.
5. Güneş HN, Bekircan-Kurt CE, Tan E, Erdem-Özdamar S. The histopathological evaluation of small fiber neuropathy in patients with vitamin B12 deficiency. *Acta Neurol Belg*. October 2017. doi:10.1007/s13760-017-0847-y.
6. Öner T, Guven B, Tavli V, Mese T, Yilmazer MM, Demirpence S. Postural orthostatic tachycardia syndrome (POTS) and vitamin B12 deficiency in adolescents. *Pediatrics*. 2014;133(1):e138–e142. doi:10.1542/peds.2012-3427.
7. Gui J, Wang R-H. Cardiovascular autonomic dysfunction in women with polycystic ovary syndrome: a systematic review and meta-analysis. *Reprod Biomed Online*. 2017;35(1):113–120. doi:10.1016/j.rbmo.2017.03.018.

CASE 19: STRAINING-INDUCED DIZZINESS

Chief complaint: Dizziness.

Case presentation: A 53-year-old woman has a history of strain-associated headaches and dizziness for several years. Usually, straining during bowel movements and heavy lifting provoked a sudden onset of severe, disabling bilateral headache or dizziness. The headaches and dizziness reach maximum within seconds and subside over several seconds or minutes after termination of straining. Because of straining-induced problems, she avoided physical activity and reduced food and fluid intake. She was referred for evaluation of suspected straining-induced dizziness.

Past medical history: Headaches.

Current medication: None.

Assessment plan: Functional autonomic tests and skin biopsy.

AUTONOMIC TESTING EVALUATION

See Table 24.1.

Heart rate: Supine heart rate was normal. Heart rate responses to deep breathing were reduced to 72.2% of normal value. Heart rate increment during the tilt (34 BPM) was exaggerated and exceeded 130 BPM.

Blood pressure:

Valsalva maneuver: Mean blood pressure failed to return to baseline at the end of Phase 2 by 27 mm Hg (i.e., 70.2% of baseline).

Tilt: Supine blood pressure was normal. Blood pressure responses to tilt were normal.

Sudomotor evaluation: Sweat output was abnormal (reduced to 48.8% of lower limit) at forearm, normal at proximal leg, normal at distal leg, and abnormal (reduced to 40% of lower limit) at foot.

Respiratory system: Respiratory frequency and end tidal CO_2 were normal in supine position and during the tilt.

Cerebral blood flow velocity (CBFv): CBFv in middle cerebral artery was normal in supine position. CBFv in middle cerebral artery was stable during the tilt.

Skin biopsy (sensory-epidermal): Epidermal nerve fiber density was normal at proximal leg and abnormal (reduced to 26.4% of normal limit) at distal leg.

Skin biopsy (sweat glands): Sweat gland nerve fiber density was normal at proximal leg and abnormal (reduced to 41.4% of normal limit) at distal leg.

Patient-reported symptoms during testing: Dizziness, headache, numb feet during the tilt.

Patient-reported symptoms for past 2 weeks:

Lightheadedness or dizziness: Occasionally
Dry eyes or mouth: None
Pale feet: Yes, minor annoyance
Cold feet: Occasionally
Reduced sweating: None
Reduced sweating after exercise: Yes, minor annoyance

TABLE 24.1 RESULTS OF AUTONOMIC TESTING

Blood pressure evaluation					
Test: Valsalva maneuver					
Pressure [mmHg]	Baseline	Phase 2			Phase 4
		Early	End		
Systolic	122	71	71		
Mean	90.7	63.7	63.7	n/a	
Diastolic	75	60	60	n/a	

Heart rate evaluation	
Test: Deep breathing	
Results	Norm*
6.5	≥9
Test: Valsalva ratio	
1.98	≥1.47

* adjusted for a gender and age

(continued)

TABLE 24.1 **CONTINUED**

Test: Tilt test										
Position		HR [BPM]	Blood pressure [mmHg]		MCA Blood flow velocity [cm/s]				Respiratory frequency [breaths/min]	End tidal CO_2 [mmHg]
			Systolic	Diastolic	Systolic	Mean	Mean drop [%]	Diastolic		
Supine		97	101	63	103	63		43	9	36
Tilt [min]	1	125	118	81	108	69.3	–10	50	14	36
	2	125	123	86						
	3	130	110	78						
	4	128	125	84						
	5	131	116	82	104	64	–1.6	44	6	39
	6	128	114	81						
	7	120	110	78						
	8	126	93	66						
	9	123	102	72						
	10	130	90	67	104	62.7	0.5	42	3	39
	15	131	105	74						
	20									
	30									
	40									

Sudomotor evaluation - functional

Test: Quantitative sudomotor axon reflex test (QSART)				
Location	Site (l/r)	Latency [min]	Volume [µl]	Norm [µl]*
Forearm	l	2.17	0.039	≥0.08
Prox. leg	l	2.11	0.155	≥0.14
Distal leg	l	1.27	0.217	≥0.07
Foot	l	4.29	0.02	≥0.05

* Normative data are adjusted for gender and age of patient.

Test: Electrochemical skin conductance (ESC)				
Location	Left [µS]	Right [µS]	Average [µS/k]	Norm [µS/kg]
Hand				≥
Feet				≥
Forehead				

For grading uses ESC [µS] adjusted for weight [µS/k].

Small fiber (sensory + sudomotor) evaluation - morphological					
Test: Skin biopsy					
Location	Site (l/r)	Nerve fibers			
		Epidermal*		Sweat glands	
		Density	Norm	Density	Norm
Proximal leg – thigh	Right	9.68	≥8.3	51.4	≥37.8
Distal leg - calf	Right	1.81	≥6.86	15.1	≥36.5
Foot	Right		≥3.11		≥34.8

* Normative data for distal leg are adjusted for gender and age of patient.

QASAT*										
Heart rate		**BP**		**CBFv**		**ET-CO2**		**Sudomotor**		**Total QASAT score**
S. bradycardia	0	Low supine	0	Low supine	0	Low supine	0	QSART	2	
S. tachycardia	0	High supine	0	High supine	0	High supine	0	ESC		
Increase tilt	6	OH	0	Tilt response	0	Tilt low	0			
Decrease tilt	0	OHTN	0	CA	1	Tilt high	0	**Skin biopsy**		21
Deep breathing	1	VM	2	CVR	0			Epidermal	3	
VR	0			VM	2			Sweat gland	4	
Total	7	Total	2	Total	3	Total	0			

*QASAT. See Novak. Quantitative Scale for Grading of Cardiovascular Autonomic Reflex Tests and Small Fibers from Skin Biopsies. *J Neurol Disord* 2015;3:2.

S, supine; Increase tilt, increased response to tilt; Decrease tilt, decreased response to tilt; BP, blood pressure; VM, Valsalva maneuver; CBFv, cerebral blood flow velocity; CA, cerebral autoregulation; MCA, middle cerebral artery; VR, Valsalva ratio; CVR, cerebral vasoreactivity.

Increased sweating: Yes, minor annoyance
Nausea: None
Diarrhea: None
Constipation: Occasionally
Urinary leaks: Yes, minor annoyance
Current pain severity: 5
Aching pain: Often, moderate
Allodynia: None
Burning pain: None
Lancinating pain: Often, moderate
Numbness: Often, moderate
Prickling sensation: Often, moderate

AUTONOMIC TESTING INTERPRETATION

- Cerebral autoregulatory failure. Dizziness and headaches associated with straining is due to cerebral hyperemia.
- Postural tachycardia syndrome (POTS), likely due to combined effect of small fiber neuropathy, volume depletion, and deconditioning.
- Small fiber neuropathy.

COMMENT

The Valsalva maneuver provoked short spells of severe dizziness and headaches and reproduced the patient's straining-related complaints (Figure 24.1). During dizziness and headache, which occurred after straining (during Phase 4), CBFv was markedly elevated and reached 195 cm/s (normal <160 cm/s). The elevated CBFv is consistent with hyperemic response due to excessive and prolonged vasodilation of cerebral vessels followed by straining.[1,2] The dizziness and headaches subsided with normalization of CBFv, further strengthening the link between hyperemia and

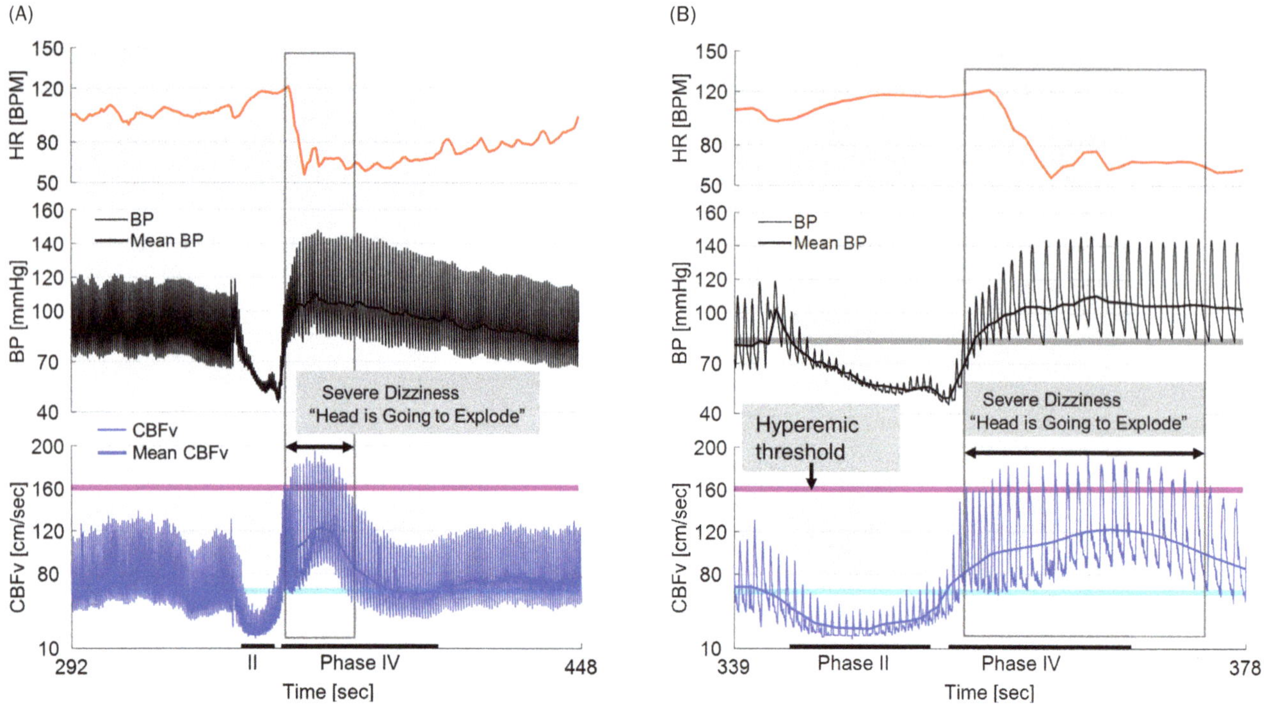

Figure 24.1 The Valsalva maneuver showed abnormal Phase 2 in blood pressure (A, B). Cerebral blood flow velocity (CBFv) exceeded the hyperemic threshold level (160 cm/s) after the strain (Phase 4). Patient was very dizzy at Phase 4.

dizziness/headaches. Straining-related headaches respond to indomethacin,[3] which is a vasoconstrictor[4] and prevents abnormal vasodilation.

The study also showed POTS and small fiber neuropathy. Deconditioning and volume depletion likely play a role in POTS, as indicated by pulse pressure collapse during Phase 2 of the Valsalva maneuver (Figure 24.1). Indeed, the patient avoided physical activity and reduced fluid and foot intake since she wanted to reduce any straining, including straining related to bowel movements, to a minimum.

TREATMENT AND FOLLOW-UP

- Indomethacin for straining-related dizziness and headaches.
- Clinical workup for small fiber neuropathy.
- Hydration and reconditioning for POTS.

CAVEATS

- Straining-related dizziness and headaches can reflect cerebral hyperemia due to abnormal cerebral autoregulation.[1]
- Indomethacin is the drug of choice for straining-induced headache and dizziness.

REFERENCES

1. Zhang R, Crandall CG, Levine BD. Cerebral hemodynamics during the Valsalva maneuver: insights from ganglionic blockade. *Stroke*. 2004;35(4):843–847. doi:10.1161/01.STR.0000120309.84666.AE.
2. Novak P. Primary headache induced by the Valsalva maneuver is associated with cerebral hyperemia due to autoregulatory failure. (P2.158). *Neurology*. 2017;88(16 Supplement). http://n.neurology.org/content/88/16_Supplement/P2.158.abstract.
3. Evers S, Goadsby P, Jensen R, et al. Treatment of miscellaneous idiopathic headache disorders (Group 4 of the IHS classification): report of an EFNS task force. *Eur J Neurol*. 2011;18(6):803–812. doi:10.1111/j.1468-1331.2011.03389.x.
4. Lucas S. The pharmacology of indomethacin. *Headache*. 2016;56(2): 436–446. doi:10.1111/head.12769.

25.

CASE 20: POSTURAL TACHYCARDIA SYNDROME VERSUS SYNCOPE WITH LOSS OF VISION

Chief complaint: Fainting spells.

Case presentation: A 31-year-old woman presents with a long history of fainting. During high school, she would faint in the shower. She was frequently nauseated and also had intermittent diarrhea. Later, she started to faint regularly and also noted chronic fatigue. She also developed brain fog and became bed bound for 9 months. A previous tilt test showed presyncope and had to be terminated at minute 3 for severe dizziness. She had an ambulatory 72-hour electroencephalogram that showed possible seizure activity. She saw a psychiatrist for postpartum depression. At present, she is dizzy and tired on most days and is unable to work. Standing and showering provokes dizziness and face twitching. She feels worse in the morning. She noted numbness in legs and arms. Mother and brother had Lyme disease. She has been bitten by a tick at a farm but she does not remember having skin rash. MRI of the brain 8 years ago was unrevealing. She was referred for autonomic testing to evaluate the cause of orthostatic intolerance.

Past medical history: Syncope, chronic fatigue, orthostatic intolerance.

Current medication: Multivitamins.

Assessment plan: Functional autonomic tests and skin biopsy.

AUTONOMIC TESTING EVALUATION

See Table 25.1.

Heart rate: Supine heart rate was normal. Heart rate responses to deep breathing were normal. Heart rate increment during the tilt (71 BPM) was exaggerated and exceeded 120 BPM at the end of tilt before syncope.

Blood pressure:

Valsalva maneuver: Blood pressure responses were normal.

Tilt: Supine blood pressure was normal. Blood pressure responses to tilt were abnormal; there was initial transient decline in blood pressure consistent with transient orthostatic hypotension and a second decline in blood pressure at minute 11 resulting in syncope.

Sudomotor evaluation: Electrochemical skin conductance was normal at hands and normal at feet.

Respiratory system: Respiratory frequency was normal in supine position and during the tilt. End tidal CO_2 was reduced in supine position and was also intermittently reduced during the tilt.

Cerebral blood flow velocity (CBFv): CBFv in middle cerebral artery was normal in supine position but was intermittently reduced during the tilt. Maximal decline in CBFv occurred during the syncope.

TABLE 25.1 **RESULTS OF AUTONOMIC TESTING**

Blood pressure evaluation					
Test: Valsalva maneuver					
Pressure [mmHg]	Baseline	Phase 2			Phase 4
		Early	End		
Systolic	79	71	79		
Mean	65	60.3	67	n/a	
Diastolic	58	55	61	n/a	

Heart rate evaluation	
Test: Deep breathing	
Results	Norm*
16	≥12
Test: Valsalva ratio	
1.56	≥1.5
* adjusted for a gender and age	

(continued)

TABLE 25.1 CONTINUED

Test: Tilt test										
Position		HR [BPM]	Blood pressure [mmHg]		MCA Blood flow velocity [cm/s]				Respiratory frequency [breaths/min]	End tidal CO_2 [mmHg]
			Systolic	Diastolic	Systolic	Mean	Mean drop [%]	Diastolic		
Supine		53	94	61	129	79		54	11	30
Tilt [min]	1	80	106	73	108	71.3	9.7	53	7	36
	2	90	102	71						
	3	86	101	71						
	4	93	91	67						
	5	87	91	70	90.3	63.6	19.5	50.2	14	32
	6	96	102	73						
	7	96	100	71						
	8	101	106	75						
	9	117	106	73						
	10	124	106	73	110	71.3	9.7	52	12	32
	15									
	20									
	30									
	40									

Sudomotor evaluation - functional

Test: Quantitative sudomotor axon reflex test (QSART)				
Location	Site (l/r)	Latency [min]	Volume [µl]	Norm [µl]*
Forearm				≥0.08
Prox. leg				≥0.14
Distal leg				≥0.15
Foot				≥0.07

* Normative data are adjusted for gender and age of patient.

Test: Electrochemical skin conductance (ESC)				
Location	Left [µS]	Right [µS]	Average [µS/k]	Norm [µS/kg]
Hand	80	82	1.1	≥1.03
Feet	88	89	1.2	≥1.14
Forehead				

For grading uses ESC [µS] adjusted for weight [µS/k].

TABLE 25.1 CONTINUED

Small fiber (sensory + sudomotor) evaluation - morphological					
Test: Skin biopsy					
Location	Site (l/r)	Nerve fibers			
		Epidermal*		Sweat glands	
		Density	Norm	Density	Norm
Proximal leg – thigh	Right	10.55	≥8.3		≥37.8
Distal leg - calf	Right	7.35	≥8.62	31.9	≥36.5
Foot	Right		≥3.11		≥34.8

* Normative data for distal leg are adjusted for gender and age of patient.

QASAT*										
Heart rate		**BP**		**CBFv**		**ET-CO2**		**Sudomotor**		**Total QASAT score**
S. bradycardia	0	Low supine	0	Low supine	0	Low supine	1	QSART		
S. tachycardia	0	High supine	0	High supine	0	High supine	0	ESC	0	
Increase tilt	1	OH	0	Tilt response	1	Tilt low	0			
Decrease tilt	0	OHTN	0	CA	0	Tilt high	0	**Skin biopsy**		5
Deep breathing	0	VM	0	CVR	0			Epidermal	1	
VR	0			VM	0			Sweat gland	1	
Total	1	Total	0	Total	1	Total	1			

*QASAT. See Novak. Quantitative Scale for Grading of Cardiovascular Autonomic Reflex Tests and Small Fibers from Skin Biopsies. *J Neurol Disord* 2015;3:2.

S, supine; Increase tilt, increased response to tilt; Decrease tilt, decreased response to tilt; BP, blood pressure; VM, Valsalva maneuver; CBFv, cerebral blood flow velocity; CA, cerebral autoregulation; MCA, middle cerebral artery; VR, Valsalva ratio; CVR, cerebral vasoreactivity.

Skin biopsy (sensory-epidermal): Epidermal nerve fiber density was normal at proximal leg and abnormal (reduced to 85.3% of normal limit) at distal leg.

Skin biopsy (sweat glands): Sweat gland nerve fiber density was abnormal (reduced to 87.4% of normal limit) at distal leg.

Patient-reported symptoms during testing: Syncope, loss of vision, and dizziness during the tilt.

Patient-reported symptoms for past 2 weeks:

Lightheadedness or dizziness: Often
Dry eyes or mouth: Occasionally
Pale feet: Often
Cold feet: Occasionally
Reduced sweating: Often
Reduced sweating after exercise: Often
Increased sweating: None
Nausea: Occasionally
Diarrhea: Occasionally
Constipation: Yes, minor annoyance
Urinary leaks: Occasionally
Current pain severity: 3
Aching pain: Often, moderate
Allodynia: None
Burning pain: None
Lancinating pain: None
Numbness: Often, severe
Prickling sensation: Often, severe

AUTONOMIC TESTING INTERPRETATION

- Syncope, neurally mediated, vasodepressor.
- Small fiber neuropathy, mixed, length-dependent.
- Hypocapnic cerebral hypoperfusion (HYCH).[1]
- Cerebral autoregulatory failure.
- Initial orthostatic hypotension.

COMMENT

The tilt showed a combination of initial orthostatic hypotension (IOH), HYCH, and vasodepressor syncope (Figure 25.1).[1,2] The heart rate increment at the end of the tilt exceeded 120 BPM, but this tachycardic response occurred during the decline in blood pressure and was part of syncopal reaction. Therefore, this is not postural tachycardia syndrome (POTS). The tilt reproduced all major patient complaints, including vision loss. Absent expected increase in systolic CBFv (Figure 25.1) is consistent with cerebral autoregulatory failure.

TREATMENT AND FOLLOW-UP

- Clinical workup for small fiber neuropathy including evaluation for Lyme disease.

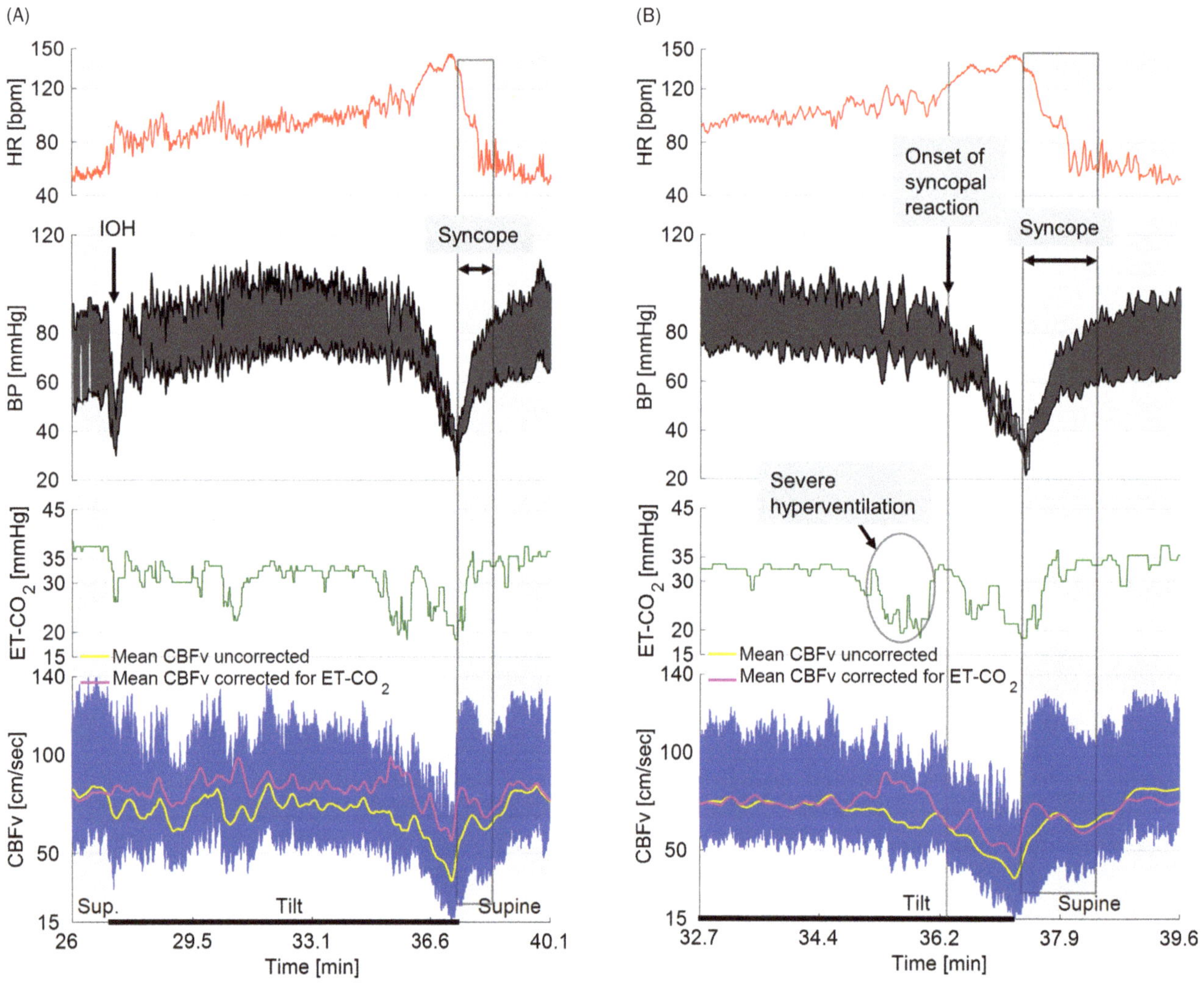

Figure 25.1 Tilt provoked initial orthostatic hypotension (IOH) within seconds of the tilt onset (A). At about minute 10 of the tilt, patient started to severely hyperventilate (*gray circle*, B). The syncopal reaction started several seconds later and was associated with persistent tachycardia (*red arrow*, C), decrease in blood pressure (*black arrow*), worsening of hypocapnia, and decrease in cerebral blood flow velocity (CBFv, *blue arrows*). Both diastolic and systolic CBFv decreased. Expected increase of systolic CBFv (*blue interrupted arrow*) was absent. A few seconds before syncope, patient lost vision (D).

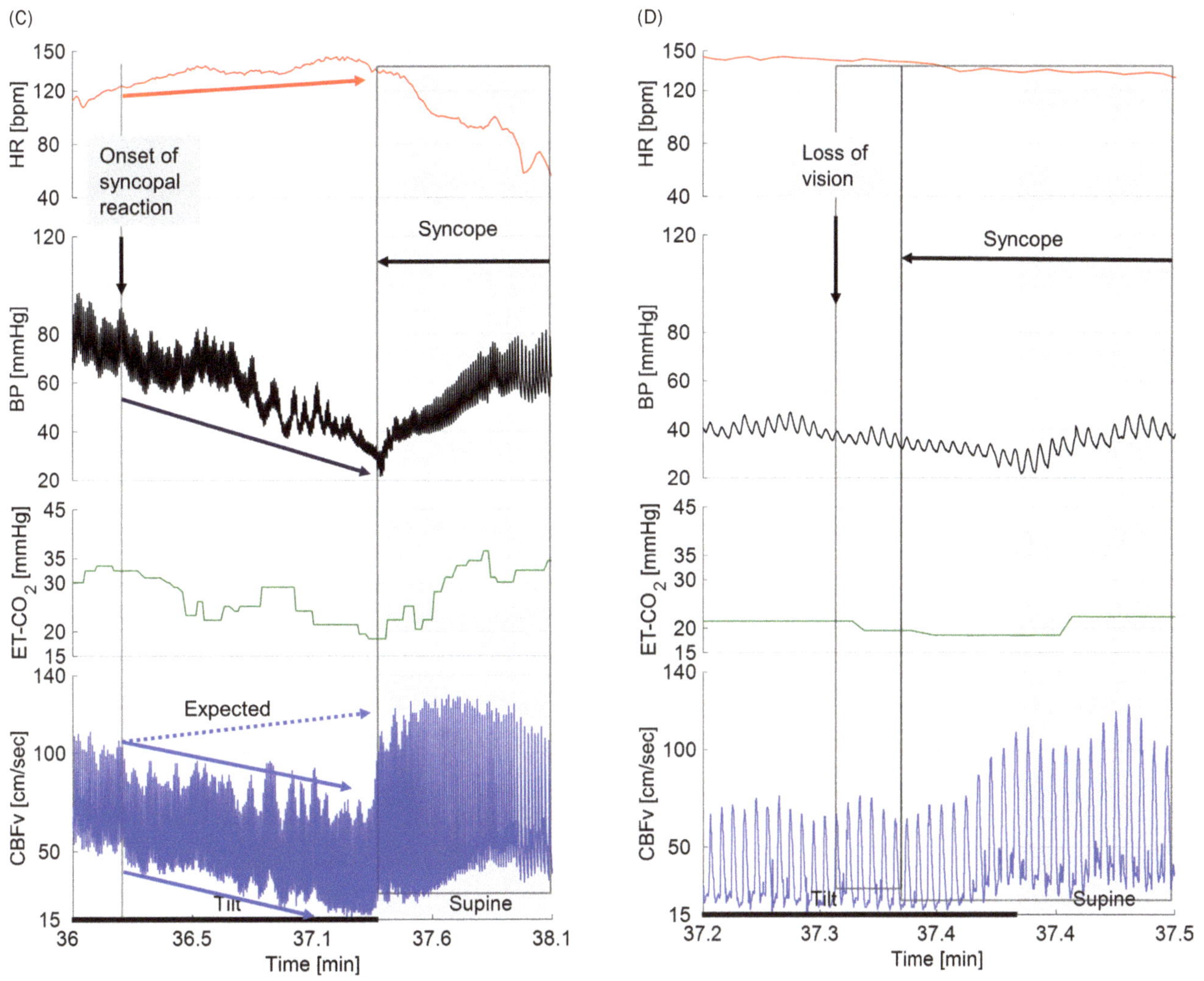

Figure 25.1 Continued

- Volume expansion through high fluid and high salt intake, exercise.

CAVEATS

- IOH, HYCH, and syncope can coexist.

REFERENCES

1. Novak P. Hypocapnic cerebral hypoperfusion: A biomarker of orthostatic intolerance. *PloS One*. 2018;*13*(9):e0204419. doi:10.1371/journal.pone.0204419.
2. Novak P. Cerebral blood flow, heart rate, and blood pressure patterns during the tilt test in common orthostatic syndromes. *Neurosci J*. 2016;2016:6127340. doi:10.1155/2016/6127340.

PART IV

ORTHOSTATIC CEREBRAL HYPOPERFUSION SYNDROME

26.

CASE 21: ORTHOSTATIC CEREBRAL HYPOPERFUSION SYNDROME, INTERMITTENT

Chief complaint: Dizziness.

Case presentation: A 28-year-old woman presents with intermittent, usually postural dizziness and headaches since a concussion 4 years ago. She was seen by several specialists; no clear diagnosis has been made. She did not improve on vestibular physical therapy. Sertraline, β-blockers, duloxetine, and nortriptyline were tried without success. Neurologic examination was unrevealing. She was suspected of having postural tachycardia syndrome (POTS).

Past medical history: Migraine, obstructive sleep apnea, concussion.

Current medication: Sertraline, magnesium.

Assessment plan: Functional autonomic tests.

AUTONOMIC TESTING EVALUATION

See Table 26.1.

Heart rate: Supine heart rate was normal. Heart rate responses to deep breathing were reduced to 70% of normal value. There was mild tachycardia during the tilt.

Blood pressure:

Valsalva maneuver: Blood pressure responses were normal.

Tilt: Supine blood pressure was within normal range. Blood pressure was elevated during the tilt.

Sudomotor evaluation: Sweat output was normal at forearm, normal at proximal leg, normal at distal leg, and normal at foot.

Respiratory system: Respiratory frequency and end tidal CO_2 were normal in supine position and during the tilt.

Cerebral blood flow velocity (CBFv): CBFv in middle cerebral artery was increased in supine position. CBFv in middle cerebral artery was mildly reduced during the tilt test.

Skin biopsy (sensory-epidermal): N/A

Skin biopsy (sweat glands): N/A

Patient-reported symptoms during testing: Dizziness and nausea during the tilt.

Patient-reported symptoms for past 2 weeks:

Lightheadedness or dizziness: Occasionally
Dry eyes or mouth: None
Pale feet: None
Cold feet: Yes, minor annoyance
Reduced sweating: None
Reduced sweating after exercise: None
Increased sweating: Yes, minor annoyance
Nausea: Occasionally

TABLE 26.1 **RESULTS OF AUTONOMIC TESTING**

Blood pressure evaluation					
Test: Valsalva maneuver					
Pressure [mmHg]	Baseline	Phase 2			Phase 4
		Early	End		
Systolic	121	125	131		
Mean	83	81.7	93.7	n/a	
Diastolic	64	60	75	n/a	

Heart rate evaluation	
Test: Deep breathing	
Results	Norm*
9.8	≥14
Test: Valsalva ratio	
1.78	≥1.46
* adjusted for a gender and age	

(continued)

TABLE 26.1 **CONTINUED**

Test: Tilt test											
Position		HR [BPM]	Blood pressure [mmHg]		MCA Blood flow velocity [cm/s]				Respiratory frequency [breaths/min]	End tidal CO_2 [mmHg]
			Systolic	Diastolic	Systolic	Mean	Mean drop [%]	Diastolic		
Supine		86	125	83	131	91		71	18	40
Tilt [min]	1	105	126	76	119	83.7	8	66	17	40
	2	109	127	94						
	3	106	132	91						
	4	112	151	81						
	5	108	131	79	121	88.3	3	72	13	36
	6	105	131	80						
	7	106	134	84						
	8	104	138	81						
	9	104	121	76						
	10	109	138	85	101	69	24.2	53	14	40
	15									
	20									
	30									
	40									

Sudomotor evaluation—functional

Test: Quantitative sudomotor axon reflex test (QSART)				
Location	Site (l/r)	Latency [min]	Volume [µl]	Norm [µl]*
Forearm	l	0.41	0.52	≥0.08
Prox. leg	l	0.45	0.638	≥0.14
Distal leg	l	0.51	1.067	≥0.24
Foot	l	2.25	0.88	≥0.09

* normative data are adjusted for a gender and age of a patient

Test: Electrochemical skin conductance (ESC)				
Location	Left [µS]	Right [µS]	Average [µS/k]	Norm [µS/kg]
Hand				≥1.03
Feet				≥1.14
Forehead				

For grading uses ESC [µS] adjusted for weight [µS/k].

Small fiber (sensory + sudomotor) evaluation—morphological					
Test: Skin biopsy					
Location	Site (l/r)	Nerve fibers			
		Epidermal*		Sweat glands	
		Density	Norm	Density	Norm
Proximal leg—thigh	Right		≥8.3		≥37.8
Distal leg—calf	Right		≥8.86		≥36.5
Foot	Right		≥3.11		≥34.8

* normative data for distal leg are adjusted for a gender and age of a patient

QASAT*											
Heart rate		**BP**		**CBFv**		**ET-CO2**		**Sudomotor**			**Total QASAT score**
S. bradycardia	0	Low supine	0	Low supine	0	Low supine	0	QSART	0		
S. tachycardia	0	High supine	0	High supine	1	High supine	0	ESC			
Increase tilt	0	OH	0	Tilt response.	2	Tilt low	0				
Decrease tilt	0	OHTN	1	CA	0	Tilt high	0	**Skin biopsy**			5
Deep breathing	1	VM	0	CVR	0			Epidermal			
VR	0			VM	0			Sweat gland			
Total	1	Total	1	Total	3	Total	0				

*QASAT. See Novak. Quantitative Scale for Grading of Cardiovascular Autonomic Reflex Tests and Small Fibers from Skin Biopsies. *J Neurol Disord* 2015;3:2.

S, supine; Increase tilt, increased response to tilt; Decrease tilt, decreased response to tilt; BP, blood pressure; VM, Valsalva maneuver; CBFv, cerebral blood flow velocity; CA, cerebral autoregulation; MCA, middle cerebral artery; VR, Valsalva ratio; CVR, cerebral vasoreactivity.

Diarrhea: None
Constipation: Yes, minor annoyance
Urinary leaks: None
Current pain severity: 7
Aching pain: None
Allodynia: Occasionally, mild
Burning pain: None
Lancinating pain: Often, severe
Numbness: None
Prickling sensation: None

AUTONOMIC TESTING INTERPRETATION

Orthostatic cerebral hypoperfusion syndrome (OCHOS).
There was no evidence of autonomic failure.

COMMENT

The tilt test showed mild OCHOS (Figure 26.1).[1] OCHOS is associated with reduced orthostatic CBFv without orthostatic hypotension, hypocapnia or arrhythmia. The proposed mechanism of OCHOS includes abnormal cerebral vasoconstriction. The decline in CBFv coincided with the symptoms of cerebral hypoperfusion (dizziness and nausea).

TREATMENT AND FOLLOW-UP

Patient was recommended to increase fluid and salt intake to expand volume, which may improve cerebral perfusion. Since diet modifications did not help, verapamil was started; verapamil dilates cerebral vessels and, in theory, may alleviate abnormal cerebral vasoconstriction, which was postulated in OCHOS.

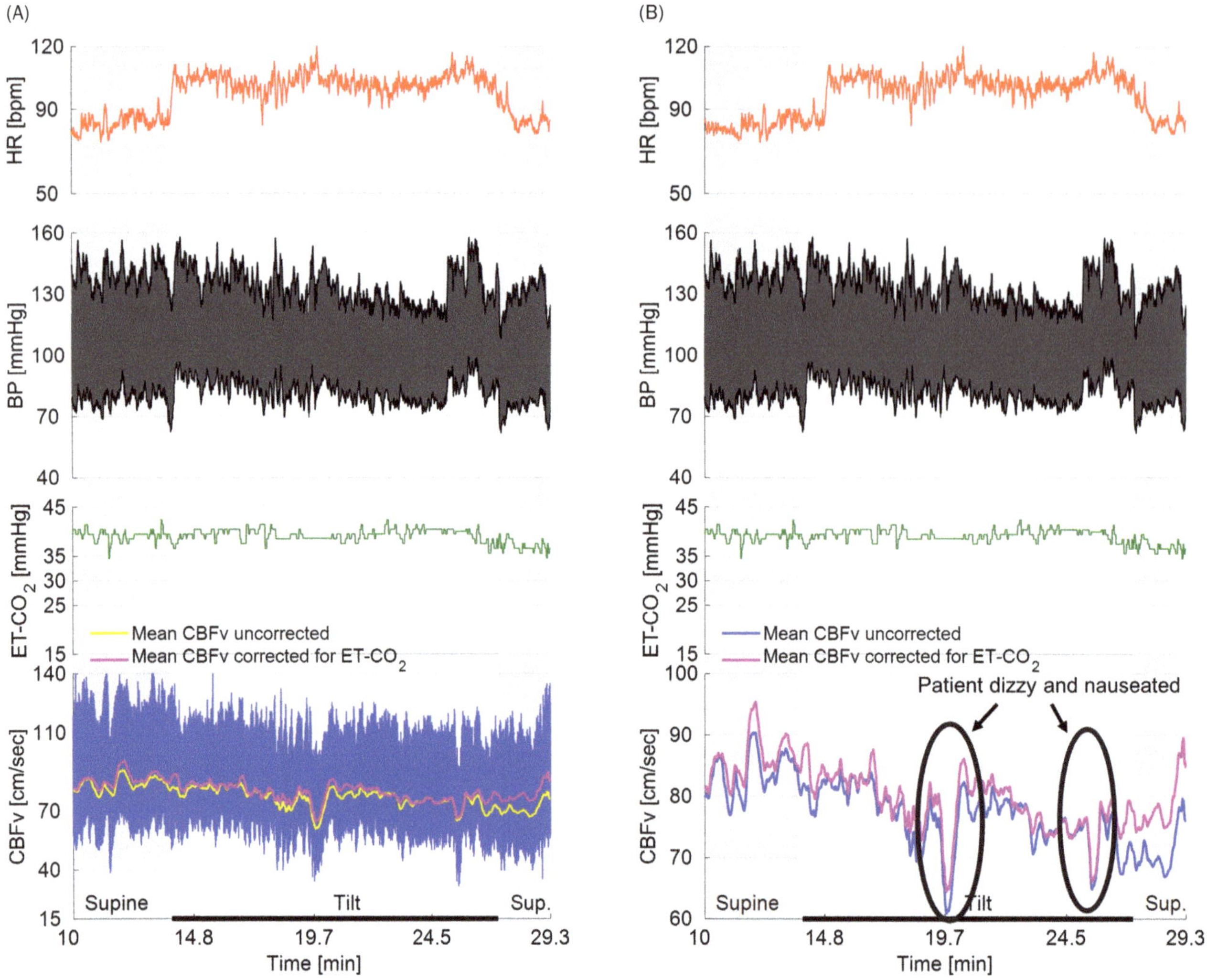

Figure 26.1 The heart rate, blood pressure, and end tidal CO_2 responses to tilt were normal (A, B). There was a progressive decline in cerebral blood flow velocity (CBFv) during the tilt with two sudden declines (*dark ovals*, B) during which patient became extremely dizzy and nauseated.

Patient was doing well at 1-year follow-up on verapamil.

CAVEATS

OCHOS can be responsible for intermittent orthostatic intolerance.
Calcium channel blockers may be helpful in OCHOS.

REFERENCE

1. Novak P. Orthostatic cerebral hypoperfusion syndrome. *Front Aging Neurosci.* 2016;8:22. doi:10.3389/fnagi.2016.00022.

27.

CASE 22: ORTHOSTATIC CEREBRAL HYPOPERFUSION SYNDROME IN ANAPHYLAXIS

Chief complaint: Dizziness.

Case presentation: A 21-year-old man presents with fatigue and intermittent orthostatic dizziness for several years. Patient has history of chronic idiopathic urticaria, anaphylaxis, and multiple food allergies. He has a history of exercise-induced anaphylactic; for example, when running or singing, he would suddenly pass out. He has episodes of dyspnea and wheezing which are triggered by infections, emotions, exercise, heat exposure, and humidity. He has chest tightness, which is relieved when he uses albuterol. Light, sun, and heat exposure triggers hives and pruritus that are relieved by diphenhydramine. He cannot be upright for more than 10 minutes without experiencing a presyncopal feeling. Proamatine improves his orthostatic intolerance. He was referred for autonomic testing to determine if episodic shortness of breath and orthostatic intolerance are related to autonomic failure.

Past medical history: Anaphylaxis, chronic idiopathic urticarial, asthma, syncope, Tourette's syndrome, Lyme disease.

Current medication: Omalizumab, omeprazole, gabapentin, albuterol.

Assessment plan: Functional autonomic tests and skin biopsy.

AUTONOMIC TESTING EVALUATION

See Table 27.1.

Heart rate: Supine heart rate was normal. Heart rate responses to deep breathing were normal. Heart rate increment during the tilt (28 BPM) was normal.

Blood pressure:

Valsalva maneuver: Blood pressure responses were normal.

Tilt: Supine blood pressure was normal. Blood pressure responses to tilt were normal.

Sudomotor evaluation: Electrochemical skin conductance was abnormal (reduced to 82.6% of normal limit) at hands and abnormal (reduced to 85.2% of normal limit) at feet.

Respiratory system: Respiratory frequency and end tidal CO_2 were normal in supine position and during the tilt.

Cerebral blood flow velocity (CBFv): CBFv in middle cerebral artery was normal in supine position but was reduced by 19% during the tilt.

Skin biopsy (sensory-epidermal): Epidermal nerve fiber density was normal at proximal leg and normal at distal leg.

Skin biopsy (sweat glands): Sweat gland nerve fiber density was abnormal (reduced to 89.6% of normal limit) at distal leg.

TABLE 27.1 **RESULTS OF AUTONOMIC TESTING**

Blood pressure evaluation					
Test: Valsalva maneuver					
Pressure [mmHg]	Baseline	Phase 2			Phase 4
		Early	End		
Systolic	126	100	128		
Mean	97.3	77.3	108	n/a	
Diastolic	83	66	98	n/a	

Heart rate evaluation	
Test: Deep breathing	
Results	Norm*
28	≥14
Test: Valsalva ratio	
2.07	≥1.59
* adjusted for a gender and age	

(continued)

TABLE 27.1 **CONTINUED**

Test: Tilt test										
Position		HR [BPM]	Blood pressure [mmHg]		MCA Blood flow velocity [cm/s]				Respiratory frequency [breaths/min]	End tidal CO_2 [mmHg]
			Systolic	Diastolic	Systolic	Mean	Mean drop [%]	Diastolic		
Supine		74	113	74	99	67.7		52	16	38
Tilt [min]	1	99	117	83	90	62	8.4	48	15	39
	2	94	115	88						
	3	91	110	81						
	4	93	115	84						
	5	94	106	82	91	65	4	52	13	37
	6	99	111	82						
	7	98	116	83						
	8	97	114	84						
	9	102	118	87						
	10	91	118	87	83	55	18.8	41	14	39
	15									
	20									
	30									
	40									

Sudomotor evaluation - functional

Test: Quantitative sudomotor axon reflex test (QSART)				
Location	Site (l/r)	Latency [min]	Volume [µl]	Norm [µl]*
Forearm				≥0.3
Prox. leg				≥0.5
Distal leg				≥0.54
Foot				≥0.34

* Normative data are adjusted for gender and age of patient.

Test: Electrochemical skin conductance (ESC)				
Location	Left [µS]	Right [µS]	Average [µS/k]	Norm [µS/kg]
Hand	76	81	0.85	≥1.03
Feet	89	90	0.98	≥1.14
Forehead				

For grading uses ESC [µS] adjusted for weight [µS/k].

TABLE 27.1 CONTINUED

Small fiber (sensory + sudomotor) evaluation - morphological					
Test: Skin biopsy					
Location	Site (l/r)	Nerve fibers			
		Epidermal*		Sweat glands	
		Density	Norm	Density	Norm
Proximal leg – thigh	Right	9.76	≥8.3		≥37.8
Distal leg - calf	Right	8.44	≥7.925	32.7	≥36.5
Foot	Right		≥3.11		≥34.8

* Normative data for distal leg are adjusted for gender and age of patient.

QASAT*												
Heart rate		BP		CBFv		ET-CO2		Sudomotor			Total QASAT score
S. bradycardia	0	Low supine	0	Low supine	0	Low supine	0	QSART			
S. tachycardia	0	High supine	0	High supine	0	High supine	0	ESC	1		
Increase tilt	0	OH	0	Tilt response	1	Tilt low	0				
Decrease tilt	0	OHTN	0	CA	0	Tilt high	0	**Skin biopsy**			3
Deep breathing	0	VM	0	CVR	0			Epidermal	0		
VR	0			VM	0			Sweat gland	1		
Total	0	Total	0	Total	1	Total	0				

*QASAT. See Novak. Quantitative Scale for Grading of Cardiovascular Autonomic Reflex Tests and Small Fibers from Skin Biopsies. *J Neurol Disord* 2015;3:2.

S, supine; Increase tilt, increased response to tilt; Decrease tilt, decreased response to tilt; BP, blood pressure; VM, Valsalva maneuver; CBFv, cerebral blood flow velocity; CA, cerebral autoregulation; MCA, middle cerebral artery; VR, Valsalva ratio; CVR, cerebral vasoreactivity.

Patient-reported symptoms during testing: Dizziness during the tilt.

Patient-reported symptoms for past 2 weeks:

Lightheadedness or dizziness: Occasionally
Dry eyes or mouth: Occasionally
Pale feet: None
Cold feet: Occasionally
Reduced sweating: None
Reduced sweating after exercise: None
Increased sweating: None
Nausea: None
Diarrhea: None
Constipation: None
Urinary leaks: None
Erection problems: None
Current pain severity: 0
Aching pain: Often, moderate
Allodynia: Occasionally, mild
Burning pain: Often, severe
Lancinating pain: Often, severe
Numbness: Often, moderate
Prickling sensation: Often, moderate

AUTONOMIC TESTING INTERPRETATION

- Orthostatic cerebral hypoperfusion syndrome (OCHOS).
- No evidence of adrenergic autonomic failure.
- Small fiber neuropathy affecting autonomic sudomotor fibers.

COMMENT

Tilt test (Figure 27.1) showed a typical OCHOS pattern with reduced orthostatic CBFv without orthostatic hypotension, tachycardia, or hypocapnia. Autonomic function tests were normal. Since patient was not hyperventilating, the corrected and uncorrected CBFv (Figure 27.1B) were similar. Second main finding was the presence of small fiber neuropathy, affecting mainly autonomic fibers.

Patients with anaphylaxis may experience dyspnea, syncope, and/or low blood pressure during acute allergic reactions,[1] which is consistent with the dysautonomia induced by a release of vasoactive mediators. This study ruled out significant dysautonomia as a cause of orthostatic intolerance;

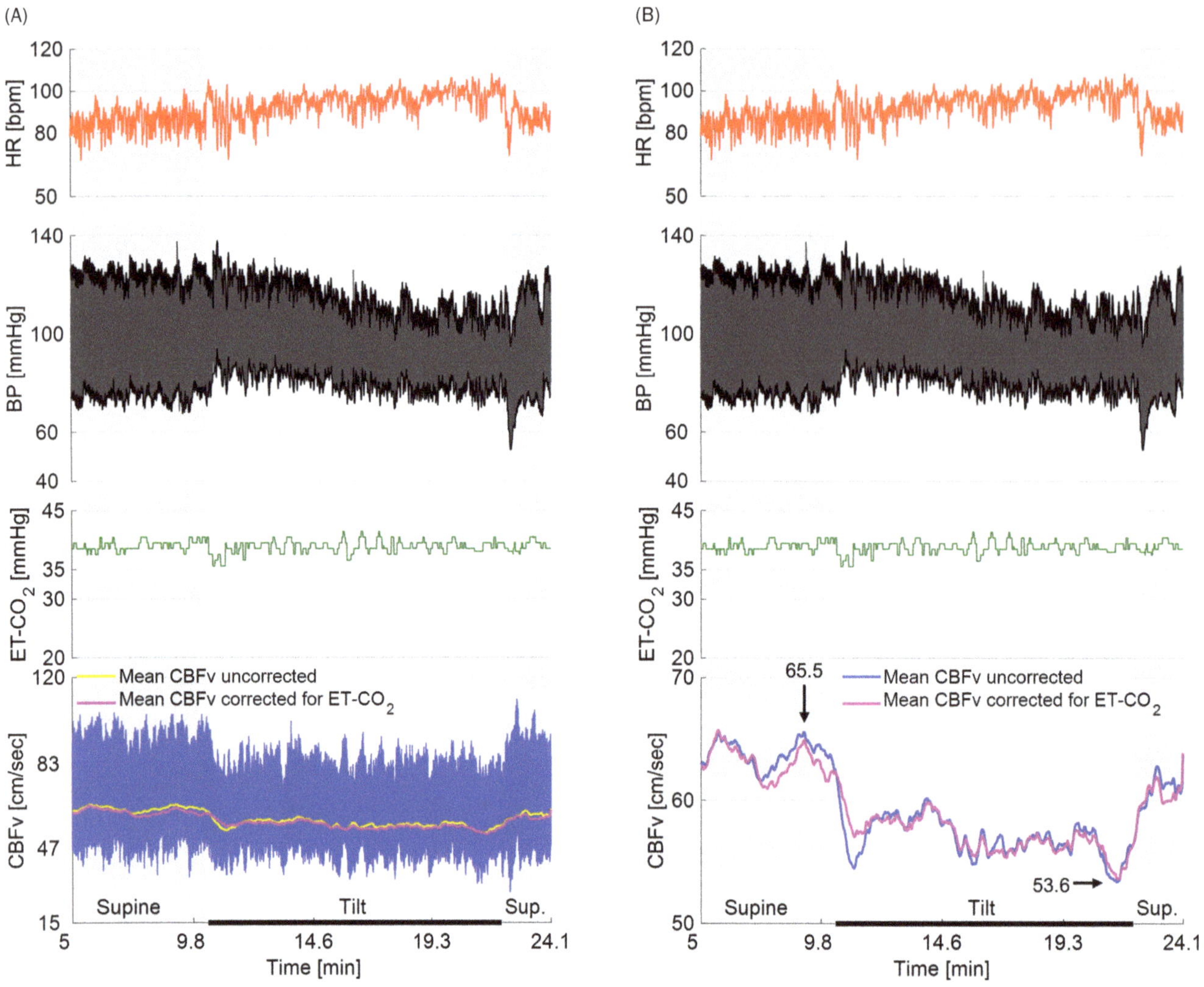

Figure 27.1 The tilt test showed decline in cerebral blood flow velocity (CBFv). All other monitored variables were stable during the tilt. The patient became mildly dizzy at the beginning of the tilt and was dizzy throughout the tilt.

therefore, the patient's acute symptoms including dyspnea, wheezing, dizziness, and even syncope are more likely due to anaphylaxis than due to primary autonomic failure.

The detected autonomic neuropathy on skin biopsy was mild and did not result in significant dysautonomia. Nevertheless, this study explains problems with prolonged standing (10 minutes or longer) that can be related to reduced cerebral blood flow due to OCHOS.

OCHOS[2] is a syndrome of orthostatic dizziness or other orthostatic symptoms associated with low orthostatic CBFv in the absence of orthostatic hypotension, arrhythmia, or hypocapnia. The postulated mechanisms include failure of cerebral autoregulation.

TREATMENT AND FOLLOW-UP

- Evaluation for small fiber neuropathy.
- Dietary volume expansion (>1.5 L/day fluids), high-salt diet (>8 g/day sodium), compression stockings. Continue proamatine; may titrate the dose upward.

CAVEATS

- OCHOS can be associated with orthostatic intolerance in anaphylaxis.
- Patients with anaphylaxis may have normal autonomic functions.

REFERENCES

1. Sampson HA, Muñoz-Furlong A, Campbell RL, et al. Second symposium on the definition and management of anaphylaxis: summary report: Second National Institute of Allergy and Infectious Disease/Food Allergy and Anaphylaxis Network symposium. *J Allergy Clin Immunol.* 2006;117(2):391–397. doi:10.1016/j.jaci.2005.12.1303.
2. Novak P. Orthostatic cerebral hypoperfusion syndrome. *Front Aging Neurosci.* 2016;8:22. doi:10.3389/fnagi.2016.00022.

28.

CASE 23: ORTHOSTATIC CEREBRAL HYPOPERFUSION SYNDROME, SEVERE

Chief complaint: Dizziness.

Case presentation: A 53-year-old man presents with orthostatic dizziness. He experienced dizziness since a young age, but the spells were usually short and not troublesome. For the past few months, the dizziness became more severe and more frequent. He notices dizziness particularly when he bends over and rises quickly. In addition, he has similar but milder symptoms every time he stands up.

Past medical history: Anxiety, asthma.

Current medication: Albuterol, trazodone, omeprazole, tramadol.

Assessment plan: Functional autonomic tests and skin biopsy.

AUTONOMIC TESTING EVALUATION

See Table 28.1.

Heart rate: Supine heart rate was normal. Heart rate responses to deep breathing were normal. Heart rate increment during the tilt (18 BPM) was normal.

Blood pressure:

Valsalva maneuver: Blood pressure responses were normal.

Tilt: Supine and orthostatic blood pressure was elevated.

Sudomotor evaluation: Electrochemical skin conductance was abnormal (reduced to 72% of normal limit) at hands and abnormal (reduced to 78.6% of normal limit) at feet.

Respiratory system: Respiratory frequency and end tidal CO_2 was normal in supine position and during the tilt.

Cerebral blood flow velocity (CBFv): CBFv in middle cerebral artery was increased in supine position. CBFv in middle cerebral artery was severely reduced during the tilt.

Skin biopsy (sensory-epidermal): Epidermal nerve fiber density was abnormal (reduced to 54.3% of normal limit) at distal leg.

Skin biopsy (sweat glands): Sweat gland nerve fiber density was abnormal (reduced to 30.1% of normal limit) at distal leg.

Patient-reported symptoms during testing: Dizziness, brain fog, and loss of vision during the tilt.

Patient-reported symptoms for past 2 weeks:

Lightheadedness or dizziness: Occasionally
Dry eyes or mouth: Occasionally
Pale feet: Occasionally
Cold feet: Occasionally
Reduced sweating: None
Reduced sweating after exercise: None
Increased sweating: None

TABLE 28.1 **RESULTS OF AUTONOMIC TESTING**

Blood pressure evaluation					
Test: Valsalva maneuver					
Pressure [mmHg]	Baseline	Phase 2			Phase 4
		Early	End		
Systolic	108	106	122		
Mean	84	93.3	108.7	n/a	
Diastolic	72	87	102	n/a	

Heart rate evaluation	
Test: Deep breathing	
Results	Norm*
11.4	≥9
Test: Valsalva ratio	
1.61	≥1.36
* adjusted for a gender and age	

(continued)

TABLE 28.1 CONTINUED

Test: Tilt test										
Position		HR [BPM]	Blood pressure [mmHg]		MCA Blood flow velocity [cm/s]				Respiratory frequency [breaths/min]	End tidal CO_2 [mmHg]
			Systolic	Diastolic	Systolic	Mean	Mean drop [%]	Diastolic		
Supine		78	133	89	110	79.3		64	11	44
Tilt [min]	1	86	144	91	91	60.3	24	45	11	44
	2	94	131	93						
	3	94	135	100						
	4	94	146	109						
	5	96	151	109	75	51	35.7	39	19	39
	6	94	142	101						
	7	92	133	95						
	8	93	132	91						
	9	94	130	96						
	10	96	128	92	74	50	36.9	38	16	38
	15									
	20									
	30									
	40									

Sudomotor evaluation - functional

Test: Quantitative sudomotor axon reflex test (QSART)				
Location	Site (l/r)	Latency [min]	Volume [µl]	Norm [µl]*
Forearm				≥0.3
Prox. leg				≥0.23
Distal leg				≥0.23
Foot				≥0.27

* Normative data are adjusted for gender and age of patient.

Test: Electrochemical skin conductance (ESC)				
Location	Left [µS]	Right [µS]	Average [µS/k]	Norm [µS/kg]
Hand	70	74	0.74	≥1.03
Feet	88	87	0.9	≥1.14
Forehead				

For grading uses ESC [µS] adjusted for weight [µS/k].

Small fiber (sensory + sudomotor) evaluation - morphological					
Test: Skin biopsy					
Location	Site (l/r)	Nerve fibers			
		Epidermal*		Sweat glands	
		Density	Norm	Density	Norm
Proximal leg – thigh	Right		≥8.3		≥37.8
Distal leg - calf	Right	3	≥5.525	11	≥36.5
Foot	Right		≥3.11		≥34.8

* Normative data for distal leg are adjusted for gender and age of patient.

QASAT*											
Heart rate		**BP**		**CBFv**		**ET-CO2**		**Sudomotor**			**Total QASAT score**
S. bradycardia	0	Low supine	0	Low supine	0	Low supine	0	QSART			
S. tachycardia	0	High supine	0	High supine	1	High supine	0	ESC	1		
Increase tilt	0	OH	0	Tilt response	8	Tilt low	0				
Decrease tilt	0	OHTN	0	CA	0	Tilt high	0	**Skin biopsy**			17
Deep breathing	0	VM	0	CVR	0			Epidermal	3		
VR	0			VM	0			Sweat gland	4		
Total	0	Total	0	Total	9	Total	0				

*QASAT. See Novak. Quantitative Scale for Grading of Cardiovascular Autonomic Reflex Tests and Small Fibers from Skin Biopsies. *J Neurol Disord* 2015;3:2.

S, supine; Increase tilt, increased response to tilt; Decrease tilt, decreased response to tilt; BP, blood pressure; VM, Valsalva maneuver; CBFv, cerebral blood flow velocity; CA, cerebral autoregulation; MCA, middle cerebral artery; VR, Valsalva ratio; CVR, cerebral vasoreactivity.

Nausea: Occasionally
Diarrhea: None
Constipation: Occasionally
Urinary leaks: None
Erection problems: None
Current pain severity: 4
Aching pain: Occasionally, mild
Allodynia: None
Burning pain: None
Lancinating pain: None
Numbness: Often, severe
Prickling sensation: Often, severe

AUTONOMIC TESTING INTERPRETATION

- Orthostatic cerebral hypoperfusion syndrome (OCHOS), severe.
- Small fiber neuropathy, severe, mixed, length-dependent.
- Supine and orthostatic hypertension.

COMMENT

The tilt test provoked the patient's typical symptoms, including dizziness and brain fog which is consistent with OCHOS (Figure 28.1).[1] CBFv declined by 37%, which is a severe reduction likely resulting in cerebral hypoperfusion. End tidal CO_2 was essentially unchanged during the tilt, and orthostatic hypotension was absent implying that the reduction in CBFv was due to cerebral autoregulatory failure.

Since OCHOS may be due to abnormal vasoconstriction, a trial of calcium channel blockers, which dilate

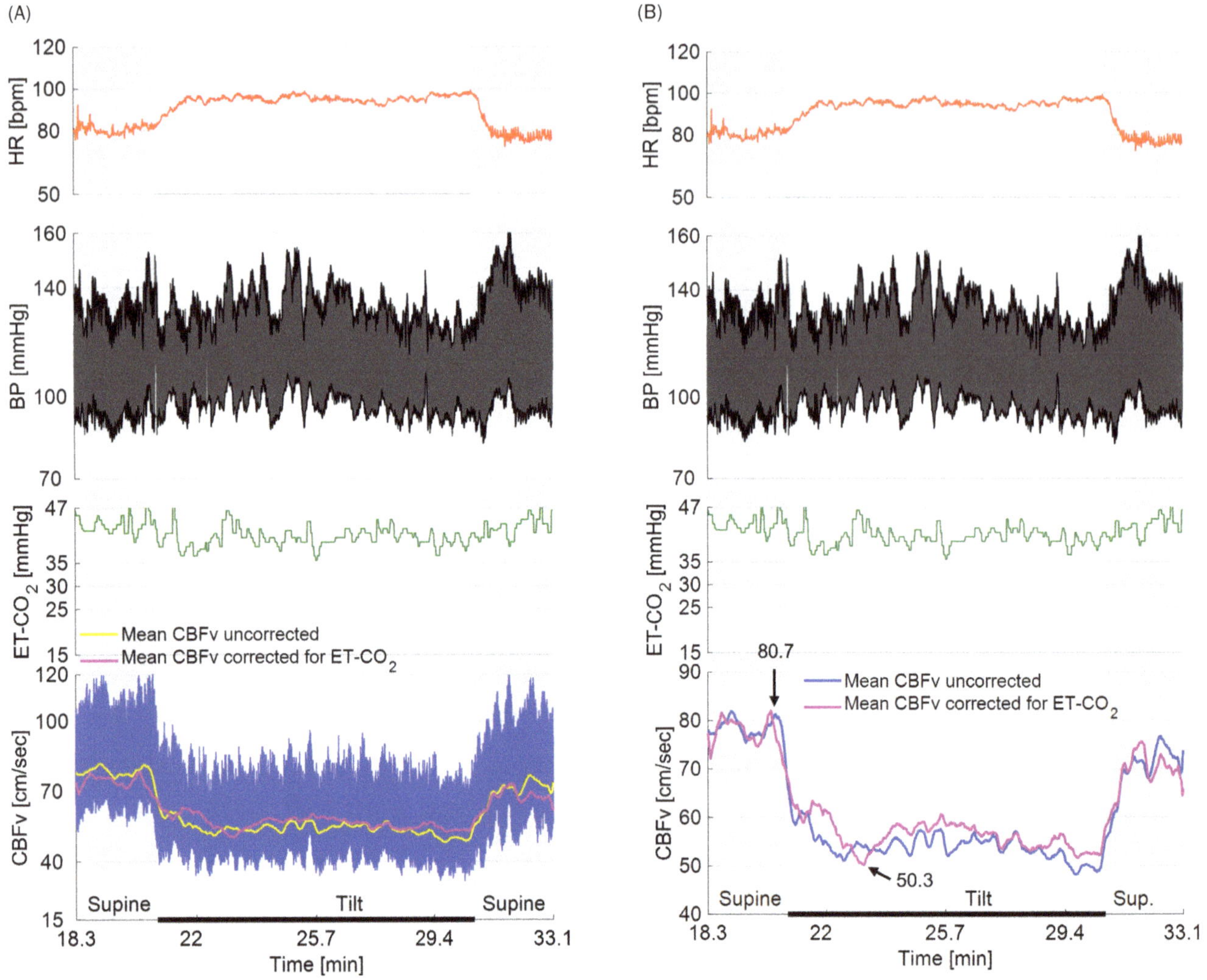

Figure 28.1 The tilt test showed severe reduction in cerebral blood flow velocity (CBFv) throughout the tilt (A, B). The blood pressure and end tidal CO_2 did not decline during the tilt; heart rate responses were also normal.

cerebral vessels, may be tried, particularly in this patient since his blood pressure has been elevated.

TREATMENT AND FOLLOW-UP

- Clinical workup for neuropathy.
- Trial of calcium channel blockers.

CAVEATS

- OCHOS can be a disabling syndrome, as described in this case.

REFERENCE

1. Novak P. Orthostatic cerebral hypoperfusion syndrome. *Front Aging Neurosci.* 2016;8:22. doi:10.3389/fnagi.2016.00022.

29.

CASE 24: ORTHOSTATIC CEREBRAL HYPOPERFUSION SYNDROME WITH VISION LOSS

Chief complaint: Intermittent loss of vision.

Case presentation: A 19-year-old man presents with intermittent vision loss for 2 years. When he stands up quickly or strains, he blacks-out for few seconds. The visual changes are causing considerable discomfort for the patient and his family. Neurological examination was entirely normal. Workup for multiple sclerosis and seizure disorder, including MRI of the brain and electroencephalogram, was unrevealing. He also has several gastrointestinal complaints such as bloating, nausea, stomach discomfort, and multiple food allergies. Extensive gastroenterology testing was unrevealing as well. The patient was referred for evaluation of suspected orthostatic intolerance.

Past medical history: None.

Current medication: None.

Assessment plan: Functional autonomic tests and skin biopsy (since GI symptoms point to involvement of enteric nervous system, which is a division of autonomic nervous system).

AUTONOMIC TESTING EVALUATION

See Table 29.1

Heart rate: Supine heart rate was normal. Heart rate responses to deep breathing were normal. There was mild tachycardia during the tilt.

Blood pressure:

Valsalva maneuver: Blood pressure responses were normal.

Tilt: Supine blood pressure was within normal range. Blood pressure responses to tilt were normal.

Sudomotor evaluation: Electrochemical skin conductance was normal at hands and normal at feet.

Respiratory system: Respiratory frequency and end tidal CO_2 were normal in supine position and during the tilt test.

Cerebral blood flow velocity (CBFv): CBFv in middle cerebral artery was normal in supine position. CBFv in middle cerebral artery was severely reduced during the tilt test.

Skin biopsy (sensory-epidermal): Epidermal nerve fiber density was normal at proximal leg and normal at distal leg.

Skin biopsy (sweat glands): Sweat gland nerve fiber density was normal at proximal leg and abnormal (reduced to 67.9% of normal limit) at distal leg.

Patient-reported symptoms during testing: Loss of vision during the tilt.

Patient-reported symptoms for past 2 weeks:

Lightheadedness or dizziness: Occasionally
Dry eyes or mouth: Occasionally
Pale feet: Occasionally

TABLE 29.1 **RESULTS OF AUTONOMIC TESTING**

Blood pressure evaluation

Test: Valsalva maneuver

Pressure [mmHg]	Baseline	Phase 2			Phase 4
		Early	End		
Systolic	93	87	101		
Mean	75	75	89	n/a	
Diastolic	66	69	83	n/a	

Heart rate evaluation

Test: Deep breathing	
Results	Norm*
21.2	≥14
Test: Valsalva ratio	
1.64	≥1.59

* adjusted for a gender and age

(continued)

Test: Tilt test										
Position		HR [BPM]	Blood pressure [mmHg]		MCA Blood flow velocity [cm/s]				Respiratory frequency [breaths/min]	End tidal CO_2 [mmHg]
			Systolic	Diastolic	Systolic	Mean	Mean drop [%]	Diastolic		
Supine		89	116	77	130	88.7		68	10	36
Tilt [min]	1	103	123	87	108	72.7	18	55	18	35
	2	111	120	86						
	3	110	122	88						
	4	108	117	87						
	5	108	118	84	108	72.7	18	55	16	36
	6	110	117	82						
	7	110	124	86						
	8	108	119	85						
	9	107	117	86						
	10	112	118	82	104	61.3	30.9	40	18	34
	15									
	20									
	30									
	40									

Sudomotor evaluation - functional

Test: Quantitative sudomotor axon reflex test (QSART)				
Location	Site (l/r)	Latency [min]	Volume [µl]	Norm [µl]*
Forearm				≥0.3
Prox. leg				≥0.5
Distal leg				≥0.54
Foot				≥0.34

* Normative data are adjusted for gender and age of patient.

Test: Electrochemical skin conductance (ESC)				
Location	Left [µS]	Right [µS]	Average [µS/k]	Norm [µS/kg]
Hand	82	78	1.41	≥1.03
Feet	94	93	1.64	≥1.14
Forehead				

For grading uses ESC [µS] adjusted for weight [µS/k].

TABLE 29.1 **CONTINUED**

Small fiber (sensory + sudomotor) evaluation - morphological					
Test: Skin biopsy					
Location	Site (l/r)	Nerve fibers			
		Epidermal*		Sweat glands	
		Density	Norm	Density	Norm
Proximal leg – thigh	Right	17.79	≥8.3	39.2	≥37.8
Distal leg - calf	Right	10.33	≥8.075	24.8	≥36.5
Foot	Right		≥3.11		≥34.8

* Normative data for distal leg are adjusted for gender and age of patient.

QASAT*										
Heart rate		**BP**		**CBFv**		**ET-CO2**		**Sudomotor**		**Total QASAT score**
S. bradycardia	0	Low supine	0	Low supine	0	Low supine	0	QSART		
S. tachycardia	0	High supine	0	High supine	0	High supine	0	ESC	0	
Increase tilt	0	OH	0	Tilt response	4	Tilt low	0			
Decrease tilt	0	OHTN	0	CA	0	Tilt high	0	**Skin biopsy**		7
Deep breathing	0	VM	0	CVR	0			Epidermal	0	
VR	0			VM	0			Sweat gland	3	
Total	0	Total	0	Total	4	Total	0			

*QASAT. See Novak. Quantitative Scale for Grading of Cardiovascular Autonomic Reflex Tests and Small Fibers from Skin Biopsies. *J Neurol Disord* 2015;3:2.

S, supine; Increase tilt, increased response to tilt; Decrease tilt, decreased response to tilt; BP, blood pressure; VM, Valsalva maneuver; CBFv, cerebral blood flow velocity; CA, cerebral autoregulation; MCA, middle cerebral artery; VR, Valsalva ratio; CVR, cerebral vasoreactivity.

Cold feet: Often
Reduced sweating: None
Reduced sweating after exercise: None
Increased sweating: None
Nausea: Occasionally
Diarrhea: Occasionally
Constipation: Occasionally
Urinary leaks: None
Erection problems: None
Current pain severity: 8
Aching pain: None
Allodynia: None
Burning pain: Occasionally, mild
Lancinating pain: Occasionally, severe
Numbness: Occasionally, moderate
Prickling sensation: Occasionally, mild

AUTONOMIC TESTING INTERPRETATION

- Orthostatic cerebral hypoperfusion syndrome (OCHOS).
- Small fiber neuropathy, length-dependent, severe, affecting predominantly autonomic sudomotor fibers; biopsy proven.
- Autonomic functions were normal; there was no evidence of orthostatic hypotension or postural tachycardia syndrome (POTS).
- Respiratory functions were normal; there was no evidence of hyperventilation or hypoventilation.

COMMENT

Orthostatic CBFv was reduced without the presence of orthostatic hypotension or hyperventilation that also reduces cerebral blood flow (Figure 29.1). This finding is consistent with OCHOS.[1] The mechanisms leading to OCHOS include abnormal cerebral vasoconstriction due to cerebral autoregulatory failure. The tilt and the Valsalva maneuver provoked the patient's typical visual loss, which correlated with the nadir in CBFv thus supporting the conclusion that the vision loss in this patient is related to cerebral flow changes.

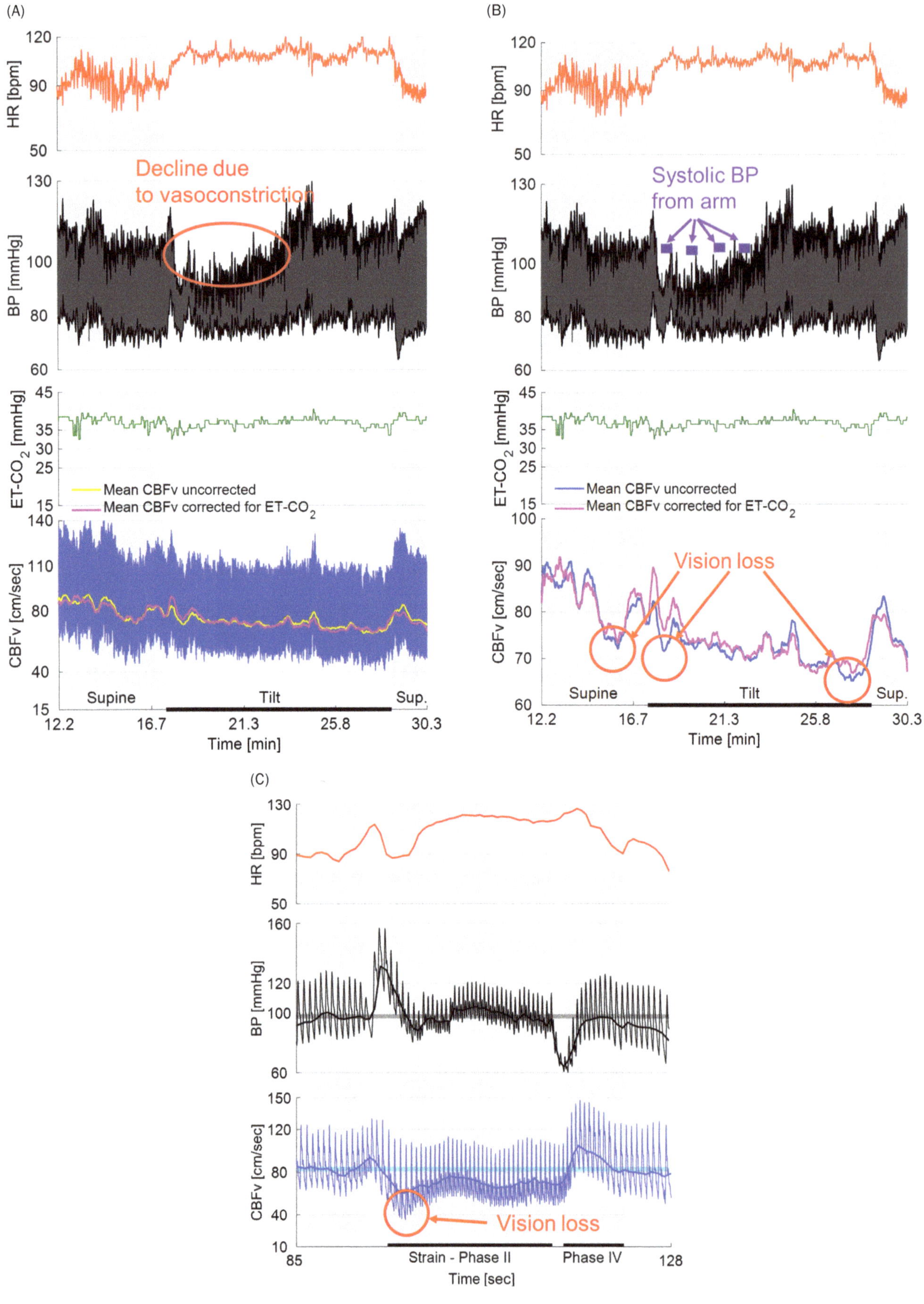

Figure 29.1 The tilt (A, B) showed normal heart rate and blood pressure responses. End tidal CO_2 was also within normal range. Cerebral blood flow velocity (CBFv) was abnormally reduced during the tilt. The tilt provoked patient's typical visual loss three times: at the tilt onset, at minute 2, and at the end of the tilt. The visual changes resolved in seconds and were accompanied by low CBFv. The Valsalva maneuver also reproduced the visual symptoms. Patient experienced visual loss during the nadir of Phase 2 of the Valsalva maneuver (C).

A second major finding of the testing was the presence of abnormal sweat gland nerve fiber density on skin biopsy, which is consistent with small fiber neuropathy affecting autonomic sudomotor fibers. The autonomic small fiber neuropathy may underlie the patient's gastrointestinal complaints.

TREATMENT AND FOLLOW-UP

- Clinical workup for neuropathy.
- Volume expansion through high fluid and high salt intake.

CAVEATS

- Postural visual disturbances may reflect reduced cerebral blood flow without the presence of orthostatic hypotension.
- Gastrointestinal complaints can be related to autonomic small fiber neuropathy.

REFERENCE

1. Novak P. Orthostatic cerebral hypoperfusion syndrome. *Front Aging Neurosci*. 2016;8:22. doi:10.3389/fnagi.2016.00022.

PART V

INAPPROPRIATE SINUS TACHYCARDIA

30.

CASE 25: INAPPROPRIATE SINUS TACHYCARDIA

Chief complaint: Tachycardia.

Case presentation: A 22-year-old woman has a history of rheumatoid arthritis. She initially presented with severe joint pain, burning leg pain, and large joint effusions. She was diagnosed with juvenile rheumatoid arthritis in childhood and was treated with methotrexate, adalimumab, etanercept, hydroxychloroquine, and meloxicam without improvement. Etanercept was discontinued because it greatly exacerbated mild baseline tachycardia and dyspnea. Despite etanercept discontinuation, tachycardia persisted. She had a tilt test at that time (2 years ago), which was normal. For the past few months, she is experiencing progressive worsening of tachycardia with dyspnea. Dyspnea occurs with minimal exertion, even during standing. Her cardiologist noted an excessive heart rate increment during standing and diagnosed postural tachycardia syndrome (POTS). At the time of this testing, she has constant tachycardia, severe leg pain, and dyspnea on minimal exertion. She was referred for evaluation of POTS versus autonomic failure.

Past medical history: POTS, rheumatoid arthritis.

Current medication: Mirtazapine, cyclobenzaprine.

Assessment plan: Functional autonomic tests and skin biopsy.

AUTONOMIC TESTING EVALUATION

See Table 30.1.

Heart rate: Supine tachycardia. Heart rate increment during the tilt (15 BPM) was normal.

Blood pressure:

Valsalva maneuver: Mean blood pressure failed to return to baseline at the end of Phase 2 by 17.4 mm Hg (i.e., 82.7% of baseline).

Tilt: Supine blood pressure was normal. Blood pressure responses to tilt were normal.

Sudomotor evaluation: Electrochemical skin conductance was abnormal (reduced to 92.4% of normal limit) at hands and abnormal (reduced to 77.4% of normal limit) at feet.

Respiratory system: Respiratory frequency was normal in supine position and during the tilt. End tidal CO_2 was reduced in supine position and during the tilt.

Cerebral blood flow velocity (CBFv): CBFv in middle cerebral artery was normal in supine position but was severely reduced during the tilt.

Skin biopsy (sensory-epidermal): Epidermal nerve fiber density was abnormal (reduced to 29.5% of normal

TABLE 30.1 **RESULTS OF AUTONOMIC TESTING**

Blood pressure evaluation					
Test: Valsalva maneuver					
Pressure [mmHg]	Baseline	Phase 2 Early	Phase 2 End		Phase 4
Systolic	126	98	100		
Mean	100.7	79.3	83.3	n/a	
Diastolic	88	70	75	n/a	

Heart rate evaluation	
Test: Deep breathing	
Results	Norm*
10.75	≥14
Test: Valsalva ratio	
1.76	≥1.46
* adjusted for a gender and age	

(continued)

TABLE 30.1 **CONTINUED**

Test: Tilt test										
Position		HR [BPM]	Blood pressure [mmHg]		MCA Blood flow velocity [cm/s]				Respiratory frequency [breaths/min]	End tidal CO_2 [mmHg]
			Systolic	Diastolic	Systolic	Mean	Mean drop [%]	Diastolic		
Supine		117	115	81	108	75.3		59	20	34
Tilt [min]	1	119	118	81	93	62.3	17.3	47	18	28
	2	129	123	86						
	3	132	120	82						
	4	116	123	85						
	5	119	109	75	82	51.3	31.9	36	13	30
	6	115	127	86						
	7	124	120	85						
	8	122	125	88						
	9	122	119	88						
	10	121	120	89	81	51	32.3	36	17	34
	15									
	20									
	30									
	40									

Sudomotor evaluation - functional

Test: Quantitative sudomotor axon reflex test (QSART)				
Location	Site (l/r)	Latency [min]	Volume [µl]	Norm [µl]*
Forearm				≥0.08
Prox. leg				≥0.14
Distal leg				≥0.24
Foot				≥0.09

* Normative data are adjusted for gender and age of patient.

Test: Electrochemical skin conductance (ESC)				
Location	Left [µS]	Right [µS]	Average [µS/k]	Norm [µS/kg]
Hand	86	78	0.95	≥1.03
Feet	77	75	0.87	≥1.14
Forehead				

For grading uses ESC [µS] adjusted for weight [µS/k].

TABLE 30.1 CONTINUED

Small fiber (sensory + sudomotor) evaluation - morphological					
Test: Skin biopsy					
Location	Site (l/r)	Nerve fibers			
		Epidermal*		Sweat glands	
		Density	Norm	Density	Norm
Proximal leg – thigh	Right	2.45	≥8.3		≥37.8
Distal leg - calf	Right	0.9	≥9.26		≥36.5
Foot	Right		≥3.11		≥34.8

* Normative data for distal leg are adjusted for gender and age of patient.

QASAT*										
Heart rate		**BP**		**CBFv**		**ET-CO2**		**Sudomotor**		**Total QASAT score**
S. bradycardia	0	Low supine	0	Low supine	0	Low supine	1	QSART		
S. tachycardia	1	High supine	0	High supine	0	High supine	0	ESC	1	
Increase tilt	0	OH	0	Tilt response	6	Tilt low	2			
Decrease tilt	0	OHTN	0	CA	0	Tilt high	0	**Skin biopsy**		18
Deep breathing	1	VM	2	CVR	0			Epidermal	4	
VR	0			VM	0			Sweat gland		
Total	2	Total	2	Total	6	Total	3			

*QASAT. See Novak. Quantitative Scale for Grading of Cardiovascular Autonomic Reflex Tests and Small Fibers from Skin Biopsies. *J Neurol Disord* 2015;3:2.

S, supine; Increase tilt, increased response to tilt; Decrease tilt, decreased response to tilt; BP, blood pressure; VM, Valsalva maneuver; CBFv, cerebral blood flow velocity; CA, cerebral autoregulation; MCA, middle cerebral artery; VR, Valsalva ratio; CVR, cerebral vasoreactivity.

limit) at proximal leg and abnormal (reduced to 9.7% of normal limit) at distal leg.

Skin biopsy (sweat glands): No sweat glands found on skin specimen

Patient-reported symptoms during testing: Dizziness and shortness of breath during the tilt.

Patient-reported symptoms for past 2 weeks:

Lightheadedness or dizziness: Often
Dry eyes or mouth: Occasionally
Pale feet: Occasionally
Cold feet: Often
Reduced sweating: Occasionally
Reduced sweating after exercise: Occasionally
Increased sweating: Occasionally
Nausea: Often
Diarrhea: Often
Constipation: None
Urinary leaks: Occasionally
Current pain severity: 6
Aching pain: continuous, severe
Allodynia: Often, mild
Burning pain: Often, moderate
Lancinating pain: Often, moderate
Numbness: Often, moderate
Prickling sensation: Often, none

AUTONOMIC TESTING INTERPRETATION

- Inappropriate sinus tachycardia (IST).
- Small fiber neuropathy, severe.

COMMENT

The tilt test was consistent with IST (Figure 30.1) because of supine tachycardia, stable blood pressure, and lack of excessive orthostatic tachycardia.[1] IST is a rare disorder. In IST, the average resting heart rate is elevated above 100 beats per minute, and the tachycardic response to activity is exaggerated.[2] There is symptomatic overlap between IST

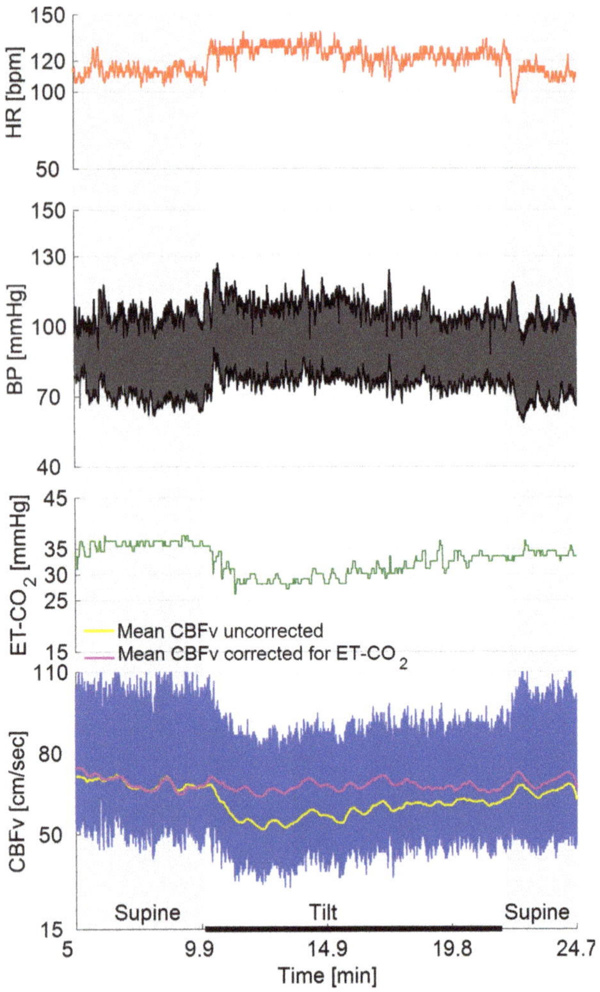

Figure 30.1 The tilt test showed supine tachycardia and normal heart rate increment to tilt. Orthostatic blood pressure was stable. Cerebral blood flow velocity (CBFv) was transiently reduced due to hypocapnia-induced cerebral vasoconstriction since CBFv adjusted for the level of end tidal CO_2 was stable. Blood pressure responses to tilt were normal.

and POTS, but IST can be induced by both physiological and emotional stresses, while POTS is typically induced by orthostatic stress (Figure 30.1).[2] IST may respond to ivabradine, which reduces the high discharge rate in the sinus node and slows down tachycardia.[3]

The patient also has severe small fiber neuropathy due to rheumatoid arthritis.

TREATMENT AND FOLLOW-UP

- Trial of ivabradine.

CAVEATS

- IST is a form of orthostatic intolerance with a presentation similar to POTS.

REFERENCES

1. Novak P. Cerebral blood flow, heart rate, and blood pressure patterns during the tilt test in common orthostatic syndromes. *Neurosci J.* 2016;2016:6127340. doi:10.1155/2016/6127340.
2. Sheldon RS, Grubb BP, Olshansky B, et al. 2015 heart rhythm society expert consensus statement on the diagnosis and treatment of postural tachycardia syndrome, inappropriate sinus tachycardia, and vasovagal syncope. *Heart Rhythm.* 2015;12(6):e41–e63. doi:10.1016/j.hrthm.2015.03.029.
3. Cappato R, Castelvecchio S, Ricci C, et al. Clinical efficacy of ivabradine in patients with inappropriate sinus tachycardia: a prospective, randomized, placebo-controlled, double-blind, crossover evaluation. *J Am Coll Cardiol.* 2012;60(15):1323–1329. doi:10.1016/j.jacc.2012.06.031.

31.

CASE 26: INAPPROPRIATE SINUS TACHYCARDIA AND ORTHOSTATIC CEREBRAL HYPOPERFUSION SYNDROME

Chief complaint: Tachycardia.

Case presentation: A 21-year-old woman presents with severe supine and orthostatic sinus tachycardia (frequently higher than 180 BPM). Since age 10, she experienced various chronic pains including headaches, arthralgia, muscular pain, and distal limb pain. She also complains on postural lightheadedness and mild intermittent right-sided weakness. She has been evaluated by neurology, cardiology, rheumatology, and psychiatry. Inappropriate sinus tachycardia (IST) has been suspected by cardiology. Neurological evaluations were unrevealing. Since no objective findings other than tachycardia were found, most complaints were attributed to somatoform disorder.

Past medical history: Somatoform disorder, chronic daily headaches, sinus tachycardia, atypical chest pain, fibromyalgia, recurrent urinary tract infections, interstitial cystitis, hypertension, asthma, anemia.

Current medication: Nadolol, verapamil, baclofen, gabapentin, amitriptyline, prednisone.

Assessment plan: Functional autonomic tests and skin biopsy

AUTONOMIC TESTING EVALUATION

See Table 31.1.

Heart rate: Supine tachycardia was present. Heart rate responses to deep breathing were reduced to 27.1% of normal value. Heart rate increment during the tilt (27 BPM) was normal.

Blood pressure:

Valsalva maneuver: Blood pressure responses were normal.

Tilt: Supine blood pressure was normal. Blood pressure responses to tilt were normal.

Sudomotor evaluation: Electrochemical skin conductance was abnormal (reduced to 97.4% of normal limit) at hands and normal at feet.

Respiratory system: Respiratory frequency was normal in supine position but was increased during the tilt. End tidal CO_2 was reduced in supine position and during the tilt.

Cerebral blood flow velocity (CBFv): CBFv in middle cerebral artery was normal in supine position but was moderately reduced during the tilt.

Skin biopsy (sensory-epidermal): Epidermal nerve fiber density was abnormal (reduced to 54.3% of normal limit) at proximal leg and normal at distal leg.

TABLE 31.1 **RESULTS OF AUTONOMIC TESTING**

Blood pressure evaluation					
Test: Valsalva maneuver					
Pressure [mmHg]	Baseline	Phase 2			Phase 4
		Early	End		
Systolic	104.8	75.9	112.2		
Mean	79.8	61.2	86.9	n/a	
Diastolic	67.3	53.9	74.21	n/a	

Heart rate evaluation	
Test: Deep breathing	
Results	Norm*
3.8	≥14
Test: Valsalva ratio	
1.72	≥1.46

* adjusted for a gender and age

(continued)

TABLE 31.1 CONTINUED

Test: Tilt test										
Position		HR [BPM]	Blood pressure [mmHg]		MCA Blood flow velocity [cm/s]				Respiratory frequency [breaths/min]	End tidal CO_2 [mmHg]
			Systolic	Diastolic	Systolic	Mean	Mean drop [%]	Diastolic		
Supine		133	120	77	121	77		55	18	27
Tilt [min]	1	151	111	77	90	59.3	23	44	20	25
	2	152	111	77						
	3	152	123	89						
	4	152	119	70						
	5	152	120	84	102	71.3	7.4	56	23	27
	6	158	115	81						
	7	158	115	81						
	8	158	118	86						
	9	158	118	86						
	10	160	114	81	91	61	20.8	46	21	27
	15									
	20									
	30									
	40									

Sudomotor evaluation - functional

Test: Quantitative sudomotor axon reflex test (QSART)				
Location	Site (l/r)	Latency [min]	Volume [µl]	Norm [µl]*
Forearm				≥0.08
Prox. leg				≥0.14
Distal leg				≥0.24
Foot				≥0.09

* Normative data are adjusted for gender and age of patient.

Test: Electrochemical skin conductance (ESC)				
Location	Left [µS]	Right [µS]	Average [µS/k]	Norm [µS/kg]
Hand	48	84	1	≥1.03
Feet	93	93	1.41	≥1.14
Forehead				

For grading uses ESC [µS] adjusted for weight [µS/k].

TABLE 31.1 CONTINUED

Small fiber (sensory + sudomotor) evaluation - morphological					
Test: Skin biopsy					
Location	Site (l/r)	Nerve fibers			
		Epidermal*		Sweat glands	
		Density	Norm	Density	Norm
Proximal leg – thigh	Right	4.51	≥8.3		≥37.8
Distal leg - calf	Right	9.83	≥9.42	37.9	≥36.5
Foot	Right		≥3.11		≥34.8

*Normative data for distal leg are adjusted for gender and age of patient.

QASAT*												
Heart rate		**BP**		**CBFv**		**ET-CO2**		**Sudomotor**			**Total QASAT score**
S. bradycardia	0	Low supine	0	Low supine	0	Low supine	1	QSART			
S. tachycardia	1	High supine	0	High supine	0	High supine	0	ESC	1		
Increase tilt	0	OH	0	Tilt response	3	Tilt low	3				
Decrease tilt	0	OHTN	0	CA	0	Tilt high	0	**Skin biopsy**			15
Deep breathing	3	VM	0	CVR	0			Epidermal	3		
VR	0			VM	0			Sweat gland	0		
Total	4	Total	0	Total	3	Total	4				

*QASAT. See Novak. Quantitative Scale for Grading of Cardiovascular Autonomic Reflex Tests and Small Fibers from Skin Biopsies. *J Neurol Disord* 2015;3:2.

S, supine; Increase tilt, increased response to tilt; Decrease tilt, decreased response to tilt; BP, blood pressure; VM, Valsalva maneuver; CBFv, cerebral blood flow velocity; CA, cerebral autoregulation; MCA, middle cerebral artery; VR, Valsalva ratio; CVR, cerebral vasoreactivity.

Skin biopsy (sweat glands): Sweat gland nerve fiber density was normal at distal leg.

Patient-reported symptoms during testing: Dizziness, shortness of breath during the tilt.

Patient-reported symptoms for past 2 weeks:

Lightheadedness or dizziness: Often
Dry eyes or mouth: Often
Pale feet: Occasionally
Cold feet: Often
Reduced sweating: Occasionally
Reduced sweating after exercise: Occasionally
Increased sweating: Occasionally
Nausea: Often
Diarrhea: Often
Constipation: Occasionally
Urinary leaks: None
Current pain severity: 8
Aching pain: Continuous, severe
Allodynia: Continuous, severe
Burning pain: Continuous, severe
Lancinating pain: Continuous, severe
Numbness: Continuous, severe
Prickling sensation: Continuous, severe

AUTONOMIC TESTING INTERPRETATION

- IST.[1]
- Orthostatic cerebral hypoperfusion syndrome (OCHOS).[2]
- Mild cardiovagal cholinergic impairment.
- Small fiber neuropathy, non–length-dependent, affecting predominantly sensory fibers.

- Hypocapnic hyperventilation in supine position and during the tilt.

COMMENT

The tilt test showed supine and orthostatic tachycardia with normal orthostatic heart rate increment (Figure 31.1). CBFv declined during the tilt, but blood pressure and end tidal CO_2 were low but unchanged during the tilt e.g. end tidal CO_2 did not decline during the tilt. This case represents a diagnostic dilemma: Is this IST, OCHOS, or combination of both? CBFv declined during the tilt due to abnormal cerebral vasoconstriction associated with cerebral autoregulatory failure since both major determinants of CFBv (e.g., blood pressure and end tidal CO_2) were stable during the tilt. This is consistent with OCHOS superimposed on IST. This reasoning assumes that the cardiac output was unchanged during the tilt. Severe tachycardia may reduce cardiac output, but then usually systemic blood pressure also declines, which was not seen in this case.

Reduction of amitriptyline did not improve tachycardia.

TREATMENT AND FOLLOW-UP

- Clinical workup for neuropathy.
- Volume expansion through high fluid and high salt intake.

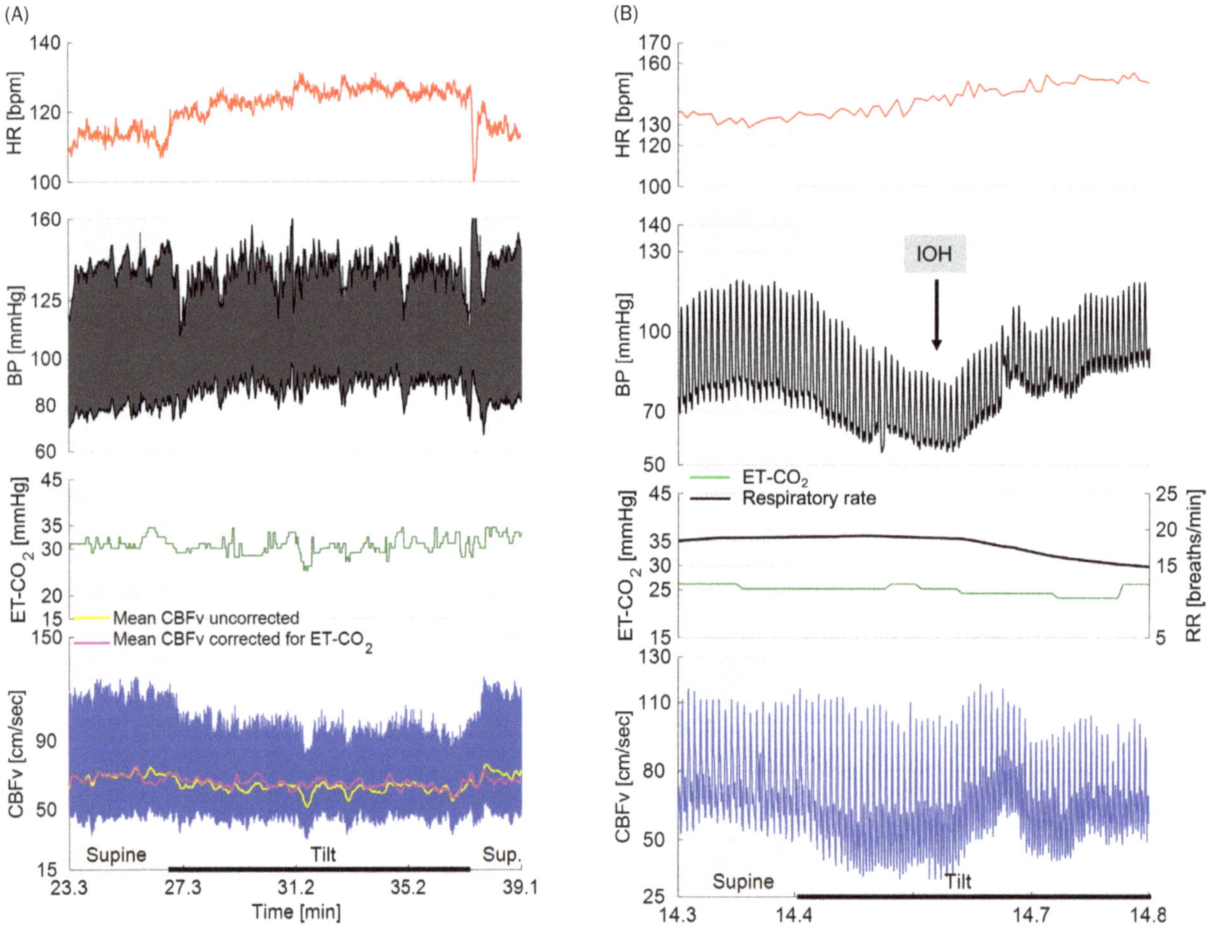

Figure 31.1 The tilt test showed supine and orthostatic tachycardia (A-C) and initial orthostatic hypotension (IOH) accompanied by decline in cerebral blood flow velocity (CBFv, B). After recovery of IOH, there was a gradual decline in CBFv, blood pressure was stable. Patient was anxious, tachypneic (RR>20 breaths/minute) and hyperventilating during the whole test, e.g. during supine position and during the tilt. RR, respiratory rate.

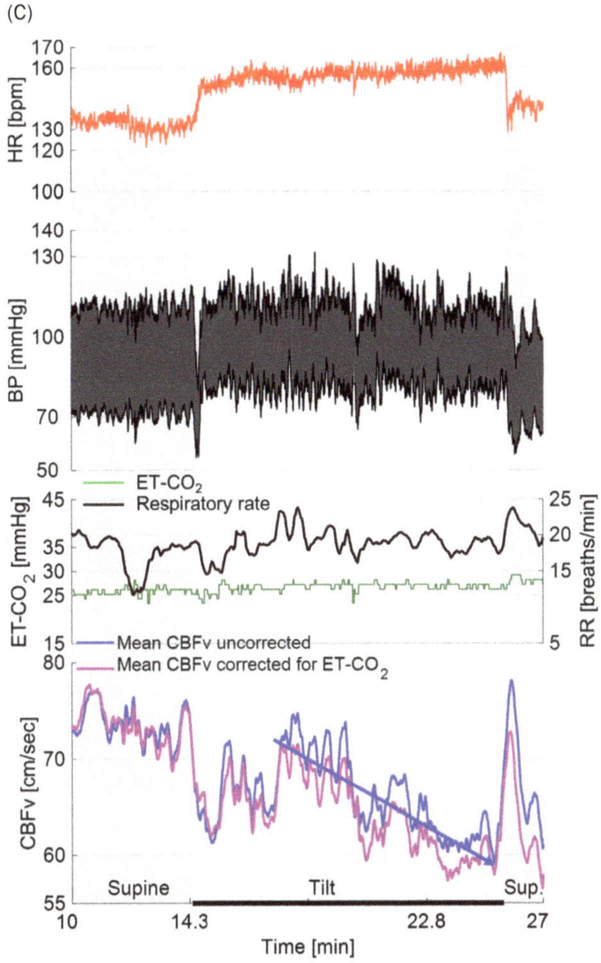

Figure 31.1 Continued

- Titration of verapamil, since in theory it may reduce cerebral vasoconstriction and also may improve tachycardia.
- Trial of ivabradine.[1]

CAVEATS

- IST and OCHOS can coexist.

REFERENCES

1. Cappato R, Castelvecchio S, Ricci C, et al. Clinical efficacy of ivabradine in patients with inappropriate sinus tachycardia: a prospective, randomized, placebo-controlled, double-blind, crossover evaluation. *J Am Coll Cardiol.* 2012;60(15):1323–1329. doi:10.1016/j.jacc.2012.06.031.
2. Novak P. Orthostatic cerebral hypoperfusion syndrome. *Front Aging Neurosci.* 2016;8:22. doi:10.3389/fnagi.2016.00022.

32.

CASE 27: INAPPROPRIATE SINUS TACHYCARDIA VERSUS POSTURAL TACHYCARDIA SYNDROME

Chief complaint: Dizziness.

Case presentation: A 40-year-old woman presents with disabling dizziness. As a child, she had frequently elevated temperature and palpitations. She was also diagnosed with supraventricular tachycardia and mitral valve prolapse. She had ablation 12 years ago with minimal improvement of tachycardia. She markedly deteriorated 2 years ago when she experienced upper respiratory infection. Subsequently, she started to pass out several times per year and noted a drop in blood pressure during standing. She thinks passing out is linked to overheating and exercise. She experienced severe heat intolerance with an increase in temperature every afternoon. Her blood pressure is low in the mornings but may be elevated during the afternoon. She continued to experience fluctuating heart rate: for example, bending forward caused severe bradycardia and standing up is causing tachycardia. She also noted intermittent skin rash, brain fog, and fatigue. She is unable to work.

Autonomic testing at other institution showed postural tachycardia syndrome (POTS). She tried fludrocortisone, propranolol, proamatine, and pyridostigmine and had some but inadequate improvement. She is being treated with intravenous hydration via a peripherally inserted central catheter (PICC line). Her resting heart rate is around 100 BPM on medications. The brain MRI was unrevealing. She was referred for evaluation of autonomic dysfunction and small fiber neuropathy.

Past medical history: Supraventricular tachycardia, POTS.

Current medication: Nortriptyline, ProAmatine, fludrocortisone, propranolol (all medications on hold for five half-lives).

Assessment plan: Functional autonomic tests and skin biopsy.

AUTONOMIC TESTING EVALUATION

See Table 32.1.

Heart rate: Supine tachycardia. Heart rate increment during the tilt (27 BPM) was normal.

Blood pressure:

Valsalva maneuver: Blood pressure responses were normal. Supine blood pressure was elevated.

Tilt: Blood pressure responses to tilt were normal.

Sudomotor evaluation: Electrochemical skin conductance was abnormal (reduced to 61.7% of normal limit) at hands and abnormal (reduced to 93% of normal limit) at feet.

Respiratory system: Respiratory frequency was normal in supine position and during the tilt. End tidal CO_2 was reduced in supine position and during the tilt.

TABLE 32.1 RESULTS OF AUTONOMIC TESTING

Blood pressure evaluation

Test: Valsalva maneuver

Pressure [mmHg]	Baseline	Phase 2			Phase 4
		Early	End		
Systolic	129	105	123		
Mean	91.7	83	101	n/a	
Diastolic	73	72	90	n/a	

Heart rate evaluation

Test: Deep breathing	
Results	Norm*
5.75	≥10
Test: Valsalva ratio	
1.97	≥1.51

* adjusted for a gender and age

TABLE 32.1 CONTINUED

Test: Tilt test											
Position		HR [BPM]	Blood pressure [mmHg]		MCA Blood flow velocity [cm/s]				Respiratory frequency [breaths/min]	End tidal CO_2 [mmHg]
			Systolic	Diastolic	Systolic	Mean	Mean drop [%]	Diastolic		
Supine		107	147	85	115	70.3		48	17	32
Tilt [min]	1	122	135	84	103	67	4.7	49	13	31
	2	122	131	83						
	3	122	149	94						
	4	122	131	83						
	5	125	133	85	93	61	13.2	45	14	29
	6	125	132	92						
	7	127	132	86						
	8	126	133	91						
	9	129	129	84						
	10	125	135	90	92	60	14.7	44	12	29
	15									
	20									
	30									
	40									

Sudomotor evaluation - functional

Test: Quantitative sudomotor axon reflex test (QSART)				
Location	Site (l/r)	Latency [min]	Volume [µl]	Norm [µl]*
Forearm				≥0.08
Prox. leg				≥0.14
Distal leg				≥0.15
Foot				≥0.07

* Normative data are adjusted for gender and age of patient.

Test: Electrochemical skin conductance (ESC)				
Location	Left [µS]	Right [µS]	Average [µS/k]	Norm [µS/kg]
Hand	48	43	0.64	≥1.03
Feet	76	75	1.06	≥1.14
Forehead				

For grading uses ESC [µS] adjusted for weight [µS/k].

(continued)

Small fiber (sensory + sudomotor) evaluation - morphological					
Test: Skin biopsy					
Location	Site (l/r)	Nerve fibers			
		Epidermal*		Sweat glands	
		Density	Norm	Density	Norm
Proximal leg – thigh	Right	7.23	≥8.3		≥37.8
Distal leg - calf	Right	6.57	≥7.9	13.5	≥36.5
Foot	Right		≥3.11		≥34.8

*normative data for distal leg are adjusted for a gender and age of a patient

QASAT*											
Heart rate		**BP**		**CBFv**		ET-CO_2		**Sudomotor**			**Total QASAT score**
S. bradycardia	0	Low supine	0	0		Low supine	1	QSART			
S. tachycardia	1	High supine	1	High supine	0	High supine		ESC	2		
Increase tilt	0	OH	0	2		Tilt low	2				
Decrease tilt	0	OHTN	0	CA	0	Tilt high	0	**Skin biopsy**			16
Deep breathing	1	VM	0	CVR	0			Epidermal	2		
VR	0			VM	0			Sweat gland	4		
Total	2	Total	1	Total	2	Total	3				

*QASAT. See Novak. Quantitative Scale for Grading of Cardiovascular Autonomic Reflex Tests and Small Fibers from Skin Biopsies. *J Neurol Disord* 2015;3:2.

S, supine; Increase tilt, increased response to tilt; Decrease tilt, decreased response to tilt; BP, blood pressure; VM, Valsalva maneuver; CBFv, cerebral blood flow velocity; CA, cerebral autoregulation; MCA, middle cerebral artery; VR, Valsalva ratio; CVR, cerebral vasoreactivity.

Cerebral blood flow velocity (CBFv): CBFv in middle cerebral artery was normal in supine position but was reduced during the tilt.

Skin biopsy (sensory-epidermal): Epidermal nerve fiber density was abnormal (reduced to 87.1% of normal limit) at proximal leg and abnormal (reduced to 83.2% of normal limit) at distal leg.

Skin biopsy (sweat glands): Sweat gland nerve fiber density was abnormal (reduced to 37% of normal limit) at distal leg.

Patient-reported symptoms during testing: Dizziness during the tilt.

Patient-reported symptoms for past 2 weeks:

Lightheadedness or dizziness: Occasionally
Dry eyes or mouth: Occasionally
Pale feet: None
Cold feet: None
Reduced sweating: Occasionally
Reduced sweating after exercise: Occasionally
Increased sweating: None
Nausea: None
Diarrhea: None
Constipation: Occasionally
Urinary leaks: Occasionally
Current pain severity: 0
Aching pain: None
Allodynia: None
Burning pain: None
Lancinating pain: None
Numbness: None
Prickling sensation: Occasionally, none

AUTONOMIC TESTING INTERPRETATION

- Inappropriate sinus tachycardia (IST).
- Orthostatic cerebral hypoperfusion syndrome (OCHOS).
- Hypocapnic hyperventilation during the supine position and during the tilt.
- Small fiber neuropathy, mixed, affecting sensory and sudomotor fibers.

COMMENT

The patient experienced symptoms of tachycardia and lightheadedness during the tilt, which was consistent with IST and OCHOS (Figure 32.1). The indwelling intravenous catheter could be replaced with high salt and fluid oral intake because of risk of infection. Twenty-four-hour blood pressure monitoring would be helpful to determine whether the diurnal pattern blood pressure variation is normal (lower in the morning, higher in the afternoons) or exaggerated.[1] In IST, ablation/modification achieves acute relief in majority of patients, but symptomatic relief decreases substantially with long-term follow-up, with a recurrence rate of 19.6%, and 29.8% of patients require antiarrhythmic therapy.[2,3]

This patient failed multiple medications for orthostatic intolerance. In theory, the patient may benefit from calcium channel blockers, which are cerebral vasodilators[4] and may improve OCHOS as well as tachycardia via the baroreflex response. Alternatively, lisinopril may be beneficial since it reduces cerebrovascular resistance and improves CBFv in hypertension.[5]

TREATMENT AND FOLLOW-UP

- Clinical workup for neuropathy
- Oral volume expansion through high fluid and high salt intake, which may reduce the need for intravenous hydration.
- Twenty-four-hour ambulatory blood pressure monitoring and antihypertensive therapy.
- Trial of verapamil or other calcium channel blockers; if ineffective, consider lisinopril.

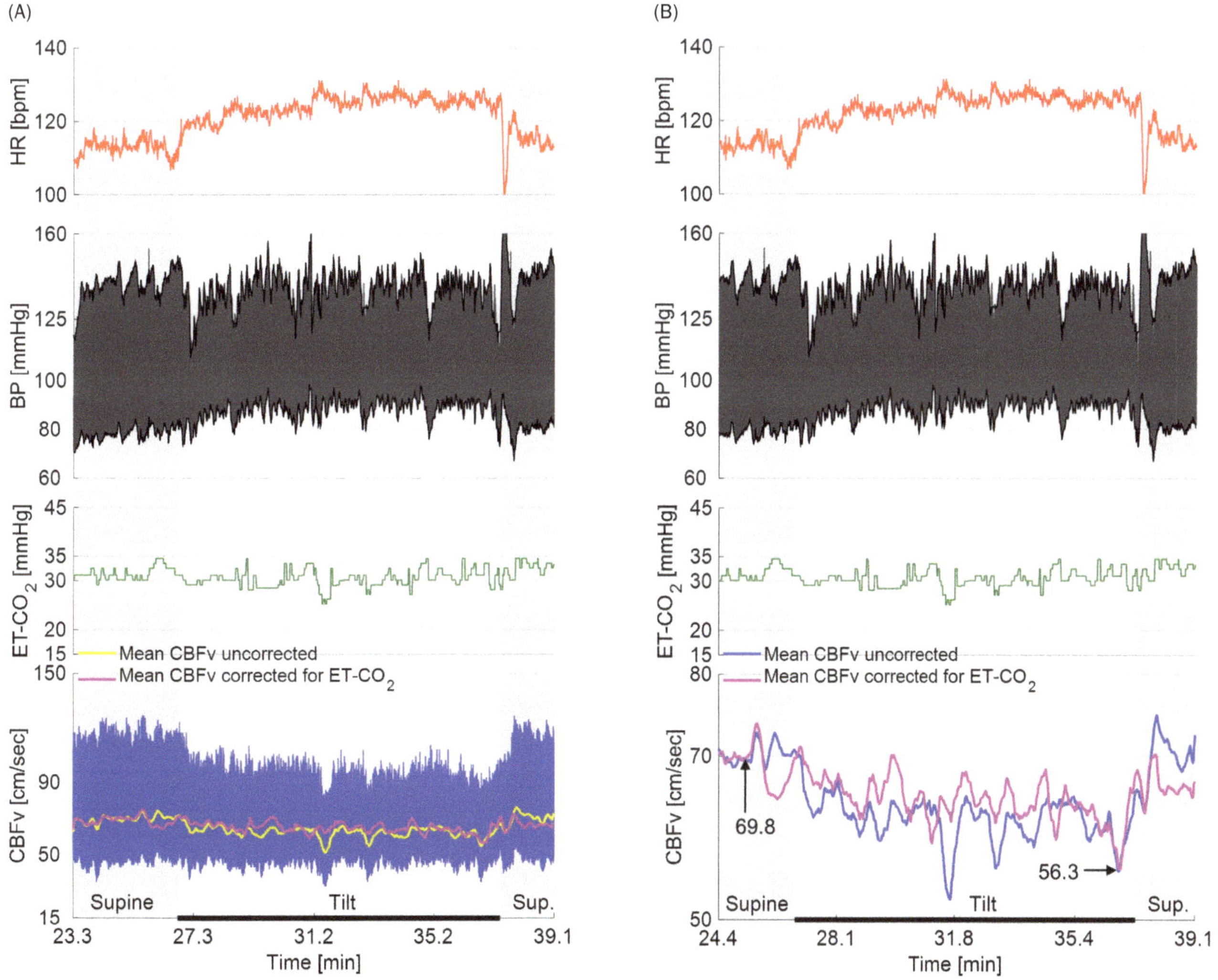

Figure 32.1 The tilt test showed supine and orthostatic tachycardia, supine and orthostatic hypocapnia and supine hypertension. Orthostatic cerebral blood flow velocity (CBFv) declined without worsening of supine hyperventilation and orthostatic hypotension (B) which is consistent with orthostatic cerebral hypoperfusion syndrome (OCHOS). Although end tidal CO_2 was mildly reduced in both supine and during the tilt, it was stable during the tilt (e.g. orthostatic end tidal CO_2 was not reduced) and therefore uncorrected and corrected CBFv are similar. The latter fact implies that decline in CBFv is not due to decline in end tidal CO_2 which is characteristic for OCHOS. The decline in orthostatic end tidal CO_2 and related decline in CBFv is seen in hypocapnic cerebral hypoperfusion (HYCH).

CAVEATS

- IST can be comorbid with OCHOS.

REFERENCES

1. Ernst ME, Bergus GR. Noninvasive 24-hour ambulatory blood pressure monitoring: overview of technology and clinical applications. *Pharmacotherapy*. 2002;22(5):597–612.
2. Rodríguez-Mañero M, Kreidieh B, Al Rifai M, et al. Ablation of inappropriate sinus tachycardia: a systematic review of the literature. *JACC Clin Electrophysiol*. 2017;3(3):253–265. doi:10.1016/j.jacep.2016.09.014.
3. Ibarra-Cortez SH, Rodríguez-Mañero M, Kreidieh B, Schurmann P, Dave AS, Valderrábano M. Strategies for phrenic nerve preservation during ablation of inappropriate sinus tachycardia. *Heart Rhythm*. 2016;13(6):1238–1245. doi:10.1016/j.hrthm.2016.01.021.
4. Lavine SD, Wang M, Etu JJ, Meyers PM, Joshi S. Augmentation of cerebral blood flow and reversal of endothelin-1-induced vasospasm: a comparison of intracarotid nicardipine and verapamil. *Neurosurgery*. 2007;60(4):742–748; discussion 748–749. doi:10.1227/01.NEU.0000255404.30904.CE.
5. Lipsitz LA, Gagnon M, Vyas M, et al. Antihypertensive therapy increases cerebral blood flow and carotid distensibility in hypertensive elderly subjects. *Hypertens Dallas Tex 1979*. 2005;45(2):216–221. doi:10.1161/01.HYP.0000153094.09615.11.

33.

CASE 28: POSTURAL TACHYCARDIA SYNDROME WITH REVERSE TILT TEST

Chief complaint: Disabling tachycardia.

Case presentation: A 19-year-old woman presents for evaluation of dizziness. She had a cerebrovascular accident as a newborn and seizures started at age 2 weeks. According to the patient, she easily becomes dehydrated. At age 14, she began to experience postural dizziness associated with darkening of vision, insomnia, and dream-like states. Head movement triggered spinning. She had pneumonia 3 years ago, Lyme disease 4 years ago. For past 2 years, she noted chronic fatigue, postural dizziness, food-induced abdominal pain and bloating, chest pain, palpitations, and shortness of breath. She was tachycardic at the office, both at supine and standing. She was referred for evaluation of postural tachycardia syndrome (POTS) versus inappropriate sinus tachycardia (IST).

Past medical history: Migraine, cerebrovascular accident, seizures, pneumonia, Lyme disease.

Current medication: Sumatriptan.

Assessment plan: Functional autonomic tests and skin biopsy.

AUTONOMIC TESTING EVALUATION

See Table 33.1.

Heart rate: There was supine tachycardia. Heart rate increment during the tilt (59 BPM) was exaggerated and exceeded 170 BPM.

Blood pressure:

Valsalva maneuver: Mean blood pressure failed to return to baseline at the end of Phase 2 by 40 mm Hg (i.e., 62.5% of baseline).

Tilt: Supine blood pressure was normal. Blood pressure responses to tilt were normal.

Sudomotor evaluation: Electrochemical skin conductance was normal at hands and normal at feet.

Respiratory system: Respiratory frequency was normal in supine position and during the tilt. End tidal CO_2 was normal in supine position but was mildly reduced during the tilt.

Cerebral blood flow velocity (CBFv): CBFv in middle cerebral artery was normal in supine position but was severely reduced during the tilt.

Skin biopsy (sensory-epidermal): Epidermal nerve fiber density was abnormal (reduced to 89.2% of normal limit) at proximal leg and abnormal (reduced to 2.8% of normal limit) at distal leg.

Skin biopsy (sweat glands): N/A

Patient-reported symptoms during testing: Dizziness, shortness of breath during the tilt.

Patient-reported symptoms for past 2 weeks:

Lightheadedness or dizziness: Often
Dry eyes or mouth: None
Pale feet: Occasionally
Cold feet: Occasionally
Reduced sweating: None

TABLE 33.1 **RESULTS OF AUTONOMIC TESTING**

Blood pressure evaluation					
Test: Valsalva maneuver					
Pressure [mmHg]	Baseline	Phase 2			Phase 4
		Early	End		
Systolic	136	74	74		
Mean	106.7	66.7	66.7	n/a	
Diastolic	92	63	63	n/a	

Heart rate evaluation	
Test: Deep breathing	
Results	Norm*
9.5	≥14
Test: Valsalva ratio	
1.53	≥1.46

* adjusted for a gender and age

(continued)

TABLE 33.1 **CONTINUED**

Test: Tilt test											
Position		HR [BPM]	Blood pressure [mmHg]		MCA Blood flow velocity [cm/s]				Respiratory frequency [breaths/min]	End tidal CO_2 [mmHg]
			Systolic	Diastolic	Systolic	Mean	Mean drop [%]	Diastolic		
Supine		120	115	82	129	95.7		79	14	36
Tilt [min]	1	154	118	83	113	70.3	26.5	49	12	31
	2	158	116	81						
	3	158	105	76						
	4	163	112	80						
	5	164	114	78	109	68.3	28.6	48	15	32
	6	169	114	78						
	7	174	112	80						
	8	173	108	76						
	9	179	107	76						
	10	172	107	76	94	54	43.6	34	9	27
	15									
	20									
	30									
	40									

Sudomotor evaluation - functional

Test: Quantitative sudomotor axon reflex test (QSART)				
Location	Site (l/r)	Latency [min]	Volume [μl]	Norm [μl]*
Forearm				≥
Prox. leg				≥
Distal leg				≥
Foot				≥

* Normative data are adjusted for gender and age of patient.

Test: Electrochemical skin conductance (ESC)				
Location	Left [μS]	Right [μS]	Average [μS/k]	Norm [μS/kg]
Hand	87	82	1.79	≥1.03
Feet	89	86	1.83	≥1.14
Forehead				

For grading uses ESC [μS] adjusted for weight [μS/k].

Small fiber (sensory + sudomotor) evaluation - morphological					
Test: Skin biopsy					
Location	Site (l/r)	Nerve fibers			
		Epidermal*		Sweat glands	
		Density	Norm	Density	Norm
Proximal leg – thigh	Right	7.4	≥8.3		≥37.8
Distal leg - calf	Right	0.27	≥9.58		≥36.5
Foot	Right		≥3.11		≥34.8

*Normative data for distal leg are adjusted for gender and age of patient.

QASAT*										
Heart rate		BP		CBFv		ET-CO2		Sudomotor		Total QASAT score
S. bradycardia	1	Low supine	0	Low supine	0	Low supine	1	QSART		
S. tachycardia	0	High supine	0	High supine	0	High supine	0	ESC	0	
Increase tilt	10	OH	0	Tilt response	7	Tilt low	2			
Decrease tilt	0	OHTN	0	CA	0	Tilt high	0	**Skin biopsy**		28
Deep breathing	1	VM	2	CVR	0			Epidermal	4	
VR	0			VM	0			Sweat gland		
Total	12	Total	2	Total	7	Total	3			

*QASAT. See Novak. Quantitative Scale for Grading of Cardiovascular Autonomic Reflex Tests and Small Fibers from Skin Biopsies. *J Neurol Disord* 2015;3:2.

S, supine; Increase tilt, increased response to tilt; Decrease tilt, decreased response to tilt; BP, blood pressure; VM, Valsalva maneuver; CBFv, cerebral blood flow velocity; CA, cerebral autoregulation; MCA, middle cerebral artery; VR, Valsalva ratio; CVR, cerebral vasoreactivity.

Reduced sweating after exercise: None
Increased sweating: Occasionally
Nausea: Often
Diarrhea: None
Constipation: None
Urinary leaks: None
Current pain severity: 4
Aching pain: Continuous, severe
Allodynia: Occasionally, mild
Burning pain: Occasionally, moderate
Lancinating pain: Often, severe
Numbness: Often, moderate
Prickling sensation: Often, moderate

AUTONOMIC TESTING INTERPRETATION

- Small fiber neuropathy, severe, length-dependent, affecting sensory fibers.
- Severe postural tachycardia syndrome (POTS). There was also evidence of mild autonomic dysfunction.
- Orthostatic cerebral blood flow was abnormal and was reduced by 43%, which was associated with hypocapnia without orthostatic hypotension.
- Hypocapnic hyperventilation the during the tilt.

COMMENT

The tilt test showed severe POTS because the heart rate increment to the tilt was exaggerated (Figure 33.1). The decline in orthostatic CBFv was driven by a decline in end tidal CO_2 since hypocapnia induces cerebral vasoconstriction and reduces cerebral blood flow (Figure 33.1). The orthostatic CBFv was markedly reduced to the level that can cause syncope in some subjects.

The cause of hypocapnia in syndromes of orthostatic intolerance is poorly understood. To differentiate between psychological causes (e.g., due to anxiety) versus physiological causes, the reverse tilt was performed. The assumption was that if the orthostatic hyperventilation was due to anxiety, the patient would be as anxious if not more so during the head-down tilt. However, during the head-down tilt,

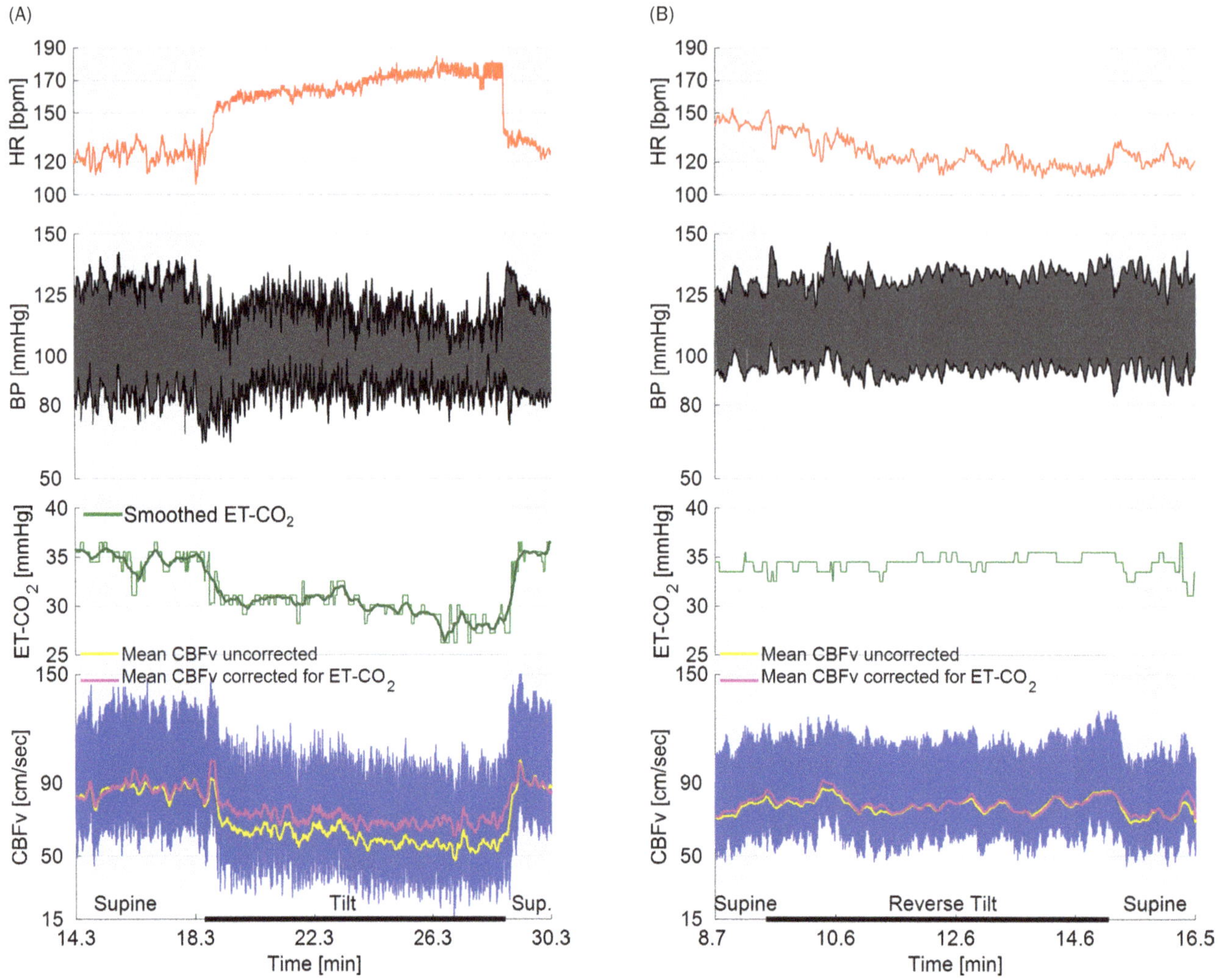

Figure 33.1 The tilt test showed supine tachycardia and exaggerated heat rate response to tilt (A). Blood pressure was stable. End tidal CO_2 and cerebral blood flow velocity (CBFv) were reduced during the tilt. Reverse tilt (head down tilt) showed improvement of tachycardia from 150 BPM to 120 BPM, normal CBFv and stable end tidal CO_2 (B). Symptoms of orthostatic intolerance were absent during the reverse tilt.

end tidal CO_2 did not decline and CBFv remained constant, indicating that anxiety did not play a role in orthostatic hyperventilation. Furthermore, the patient felt subjectively much better during the reverse tilt: there was no dizziness and severe orthostatic shortness of breath disappeared.

She is being treated with sumatriptan for her headaches, which may further affect regulation of cerebral perfusion.[1] Sumatriptan can also cause hyperventilation.[2]

TREATMENT AND FOLLOW-UP

- Clinical workup for neuropathy.
- Volume expansion through high fluid and high salt intake.
- Discontinue sumatriptan.

CAVEATS

- Reverse tilt may differentiate between psychogenic and physiologic hypocapnia.
- Hyperventilation in POTS may be due to physiological mechanisms in certain patients.

REFERENCES

1. Benemei S, Cortese F, Labastida-Ramírez A, et al. Triptans and CGRP blockade—impact on the cranial vasculature. *J Headache Pain*. 2017;18(1):103. doi:10.1186/s10194-017-0811-5.
2. Will you have hyperventilation with sumatriptan—from FDA reports—eHealthMe. https://www.ehealthme.com/ds/sumatriptan/hyperventilation/. Accessed July 2, 2018.

PART VI

HYPOCAPNIC CEREBRAL HYPOPERFUSION

34.

CASE 29: HYPOCAPNIC CEREBRAL HYPOPERFUSION

Chief complaint: Fatigue.

Case presentation: A 40-year-old women presents with extreme fatigue for several years. She sleeps sometimes 3–4 days in a row. She also notes intermittent tachycardia with little exertion that worsens with standing and improves with lying down. She feels too hot and dizzy when standing. She has purple skin at feet with prolonged standing. She was referred for evaluation of orthostatic intolerance.

Past medical history: Migraine, anxiety.

Current medication: Fluoxetine, topiramate, diazepam, levothyroxine, quetiapine, gabapentin, ibuprofen, multivitamins.

Assessment plan: Functional autonomic tests and skin biopsy.

AUTONOMIC TESTING EVALUATION

See Table 34.1.

Heart rate: Supine heart rate was normal. Heart rate responses to deep breathing were reduced to 80% of normal value. Heart rate increment during the tilt (24 BPM) was normal (Figure 34.1).

Blood pressure:

Valsalva maneuver: Mean blood pressure failed to return to baseline at the end of Phase 2 by 11.3 mm Hg (i.e., 83.9% of baseline).

Tilt: Supine blood pressure was normal. Blood pressure responses to tilt were normal.

Sudomotor evaluation: Electrochemical skin conductance was abnormal (reduced to 91.7% of normal limit) at hands and normal at feet.

Respiratory system: Respiratory frequency was normal in supine position and during the tilt. End tidal CO_2 was reduced in supine position and was further reduced during the tilt.

Cerebral blood flow velocity (CBFv): CBFv in middle cerebral artery was normal in supine position but was severely reduced during the tilt.

Skin biopsy (sensory-epidermal): Epidermal nerve fiber density was normal at proximal leg and normal at distal leg.

Skin biopsy (sweat glands): Sweat gland nerve fiber density was abnormal (reduced to 88.2% of normal limit) at distal leg.

Patient-reported symptoms during testing: Dizziness, shortness of breath during the tilt.

Patient-reported symptoms for past 2 weeks:

Lightheadedness or dizziness: Occasionally
Dry eyes or mouth: Occasionally
Pale feet: None
Cold feet: Often
Reduced sweating: Occasionally
Reduced sweating after exercise: None

TABLE 34.1 RESULTS OF AUTONOMIC TESTING

Blood pressure evaluation					
Test: Valsalva maneuver					
Pressure [mmHg]	Baseline	Phase 2			Phase 4
		Early	End		
Systolic	91	74	75		
Mean	70.3	58	59	n/a	
Diastolic	60	50	51	n/a	

Heart rate evaluation	
Test: Deep breathing	
Results	Norm*
8	≥10
Test: Valsalva ratio	
1.24	≥1.51
* adjusted for a gender and age	

(continued)

Test: Tilt test										
Position		HR [BPM]	Blood pressure [mmHg]		MCA Blood flow velocity [cm/s]				Respiratory frequency [breaths/min]	End tidal CO_2 [mmHg]
			Systolic	Diastolic	Systolic	Mean	Mean drop [%]	Diastolic		
Supine		84	105	72	117	69		45	12	29
Tilt [min]	1	97	107	72	86	54	21.7	38	14	19
	2	104	113	80						
	3	108	112	78						
	4	108	112	78						
	5	103	97	70	91	53.7	22.2	35	15	15
	6	95	107	75						
	7	98	111	79						
	8	91	112	77						
	9	92	114	80						
	10	87	109	77	90	52.7	23.6	34	15	22
	15									
	20									
	30									
	40									

Sudomotor evaluation - functional

Test: Quantitative sudomotor axon reflex test (QSART)				
Location	Site (l/r)	Latency [min]	Volume [µl]	Norm [µl]*
Forearm				≥0.08
Prox. leg				≥0.14
Distal leg				≥0.15
Foot				≥0.07

* Normative data are adjusted for gender and age of patient.

Test: Electrochemical skin conductance (ESC)				
Location	Left [µS]	Right [µS]	Average [µS/k]	Norm [µS/kg]
Hand	63	58	0.94	≥1.03
Feet	79	77	1.21	≥1.14
Forehead				

For grading uses ESC [µS] adjusted for weight [µS/k].

TABLE 34.1 CONTINUED

Small fiber (sensory + sudomotor) evaluation - morphological					
Test: Skin biopsy					
Location	Site (l/r)	Nerve fibers			
		Epidermal*		Sweat glands	
		Density	Norm	Density	Norm
Proximal leg – thigh	Right	10.12	≥8.3		≥37.8
Distal leg - calf	Right	8.93	≥7.9	32.2	≥36.5
Foot	Right		≥3.11		≥34.8

*Normative data for distal leg are adjusted for gender and age of patient.

QASAT*											
Heart rate		**BP**		**CBFv**		**ET-CO2**		**Sudomotor**			**Total QASAT score**
S. bradycardia	0	Low supine	0	Low supine	0	Low supine	1	QSART			
S. tachycardia	0	High supine	0	High supine	0	High supine	0	ESC	1		
Increase tilt	0	OH	0	Tilt respons.	6	Tilt low	8				
Decrease tilt	0	OHTN	0	CA	0	Tilt high	0	**Skin biopsy**			21
Deep breathing	1	VM	2	CVR	0			Epidermal	0		
VR	1			VM	0			Sweat gland	1		
Total	2	Total	2	Total	6	Total	9				

*QASAT. See Novak. Quantitative Scale for Grading of Cardiovascular Autonomic Reflex Tests and Small Fibers from Skin Biopsies. *J Neurol Disord* 2015;3:2.

S, supine; Increase tilt, increased response to tilt; Decrease tilt, decreased response to tilt; BP, blood pressure; VM, Valsalva maneuver; CBFv, cerebral blood flow velocity; CA, cerebral autoregulation; MCA, middle cerebral artery; VR, Valsalva ratio; CVR, cerebral vasoreactivity.

Increased sweating: None
Nausea: Occasionally
Diarrhea: None
Constipation: Occasionally
Urinary leaks: None
Current pain severity: 3
Aching pain: Occasionally, mild
Allodynia: Occasionally, mild
Burning pain: None
Lancinating pain: Occasionally, moderate
Numbness: None
Prickling sensation: Often, moderate

AUTONOMIC TESTING INTERPRETATION

- Hypocapnic cerebral hypoperfusion (HYCH).[1]
- Small fiber neuropathy affecting predominantly autonomic fibers associated with mild autonomic dysfunction.

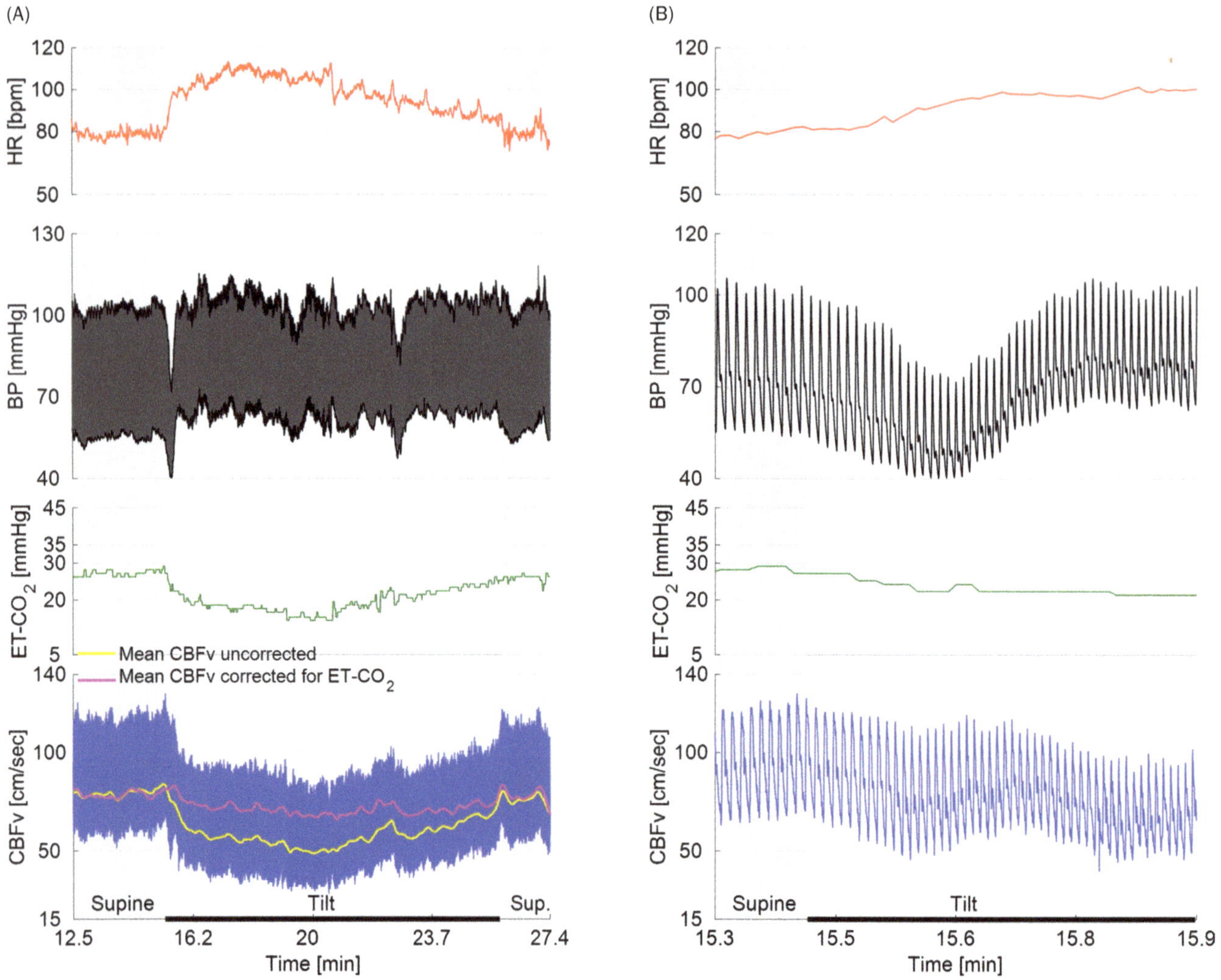

Figure 34.1 The tilt test provoked decline in cerebral blood flow velocity (CBFv) associated with decline in end tidal CO_2 (A). Heart rate and blood pressure responses to tilt were normal Patient was minimally short of breath at supine but she complained on severe shortness of breath during the tilt. Initially, blood pressure declined with the tilt up but recovered within the first minute (B).

COMMENT

The testing showed characteristic HYCH (Figure 34.1). CBFv monitoring is necessary to detect abnormality in patients with orthostatic intolerance without postural tachycardia.

TREATMENT AND FOLLOW-UP

- Clinical workup for neuropathy.
- Volume expansion through high fluid and high salt intake.

CAVEATS

- HYCH is associated with orthostatic intolerance.
- HYCH is POTS without the "T."

REFERENCE

1. Novak P. Hypocapnic cerebral hypoperfusion: A biomarker of orthostatic intolerance. *PloS One*. 2018;13(9):e0204419. doi:10.1371/journal.pone.0204419

35.

CASE 30: HYPOCAPNIC CEREBRAL HYPOPERFUSION WITH PACED BREATHING

Chief complaint: Dizziness.

Case presentation: A 32-year-old woman presents with unexplained, usually orthostatic dizziness for 3 years. She also experienced shortness of breath and chest tightness. Shortness of breath is the most distressing problem. Pulmonary evaluations including computed tomography (CT) of the chest, pulmonary, and function tests were normal. Patient was referred for evaluation of autonomic functions.

Past medical history: Traumatic brain injury 3 years ago, low vitamin D, migraine, pneumonia, sinus infections, chronic fatigue syndrome.

Current medication: Naproxen, gabapentin.

Assessment plan: Functional autonomic tests.

AUTONOMIC TESTING EVALUATION

See Table 35.1.

Heart rate: Supine heart rate was normal. Heart rate responses to deep breathing were normal. Heart rate increment during the tilt (18 BPM) was normal.

Blood pressure:

Valsalva maneuver: Mean blood pressure failed to return to baseline at the end of Phase 2 by 0.4 mm Hg (i.e., 99.5% of baseline).

Tilt: Supine blood pressure was normal. Blood pressure responses to tilt were abnormal and consistent with moderate orthostatic hypotension.

Sudomotor evaluation: Electrochemical skin conductance was normal at hands and normal at feet.

Respiratory system: Respiratory frequency was normal in supine position and during the tilt. End tidal CO_2 was minimally reduced in supine position but was severely reduced during the tilt.

Cerebral blood flow velocity (CBFv): CBFv in middle cerebral artery was normal in supine position but was severely reduced during the tilt.

Skin biopsy (sensory-epidermal): N/A

Skin biopsy (sweat glands): N/A

Patient-reported symptoms during testing: Dizziness, shortness of breath, confusion during the tilt.

Patient-reported symptoms for past 2 weeks:

Lightheadedness or dizziness: Often
Dry eyes or mouth: Occasionally
Pale feet: Occasionally
Cold feet: Occasionally
Reduced sweating: None
Reduced sweating after exercise: Occasionally
Increased sweating: None
Nausea: Occasionally

TABLE 35.1 RESULTS OF AUTONOMIC TESTING

Blood pressure evaluation					
Test: Valsalva maneuver					
Pressure [mmHg]	Baseline	Phase 2			Phase 4
		Early	End		
Systolic	105	82	102		
Mean	81.7	68.7	81.3	n/a	
Diastolic	70	62	71	n/a	

Heart rate evaluation	
Test: Deep breathing	
Results	Norm*
23.3	≥12
Test: Valsalva ratio	
1.11	≥1.5
* adjusted for a gender and age	

(continued)

TABLE 35.1 **CONTINUED**

Test: Tilt test										
Position		HR [BPM]	Blood pressure [mmHg]		MCA Blood flow velocity [cm/s]				Respiratory frequency [breaths/min]	End tidal CO_2 [mmHg]
			Systolic	Diastolic	Systolic	Mean	Mean drop [%]	Diastolic		
Supine		89	110	70	134	86.7		63	9	31
Tilt [min]	1	105	108	71	103	53.7	38.1	29	13	23
	2	101	102	70						
	3	105	109	74						
	4	98	99	68						
	5	106	100	66	107	59	31.9	35	14	23
	6	107	103	71						
	7	104	94	64						
	8	92	87	55						
	9	101	89	60						
	10	105	86	57	107	58.3	32.8	34	13	22
	15									
	20									
	30									
	40									

Sudomotor evaluation – functional

Test: Quantitative sudomotor axon reflex test (QSART)				
Location	Site (l/r)	Latency [min]	Volume [μl]	Norm [μl]*
Forearm				≥0.08
Prox. leg				≥0.14
Distal leg				≥0.15
Foot				≥0.07

* Normative data are adjusted for gender and age of patient.

Test: Electrochemical skin conductance (ESC)				
Location	Left [μS]	Right [μS]	Average [μS/k]	Norm [μS/kg]
Hand	79	76	1.36	≥1.03
Feet	81	82	1.45	≥1.14
Forehead				

For grading uses ESC [μS] adjusted for weight [μS/k].

TABLE 35.1 CONTINUED

Small fiber (sensory + sudomotor) evaluation - morphological					
Test: Skin biopsy					
Location	Site (l/r)	Nerve fibers			
		Epidermal*		Sweat glands	
		Density	Norm	Density	Norm
Proximal leg – thigh	Right		≥8.3		≥37.8
Distal leg - calf	Right		≥8.54		≥36.5
Foot	Right		≥3.11		≥34.8

*Normative data for distal leg are adjusted for gender and age of patient.

QASAT*											
Heart rate		**BP**		**CBFv**		**ET-CO2**		**Sudomotor**			**Total QASAT score**
S. bradycardia	0	Low supine	0	Low supine	0	Low supine	1	QSART			
S. tachycardia	0	High supine	0	High supine	0	High supine	0	ESC	0		
Increase tilt	0	OH	3	Tilt respons.	8	Tilt low	6				
Decrease tilt	0	OHTN	0	CA	0	Tilt high	0	**Skin biopsy**			20
Deep breathing	0	VM	1	CVR	0			Epidermal			
VR	1			VM	0			Sweat gland			
Total	1	Total	4	Total	8	Total	7				

*QASAT. See Novak. Quantitative Scale for Grading of Cardiovascular Autonomic Reflex Tests and Small Fibers from Skin Biopsies. *J Neurol Disord* 2015;3:2.

S, supine; Increase tilt, increased response to tilt; Decrease tilt, decreased response to tilt; BP, blood pressure; VM, Valsalva maneuver; CBFv, cerebral blood flow velocity; CA, cerebral autoregulation; MCA, middle cerebral artery; VR, Valsalva ratio; CVR, cerebral vasoreactivity.

Diarrhea: Occasionally
Constipation: Occasionally
Urinary leaks: None
Current pain severity: 0
Aching pain: None
Allodynia: None
Burning pain: None
Lancinating pain: None
Numbness: None
Prickling sensation: None

AUTONOMIC TESTING INTERPRETATION

- Hypovolemia associated with orthostatic hypotension.
- Hypocapnic cerebral hypoperfusion (HYCH).[1]
- There was no evidence of significant autonomic failure.

COMMENT

CBFv was reduced by 38% during the tilt (Figure 35.1). The reduction in the blood flow velocity was due to hypocapnia-induced cerebral vasoconstriction and not due to orthostatic hypotension since velocity adjusted for the effect of end tidal CO_2 was not reduced during the tilt. Repeat tilt with paced breathing at a 10-second cycle (5-second inhalation and 5-second exhalation) gave similar results, with severe hypocapnia (~20 mm Hg) and markedly reduced CBFv (from baseline 72 cm/s to 52 cm/s at the end of the tilt). Persistent hypocapnia with paced breathing suggests that the hypocapnia is physiological and not psychological.

TREATMENT AND FOLLOW-UP

- Volume expansion through high fluid and high salt intake.
- Behavioral therapy, including relaxation and breathing exercises.

CAVEATS

Postural dizziness usually reflects cerebral hypoperfusion and may be related to reduced CBFv. Patients with symptomatic orthostatic hypotension are assumed to have reduced cerebral perfusion. Decline in perfusion can be due to the effect of orthostatic hypotension when the hypotension is below the autoregulatory range or when cerebral autoregulation fails. The hypocapnia may also induce low cerebral flow with signs of cerebral hypoperfusion. In this patient, the low CBFv was

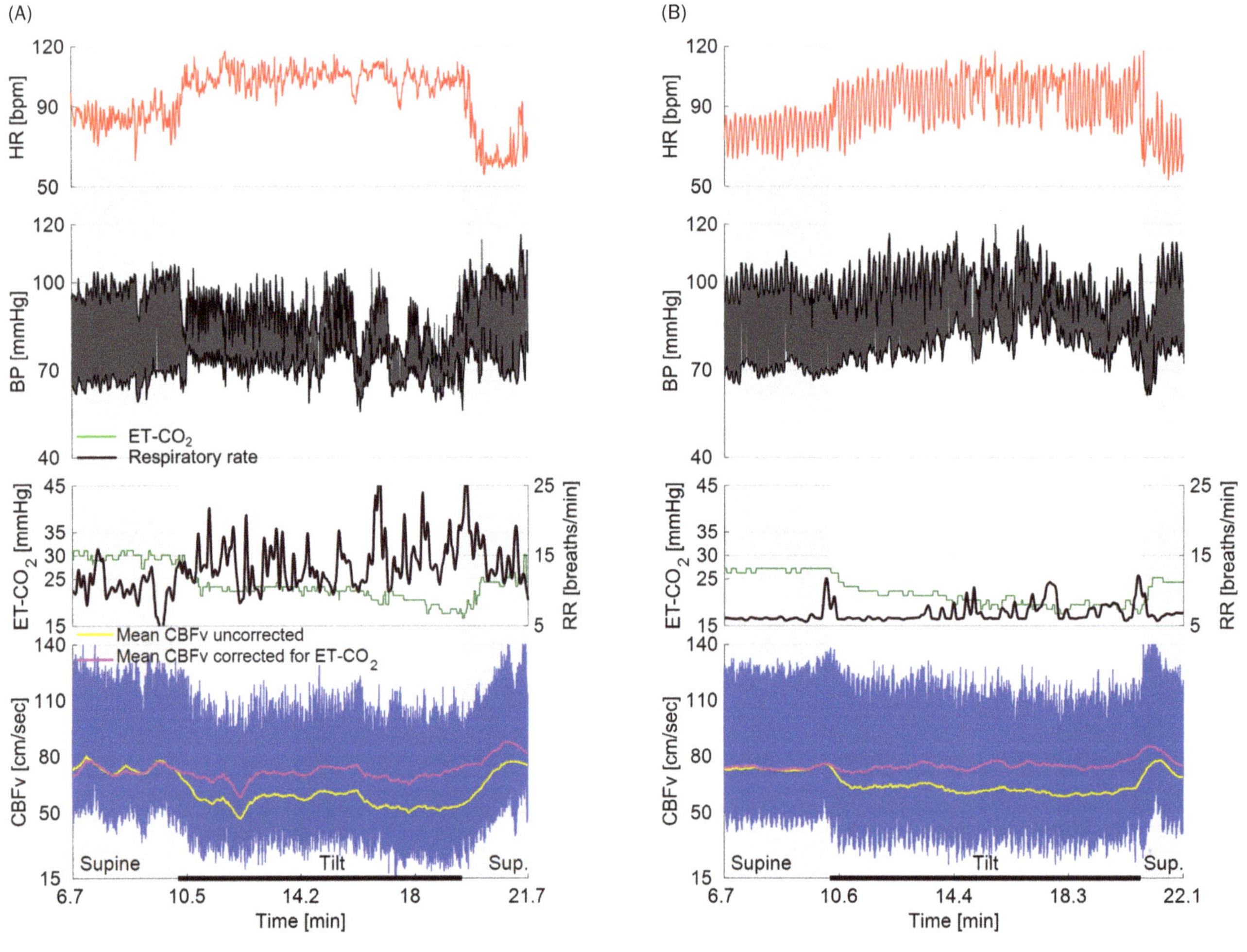

Figure 35.1 The regular tilt test with spontaneous breathing (A,C) showed normal heart rate and prominent blood pressure oscillations with mild decrease of mean blood pressure at the second half of the tilt. End tidal CO_2 was severely reduced during the tilt that also induced decline in cerebral blood flow velocity (CBFv, A,C). The tilt was repeated and the patient was ask to breathe at paced rate (cycles 6 per minute, B,D). Even with much slower paced frequency compared to the first tilt test, the end tidal CO_2 remained low. RR, respiratory rate.

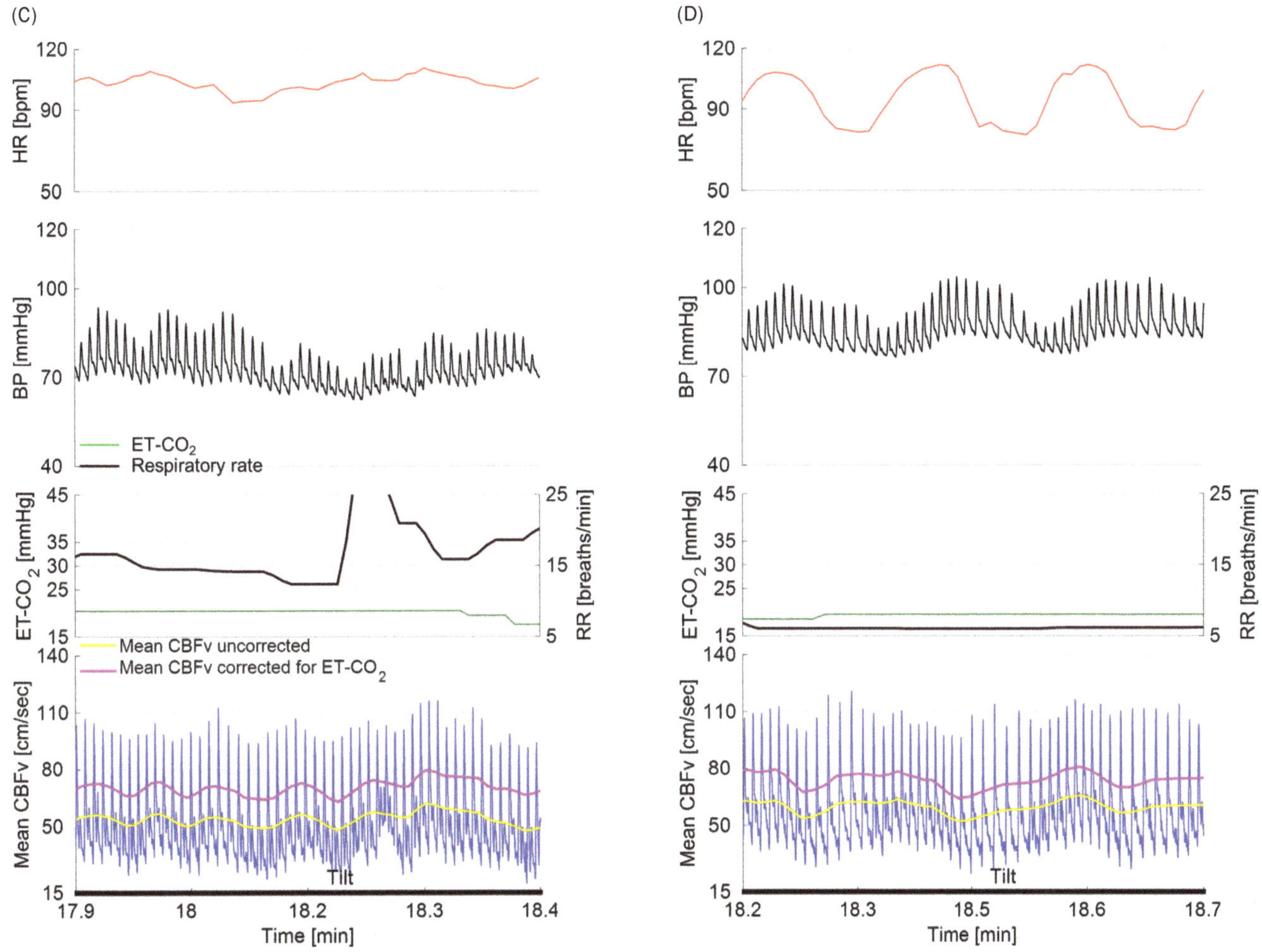

Figure 35.1 Continued

induced by hypocapnia and not by orthostatic hypotension. Simultaneous measurement of CBFv and end tidal CO_2 can help to differentiate symptoms of orthostatic intolerance

REFERENCE

1. Novak P. Hypocapnic cerebral hypoperfusion: A biomarker of orthostatic intolerance. *PloS One*. 2018;13(9):e0204419. doi:10.1371/journal.pone.0204419

36.

CASE 31: HYPOCAPNIC CEREBRAL HYPOPERFUSION WITH AN ARTIFACT

Chief complaint: Palpitations.

Case presentation: A 45-year-old woman presents with palpitations. Two years ago, she experienced a viral illness associated with fatigue, shortness of breath, abdominal cramps, chest tightness, swelling of the neck, and low grade fever. Since then, she has not felt well, and she continues to have the aforementioned symptoms. She has been evaluated by multiple specialists, including cardiology, allergy/immunology, gastroenterology, and endocrinology. Previous autonomic testing was inconclusive. Over the past year, symptoms worsened. She has chest tightness, shortness of breath, facial flushing, disabling abdominal cramping, and daily diarrhea. She has been losing weight. Evaluation for carcinoid tumor and mast cell activation syndrome/mastocytosis was negative. Patient was referred for autonomic testing to determine if dysautonomia is responsible for patient's symptoms.

Past medical history: Chronic fatigue syndrome.

Current medication: None.

Assessment plan: Functional autonomic tests and skin biopsy.

AUTONOMIC TESTING EVALUATION

See Table 36.1.

Heart rate: Supine tachycardia. Heart rate responses to deep breathing were normal. Heart rate increment during the tilt (13 BPM) was normal.

Blood pressure:

Valsalva maneuver: Blood pressure responses were normal.

Tilt: Supine blood pressure was normal. Blood pressure responses to tilt were normal.

Sudomotor evaluation: Electrochemical skin conductance was normal at hands and normal at feet.

Respiratory system: Respiratory frequency was normal in supine position and during the tilt. End tidal CO_2 was normal in supine position but was reduced during the tilt.

Cerebral blood flow velocity (CBFv): CBFv in middle cerebral artery was normal in supine position but was severely reduced during the tilt.

Skin biopsy (sensory-epidermal): Epidermal nerve fiber density was normal at proximal leg and normal at distal leg.

Skin biopsy (sweat glands): Sweat gland nerve fiber density was normal at proximal leg and normal at distal leg.

Patient-reported symptoms during testing: Dizziness during the tilt.

Patient-reported symptoms for past 2 weeks:

Lightheadedness or dizziness: Occasionally
Dry eyes or mouth: Occasionally
Pale feet: Occasionally
Cold feet: Occasionally
Reduced sweating: None
Reduced sweating after exercise: None
Increased sweating: None

TABLE 36.1 RESULTS OF AUTONOMIC TESTING

Blood pressure evaluation					
Test: Valsalva maneuver					
Pressure [mmHg]	Baseline	Phase 2			Phase 4
		Early	End		
Systolic	120	102	116		
Mean	90	85.3	99.3	n/a	
Diastolic	75	77	91	n/a	

Heart rate evaluation	
Test: Deep breathing	
Results	Norm*
16	≥10
Test: Valsalva ratio	
1.68	≥1.51
* adjusted for a gender and age	

TABLE 36.1 **CONTINUED**

Test: Tilt test											
Position		HR [BPM]	Blood pressure [mmHg]		MCA Blood flow velocity [cm/s]				Respiratory frequency [breaths/min]	End tidal CO_2 [mmHg]
			Systolic	Diastolic	Systolic	Mean	Mean drop [%]	Diastolic		
Supine		105	109	74	105	73		57	10	38
Tilt [min]	1	116	107	75	79	46.3	36.6	30	8	36
	2	105	110	74						
	3	118	103	70						
	4	117	111	78						
	5	111	105	72	77	48.3	33.8	34	17	30
	6	114	94	70						
	7	116	100	70						
	8	111	93	68						
	9	107	99	70						
	10	109	104	73	80	48.7	33.3	33	19	31
	15									
	20									
	30									
	40									

Sudomotor evaluation - functional

Test: Quantitative sudomotor axon reflex test (QSART)				
Location	Site (l/r)	Latency [min]	Volume [µl]	Norm [µl]*
Forearm				≥0.08
Prox. leg				≥0.14
Distal leg				≥0.15
Foot				≥0.07

* Normative data are adjusted for gender and age of patient.

Test: Electrochemical skin conductance (ESC)				
Location	Left [µS]	Right [µS]	Average [µS/k]	Norm [µS/kg]
Hand	75	73	1.39	≥1.03
Feet	89	89	1.68	≥1.14
Forehead				

For grading uses ESC [µS] adjusted for weight [µS/k].

(continued)

TABLE 36.1 **CONTINUED**

Small fiber (sensory + sudomotor) evaluation - morphological					
Test: Skin biopsy					
Location	Site (l/r)	Nerve fibers			
		Epidermal*		Sweat glands	
		Density	Norm	Density	Norm
Proximal leg – thigh	Right	9.77	≥8.3	42.5	≥37.8
Distal leg - calf	Right	7.73	≥7.5	41.2	≥36.5
Foot	Right		≥3.11		≥34.8

*Normative data for distal leg are adjusted for gender and age of patient.

QASAT*										
Heart rate		**BP**		**CBFv**		**ET-CO2**		**Sudomotor**		**Total QASAT score**
S. bradycardia	0	Low supine	0	Low supine	0	Low supine	0	QSART		
S. tachycardia	1	High supine	0	High supine	0	High supine	0	ESC	0	
Increase tilt	0	OH	0	Tilt response	9	Tilt low	1			
Decrease tilt	0	OHTN	0	CA	0	Tilt high	0	**Skin biopsy**		12
Deep breathing	0	VM	0	CVR	0			Epidermal	0	
VR	0			VM	0			Sweat gland	0	
Total	1	Total	0	Total	9	Total	1			

*QASAT. See Novak. Quantitative Scale for Grading of Cardiovascular Autonomic Reflex Tests and Small Fibers from Skin Biopsies. *J Neurol Disord* 2015;3:2.

S, supine; Increase tilt, increased response to tilt; Decrease tilt, decreased response to tilt; BP, blood pressure; VM, Valsalva maneuver; CBFv, cerebral blood flow velocity; CA, cerebral autoregulation; MCA, middle cerebral artery; VR, Valsalva ratio; CVR, cerebral vasoreactivity.

Nausea: Occasionally
Diarrhea: Occasionally
Constipation: Yes, minor annoyance
Urinary leaks: Yes, minor annoyance
Current pain severity: 5
Aching pain: Often, moderate
Allodynia: Occasionally, mild
Burning pain: Occasionally, mild
Lancinating pain: Occasionally, mild
Numbness: Often, moderate
Prickling sensation: Often, moderate

AUTONOMIC TESTING INTERPRETATION

- Hypocapnic cerebral hypoperfusion (HYCH).[1]
- No evidence of autonomic failure or paroxysmal dysautonomia.
- No evidence of small fiber neuropathy.

COMMENT

The testing revealed normal autonomic functions (Figure 36.1). It is important always to check the raw data. Blood pressure from the finger cuff is not always accurate. The oscillometric brachial cuff device should be used for calibration of finger blood pressure.

TREATMENT AND FOLLOW-UP

- Volume expansion through high fluid and high salt intake, exercise.

CAVEATS

- It is important to recognize artifacts in recordings. Continuous blood pressure obtained from the finger cuff may exaggerate or underrate the blood pressure.[2,3]

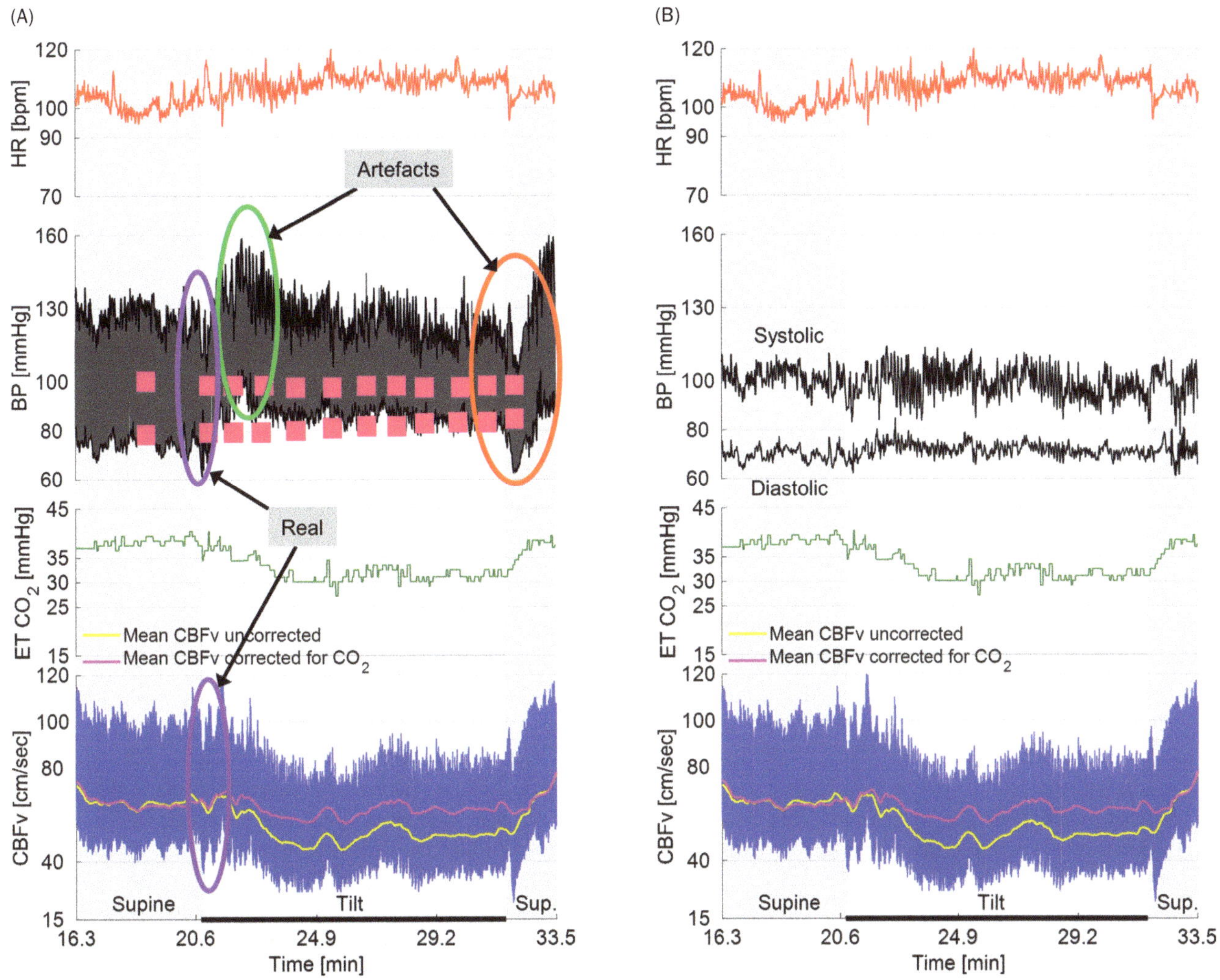

Figure 36.1 Initial decline in blood pressure at the tilt onset was real since it was accompanied by the decline in cerebral blood flow velocity and heart rate responses ("Real," magenta oval, A). Subsequent increases in blood pressure ("Artefacts," green oval) was artificial since there was no corresponding changes in cerebral blood flow velocity, heart rate or end tidal CO_2. Pink squares indicate blood pressure obtained from arm. A decline in blood pressure at the end in tilt ("Artefacts," red oval) was also an artifact since there was no corresponding change in other signals. The continuous systolic and diastolic blood pressure calibrated for the arm blood pressure showed normal response to tilt (B).

REFERENCES

1. Novak P. Hypocapnic cerebral hypoperfusion: A biomarker of orthostatic intolerance. *PloS One.* 2018;13(9):e0204419. doi:10.1371/journal.pone.0204419
2. Novak V, Novak P, Schondorf R. Accuracy of beat-to-beat noninvasive measurement of finger arterial pressure using the Finapres: a spectral analysis approach. *J Clin Monit.* 1994;10(2):118–126.
3. Lakhal K, Martin M, Faiz S, et al. The CNAP™ finger cuff for noninvasive beat-to-beat monitoring of arterial blood pressure: an evaluation in intensive care unit patients and a comparison with 2 intermittent devices. *Anesth Analg.* 2016;123(5):1126–1135. doi:10.1213/ANE.0000000000001324.

37.

CASE 32: SMALL FIBER NEUROPATHY, ORTHOSTATIC HYPERTENSION, AND HYPOCAPNIC CEREBRAL HYPOPERFUSION

Chief complaint: Labile blood pressure and chronic pain.

Case presentation: A 52-year-old woman has a history of complex regional pain syndrome after being struck by lightning 22 years ago. For the past few months, she experienced intermittent dizziness associated with hypertension. Pheochromocytoma has been considered given her history of labile blood pressures, but serum metanephrines and adrenal imaging were normal. Patient was referred for evaluation of suspected dysautonomia.

Past medical history: Complex regional pain syndrome, dyslipidemia, headaches, hypertension, chronic pain syndrome, depression, anxiety.

Current medication: Morphine, valium.

Assessment plan: Functional autonomic tests and skin biopsy.

AUTONOMIC TESTING EVALUATION

See Table 37.1.

Heart rate: Supine heart rate was normal. Heart rate responses to deep breathing were reduced to 82.5% of normal value. Heart rate increment during the tilt (23 BPM) was normal.

Blood pressure:

Valsalva maneuver: Mean blood pressure failed to return to baseline at the end of Phase 2 by 2 mm Hg (i.e., 98.6% of baseline). Supine blood pressure was normal.

Tilt: Blood pressure responses to tilt were normal.

Sudomotor evaluation: Electrochemical skin conductance was normal at hands and normal at feet.

Respiratory system: Respiratory frequency was normal in supine position. Respiratory frequency was normal during the tilt. End tidal CO_2 was normal in supine position. End tidal CO_2 was moderately reduced during the tilt.

Cerebral blood flow velocity (CBFv): CBFv in middle cerebral artery was normal in supine position. CBFv in middle cerebral artery was severely reduced during the tilt.

Skin biopsy (sensory-epidermal): Epidermal nerve fiber density was normal at proximal leg and abnormal (reduced to 69.2% of normal limit) at distal leg.

Skin biopsy (sweat glands): Sweat gland nerve fiber density was normal at proximal leg and abnormal (reduced to 84.1% of normal limit) at distal leg.

Patient-reported symptoms during testing: Dizziness, shortness of breath, and chest pain during the tilt.

Patient-reported symptoms for past 2 weeks:

Lightheadedness or dizziness: Occasionally
Dry eyes or mouth: Occasionally
Pale feet: Occasionally
Cold feet: Often
Reduced sweating: Occasionally
Reduced sweating after exercise: None
Increased sweating: Occasionally

TABLE 37.1 **RESULTS OF AUTONOMIC TESTING**

Blood pressure evaluation					
Test: Valsalva maneuver					
Pressure [mmHg]	Baseline	Phase 2			Phase 4
		Early	End		
Systolic	173	141	159		
Mean	145.7	125.7	143.7	n/a	
Diastolic	132	118	136	n/a	

Heart rate evaluation	
Test: Deep breathing	
Results	Norm*
7.43	≥9
Test: Valsalva ratio	
1.5	≥1.47
* adjusted for a gender and age	

TABLE 37.1 CONTINUED

Test: Tilt test											
Position		HR [BPM]	Blood pressure [mmHg]		MCA Blood flow velocity [cm/s]				Respiratory frequency [breaths/min]	End tidal CO_2 [mmHg]
			Systolic	Diastolic	Systolic	Mean	Mean drop [%]	Diastolic		
Supine		63	122	81	106	66		46	9	43
Tilt [min]	1	59	133	85	95	64.3	2.6	49	11	42
	2	65	145	85						
	3	71	132	86						
	4	84	134	89						
	5	82	119	90	78	41.3	37.4	23	15	30
	6	86	140	97						
	7	78	129	90						
	8	83	138	91						
	9	86	127	87						
	10	82	134	89	79	44.3	32.9	27	13	25
	15									
	20									
	30									
	40									

Sudomotor evaluation - functional

Test: Quantitative sudomotor axon reflex test (QSART)				
Location	Site (l/r)	Latency [min]	Volume [µl]	Norm [µl]*
Forearm				≥0.08
Prox. leg				≥0.14
Distal leg				≥0.07
Foot				≥0.05

* Normative data are adjusted for gender and age of patient.

Test: Electrochemical skin conductance (ESC)				
Location	Left [µS]	Right [µS]	Average [µS/k]	Norm [µS/kg]
Hand	85	85	1.8	≥1.03
Feet	94	93	1.97	≥1.14
Forehead				

For grading uses ESC [µS] adjusted for weight [µS/k].

(continued)

Small fiber (sensory + sudomotor) evaluation - morphological					
Test: Skin biopsy					
Location	Site (l/r)	Nerve fibers			
		Epidermal*		Sweat glands	
		Density	Norm	Density	Norm
Proximal leg – thigh	Right	8.4	≥8.3	47.7	≥37.8
Distal leg - calf	Right	4.8	≥6.94	30.7	≥36.5
Foot	Right		≥3.11		≥34.8

*Normative data for distal leg are adjusted for gender and age of patient.

QASAT*											
Heart rate		**BP**		**CBFv**		**ET-CO2**		**Sudomotor**			**Total QASAT score**
S. bradycardia	0	Low supine	0	Low supine	0	Low supine	0	QSART			
S. tachycardia	0	High supine	0	High supine	0	High supine	0	ESC	0		
Increase tilt	0	OH	0	Tilt response	5	Tilt low	3				
Decrease tilt	0	OHTN	1	CA	0	Tilt high	0	**Skin biopsy**			17
Deep breathing	1	VM	1	CVR	0			Epidermal	3		
VR	0			VM	0			Sweat gland	3		
Total	1	Total	2	Total	5	Total	3				

*QASAT. See Novak. Quantitative Scale for Grading of Cardiovascular Autonomic Reflex Tests and Small Fibers from Skin Biopsies. *J Neurol Disord* 2015;3:2.

S, supine; Increase tilt, increased response to tilt; Decrease tilt, decreased response to tilt; BP, blood pressure; VM, Valsalva maneuver; CBFv, cerebral blood flow velocity; CA, cerebral autoregulation; MCA, middle cerebral artery; VR, Valsalva ratio; CVR, cerebral vasoreactivity.

Nausea: Often
Diarrhea: None
Constipation: None
Urinary leaks: None
Current pain severity: 8
Aching pain: Continuous, severe
Allodynia: Often, moderate
Burning pain: Often, severe
Lancinating pain: Often, severe
Numbness: Often, moderate
Prickling sensation: Often, severe

AUTONOMIC TESTING INTERPRETATION

- Small fiber neuropathy, painful, mixed, length-dependent, affecting sensory and autonomic fibers.
- Orthostatic hypertension.
- Mild autonomic dysfunction affecting cardiovagal and adrenergic systems.
- Orthostatic hypertension
- Hypocapnic cerebral hypoperfusion (HYCH).[1]
- Hypocapnic hyperventilation during the tilt.

COMMENT

The testing showed several findings including small fiber neuropathy, orthostatic hypertension, and hypocapnic cerebral hypoperfusion (Figure 37.1). Elevated orthostatic blood pressure is commonly seen in painful neuropathies.[2] Indeed, the level of pain in this patient was 8 out of 10 during the tilt test.

Patient is being treated with morphine, which has numerous side effects including labile blood pressure, orthostatic intolerance, dizziness, and fainting. Therefore, alternative pain management may be needed.[3]

In spite of elevated orthostatic blood pressure, orthostatic CBFv was reduced. The entire drop in CBFv (37%

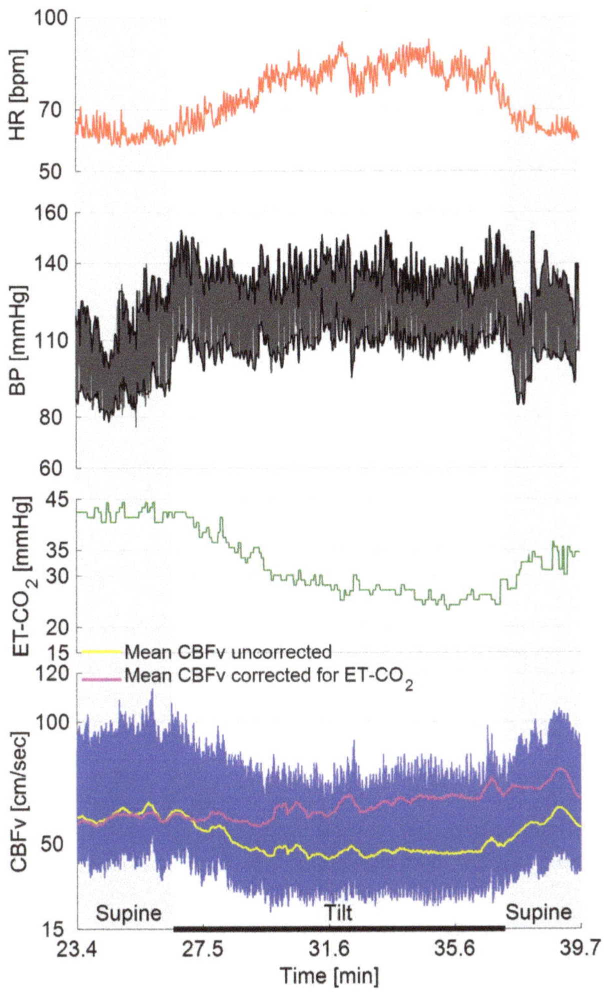

Figure 37.1 Tilt test showed elevated blood pressure consistent with orthostatic hypertension. Heart rate responses were normal. Orthostatic cerebral blood flow velocity (CBFv) declined due to vasoconstrictive effect of CO_2 since adjusted CBFv was stable.

in this case) can be explained by the vasoconstrictive effect of CO_2. This finding is consistent with hypocapnic cerebral hypoperfusion.

TREATMENT AND FOLLOW-UP

- Pain control with alternative to morphine.
- Evaluation for neuropathy.
- Ambulatory 24-hour blood pressure monitoring may be helpful to assess blood pressure lability.

CAVEATS

- Elevated orthostatic blood pressure may be seen in severe pain.
- This patient has small fiber neuropathy, which can be a reason for her chronic pain.

REFERENCES

1. Novak P. Hypocapnic cerebral hypoperfusion: A biomarker of orthostatic intolerance. *PloS One.* 2018;13(9):e0204419. doi:10.1371/journal.pone.0204419
2. Novak V, Freimer ML, Kissel JT, et al. Autonomic impairment in painful neuropathy. *Neurology.* 2001;56(7):861–868.
3. Cruccu G, Truini A. A review of neuropathic pain: from guidelines to clinical practice. *Pain Ther.* 2017;6(Suppl 1):35–42. doi:10.1007/s40122-017-0087-0.

38.

CASE 33: HYPOCAPNIC CEREBRAL HYPOPERFUSION WITH CHOLINERGIC SMALL FIBER NEUROPATHY

Chief complaint: Dizziness and gastrointestinal complaints.

Case presentation: A 33-year-old woman presents with dizziness, abdominal pain, and nausea. She was healthy until her 20s, when she started passing out frequently. Since then, she has been complaining of lightheadedness and dizziness with postural changes. She complaints of numbness in the lateral aspect of her right foot; intermittent pins-and-needles on the right side of her face and hand; and midline back pain in the thoracic region with no radicular symptoms; this occurs about twice a week. Autonomic testing done 10 years ago was normal. Later, she was treated for postural tachycardia syndrome (POTS) and was doing relatively well on β-blockers except for intermittent hypotension. She has a long history (many years) of disabling gastrointestinal symptoms, including epigastric pain, nausea. She was diagnosed with enteric neuropathy and has a j-tube for feeding. She had severe endometriosis and has had multiple procedures to treat this, including intra-abdominal and pelvic procedures during which loose bowels with adhesions were found. She feels as if she is "always swimming all the time." Patient was referred for evaluation of small fiber neuropathy and suspected autonomic failure.

Past medical history: Migraine, cervical syrinx, hysterectomy, endometriosis, postural tachycardia syndrome.

Current medication: Total parenteral nutrition.

Assessment plan: Functional autonomic tests and skin biopsy.

AUTONOMIC TESTING EVALUATION

See Table 38.1.

Heart rate: Supine heart rate was normal. Heart rate responses to deep breathing were reduced to 85.4% of normal value. Heart rate increment during the tilt (23 BPM) was normal.

Blood pressure:

Valsalva maneuver: Blood pressure responses were normal.

Tilt: Supine blood pressure was normal. Blood pressure responses to tilt were normal.

Sudomotor evaluation: Electrochemical skin conductance was abnormal (reduced to 87.4% of normal limit) at hands and normal at feet.

Respiratory system: Respiratory frequency was normal in supine position but was increased during the tilt. End tidal CO_2 was reduced in supine position and declined further during the tilt.

Cerebral blood flow velocity (CBFv): CBFv in middle cerebral artery was normal in supine position but was transiently reduced by 20% during the tilt.

Skin biopsy (sensory-epidermal): Epidermal nerve fiber density was normal at proximal leg and normal at distal leg.

Skin biopsy (sweat glands): Sweat gland nerve fiber density was abnormal (reduced to 75.7% of normal limit) at proximal leg.

TABLE 38.1 RESULTS OF AUTONOMIC TESTING

Blood pressure evaluation					
Test: Valsalva maneuver					
Pressure [mmHg]	Baseline	Phase 2			Phase 4
		Early	End		
Systolic	104	79	83		
Mean	63.3	59.7	63.7	n/a	
Diastolic	43	50	54	n/a	

Heart rate evaluation	
Test: Deep breathing	
Results	Norm*
10.25	≥12
Test: Valsalva ratio	
1.95	≥1.5
* adjusted for a gender and age	

TABLE 38.1 **CONTINUED**

Test: Tilt test										
Position		HR [BPM]	Blood pressure [mmHg]		MCA Blood flow velocity [cm/s]				Respiratory frequency [breaths/min]	End tidal CO_2 [mmHg]
			Systolic	Diastolic	Systolic	Mean	Mean drop [%]	Diastolic		
Supine		76	100	65	120	67.3		41	16	33
Tilt [min]	1	86	108	70	98	54	19.8	32	23	23
	2	92	108	73						
	3	96	106	73						
	4	90	105	72						
	5	98	102	71	100	60.7	9.8	41	21	20
	6	96	106	72						
	7	98	112	78						
	8	99	102	70						
	9	97	109	73						
	10	93	104	68	100	59.3	11.9	39	23	24
	15									
	20									
	30									
	40									

Sudomotor evaluation - functional

Test: Quantitative sudomotor axon reflex test (QSART)				
Location	Site (l/r)	Latency [min]	Volume [µl]	Norm [µl]*
Forearm				≥0.08
Prox. leg				≥0.14
Distal leg				≥0.15
Foot				≥0.07

* Normative data are adjusted for gender and age of patient.

Test: Electrochemical skin conductance (ESC)				
Location	Left [µS]	Right [µS]	Average [µS/k]	Norm [µS/kg]
Hand	48	51	0.9	≥1.03
Feet	90	87	1.6	≥1.14
Forehead				
For grading uses ESC [µS] adjusted for weight [µS/k].				

(continued)

TABLE 38.1 CONTINUED

Small fiber (sensory + sudomotor) evaluation - morphological					
Test: Skin biopsy					
Location	Site (l/r)	Nerve fibers			
		Epidermal*		Sweat glands	
		Density	Norm	Density	Norm
Proximal leg – thigh	Right	13.73	≥8.3	28.6	≥37.8
Distal leg - calf	Right	9.86	≥8.46		≥36.5
Foot	Right		≥3.11		≥34.8

*Normative data for distal leg are adjusted for gender and age of patient.

QASAT*											
Heart rate		**BP**		**CBFv**		**ET-CO2**		**Sudomotor**			**Total QASAT score**
S. bradycardia	0	Low supine	0	Low supine	0	Low supine	1	QSART			
S. tachycardia	0	High supine	0	High supine	0	High supine	0	ESC	1		
Increase tilt	0	OH	0	Tilt response	1	Tilt low	7				
Decrease tilt	0	OHTN	0	CA	0	Tilt high	0	**Skin biopsy**			14
Deep breathing	1	VM	0	CVR	0			Epidermal	0		
VR	0			VM	0			Sweat gland	3		
Total	1	Total	0	Total	1	Total	8				

*QASAT. See Novak. Quantitative Scale for Grading of Cardiovascular Autonomic Reflex Tests and Small Fibers from Skin Biopsies. *J Neurol Disord* 2015;3:2.

S, supine; Increase tilt, increased response to tilt; Decrease tilt, decreased response to tilt; BP, blood pressure; VM, Valsalva maneuver; CBFv, cerebral blood flow velocity; CA, cerebral autoregulation; MCA, middle cerebral artery; VR, Valsalva ratio; CVR, cerebral vasoreactivity.

Patient-reported symptoms during testing: Dizziness during the tilt.

Patient-reported symptoms for past 2 weeks:

Lightheadedness or dizziness: Often
Dry eyes or mouth: Occasionally
Pale feet: Occasionally
Cold feet: Occasionally
Reduced sweating: Occasionally
Reduced sweating after exercise: Occasionally
Increased sweating: Occasionally
Nausea: Often
Diarrhea: Occasionally
Constipation: Often
Urinary leaks: Occasionally
Current pain severity: 7
Aching pain: Often, moderate
Allodynia: Often, moderate
Burning pain: Occasionally, moderate
Lancinating pain: Often, moderate
Numbness: Continuous, moderate
Prickling sensation: Occasionally, none

AUTONOMIC TESTING INTERPRETATION

- Small fiber neuropathy, affecting predominantly autonomic fibers.
- Mild autonomic dysfunction. Orthostatic hypotension, a marker of more severe adrenergic sympathetic failure was absent.
- Hypocapnic cerebral hypoperfusion (HYCH).[1]
- Severe hypocapnic hyperventilation during the supine position and during the tilt.

COMMENT

Patient experienced symptoms of orthostatic intolerance, most likely due to mild cerebral hypoperfusion due to hypocapnia but with normal orthostatic heart rate responses, which is typical for HYCH (Figure 38.1).

The testing was consistent with cholinergic small fiber neuropathy since the patient had abnormal parasympathetic

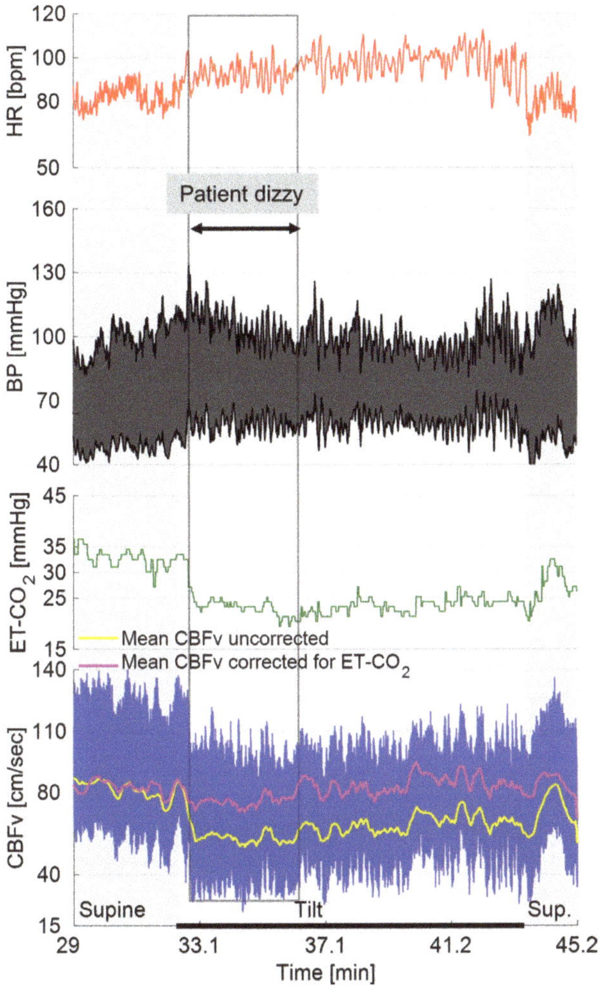

Figure 38.1 Heart rate and blood pressure responses to the tilt were normal. The tilt test showed hypocapnic hyperventilation with a decline in end tidal CO_2 and cerebral blood flow velocity (CBFv).

cardiovagal functions and abnormal sweat gland nerve fiber density. Acetylcholine is a principal neurotransmitter in both tests. Cholinergic small fiber neuropathy can be seen in enteric neuropathy.

Enteric neuropathy with cholinergic and sympathetic dysregulation is a disorder characterized by degradation of the nerves and muscles in the digestive system.[2] Enteric neuropathies can be serious and life-threatening conditions because of their effects on fluid and nutrient absorption, smooth muscle degradation, and altered feedback to the central nervous and endocrine systems for the regulation fluid intake.

TREATMENT AND FOLLOW-UP

- Evaluation for inflammatory neuropathy.
- Continue total parenteral nutrition.

CAVEATS

- Cholinergic small fiber neuropathy can be associated with enteric neuropathy.

REFERENCES

1. Novak P. Hypocapnic cerebral hypoperfusion: A biomarker of orthostatic intolerance. *PloS One.* 2018;13(9):e0204419. doi:10.1371/journal.pone.0204419
2. Furness JB. The enteric nervous system and neurogastroenterology. *Nat Rev Gastroenterol Hepatol.* 2012;9(5):286–294. doi:10.1038/nrgastro.2012.32.

39.

CASE 34: HYPOCAPNIC CEREBRAL HYPOPERFUSION AND EFFECT OF END TIDAL CO_2

Chief complaint: Dizziness.

Case presentation: A 25-year-old woman presents with unexplained dizziness. She was healthy until 5 years ago, when she experienced several viral infections. She also tested positive for Lyme disease and was treated with oral doxycycline. Since then, she has experienced fainting, orthostatic dizziness, fatigue, visual changes, and excessive sweating, and she was diagnosed with postural tachycardia syndrome (POTS). She responded poorly to β-blockers, promatine, and fludrocortisone. She only benefits from intravenous hydration. She also experienced several pain syndromes including distal skin burning sensation and joint pain. Skin biopsy confirmed small fiber neuropathy. Patient reported progression of symptoms, particularly worsening of numbness, fatigue, dizziness, orthostatic tremor, mental fog, and headaches during the past year.

Past medical history: POTS, small fiber neuropathy.

Current medication: None.

Assessment plan: Functional autonomic tests and skin biopsy.

AUTONOMIC TESTING EVALUATION

See Table 39.1.

Heart rate: Supine heart rate was normal. Heart rate responses to deep breathing were normal. Heart rate increment during the tilt (14 BPM) was normal.

Blood pressure:

Valsalva maneuver: Blood pressure responses were normal.

Tilt: Supine blood pressure was normal. Blood pressure responses to tilt were normal.

Sudomotor evaluation: Electrochemical skin conductance was normal at hands and normal at feet.

Respiratory system: Respiratory frequency was normal in supine position but was increased during the tilt. End tidal CO_2 was reduced in supine position and during the tilt.

Cerebral blood flow velocity (CBFv): CBFv in middle cerebral artery was normal in supine position but was severely reduced during the tilt.

Skin biopsy (sensory-epidermal): Epidermal nerve fiber density was normal at proximal leg and abnormal (reduced to 96.3% of normal limit) at distal leg.

Skin biopsy (sweat glands): Sweat gland nerve fiber density was normal at proximal leg and normal at distal leg.

Patient-reported symptoms during testing: Dizziness, feels loopy during the tilt.

Patient-reported symptoms for past 2 weeks:

Lightheadedness or dizziness: Occasionally
Dry eyes or mouth: Yes, minor annoyance
Pale feet: Occasionally
Cold feet: Occasionally

TABLE 39.1 RESULTS OF AUTONOMIC TESTING

Blood pressure evaluation					
Test: Valsalva maneuver					
Pressure [mmHg]	Baseline	Phase 2			Phase 4
		Early	End		
Systolic	160	143	148		
Mean	117.3	113	118	n/a	
Diastolic	96	98	103	n/a	

Heart rate evaluation	
Test: Deep breathing	
Results	Norm*
15	≥14
Test: Valsalva ratio	
1.68	≥1.46
* adjusted for a gender and age	

TABLE 39.1 **CONTINUED**

Test: Tilt test										
Position		HR [BPM]	Blood pressure [mmHg]		MCA Blood flow velocity [cm/s]				Respiratory frequency [breaths/min]	End tidal CO_2 [mmHg]
			Systolic	Diastolic	Systolic	Mean	Mean drop [%]	Diastolic		
Supine		62	119	81	142	90		64	12	31
Tilt [min]	1	70	114	79	89	51.7	42.6	33	21	23
	2	74	110	71						
	3	76	106	72						
	4	72	106	71						
	5	67	103	70	93	57.7	35.9	40	21	27
	6	70	104	70						
	7	66	108	73						
	8	63	104	73						
	9	68	101	70						
	10	70	104	72	125	79.7	11.4	57	26	30
	15									
	20									
	30									
	40									

Sudomotor evaluation - functional

Test: Quantitative sudomotor axon reflex test (QSART)				
Location	Site (l/r)	Latency [min]	Volume [µl]	Norm [µl]*
Forearm				≥0.08
Prox. leg				≥0.14
Distal leg				≥0.24
Foot				≥0.09

* Normative data are adjusted for gender and age of patient.

Test: Electrochemical skin conductance (ESC)				
Location	Left [µS]	Right [µS]	Average [µS/k]	Norm [µS/kg]
Hand	76	76	1.35	≥1.03
Feet	83	87	1.55	≥1.14
Forehead				

For grading uses ESC [µS] adjusted for weight [µS/k].

(continued)

TABLE 39.1 **CONTINUED**

Small fiber (sensory + sudomotor) evaluation - morphological					
Test: Skin biopsy					
Location	Site (l/r)	Nerve fibers			
		Epidermal*		Sweat glands	
		Density	Norm	Density	Norm
Proximal leg – thigh	Right	12.03	≥8.3	69	≥37.8
Distal leg - calf	Right	8.76	≥9.1	61.6	≥36.5
Foot	Right		≥3.11		≥34.8

*Normative data for distal leg are adjusted for gender and age of patient.

QASAT*											
Heart rate		**BP**		**CBFv**		**ET-CO2**		**Sudomotor**		**Total QASAT score**	
S. bradycardia	0	Low supine	0	Low supine	0	Low supine	1	QSART			
S. tachycardia	0	High supine	0	High supine	0	High supine	0	ESC	0		
Increase tilt	0	OH	0	Tilt response	6	Tilt low	3				
Decrease tilt	0	OHTN	0	CA	0	Tilt high	0	**Skin biopsy**		11	
Deep breathing	0	VM	0	CVR	0			Epidermal	1		
VR	0			VM	0			Sweat gland	0		
Total	0	Total	0	Total	6	Total	4				

*QASAT. See Novak. Quantitative Scale for Grading of Cardiovascular Autonomic Reflex Tests and Small Fibers from Skin Biopsies. *J Neurol Disord* 2015;3:2.

S, supine; Increase tilt, increased response to tilt; Decrease tilt, decreased response to tilt; BP, blood pressure; VM, Valsalva maneuver; CBFv, cerebral blood flow velocity; CA, cerebral autoregulation; MCA, middle cerebral artery; VR, Valsalva ratio; CVR, cerebral vasoreactivity.

Reduced sweating: Occasionally
Reduced sweating after exercise: Occasionally
Increased sweating: Occasionally
Nausea: Occasionally
Diarrhea: None
Constipation: None
Urinary leaks: Occasionally
Current pain severity: 0
Aching pain: Often, moderate
Allodynia: Often, moderate
Burning pain: Often, severe
Lancinating pain: Occasionally, severe
Numbness: Continuous, moderate
Prickling sensation: Often, moderate

AUTONOMIC TESTING INTERPRETATION

- Small fiber neuropathy, length-dependent, affecting sensory fibers.
- Hypocapnic cerebral hypoperfusion (HYCH).[1]

COMMENT

The patient experienced symptoms of dizziness associated with hypocapnic cerebral vasoconstriction and hypoperfusion (HYCH) without tachycardia (Figure 39.1). The decline in CBFv is due to hypocapnic hyperventilation, as demonstrated by voluntary hyperventilation in supine position (Figure 39.1C).

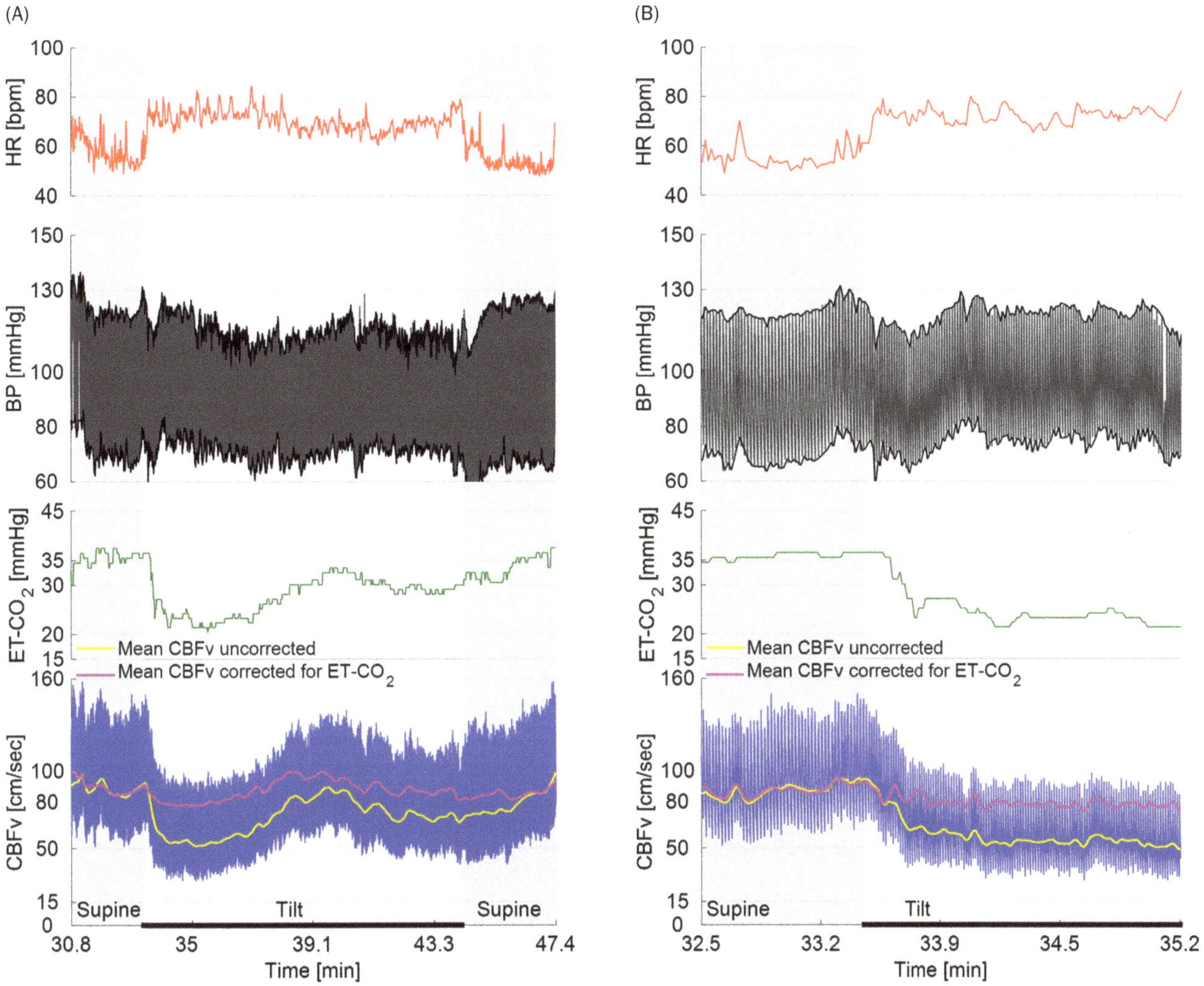

Figure 39.1 Heart rate and blood pressure responses to the tilt were normal. The tilt test showed hypocapnic hyperventilation with a severe decline in end tidal CO_2 and cerebral blood flow velocity (CBFv) (A, B). The patient complained of dizziness. Voluntary hyperventilation at supine position reproduced the CBFv decline and dizziness (C).

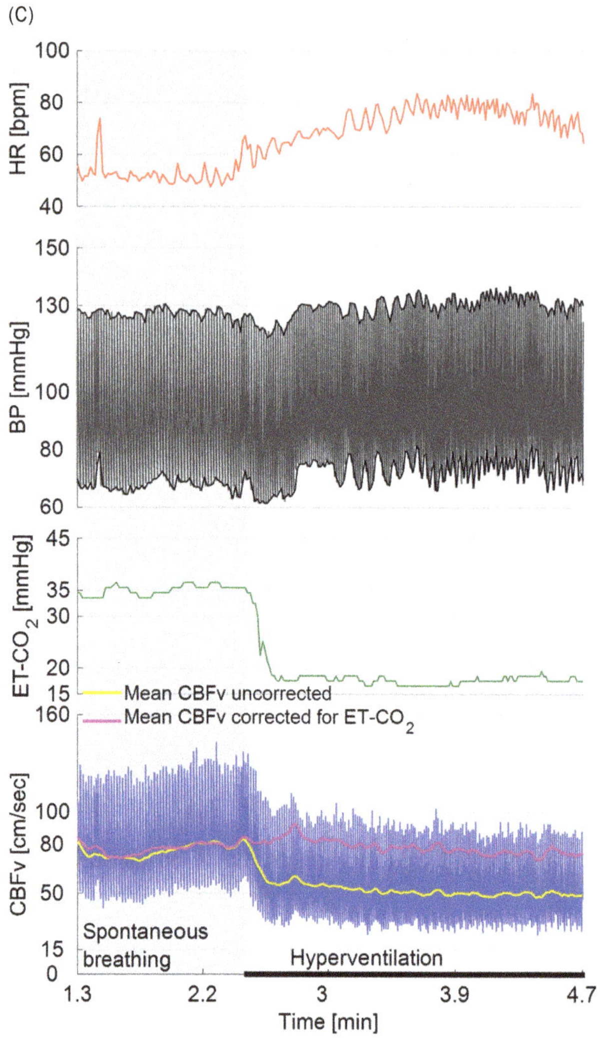

Figure 39.1 Continued

TREATMENT AND FOLLOW-UP

- Clinical workup for neuropathy.
- Relaxation and breathing therapy.

CAVEATS

Hypocapnic cerebral vasoconstriction and hypoperfusion (HYCH) can reproduce symptoms of orthostatic intolerance without tachycardia. POTS, however, is also often associated with hyperventilation,[2] so there is a considerable overlap in cerebral blood flow responses to orthostatic intolerance in these disorders, e.g. between HYCH and POTS.

REFERENCES

1. Novak P. Hypocapnic cerebral hypoperfusion: A biomarker of orthostatic intolerance. *PloS One*. 2018;13(9):e0204419. doi:10.1371/journal.pone.0204419
2. Novak V, Spies JM, Novak P, McPhee BR, Rummans TA, Low PA. Hypocapnia and cerebral hypoperfusion in orthostatic intolerance. *Stroke*. 1998;29(9):1876–1881.

40.

CASE 35: INITIAL ORTHOSTATIC HYPOTENSION

Chief complaint: Dizziness.

Case presentation: A 62-year-old woman presents with postural dizziness. She has gastrointestinal problems and irritable bowel syndrome with alternating diarrhea and constipation for 30 years. The digestive complaints worsened during the past 2 years. After starting to eat, her heart rate increases and she feels dizzy and may sweat profusely. She avoids many foods. She was diagnosed with multiple food allergies. She was referred for autonomic testing to characterize her autonomic functions.

Past medical history: Migraine, irritable bowel syndrome, Lyme disease.

Current medication: Levothyroxine, ranitidine.

Assessment plan: Functional autonomic tests and skin biopsy.

AUTONOMIC TESTING EVALUATION

See Table 40.1.

Heart rate: Supine heart rate was normal. Heart rate responses to deep breathing were normal. Heart rate increment during the tilt (26 BPM) was normal (Figure 40.1).

Blood pressure:

Valsalva maneuver: Mean blood pressure failed to return to baseline at the end of Phase 2 by 23.7 mm Hg (i.e., 75% of baseline).

Tilt: Supine blood pressure was normal. Blood pressure responses to tilt were normal.

Sudomotor evaluation: Electrochemical skin conductance was normal at hands and normal at feet.

Respiratory system: Respiratory frequency and end tidal CO_2 were normal in supine position and during the tilt.

Cerebral blood flow velocity (CBFv): CBFv in middle cerebral artery was normal in supine position and was transiently reduced during the tilt.

Skin biopsy (sensory-epidermal): Epidermal nerve fiber density was normal at proximal leg and normal at distal leg.

Skin biopsy (sweat glands): Sweat gland nerve fiber density was normal at proximal leg.

Patient-reported symptoms during testing: Dizziness, shortness of breath during the tilt.

Patient-reported symptoms for past 2 weeks:

Lightheadedness or dizziness: None
Dry eyes or mouth: Occasionally
Pale feet: Often
Cold feet: Occasionally
Reduced sweating: Occasionally
Reduced sweating after exercise: None
Increased sweating: Yes, minor annoyance
Nausea: Often

TABLE 40.1 **RESULTS OF AUTONOMIC TESTING**

Blood pressure evaluation						Heart rate evaluation	
Test: Valsalva maneuver						Test: Deep breathing	
Pressure [mmHg]	Baseline	Phase 2			Phase 4	Results	Norm*
		Early	End			14.25	≥7
Systolic	138	76	83			Test: Valsalva ratio	
Mean	94.7	66	71	n/a		1.8	≥1.39
Diastolic	73	61	65	n/a		* adjusted for a gender and age	

(continued)

Test: Tilt test										
Position		HR [BPM]	Blood pressure [mmHg]		MCA Blood flow velocity [cm/s]				Respiratory frequency [breaths/min]	End tidal CO_2 [mmHg]
			Systolic	Diastolic	Systolic	Mean	Mean drop [%]	Diastolic		
Supine		77	122	74	93	64.3		50	13	38
Tilt [min]	1	86	112	75	92	62	3.6	47	14	32
	2	97	111	76						
	3	103	120	79						
	4	97	113	78						
	5	99	111	76	91	61.7	4	47	12	34
	6	95	118	78						
	7	96	113	77						
	8	100	113	76						
	9	97	114	76						
	10	99	114	80	94	58.7	8.7	41	19	32
	15									
	20									
	30									
	40									

Sudomotor evaluation - functional

Test: Quantitative sudomotor axon reflex test (QSART)				
Location	Site (l/r)	Latency [min]	Volume [μl]	Norm [μl]*
Forearm				≥0.08
Prox. leg				≥0.14
Distal leg				≥0.07
Foot				≥0.05

* Normative data are adjusted for gender and age of patient.

Test: Electrochemical skin conductance (ESC)				
Location	Left [μS]	Right [μS]	Average [μS/k]	Norm [μS/kg]
Hand	61	62	1.27	≥1.03
Feet	83	83	1.73	≥1.14
Forehead				

For grading uses ESC [μS] adjusted for weight [μS/k].

TABLE 40.1 CONTINUED

Small fiber (sensory + sudomotor) evaluation - morphological					
Test: Skin biopsy					
Location	Site (l/r)	Nerve fibers			
		Epidermal*		Sweat glands	
		Density	Norm	Density	Norm
Proximal leg – thigh	Right	17.33	≥8.3	60.3	≥37.8
Distal leg – calf	Right	13.42	≥6.14		≥36.5
Foot	Right		≥3.11		≥34.8

*Normative data for distal leg are adjusted for gender and age of patient.

QASAT*										
Heart rate		**BP**		**CBFv**		**ET-CO2**		**Sudomotor**		**Total QASAT score**
S. bradycardia	0	Low supine	0	Low supine	0	Low supine	0	QSART		
S. tachycardia	0	High supine	0	High supine	0	High supine	0	ESC	0	
Increase tilt	0	OH	0	Tilt response	0	Tilt low	0			
Decrease tilt	0	OHTN	0	CA	0	Tilt high	0	**Skin biopsy**		2
Deep breathing	0	VM	2	CVR	0			Epidermal	0	
VR	0			VM	0			Sweat gland	0	
Total	0	Total	2	Total	0	Total	0			

*QASAT. See Novak. Quantitative Scale for Grading of Cardiovascular Autonomic Reflex Tests and Small Fibers from Skin Biopsies. *J Neurol Disord* 2015;3:2.

S, supine; Increase tilt, increased response to tilt; Decrease tilt, decreased response to tilt; BP, blood pressure; VM, Valsalva maneuver; CBFv, cerebral blood flow velocity; CA, cerebral autoregulation; MCA, middle cerebral artery; VR, Valsalva ratio; CVR, cerebral vasoreactivity.

Diarrhea: Occasionally
Constipation: Often
Urinary leaks: Occasionally
Current pain severity: 0
Aching pain: Occasionally, mild
Allodynia: None
Burning pain: None
Lancinating pain: Occasionally, moderate
Numbness: Occasionally, mild
Prickling sensation: Occasionally, mild

AUTONOMIC TESTING INTERPRETATION

- Initial orthostatic hypotension (IOH).
- Mild adrenergic dysfunction without evidence of orthostatic hypotension.
- No evidence of small fiber neuropathy.
- Orthostatic cerebral hypoperfusion syndrome (OCHOS), mild.

COMMENT

The tilt test provoked IOH (Figure 40.1).[1] IOH is characterized by a rapid decrease in blood pressure in response to standing up quickly. It is characterized by immediacy and is transient in nature, with restoration of blood pressure in less than a minute. The tilt test reproduced the dizziness. However, the dizziness did not occur at the nadir of the initial orthostatic hypotension but was observed seconds later and correlated with the decline in CBFv. The transient decline in CBFv is indicative of cerebral autoregulatory failure associated with OCHOS.

Although the testing was abnormal, the abnormalities were mild (QASAT total score of only 2) and of questionable clinical significance. Patients with multiple food allergies may experience signs of dysautonomia after exposure to the food trigger.[2–4] Autonomic testing in this patient was, however, negative for major evidence of autonomic failure, implying that autonomic symptoms triggered by food are likely due to an allergic reaction.

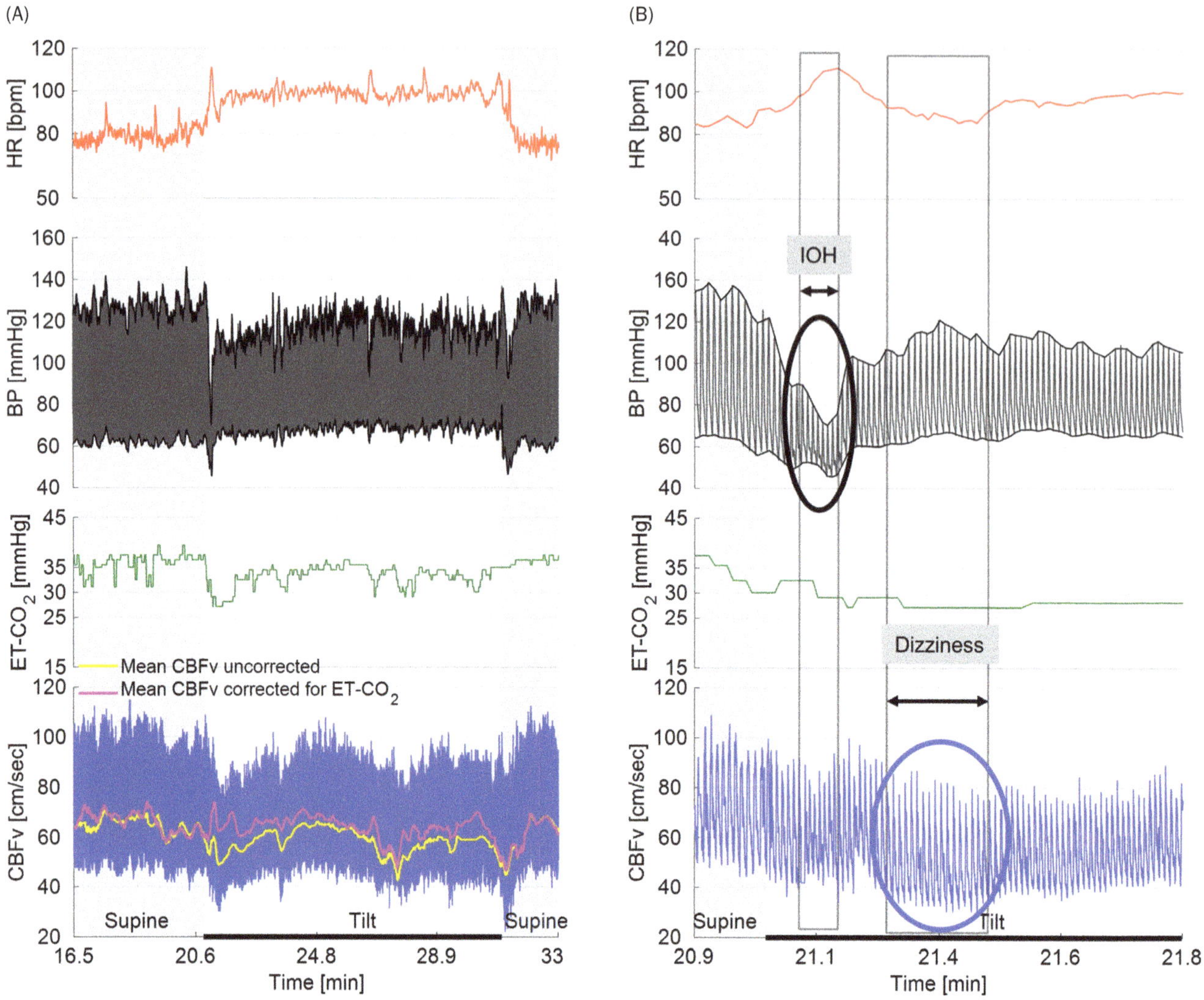

Figure 40.1 The tilt test provoked immediate decline in blood pressure which was consistent with initial orthostatic hypotension (A,B). However, the patient became dizzy later which corresponded to decline in cerebral blood flow velocity (CBFv). CBFv declined several times during the tilt.

TREATMENT AND FOLLOW-UP

- Reassurance.

CAVEATS

- IOH may be asymptomatic; the orthostatic symptoms correlate better with changes in CBFv than in blood pressure.
- Multiple food allergies may be associated with mild dysautonomia.

REFERENCES

1. Wieling W, Krediet CTP, van Dijk N, Linzer M, Tschakovsky ME. Initial orthostatic hypotension: review of a forgotten condition. *Clin Sci Lond Engl 1979*. 2007;112(3):157–165. doi:10.1042/CS20060091.
2. Wang J. Management of the patient with multiple food allergies. *Curr Allergy Asthma Rep*. 2010;10(4):271–277. doi:10.1007/s11882-010-0116-0.
3. Iweala OI, Choudhary SK, Commins SP. Food allergy. *Curr Gastroenterol Rep*. 2018;20(5):17. doi:10.1007/s11894-018-0624-y.
4. De Luca L, Foggia L, Chiummariello S. [A correlation between food allergy, the autonomic nervous system and the central nervous system: a study of 8 patients in childhood]. *Pediatr Medica E Chir Med Surg Pediatr*. 1996;18(6):565–571.

41.

CASE 36: ORTHOSTATIC HYPERTENSION

Chief complaint: Dizziness and headaches.

Case presentation: A 52-year-old man presents with dizziness associated with severe headaches for 1 year. Both dizziness and headaches are worse in the morning after awakening around 8 AM and in the early afternoon around 4 PM. He has history of essential hypertension; previous evaluations for secondary hypertension were unrevealing. Thorough neurological examination was normal. MRI of the brain was normal.

Past medical history: Obstructive sleep apnea, essential hypertension, dyslipidemia.

Current medication: Simvastatin, lisinopril, fluoxetine.

Assessment plan: Functional autonomic tests.

AUTONOMIC TESTING EVALUATION

See Table 41.1.

Heart rate: Supine heart rate was normal. Heart rate responses to deep breathing were reduced to 38.9% of normal value. Heart rate increment during the tilt (12 BPM) was normal.

Blood pressure:

Valsalva maneuver: Blood pressure responses were normal.

Tilt: Supine blood pressure was normal. Blood pressure was elevated during the tilt.

Sudomotor evaluation: Sweat output was normal at forearm, normal at proximal leg, normal at distal leg, and normal at foot.

Respiratory system: Respiratory frequency and end tidal CO_2 were normal in supine and during the tilt.

Cerebral blood flow velocity (CBFv): CBFv in middle cerebral artery was reduced in supine position (mean CBFv 44.7 cm/s, age and gender adjusted range of normal value 46.9 – 76.1 cm/s) and was further reduced during the tilt.

Skin biopsy (sensory-epidermal): N/A

Skin biopsy (sweat glands): N/A

Patient-reported symptoms during testing: Headache, feeling hot, and dry mouth during the tilt.

Patient-reported symptoms for past 2 weeks:

Lightheadedness or dizziness: Occasionally
Dry eyes or mouth: Occasionally
Pale feet: None
Cold feet: None
Reduced sweating: Yes, minor annoyance
Reduced sweating after exercise: Occasionally
Increased sweating: None
Nausea: None
Diarrhea: None
Constipation: Yes, minor annoyance
Urinary leaks: None
Erection problems: None
Aching pain: Often, moderate

TABLE 41.1 **RESULTS OF AUTONOMIC TESTING**

Blood pressure evaluation					
Test: Valsalva maneuver					
Pressure [mmHg]	Baseline	Phase 2			Phase 4
		Early	End		
Systolic	133	113	123		
Mean	90.3	89.7	99.7	n/a	
Diastolic	69	78	88	n/a	

Heart rate evaluation	
Test: Deep breathing	
Results	Norm*
3.5	≥9
Test: Valsalva ratio	
1.29	≥1.36
* adjusted for a gender and age	

(continued)

TABLE 41.1 **CONTINUED**

Test: Tilt test											
Position		HR [BPM]	Blood pressure [mmHg]		MCA Blood flow velocity [cm/s]				Respiratory frequency [breaths/min]	End tidal CO_2 [mmHg]
			Systolic	Diastolic	Systolic	Mean	Mean drop [%]	Diastolic		
Supine		68	137	87	64	44.7		35	16	35
Tilt [min]	1	75	151	92	77	49	-9.6	35	18	38
	2	74	156	96						
	3	71	155	92						
	4	73	153	93						
	5	68	151	96	66	40.7	8.9	28	15	40
	6	72	159	92						
	7	72	153	92						
	8	73	146	93						
	9	73	150	94						
	10	75	147	94	62	39.3	12.1	28	18	38
	15	73	150	93						
	20	74	150	95						
	30	75	156	106						
	40	80	158	108						

Sudomotor evaluation - functional

Test: Quantitative sudomotor axon reflex test (QSART)				
Location	Site (l/r)	Latency [min]	Volume [µl]	Norm [µl]*
Forearm	l	2.51	0.663	≥0.3
Prox. leg	l	2.4	0.42	≥0.23
Distal leg	l	1.47	1.085	≥0.23
Foot	l	1.5	0.56	≥0.27

* Normative data are adjusted for gender and age of patient.

Test: Electrochemical skin conductance (ESC)				
Location	Left [µS]	Right [µS]	Average [µS/k]	Norm [µS/kg]
Hand				≥
Feet				≥
Forehead				

For grading uses ESC [µS] adjusted for weight [µS/k].

TABLE 41.1 CONTINUED

Small fiber (sensory + sudomotor) evaluation - morphological					
Test: Skin biopsy					
Location	Site (l/r)	Nerve fibers			
		Epidermal*		Sweat glands	
		Density	Norm	Density	Norm
Proximal leg – thigh	Right		≥8.3		≥37.8
Distal leg - calf	Right		≥		≥36.5
Foot	Right		≥3.11		≥34.8

*Normative data for distal leg are adjusted for gender and age of patient.

QASAT*											
Heart rate		BP		CBFv		ET-CO2		Sudomotor			Total QASAT score
S. bradycardia	0	Low supine	0	Low supine	1	Low supine	0	QSART	0		
S. tachycardia	0	High supine	0	High supine	0	High supine	0	ESC			
Increase tilt	0	OH	0	Tilt response	0	Tilt low	0				
Decrease tilt	0	OHTN	2	CA	0	Tilt high	0	**Skin biopsy**			6
Deep breathing	2	VM	0	CVR	0			Epidermal			
VR	1			VM	0			Sweat gland			
Total	3	Total	2	Total	1	Total	0				

*QASAT. See Novak. Quantitative Scale for Grading of Cardiovascular Autonomic Reflex Tests and Small Fibers from Skin Biopsies. *J Neurol Disord* 2015;3:2.

S, supine; Increase tilt, increased response to tilt; Decrease tilt, decreased response to tilt; BP, blood pressure; VM, Valsalva maneuver; CBFv, cerebral blood flow velocity; CA, cerebral autoregulation; MCA, middle cerebral artery; VR, Valsalva ratio; CVR, cerebral vasoreactivity.

Allodynia: None
Burning pain: None
Lancinating pain: Occasionally, moderate
Numbness: Occasionally, mild
Prickling sensation: Occasionally, mild

AUTONOMIC TESTING INTERPRETATION

- Orthostatic hypertension.
- Cerebral autoregulatory failure.
- Mild parasympathetic dysfunction.

COMMENT

Orthostatic hypertension is a syndrome associated with a rise in orthostatic blood pressure (Figure 41.1).[1] It can be seen in patients with a history of a variety of conditions including essential hypertension, diabetes, and dysautonomia. Sometimes orthostatic hypertension can be present during labile hypertension before developing sustained hypertension. Potential mechanisms include vascular adrenergic hypersensitivity, baroreflex dysfunction associated with excessive sympathetic stimulation, and excessive release of catecholamines from adrenergic terminals on standing.

This patient had low supine CBFv due to hypertension-induced cerebral vasoconstriction. In spite of elevated orthostatic systemic blood pressure, orthostatic CBFv was reduced in this patient, which is consistent with absent compensatory cerebral vasodilation due to cerebral autoregulatory failure (CAF).[2] In CAF, the cerebral vasoconstriction/vasodilation occurs at the level of cerebral arterioles, which contrasts with reversible vasoconstriction syndrome where the constriction affects large cerebral arteries and increases CBFv.[3] Note that hypocapnia, which also causes cerebral vasoconstriction, was absent in this patient.

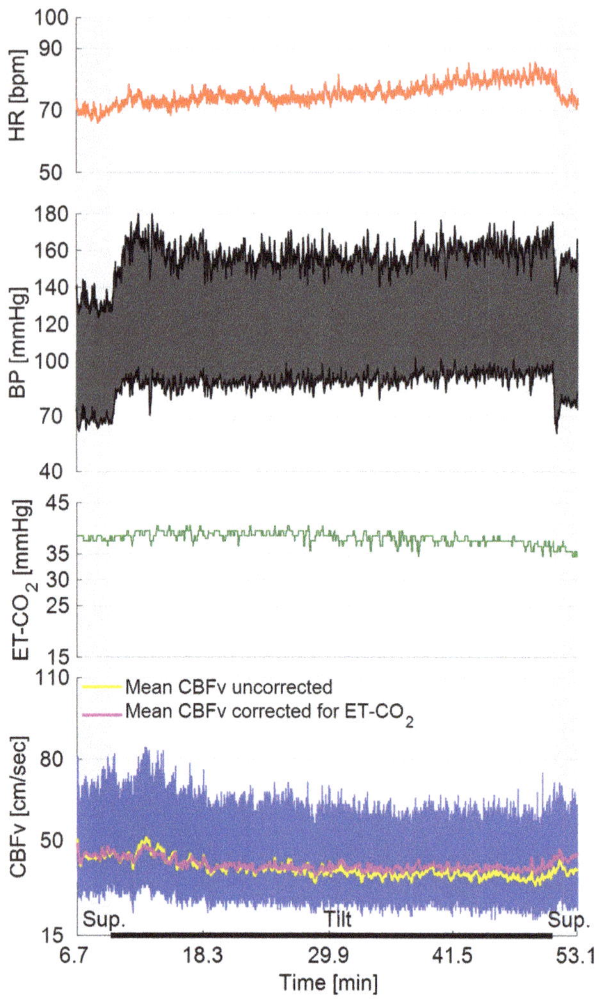

Figure 41.1 The tilt test showed elevated orthostatic blood pressure. Heart rate and end tidal CO_2 responses to the tilt were normal. Cerebral blood flow velocity was reduced during the supine position and was further reduced during the tilt.

TREATMENT AND FOLLOW-UP

- Consider therapy with calcium channel blockers that may reduce hypertension and also may improve cerebral perfusion since they dilate cerebral vessels.[4]

CAVEATS

- Orthostatic dizziness associated with cerebral hypoperfusion can be seen even when the systemic blood pressure is elevated.
- CBFv can be reduced due to abnormal vasoconstriction associated with cerebral autoregulatory failure.

REFERENCES

1. Fessel J, Robertson D. Orthostatic hypertension: when pressor reflexes overcompensate. *Nat Clin Pract Nephrol.* 2006;2(8):424–431. doi:10.1038/ncpneph0228.
2. Novak P. Cerebral blood flow, heart rate, and blood pressure patterns during the tilt test in common orthostatic syndromes. *Neurosci J.* 2016;2016:6127340. doi:10.1155/2016/6127340.
3. Ducros A, Bousser M-G. Reversible cerebral vasoconstriction syndrome. *Pract Neurol.* 2009;9(5):256–267. doi:10.1136/jnnp.2009.187856.
4. Nowak DA, Rodiek SO, Henneken S, et al. Reversible segmental cerebral vasoconstriction (Call-Fleming syndrome): are calcium channel inhibitors a potential treatment option? *Cephalalgia Int J Headache.* 2003;23(3):218–222. doi:10.1046/j.1468-2982.2003.00507.x.

42.

CASE 37: SEVERE DYSPNEA AND PRELOAD FAILURE

Chief complaint: Dyspnea.

Case presentation: A 65-year-old woman presents with fatigue, exertional dyspnea, exertional chest tightness, and palpitations. All complaints started after resolution of bronchitis 2 years ago. Invasive cardiopulmonary exercise testing (CPET) showed preload failure. She was referred for evaluation of autonomic functions.

Past medical history: Depression, hypertension.

Current medication: Synthroid, lisinopril, lorazepam, multivitamins.

Assessment plan: Functional autonomic tests and skin biopsy.

AUTONOMIC TESTING EVALUATION

See Table 42.1.

Heart rate: Supine heart rate was normal. Heart rate responses to deep breathing were normal. Heart rate increment during the tilt (23 BPM) was normal.

Blood pressure:

Valsalva maneuver: Mean blood pressure failed to return to baseline at the end of Phase 2 by 4.7 mm Hg (i.e., 94.6% of baseline).

Tilt: Supine blood pressure was normal. Blood pressure responses to tilt were normal.

Sudomotor evaluation: Electrochemical skin conductance was abnormal (reduced to 91.7% of normal limit) at hands and abnormal (reduced to 93.9% of normal limit) at feet.

Respiratory system: Respiratory frequency was normal in supine position and during the tilt. End tidal CO_2 was reduced in supine position and declined further during the tilt.

Cerebral blood flow velocity (CBFv): CBFv in middle cerebral artery was normal in supine position but was reduced by 26% during the tilt.

Skin biopsy (sensory-epidermal): Epidermal nerve fiber density was abnormal (reduced to 6.8% of normal limit) at distal leg.

Skin biopsy (sweat glands): No sweat glands found on the specimen.

Patient-reported symptoms during testing: Dizziness and shortness of breath during the tilt.

Patient-reported symptoms for past 2 weeks:

Lightheadedness or dizziness: Occasionally
Dry eyes or mouth: Occasionally
Pale feet: Often
Cold feet: Occasionally
Reduced sweating: Occasionally
Reduced sweating after exercise: None
Increased sweating: None
Nausea: None
Diarrhea: Occasionally
Constipation: None

TABLE 42.1 **RESULTS OF AUTONOMIC TESTING**

Blood pressure evaluation					
Test: Valsalva maneuver					
Pressure [mmHg]	Baseline	Phase 2			Phase 4
		Early	End		
Systolic	105	89	97		
Mean	87.7	78.3	83	n/a	
Diastolic	79	73	76	n/a	

Heart rate evaluation	
Test: Deep breathing	
Results	Norm*
11.5	≥7
Test: Valsalva ratio	
1.41	≥1.39
* adjusted for a gender and age	

(continued)

TABLE 42.1 **CONTINUED**

Test: Tilt test											
Position		HR [BPM]	Blood pressure [mmHg]		MCA Blood flow velocity [cm/s]				Respiratory frequency [breaths/min]	End tidal CO_2 [mmHg]
			Systolic	Diastolic	Systolic	Mean	Mean drop [%]	Diastolic		
Supine		98	119	80	94	60		43	18	30
Tilt [min]	1	107	115	69	88	54.7	8.8	38	18	24
	2	112	118	81						
	3	118	122	81						
	4	120	114	78						
	5	118	121	81	70	46.7	22.2	35	15	22
	6	116	110	79						
	7	114	115	78						
	8	119	115	81						
	9	120	115	82						
	10	121	113	76	67	44.3	26.2	33	13	21
	15									
	20									
	30									
	40									

Sudomotor evaluation - functional

Test: Quantitative sudomotor axon reflex test (QSART)				
Location	Site (l/r)	Latency [min]	Volume [µl]	Norm [µl]*
Forearm				≥0.08
Prox. leg				≥0.14
Distal leg				≥0.07
Foot				≥0.05

* Normative data are adjusted for gender and age of patient.

Test: Electrochemical skin conductance (ESC)				
Location	Left [µS]	Right [µS]	Average [µS/k]	Norm [µS/kg]
Hand	79	72	0.94	≥1.03
Feet	85	86	1.08	≥1.14
Forehead				

For grading uses ESC [µS] adjusted for weight [µS/k].

TABLE 42.1 CONTINUED

Small fiber (sensory + sudomotor) evaluation - morphological					
Test: Skin biopsy					
Location	Site (l/r)	Nerve fibers			
		Epidermal*		Sweat glands	
		Density	Norm	Density	Norm
Proximal leg – thigh	Right		≥8.3		≥37.8
Distal leg - calf	Right	0.4	≥5.9		≥36.5
Foot	Right		≥3.11		≥34.8

*Normative data for distal leg are adjusted for gender and age of patient.

QASAT*											
Heart rate		BP		CBFv		ET-CO2		Sudomotor			Total QASAT score
S. bradycardia	0	Low supine	0	Low supine	0	Low supine	1	QSART			
S. tachycardia	0	High supine	0	High supine	0	High supine	0	ESC	1		
Increase tilt	0	OH	0	Tilt response	4	Tilt low	7				
Decrease tilt	0	OHTN	0	CA	0	Tilt high	0	**Skin biopsy**			18
Deep breathing	0	VM	1	CVR	0			Epidermal	4		
VR	0			VM	0			Sweat gland			
Total	0	Total	1	Total	4	Total	8				

*QASAT. See Novak. Quantitative Scale for Grading of Cardiovascular Autonomic Reflex Tests and Small Fibers from Skin Biopsies. *J Neurol Disord* 2015;3:2.

S, supine; Increase tilt, increased response to tilt; Decrease tilt, decreased response to tilt; BP, blood pressure; VM, Valsalva maneuver; CBFv, cerebral blood flow velocity; CA, cerebral autoregulation; MCA, middle cerebral artery; VR, Valsalva ratio; CVR, cerebral vasoreactivity.

Urinary leaks: None
Current pain severity: 0
Aching pain: Occasionally, mild
Allodynia: None
Burning pain: Occasionally, moderate
Lancinating pain: Occasionally, moderate
Numbness: Occasionally, none
Prickling sensation: Continuous, moderate

AUTONOMIC TESTING INTERPRETATION

- Small fiber neuropathy, mixed, length-dependent.
- Hypocapnic cerebral hypoperfusion (HYCH)
- Mild adreneregic dysfunction

COMMENT

Patient had invasive CPET, which evaluates the causes of unexplained dyspnea.[1] CPET showed low biventricular filling pressure and poor peripheral oxygen extraction as a cause of dyspnea, consistent with preload failure. Autonomic testing showed HYCH[2]. In HYCH, hypocapnia induces cerebral arterioral vasoconstrition and reduces cerebral blood flow. HYCH patients frequently complaint on dyspnea. This case shows that preload failure, in addition to being linked to dyspnea, also may play a role in HYCH. CPET evaluates preload functions in contrast to established autonomic testing that evaluates afterload functions. Thus, CPET and autonomic testing complement each other.

TREATMENT AND FOLLOW-UP

- Clinical workup for neuropathy.
- Trial of pyridostigmine, which can reduce dyspnea.

CAVEATS

- CPET complements autonomic testing.
- HYCH can be associated with preload failure.

REFERENCE

1. Huang W, Resch S, Oliveira RK, Cockrill BA, Systrom DM, Waxman AB. Invasive cardiopulmonary exercise testing in the evaluation of unexplained dyspnea: Insights from a multidisciplinary dyspnea center. *Eur J Prev Cardiol.* 2017;24(11):1190–1199. doi:10.1177/2047487317709605.

2. Novak P. Hypocapnic cerebral hypoperfusion: A biomarker of orthostatic intolerance. *PloS One.* 2018;13(9):e0204419. doi:10.1371/journal.pone.0204419

43.

CASE 38: DIZZINESS AND ELEVATED CEREBRAL BLOOD FLOW VELOCITY

Chief complaint: Dizziness.

Case presentation: A 22-year-old woman presents with dizziness. She has a history of chronic constipation since childhood. Dysautonomia has been suspected since gastrointestinal evaluations were consistent with gastroparesis. She also experienced tachycardia and lightheadedness and has been diagnosed with postural tachycardia syndrome (POTS). She frequently develops lightheadedness and dizziness after straining during defecation and presyncopal feelings after getting up from the toilet. Her father has mixed small fiber neuropathy.

Past medical history: Seizure disorder, chronic constipation, POTS.

Current medication: Linaclotide.

Assessment plan: Functional autonomic tests and skin biopsy.

AUTONOMIC TESTING EVALUATION

See Table 43.1.

Heart rate: Supine heart rate was normal. Heart rate responses to deep breathing were reduced to 47.6% of normal value. Heart rate increment during the tilt (8 BPM) was normal.

Blood pressure:

Valsalva maneuver: Blood pressure responses were normal.

Tilt: Supine blood pressure was normal. Variability of blood pressure increased during the tilt but average blood pressure responses to tilt were normal.

Sudomotor evaluation: Electrochemical skin conductance was abnormal (reduced to 76.4% of normal limit) at hands and abnormal (reduced to 92.4% of normal limit) at feet.

Respiratory system: Respiratory frequency was normal in supine position. Respiratory frequency was normal during the tilt. End tidal CO_2 was normal in supine position. End tidal CO_2 was normal during the tilt.

Cerebral blood flow velocity (CBFv): CBFv in middle cerebral artery was normal in supine position. Mean CBFv in middle cerebral artery was stable during the tilt but CBFv was intermittently elevated and abnormally oscillated between (systolic/diastolic) 107/49–131/80 cm/s within seconds.

Skin biopsy (sensory-epidermal): Epidermal nerve fiber density was normal at proximal leg and abnormal (reduced to 77% of normal limit) at distal leg.

TABLE 43.1 **RESULTS OF AUTONOMIC TESTING**

Blood pressure evaluation					
Test: Valsalva maneuver					
Pressure [mmHg]	Baseline	Phase 2			Phase 4
		Early	End		
Systolic	88	87	86		
Mean	70.7	75.7	83.3	n/a	
Diastolic	62	70	82	n/a	

Heart rate evaluation	
Test: Deep breathing	
Results	Norm*
6.7	≥14
Test: Valsalva ratio	
1.75	≥1.46

* adjusted for a gender and age

(continued)

TABLE 43.1 **CONTINUED**

Test: Tilt test										
Position		HR [BPM]	Blood pressure [mmHg]		MCA Blood flow velocity [cm/s]				Respiratory frequency [breaths/min]	End tidal CO_2 [mmHg]
			Systolic	Diastolic	Systolic	Mean	Mean drop [%]	Diastolic		
Supine		96	125	84	118	84		67	19	36
Tilt [min]	1	98	137	86	116	82	2.4	65	14	34
	2	103	127	92						
	3	91	122	88						
	4	99	112	80						
	5	102	113	79	110	77.3	8	61	18	35
	6	100	124	86						
	7	104	122	74						
	8	101	109	78						
	9	96	120	84						
	10	104	114	83	114	74.7	11.1	55	14	36
	15									
	20									
	30									
	40									

Sudomotor evaluation - functional

Test: Quantitative sudomotor axon reflex test (QSART)				
Location	Site (l/r)	Latency [min]	Volume [μl]	Norm [μl]*
Forearm				≥0.08
Prox. leg				≥0.14
Distal leg				≥0.24
Foot				≥0.09

* Normative data are adjusted for gender and age of patient.

Test: Electrochemical skin conductance (ESC)				
Location	Left [μS]	Right [μS]	Average [μS/k]	Norm [μS/kg]
Hand	60	71	0.79	≥1.03
Feet	87	87	1.05	≥1.14
Forehead				

For grading uses ESC [μS] adjusted for weight [μS/k].

TABLE 43.1 CONTINUED

Small fiber (sensory + sudomotor) evaluation - morphological					
Test: Skin biopsy					
Location	Site (l/r)	Nerve fibers			
		Epidermal*		Sweat glands	
		Density	Norm	Density	Norm
Proximal leg – thigh	Right	9.84	≥8.3	65.4	≥37.8
Distal leg - calf	Right	7.07	≥9.18	45.5	≥36.5
Foot	Right		≥3.11		≥34.8

*Normative data for distal leg are adjusted for gender and age of patient.

QASAT*										
Heart rate		**BP**		**CBFv**		**ET-CO2**		**Sudomotor**		**Total QASAT score**
S. bradycardia	0	Low supine	0	Low supine	0	Low supine	0	QSART		
S. tachycardia	0	High supine	0	High supine	0	High supine	0	ESC	1	
Increase tilt	0	OH	0	Tilt response	0	Tilt low	0			
Decrease tilt	1	OHTN	0	CA	0	Tilt high	0	**Skin biopsy**		5
Deep breathing	2	VM	0	CVR	0			Epidermal	1	
VR	0			VM	0			Sweat gland	0	
Total	3	Total	0	Total	0	Total	0			

*QASAT. See Novak. Quantitative Scale for Grading of Cardiovascular Autonomic Reflex Tests and Small Fibers from Skin Biopsies. *J Neurol Disord* 2015;3:2.

S, supine; Increase tilt, increased response to tilt; Decrease tilt, decreased response to tilt; BP, blood pressure; VM, Valsalva maneuver; CBFv, cerebral blood flow velocity; CA, cerebral autoregulation; MCA, middle cerebral artery; VR, Valsalva ratio; CVR, cerebral vasoreactivity.

Skin biopsy (sweat glands): Sweat gland nerve fiber density was normal at proximal leg and normal at distal leg.

Patient-reported symptoms during testing: Dizziness during the tilt.

Patient-reported symptoms for past 2 weeks:

Lightheadedness or dizziness: Often
Dry eyes or mouth: None
Pale feet: None
Cold feet: None
Reduced sweating: None
Reduced sweating after exercise: None
Increased sweating: None
Nausea: Often
Diarrhea: None
Constipation: Often
Urinary leaks: None
Current pain severity: 9
Aching pain: Occasionally, mild
Allodynia: None
Burning pain: None
Lancinating pain: None
Numbness: None
Prickling sensation: None

AUTONOMIC TESTING INTERPRETATION

- Small fiber neuropathy, length-dependent.
- Mild parasympathetic dysfunction, There was no evidence of POTS.
- Cerebral autoregulatory failure.

COMMENT

The tilt test reproduced several of the patient's complaints, including dizziness and palpitations (Figure 43.1). During

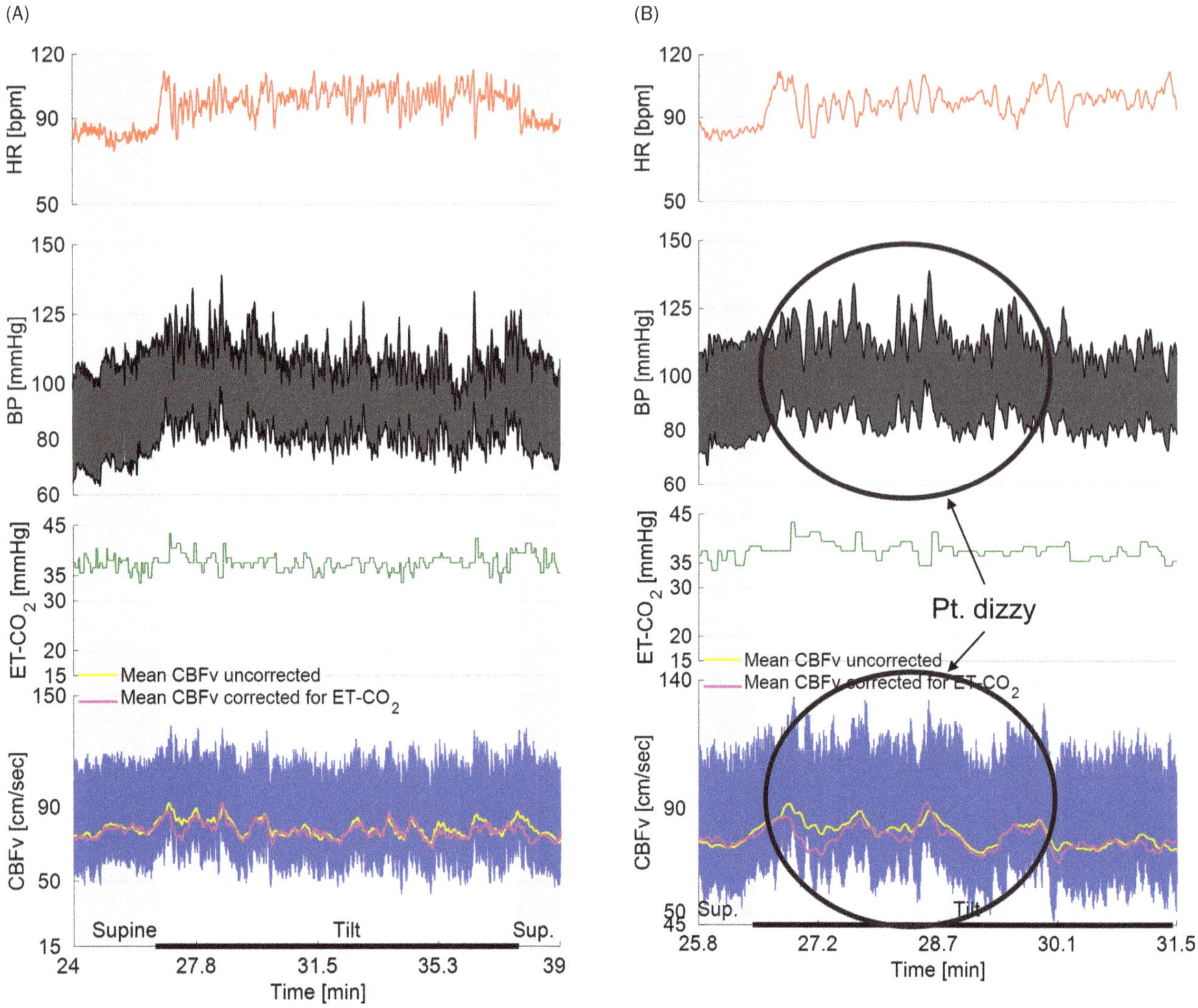

Figure 43.1 The tilt showed fluctuated and transiently elevated cerebral blood flow velocity (CBFv) associated with dizziness. For example, supine CBFv (systolic/mean/diastolic, 109/73.7/56 cm/s just before the tilt) increased within 15 seconds to 133/99.7/83 cm/s at the tilt onset and caused considerable dizziness. Blood pressure and heart rate responses were normal.

her symptoms, she was neither tachycardic nor hypotensive but CBFv was intermittently elevated up 25% (Figure 43.1) and fluctuated. Brain is sensitive to blood flow and it is our experience that even mild changes in CBFv, either increases or decreases, can be symptomatic. Since all parameters that affect CBFv were stable (heart rate, blood pressure, and end tidal CO_2), CBFv changes are indicative of cerebral autoregulatory failure.[1]

TREATMENT AND FOLLOW-UP

- Clinical workup for neuropathy.
- Volume expansion through high fluid and high salt intake.

CAVEATS

- Orthostatic dizziness can be associated with elevated and fluctuating CBFv.

REFERENCE

1. Panerai RB. Transcranial Doppler for evaluation of cerebral autoregulation. *Clin Auton Res Off J Clin Auton Res Soc*. 2009;19(4): 197–211. doi:10.1007/s10286-009-0011-8.

PART VII

NEURODEGENERATIVE DISORDERS

44.

CASE 39: HYPOTHERMIA IN FRONTOTEMPORAL DEMENTIA

Chief complaint: Intermittent hypothermia.

Case presentation: A 74-year-old man presents with a history of hypothermia. Previously, he was very active, visiting the gym regularly. He noted word finding difficulties starting 5 years ago. He fell and hurt his knee 4 years ago, requiring three surgeries complicated by infections. Subsequently, he deteriorated. Family noted progressive balance problems with falls, intermittent confusion, and worrisome hypothermic episodes (which started last year), with a fall in body temperature to below 32.2°C (90°F). Family noted confusion and transient cognitive worsening with decline in temperature and improvement with body temperature rise. On a usual day, he may have a temperature of 33.3°C (92°F) in the morning, then a normal temperature during the day. The lowest core temperature was 28.3°C (83°F). Last year, the patient was diagnosed with frontotemporal dementia (FTD). Patient did not benefit from memantine and rivastigmine. More recently, he has been sleepy and tired during the daytime and frequently falls asleep after meals. He was found to be bradycardic and placed on pilocarpine. He was referred for evaluation of suspected autonomic failure.

Past medical history: FTD, macrocytic anemia due to myelodysplastic syndrome.

Current medication: Pilocarpine, melatonin.

Assessment plan: Functional autonomic tests.

AUTONOMIC TESTING EVALUATION

See Table 44.1.

Heart rate: Supine heart rate was normal. Heart rate responses to deep breathing were reduced to 54.3% of normal value. Heart rate increment during the tilt (12 BPM) was normal.

Blood pressure:

Valsalva maneuver: Mean blood pressure failed to return to baseline at the end of Phase 2 by 14.4 mm Hg (i.e., 84.1% of baseline).

Tilt: Supine blood pressure was normal. Blood pressure responses to tilt were abnormal and consistent with marked orthostatic hypotension.

Sudomotor evaluation: Sweat output was normal at forearm, abnormal (reduced to 27% of lower limit) at proximal leg, abnormal (reduced to 17.4% of lower limit) at distal leg, and abnormal (reduced to 88.5% of lower limit) at foot. QSART showed length-dependent pattern with a decrease of sweat output distally of at least 33%.

Respiratory system: Respiratory frequency and end tidal CO_2 were normal in supine position and during the tilt.

Cerebral blood flow velocity (CBFv): CBFv in middle cerebral artery was normal in supine position but was severely reduced during the tilt.

TABLE 44.1 RESULTS OF AUTONOMIC TESTING

Blood pressure evaluation					
Test: Valsalva maneuver					
Pressure [mmHg]	Baseline	Phase 2			Phase 4
		Early	End		
Systolic	140	89	89		
Mean	90.7	76.3	76.3	n/a	
Diastolic	66	70	70	n/a	

Heart rate evaluation	
Test: Deep breathing	
Results	Norm*
3.8	≥7
Test: Valsalva ratio	
1.24	≥1.29
* adjusted for a gender and age	

(continued)

TABLE 44.1 **CONTINUED**

Test: Tilt test

Position		HR [BPM]	Blood pressure [mmHg]		MCA Blood flow velocity [cm/s]				Respiratory frequency [breaths/min]	End tidal CO_2 [mmHg]
			Systolic	Diastolic	Systolic	Mean	Mean drop [%]	Diastolic		
Supine		50	131	76	105.3	63.9		43.2	11	38
Tilt [min]	1	52	100	66	93.5	56.9	11	38.6	13	36
	2	57	97	52						
	3	62	100	65						
	4	59	99	63						
	5	59	101	65	86.5	46.8	26.8	26.9	9	34
	6	59	106	59						
	7	60	96	61						
	8	60	96	62						
	9	57	97	62						
	10	55	99	63	84.2	49.1	23.2	31.5	9	34
	15									
	20									
	30									
	40									

Sudomotor evaluation - functional

Test: Quantitative sudomotor axon reflex test (QSART)

Location	Site (l/r)	Latency [min]	Volume [μl]	Norm [μl]*
Forearm	l	1.22	0.724	≥0.3
Prox. leg	l	2.18	0.062	≥0.23
Distal leg	l	2.27	0.04	≥0.23
Foot	l	1.41	0.239	≥0.27

* Normative data are adjusted for gender and age of patient.

Test: Electrochemical skin conductance (ESC)

Location	Left [μS]	Right [μS]	Average [μS/k]	Norm [μS/kg]
Hand				≥
Feet				≥
Forehead				

For grading uses ESC [μS] adjusted for weight [μS/k].

TABLE 44.1 **CONTINUED**

Small fiber (sensory + sudomotor) evaluation - morphological					
Test: Skin biopsy					
Location	Site (l/r)	Nerve fibers			
		Epidermal*		Sweat glands	
		Density	Norm	Density	Norm
Proximal leg – thigh	Right		≥8.3		≥37.8
Distal leg - calf	Right		≥		≥36.5
Foot	Right		≥3.11		≥34.8

*Normative data for distal leg are adjusted for gender and age of patient.

QASAT*											
Heart rate		BP		CBFv		ET-CO2		Sudomotor			Total QASAT score
S. bradycardia	0	Low supine	0	Low supine	0	Low supine	0	QSART	2		
S. tachycardia	0	High supine	0	High supine	0	High supine	0	ESC			
Increase tilt	0	OH	10	Tilt response	5	Tilt low	0				
Decrease tilt	0	OHTN	0	CA	0	Tilt high	0	**Skin biopsy**			21
Deep breathing	1	VM	2	CVR	0			Epidermal			
VR	1			VM	0			Sweat gland			
Total	2	Total	12	Total	5	Total	0				

*QASAT. See Novak. Quantitative Scale for Grading of Cardiovascular Autonomic Reflex Tests and Small Fibers from Skin Biopsies. *J Neurol Disord* 2015;3:2.

S, supine; Increase tilt, increased response to tilt; Decrease tilt, decreased response to tilt; BP, blood pressure; VM, Valsalva maneuver; CBFv, cerebral blood flow velocity; CA, cerebral autoregulation; MCA, middle cerebral artery; VR, Valsalva ratio; CVR, cerebral vasoreactivity.

Skin biopsy (sensory-epidermal): N/A

Skin biopsy (sweat glands): N/A

Patient-reported symptoms during testing: Feeling chilly and dizzy during the tilt.

Patient-reported symptoms for past 2 weeks:

Lightheadedness or dizziness: Yes, minor annoyance
Dry eyes or mouth: Occasionally
Pale feet: Occasionally
Cold feet: Occasionally
Reduced sweating: Yes, minor annoyance
Reduced sweating after exercise: Occasionally
Increased sweating: Yes, minor annoyance
Nausea: Occasionally
Diarrhea: Occasionally
Constipation: Occasionally
Urinary leaks: Occasionally
Erection problems: Occasionally
Current pain severity: 0
Aching pain: Occasionally, mild
Allodynia: Occasionally, mild
Burning pain: None
Lancinating pain: Occasionally, moderate
Numbness: Occasionally, moderate
Prickling sensation: Occasionally, mild

AUTONOMIC TESTING INTERPRETATION

- Generalized autonomic failure.

COMMENT

Autonomic testing was consistent with severe autonomic failure (Figure 44.1). This patient has FTD and a history of hypothermia. Thermoregulation is a vital function of autonomic nervous system. The primary thermoregulatory center is the preoptic area and posterior hypothalamus. Temperature is maintained within a narrow range (36.1–37°C).[1] Hypothermia, defined as a core temperature

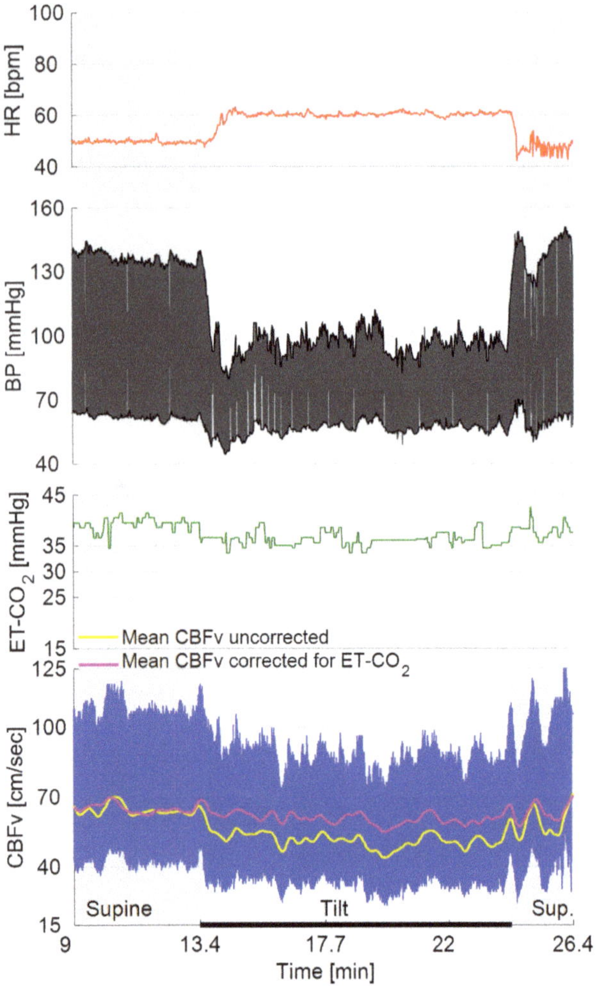

Figure 44.1 The tilt test provoked severe sustained orthostatic hypotension associated with reduced heart rate response and decline in cerebral blood flow velocity (CBFv). Patient was symptomatic.

of less than 35°C (<95°F) may impair mental function. In addition to cold injuries, hypothermia accompanies disorders that affect thermoregulatory autonomic pathways including diabetes, stroke, Parkinson's disease, spinal cord injuries, and dementia. In this patient, hypothermia can be associated with hypothalamic degeneration as seen in FTD.[2]

Prevention of hypothermia includes wearing warm clothing and avoiding dehydration. Mild hypothermia can be managed with external passive or active core warming. If patients are dehydrated, they should receive supplemental fluids.

TREATMENT AND FOLLOW-UP

- Volume expansion through high fluid and high salt intake. Trial of proamatine.
- Passive rewarming of hypothermic episodes.

CAVEATS

- Hypothermia can be part of generalized autonomic failure.
- FTD can be accompanied by severe generalized autonomic failure and hypothermia.
- Hypothermia can be a medical emergency and should be treated urgently.

REFERENCES

1. Cheshire WP. Thermoregulatory disorders and illness related to heat and cold stress. *Auton Neurosci Basic Clin*. 2016;196:91–104. doi:10.1016/j.autneu.2016.01.001.
2. Vercruysse P, Vieau D, Blum D, Petersén Å, Dupuis L. Hypothalamic alterations in neurodegenerative diseases and their relation to abnormal energy metabolism. *Front Mol Neurosci*. 2018;11:2. doi:10.3389/fnmol.2018.00002.

45.

CASE 40: PARKINSON'S DISEASE WITH COMPENSATED ORTHOSTATIC HYPOTENSION

Chief complaint: Dizziness.

Case presentation: A 59-year-old man with history of Parkinson's disease for 4 years initially presented with left arm and leg rigidity, limb tremor, and bradykinesia. For the past 2 years, he experienced orthostatic dizziness and balance problems. His parkinsonism is responding well to levodopa. For the past several months, the patient experienced deterioration of balance with frequent falls and increased urinary frequency. He was referred for autonomic testing for evaluation of suspected autonomic failure to determine if autonomic failure is a factor in his falls.

Past medical history: Parkinson's disease, hypertension, dyslipidemia.

Current medication: Levodopa, lisinopril.

Assessment plan: Functional autonomic tests and skin biopsy.

AUTONOMIC TESTING EVALUATION

See Table 45.1.

Heart rate: Supine tachycardia. There was mild tachycardia during the tilt.

Blood pressure:

Valsalva maneuver: Mean blood pressure failed to return to baseline at the end of Phase 2 by 35 mm Hg (i.e., 70.3% of baseline).

Tilt: Supine blood pressure was elevated. Blood pressure responses to tilt were abnormal and consistent with marked orthostatic hypotension (OH).

Sudomotor evaluation: Sweat output was normal at proximal leg.

Respiratory system: Respiratory frequency and end tidal CO_2 were normal in supine position and during the tilt.

Cerebral blood flow velocity (CBFv): CBFv in middle cerebral artery was normal in supine position and was stable during the tilt.

Skin biopsy (sensory-epidermal): Epidermal nerve fiber density was abnormal (reduced to 27.2% of normal limit) at proximal leg and abnormal (reduced to 2.8% of normal limit) at distal leg.

Skin biopsy (sweat glands): Sweat gland nerve fiber density was normal at distal leg.

Patient-reported symptoms during testing: Dizziness during the tilt.

Patient-reported symptoms for past 2 weeks:

Lightheadedness or dizziness: Occasionally
Dry eyes or mouth: None
Pale feet: None
Cold feet: Occasionally
Reduced sweating: Yes, minor annoyance
Reduced sweating after exercise: Yes, minor annoyance

TABLE 45.1 **RESULTS OF AUTONOMIC TESTING**

Blood pressure evaluation					
Test: Valsalva maneuver					
Pressure [mmHg]	Baseline	Phase 2			Phase 4
		Early	End		
Systolic	167	104	104		
Mean	117.7	82.7	82.7	n/a	
Diastolic	93	72	72	n/a	

Heart rate evaluation	
Test: Deep breathing	
Results	Norm*
4.6	≥9
Test: Valsalva ratio	
1.09	≥1.36
* adjusted for a gender and age	

(continued)

TABLE 45.1 CONTINUED

Test: Tilt test

Position		HR [BPM]	Blood pressure [mmHg]		MCA Blood flow velocity [cm/s]				Respiratory frequency [breaths/min]	End tidal CO_2 [mmHg]
			Systolic	Diastolic	Systolic	Mean	Mean drop [%]	Diastolic		
Supine		101	179	122	77	47		32	15	42
Tilt [min]	1	102	121	90	73	43.7	7	29	14	34
	2	114	113	80						
	3	110	118	83						
	4	107	117	82						
	5	105	115	83	72.5	43.5	7.4	29	12	37
	6	103	125	84						
	7	104	123	83						
	8	105	122	85						
	9	104	114	82						
	10	106	114	82	68	41.3	12.1	28	15	36
	15									
	20									
	30									
	40									

Sudomotor evaluation - functional

Test: Quantitative sudomotor axon reflex test (QSART)

Location	Site (l/r)	Latency [min]	Volume [μl]	Norm [μl]*
Forearm				≥0.3
Prox. leg	l	1.47	0.573	≥0.23
Distal leg				≥0.23
Foot				≥0.27

* Normative data are adjusted for gender and age of patient.

Test: Electrochemical skin conductance (ESC)

Location	Left [μS]	Right [μS]	Average [μS/k]	Norm [μS/kg]
Hand				≥
Feet				≥
Forehead				

For grading uses ESC [μS] adjusted for weight [μS/k].

Small fiber (sensory + sudomotor) evaluation - morphological					
Test: Skin biopsy					
Location	Site (l/r)	Nerve fibers			
		Epidermal*		Sweat glands	
		Density	Norm	Density	Norm
Proximal leg – thigh	Right	2.26	≥8.3		≥37.8
Distal leg - calf	Right	0.14	≥5.075	37.4	≥36.5
Foot	Right		≥3.11		≥34.8

*Normative data for distal leg are adjusted for gender and age of patient.

QASAT*											
Heart rate		**BP**		**CBFv**		**ET-CO2**		**Sudomotor**			**Total QASAT score**
S. bradycardia	0	Low supine	0	Low supine	0	Low supine	0	QSART			
S. tachycardia	1	High supine	3	High supine	0	High supine	0	ESC			
Increase tilt	0	OH	10	Tilt response	0	Tilt low	0				
Decrease tilt	0	OHTN	0	CA	0	Tilt high	0	**Skin biopsy**			22
Deep breathing	1	VM	2	CVR	0			Epidermal	4		
VR	1			VM	0			Sweat gland	0		
Total	3	Total	15	Total	0	Total	0				

*QASAT. See Novak. Quantitative Scale for Grading of Cardiovascular Autonomic Reflex Tests and Small Fibers from Skin Biopsies. *J Neurol Disord* 2015;3:2.

S, supine; Increase tilt, increased response to tilt; Decrease tilt, decreased response to tilt; BP, blood pressure; VM, Valsalva maneuver; CBFv, cerebral blood flow velocity; CA, cerebral autoregulation; MCA, middle cerebral artery; VR, Valsalva ratio; CVR, cerebral vasoreactivity.

Increased sweating: None
Nausea: None
Diarrhea: None
Constipation: Occasionally
Urinary leaks: Occasionally
Erection problems: Occasionally
Current pain severity: 2
Aching pain: Occasionally, mild
Allodynia: None
Burning pain: Occasionally, mild
Lancinating pain: None
Numbness: Often, mild
Prickling sensation: Occasionally, mild

AUTONOMIC TESTING INTERPRETATION

- Autonomic failure, generalized, severe, associated with neurogenic OH and supine hypertension.
- Small fiber neuropathy.
- Stable CBFv.

COMMENT

Although this patient had neurogenic OH, the orthostatic CBFv was stable, indicating effective cerebral autoregulation that compensates for the blood pressure drop by cerebral vasodilation (Figure 45.1). Indeed, there was no evidence of cerebral hypoperfusion as the patient was asymptomatic. As such, it is unlikely that orthostatic hypoperfusion is a major determinant of the patient's falls.

Autonomic failure manifesting as neurogenic OH and supine hypertension are common manifestations of cardiovascular dysautonomia in Parkinson's disease.[1] Whereas neurogenic OH poses a risk for falls and can be associated with cognitive impairment, chronic supine hypertension

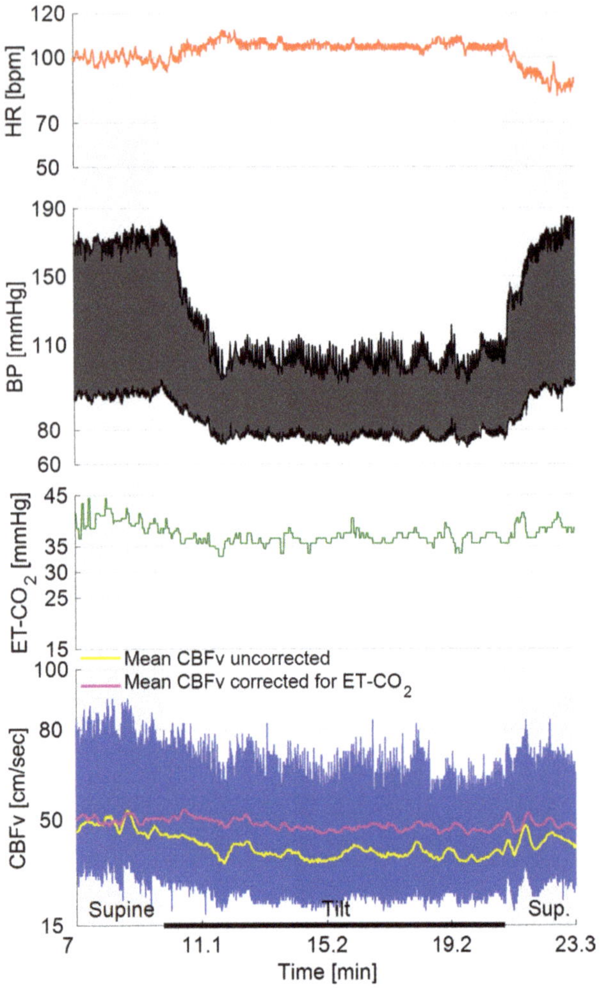

Figure 45.1 The tilt test showed sustained orthostatic hypotension. Orthostatic cerebral blood flow velocity was stable, minor decrease was within normal range. There was supine tachycardia with preserved heart rate increment during the tilt. Patient was asymptomatic.

can be associated with stroke and myocardial infarction in the long term.

TREATMENT AND FOLLOW-UP

- Volume expansion through high fluid and high salt intake.
- Avoid supine position during the day since patient has supine hypertension. Sleep with the head of the bed elevated at least 35 degree to reduce supine hypertension.
- Consider gently increasing lisinopril at night to reduce supine hypertension.

CAVEATS

- Depending on cerebral blood flow, neurogenic OH can be either compensated (with stable orthostatic cerebral blood flow) or noncompensated (with reduced flow). Compensated OH needs less aggressive treatment.
- CBFv monitoring is useful in managing autonomic failure.

REFERENCE

1. Espay AJ, LeWitt PA, Hauser RA, Merola A, Masellis M, Lang AE. Neurogenic orthostatic hypotension and supine hypertension in Parkinson's disease and related synucleinopathies: prioriti sation of treatment targets. *Lancet Neurol.* 2016;15(9):954–966. doi:10.1016/S1474-4422(16)30079-5.

46.

CASE 41: ATYPICAL PARKINSONISM

Chief complaint: Unsteady gait.

Case presentation: A 56-year-old woman presented with unsteady gait. About 10 years ago, she began to develop visual problems including focusing difficulties, decreased smell, and insomnia. For the past 6 years, she noticed involuntary jerking movements that happen randomly anywhere in her body. She became stiffer in her legs, particularly her calves, and her legs became difficult to bend. She also noted slowness, including when talking, writing, opening things with her hands, and walking. She experienced tremor when holding objects but not resting tremor. She did respond only modestly to levodopa, rasagiline, and pramipexole; therefore she was diagnosed with atypical parkinsonism. A nerve conduction study showed sensorimotor polyneuropathy, which was attributed to B_{12} deficiency. More recently, she experienced heat intolerance and fullness after meals, and she is unable to work. She was referred for an evaluation of autonomic failure.

Past medical history: Atypical parkinsonism, vitamin B_{12} deficiency, migraine.

Current medication: Levodopa, rasagiline, pramipexole, B_{12} supplements, trazodone.

Assessment plan: Functional autonomic tests and skin biopsy.

AUTONOMIC TESTING EVALUATION

See Table 46.1.

Heart rate: Supine heart rate was normal. Heart rate responses to deep breathing were reduced to 90.8% of normal value. Heart rate increment during the tilt (18 BPM) was normal.

Blood pressure:

Valsalva maneuver: Blood pressure responses were normal.

Tilt: Supine blood pressure was normal. Blood pressure responses to tilt were normal.

Sudomotor evaluation: Electrochemical skin conductance was abnormal (reduced to 93.9% of normal limit) at hands and abnormal (reduced to 89.8% of normal limit) at feet.

Respiratory system: Respiratory frequency and end tidal CO_2 were normal in supine position and during the tilt.

Cerebral blood flow velocity (CBFv): CBFv in middle cerebral artery was normal in supine position but was moderately reduced during the tilt (24% at the end of the tilt. In our lab normal orthostatic drop is up 14% at the minute 10 of the tilt assuming that the end tidal CO_2 remains unchanged.

TABLE 46.1 RESULTS OF AUTONOMIC TESTING

Blood pressure evaluation					
Test: Valsalva maneuver					
Pressure [mmHg]	Baseline	Phase 2			Phase 4
		Early	End		
Systolic	109	77	104		
Mean	76.3	61.7	85.3	n/a	
Diastolic	60	54	76	n/a	

Heart rate evaluation	
Test: Deep breathing	
Results	Norm*
8.17	≥9
Test: Valsalva ratio	
1.43	≥1.47
* adjusted for a gender and age	

(continued)

TABLE 46.1 **CONTINUED**

Test: Tilt test										
Position		HR [BPM]	Blood pressure [mmHg]		MCA Blood flow velocity [cm/s]				Respiratory frequency [breaths/min]	End tidal CO_2 [mmHg]
			Systolic	Diastolic	Systolic	Mean	Mean drop [%]	Diastolic		
Supine		71	107	70	107	67		47	15	36
Tilt [min]	1	79	125	82	95	60.3	10	43	11	36
	2	82	124	84						
	3	79	126	83						
	4	79	130	85						
	5	76	124	86	97	59	11.9	40	10	36
	6	82	130	82						
	7	79	127	85						
	8	76	129	83						
	9	78	127	87						
	10	89	130	79	87	51	23.9	33	12	35
	15									
	20									
	30									
	40									

Sudomotor evaluation - functional

Test: Quantitative sudomotor axon reflex test (QSART)				
Location	Site (l/r)	Latency [min]	Volume [μl]	Norm [μl]*
Forearm				≥0.08
Prox. leg				≥0.14
Distal leg				≥0.07
Foot				≥0.05

* Normative data are adjusted for gender and age of patient.

Test: Electrochemical skin conductance (ESC)				
Location	Left [μS]	Right [μS]	Average [μS/k]	Norm [μS/kg]
Hand	87	85	0.97	≥1.03
Feet	92	91	1.02	≥1.14
Forehead				

For grading uses ESC [μS] adjusted for weight [μS/k].

Small fiber (sensory + sudomotor) evaluation - morphological					
Test: Skin biopsy					
Location	Site (l/r)	Nerve fibers			
		Epidermal*		Sweat glands	
		Density	Norm	Density	Norm
Proximal leg – thigh	Right	12.99	≥8.3	44.4	≥37.8
Distal leg - calf	Right	3.37	≥6.54		≥36.5
Foot	Right		≥3.11		≥34.8

*Normative data for distal leg are adjusted for gender and age of patient.

QASAT*											
Heart rate		BP		CBFv		ET-CO2		Sudomotor			Total QASAT score
S. bradycardia	0	Low supine	0	Low supine	0	Low supine	0	QSART			
S. tachycardia	0	High supine	0	High supine	0	High supine	0	ESC	1		
Increase tilt	0	OH	0	Tilt response	3	Tilt low	0				
Decrease tilt	0	OHTN	0	CA	0	Tilt high	0	**Skin biopsy**			9
Deep breathing	1	VM	0	CVR	0			Epidermal	3		
VR	1			VM	0			Sweat gland	0		
Total	2	Total	0	Total	3	Total	0				

*QASAT. See Novak. Quantitative Scale for Grading of Cardiovascular Autonomic Reflex Tests and Small Fibers from Skin Biopsies. *J Neurol Disord* 2015;3:2.

S, supine; Increase tilt, increased response to tilt; Decrease tilt, decreased response to tilt; BP, blood pressure; VM, Valsalva maneuver; CBFv, cerebral blood flow velocity; CA, cerebral autoregulation; MCA, middle cerebral artery; VR, Valsalva ratio; CVR, cerebral vasoreactivity.

Skin biopsy (sensory-epidermal): Epidermal nerve fiber density was normal at proximal leg and abnormal (reduced to 51.5% of normal limit) at distal leg.

Skin biopsy (sweat glands): Sweat gland nerve fiber density was normal at proximal leg.

Patient-reported symptoms during testing: Dizziness during the tilt.

Patient-reported symptoms for past 2 weeks:

Lightheadedness or dizziness: Occasionally
Dry eyes or mouth: Often
Pale feet: None
Cold feet: Occasionally
Reduced sweating: None
Reduced sweating after exercise: Often
Increased sweating: Occasionally
Nausea: Occasionally
Diarrhea: Occasionally
Constipation: Often
Urinary leaks: Occasionally
Current pain severity: 5
Aching pain: Continuous, severe
Allodynia: None
Burning pain: Occasionally, mild
Lancinating pain: Occasionally, mild
Numbness: Continuous, moderate
Prickling sensation: Continuous, moderate

AUTONOMIC TESTING INTERPRETATION

- Small fiber neuropathy, length-dependent, affecting predominantly sensory fibers, biopsy-proven.
- Mild autonomic dysfunction. Orthostatic hypotension, a marker of more advanced adrenergic failure, was not seen in this patient.
- Orthostatic cerebral hypoperfusion syndrome (OCHOS).[1]
- Respiratory functions were normal; there was no evidence of hyperventilation or hypoventilation.

COMMENT

The testing showed minimal dysautonomia, small fiber neuropathy, and OCHOS (Figure 46.1). Small fiber neuropathy can be due to vitamin B_{12} deficiency. Mild

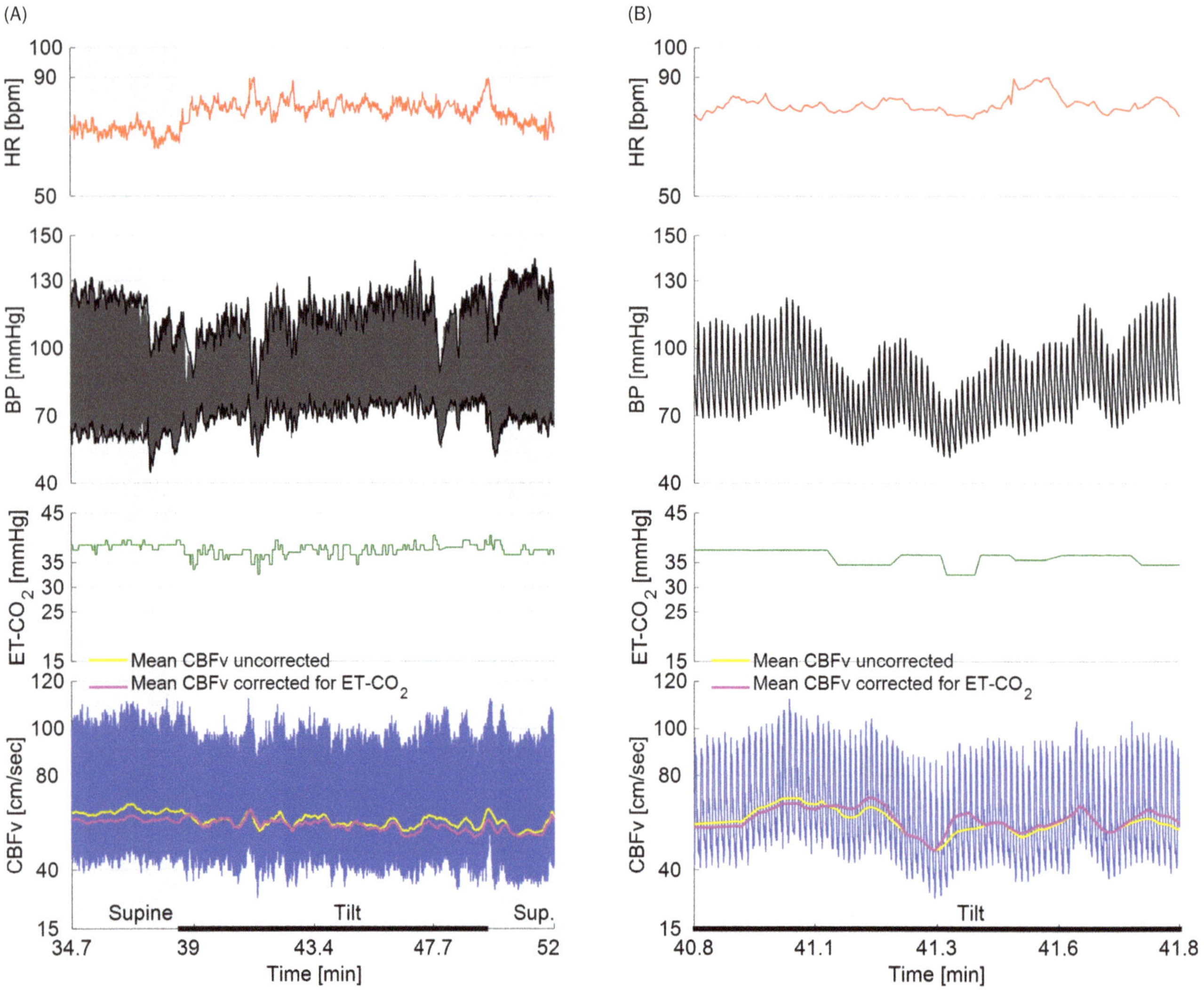

Figure 46.1 The tilt test showed reduced orthostatic cerebral blood flow velocity. While heart rate, blood pressure and end tidal CO_2 responses to tilt were normal (A,B).

dysautonomia speaks against Parkinson's disease and also against multiple system atrophy.[2]

Atypical parkinsonism may be related to OCHOS. Measurements of CBFv and cerebral autoregulation provide important insights into the pathophysiology of hypoperfusion syndromes.[3]

TREATMENT AND FOLLOW-UP

- Small fiber neuropathy can be due to B_{12} deficiency.
- Pyridostigmine for gastroparesis.

CAVEATS

- Atypical parkinsonism can be associated with OCHOS.

REFERENCES

1. Novak P. Orthostatic cerebral hypoperfusion syndrome. *Front Aging Neurosci*. 2016;8:22. doi:10.3389/fnagi.2016.00022.
2. Gilman S, Wenning GK, Low PA, et al. Second consensus statement on the diagnosis of multiple system atrophy. *Neurology*. 2008;71(9):670–676. doi:10.1212/01.wnl.0000324625.00404.15.
3. Panerai RB. Transcranial Doppler for evaluation of cerebral autoregulation. *Clin Auton Res Off J Clin Auton Res Soc*. 2009;19(4):197–211. doi:10.1007/s10286-009-0011-8.

47.

CASE 42: MULTIPLE SYSTEM ATROPHY VERSUS PARKINSON'S DISEASE?

Chief complaint: Parkinsonism.

Case presentation: A 49-year-old woman presents with a history of balance and coordination difficulties for 2 years. She also noticed right-sided hand resting tremor for 1 year. Neurologic examination was consistent with asymmetric parkinsonism. Patient noted benefit from levodopa. Nevertheless, patient had prominent axial symptoms, and therefore she was referred for evaluation of dysautonomia, which can be helpful in evaluation of atypical parkinsonism or multiple system atrophy.

Past medical history: Parkinsonism, depression, insomnia, breast cancer.

Current medication: Levodopa.

Assessment plan: Functional autonomic tests and skin biopsy.

AUTONOMIC TESTING EVALUATION

See Table 47.1.

Heart rate: Supine heart rate was normal. Heart rate responses to deep breathing were reduced to 55% of normal value. Heart rate increment during the tilt (28 BPM) was normal.

Blood pressure:

Valsalva maneuver: Mean blood pressure failed to return to baseline at the end of Phase 2 by 48.6 mm Hg (i.e., 53.8% of baseline).

Tilt: Supine blood pressure was normal. Blood pressure was elevated during the tilt.

Sudomotor evaluation: Electrochemical skin conductance was abnormal (reduced to 68% of normal limit) at hands and normal at feet.

Respiratory system: Respiratory frequency was normal in supine position and during the tilt. End tidal CO_2 was normal in supine position but was mildly reduced during the tilt.

Cerebral blood flow velocity (CBFv): CBFv in middle cerebral artery was normal in supine position and stable during the tilt.

Skin biopsy (sensory-epidermal): Epidermal nerve fiber density was normal at proximal leg and normal at distal leg.

Skin biopsy (sweat glands): Sweat gland nerve fiber density was normal at distal leg.

Patient-reported symptoms during testing: Dizziness during the tilt.

TABLE 47.1 **RESULTS OF AUTONOMIC TESTING**

Blood pressure evaluation							Heart rate evaluation	
Test: Valsalva maneuver							Test: Deep breathing	
Pressure [mmHg]	Baseline	Phase 2			Phase 4		Results	Norm*
		Early	End				5.5	≥10
Systolic	154	70	70				Test: Valsalva ratio	
Mean	105.3	56.7	56.7	n/a			1.3	≥1.51
Diastolic	81	50	50	n/a			* adjusted for a gender and age	

(continued)

TABLE 47.1 **CONTINUED**

Test: Tilt test											
Position		HR [BPM]	Blood pressure [mmHg]		MCA Blood flow velocity [cm/s]				Respiratory frequency [breaths/min]	End tidal CO_2 [mmHg]
			Systolic	Diastolic	Systolic	Mean	Mean drop [%]	Diastolic		
Supine		73	122	78	111	65		42	18	36
Tilt [min]	1	92	130	82	90	60	7.7	45	10	35
	2	91	129	80						
	3	93	130	81						
	4	93	130	81						
	5	95	135	90	104	64.7	0.5	45	20	29
	6	95	135	90						
	7	101	126	91						
	8	97	131	71						
	9	91	128	79						
	10	98	125	82	103	63.7	2	44	18	36
	15									
	20									
	30									
	40									

Sudomotor evaluation - functional

Test: Quantitative sudomotor axon reflex test (QSART)				
Location	Site (l/r)	Latency [min]	Volume [µl]	Norm [µl]*
Forearm				≥0.08
Prox. leg				≥0.14
Distal leg				≥0.15
Foot				≥0.07

* Normative data are adjusted for gender and age of patient.

Test: Electrochemical skin conductance (ESC)				
Location	Left [µS]	Right [µS]	Average [µS/k]	Norm [µS/kg]
Hand	51	44	0.7	≥1.03
Feet	89	90	1.34	≥1.14
Forehead				

For grading uses ESC [µS] adjusted for weight [µS/k].

TABLE 47.1 **CONTINUED**

Small fiber (sensory + sudomotor) evaluation - morphological					
Test: Skin biopsy					
Location	Site (l/r)	Nerve fibers			
		Epidermal*		Sweat glands	
		Density	Norm	Density	Norm
Proximal leg – thigh	Right	12.67	≥8.3		≥37.8
Distal leg - calf	Right	8.93	≥7.18	39.3	≥36.5
Foot	Right		≥3.11		≥34.8

*Normative data for distal leg are adjusted for gender and age of patient.

QASAT*												
Heart rate		**BP**		**CBFv**		**ET-CO2**		**Sudomotor**			**Total QASAT score**
S. bradycardia	0	Low supine	0	Low supine	0	Low supine	0	QSART			
S. tachycardia	0	High supine	0	High supine	0	High supine	0	ESC	1		
Increase tilt	0	OH	0	Tilt response	0	Tilt low	1				
Decrease tilt	0	OHTN	0	CA	0	Tilt high	0	**Skin biopsy**			7
Deep breathing	1	VM	3	CVR	0			Epidermal	0		
VR	1			VM	0			Sweat gland	0		
Total	2	Total	3	Total	0	Total	1				

*QASAT. See Novak. Quantitative Scale for Grading of Cardiovascular Autonomic Reflex Tests and Small Fibers from Skin Biopsies. *J Neurol Disord* 2015;3:2.

S, supine; Increase tilt, increased response to tilt; Decrease tilt, decreased response to tilt; BP, blood pressure; VM, Valsalva maneuver; CBFv, cerebral blood flow velocity; CA, cerebral autoregulation; MCA, middle cerebral artery; VR, Valsalva ratio; CVR, cerebral vasoreactivity.

Patient-reported symptoms for past 2 weeks:

Lightheadedness or dizziness: Occasionally
Dry eyes or mouth: Occasionally
Pale feet: Occasionally
Cold feet: None
Reduced sweating: None
Reduced sweating after exercise: None
Increased sweating: Occasionally
Nausea: None
Diarrhea: Often
Constipation: Occasionally
Urinary leaks: Occasionally
Current pain severity: 0
Aching pain: Often, moderate
Allodynia: None
Burning pain: None
Lancinating pain: None
Numbness: None
Prickling sensation: None

AUTONOMIC TESTING INTERPRETATION

- Generalized but mild autonomic failure. Orthostatic hypotension, a marker of more advanced autonomic failure, was not seen in this study.
- Minimal sudomotor dysfunction can be seen in mild or early small fiber neuropathy even skin biopsy was normal.
- Cerebral blood flow was normal in supine position. Orthostatic cerebral blood flow was stable.

COMMENT

Overall, there was no evidence of the severe generalized autonomic failure that is seen in a typical case of multiple system atrophy (Figure. 47.1).[1,2] There was evidence of mild but widespread autonomic dysfunction. This finding

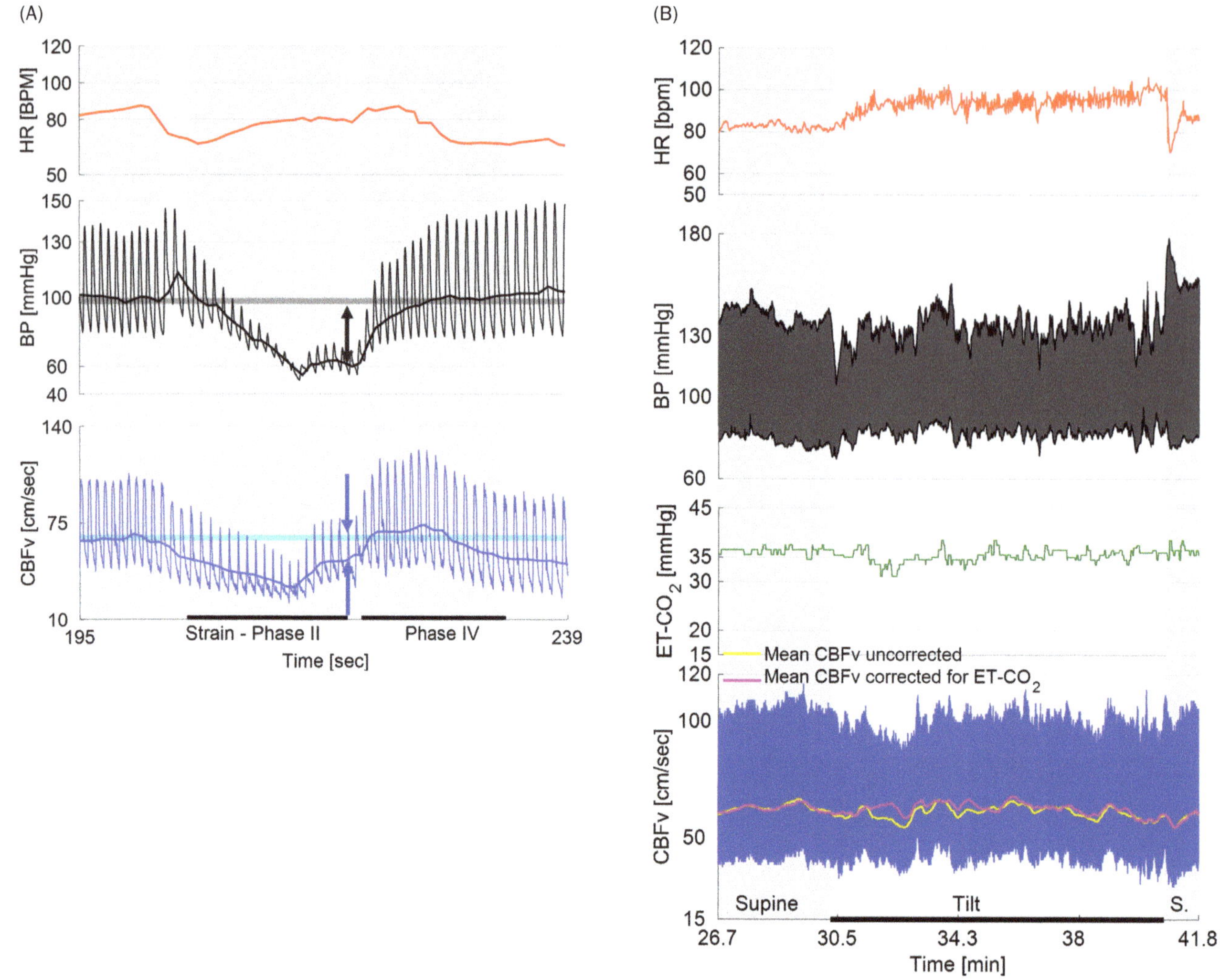

Figure 47.1 The Valsalva maneuver was abnormal and showed reduction of Phase 2 with partial recovery in blood pressure (black arrows) and cerebral blood flow velocity (blue arrows, A). Tilt test was normal (B).

is nonspecific and can be seen in variety of central (α-synucleinopathies) and peripheral (autonomic neuropathy/ganglionopathy) disorders. The sudomotor dysfunction localizes the lesion to postganglionic system and therefore the autonomic dysfunction in this patient is probably due to peripheral small fiber autonomic neuropathy.

TREATMENT AND FOLLOW-UP

- Clinical workup for neuropathy showed elevated acetylcholine ganglionic neuronal antibodies (titer 0.14, normal ≤0.02 nmol/L).
- Cancer screening was negative.
- Patient was recommended to start immunotherapy with intravenous immunoglobulins for suspected autoimmune autonomic neuropathy.[3]

CAVEATS

- Autonomic testing together with autoimmune evaluation may reveal unexpected diagnosis, as in this case, which showed autoimmune autonomic neuropathy.

REFERENCES

1. Iodice V, Low DA, Vichayanrat E, Mathias CJ. Cardiovascular autonomic dysfunction in MSA and Parkinson's disease: similarities and differences. *J Neurol Sci*. 2011;310(1-2):133–138. doi:10.1016/j.jns.2011.07.014.
2. Gilman S, Wenning GK, Low PA, et al. Second consensus statement on the diagnosis of multiple system atrophy. *Neurology*. 2008;71(9):670–676. doi:10.1212/01.wnl.0000324625.00404.15.
3. Iodice V, Sandroni P. Autonomic neuropathies. *Contin Minneap Minn*. 2014;20(5 Peripheral Nervous System Disorders):1373–1397. doi:10.1212/01.CON.0000455875.76179.b1.

48.

CASE 44: MULTIPLE SYSTEM ATROPHY

Chief complaint: Orthostatic dizziness.

Case presentation: A 53-year-old man, previously healthy, presents with a progressive deterioration of his functioning for past 2 years. Initially, he experienced difficulties with fine finger movement, as when typing or writing. Subsequently, he developed slowness of movement, balance problems, disabling orthostatic dizziness (can stand for 1 minute only), and fatigue. Neurological examination showed a combination of symmetrical parkinsonism with prominent rigidity and bradykinesia, cerebellar syndrome, and orthostatic hypotension. MRI of the brain was unrevealing. Patient was referred for assessment of autonomic failure that is part of suspected multiple system atrophy (MSA).

Past medical history: Suspected MSA.

Current medication: Lorazepam, venlafaxine, buspirone.

Assessment plan: Functional autonomic tests and skin biopsy.

AUTONOMIC TESTING EVALUATION

See Table 48.1.

Heart rate: Supine heart rate was normal. Heart rate responses to deep breathing were reduced to 80% of normal value. Heart rate increment during the tilt (17 BPM) was normal.

Blood pressure:

Valsalva maneuver: Mean blood pressure failed to return to baseline at the end of Phase 2 by 48.7 mm Hg (i.e., 54.9% of baseline).

Tilt: Supine blood pressure was elevated. Blood pressure responses to tilt were abnormal and consistent with marked orthostatic hypotension.

Sudomotor evaluation: Sweat output was normal at forearm, normal at proximal leg, normal at distal leg, and normal at foot.

Respiratory system: Respiratory frequency was normal in supine position and during the tilt. End tidal CO_2 was normal in supine position but was reduced during the tilt.

Cerebral blood flow velocity (CBFv): CBFv in middle cerebral artery was normal in supine position but was severely reduced during the tilt.

Skin biopsy (sensory-epidermal): Epidermal nerve fiber density was normal at proximal leg and normal at distal leg.

Skin biopsy (sweat glands): Sweat gland nerve fiber density was normal at proximal leg and normal at distal leg.

Patient-reported symptoms during testing: Dizziness during the tilt.

TABLE 48.1 **RESULTS OF AUTONOMIC TESTING**

Blood pressure evaluation					
Test: Valsalva maneuver					
Pressure [mmHg]	Baseline	Phase 2			Phase 4
		Early	End		
Systolic	148	74	74		
Mean	108	59.3	59.3	n/a	
Diastolic	88	52	52	n/a	

Heart rate evaluation	
Test: Deep breathing	
Results	Norm*
7.2	≥9
Test: Valsalva ratio	
1.16	≥1.36
* adjusted for a gender and age	

(continued)

TABLE 48.1 **CONTINUED**

Test: Tilt test											
Position		HR [BPM]	Blood pressure [mmHg]		MCA Blood flow velocity [cm/s]				Respiratory frequency [breaths/min]	End tidal CO_2 [mmHg]
			Systolic	Diastolic	Systolic	Mean	Mean drop [%]	Diastolic		
Supine		81	153	88	83	51		35	15	37
Tilt [min]	1	98	95	64	68	40.7	20.2	27	16	29
	2	94	92	61						
	3	93	90	58						
	4	89	89	57						
	5	93	84	55	68	38	25.5	23	15	28
	6	91	84	52						
	7	90	84	52						
	8	90	84	52						
	9	90	84	52						
	10	90	84	52	60	34	33.3	21	17	28
	15									
	20									
	30									
	40									

Sudomotor evaluation - functional

Test: Quantitative sudomotor axon reflex test (QSART)				
Location	Site (l/r)	Latency [min]	Volume [µl]	Norm [µl]*
Forearm	l	2.5	0.67	≥0.3
Prox. leg	l	1.38	0.712	≥0.23
Distal leg	l	1.56	0.6	≥0.23
Foot	l	2.22	0.5	≥0.27

* Normative data are adjusted for gender and age of patient.

Test: Electrochemical skin conductance (ESC)				
Location	Left [µS]	Right [µS]	Average [µS/k]	Norm [µS/kg]
Hand				≥1.03
Feet				≥1.14
Forehead				

For grading uses ESC [µS] adjusted for weight [µS/k].

TABLE 48.1 **CONTINUED**

Small fiber (sensory + sudomotor) evaluation - morphological					
Test: Skin biopsy					
Location	Site (l/r)	Nerve fibers			
		Epidermal*		Sweat glands	
		Density	Norm	Density	Norm
Proximal leg – thigh	Right	9.68	≥8.3	58.6	≥37.8
Distal leg - calf	Right	7.48	≥5.525	39.7	≥36.5
Foot	Right		≥3.11		≥34.8

*Normative data for distal leg are adjusted for gender and age of patient.

QASAT*											
Heart rate		**BP**		**CBFv**		**ET-CO2**		**Sudomotor**			**Total QASAT score**
S. bradycardia	0	Low supine	0	Low supine	0	Low supine	0	QSART	0		
S. tachycardia	0	High supine	1	High supine	0	High supine	0	ESC			
Increase tilt	0	OH	10	Tilt response	7	Tilt low	2				
Decrease tilt	0	OHTN	0	CA	0	Tilt high	0	**Skin biopsy**			25
Deep breathing	1	VM	3	CVR	0			Epidermal	0		
VR	1			VM	0			Sweat gland	0		
Total	2	Total	14	Total	7	Total	2				

*QASAT. See Novak. Quantitative Scale for Grading of Cardiovascular Autonomic Reflex Tests and Small Fibers from Skin Biopsies. *J Neurol Disord* 2015;3:2.

S, supine; Increase tilt, increased response to tilt; Decrease tilt, decreased response to tilt; BP, blood pressure; VM, Valsalva maneuver; CBFv, cerebral blood flow velocity; CA, cerebral autoregulation; MCA, middle cerebral artery; VR, Valsalva ratio; CVR, cerebral vasoreactivity.

Patient-reported symptoms for past 2 weeks:

Lightheadedness or dizziness: Occasionally
Dry eyes or mouth: None
Pale feet: None
Cold feet: Occasionally
Reduced sweating: Occasionally
Reduced sweating after exercise: Occasionally
Increased sweating: None
Nausea: None
Diarrhea: None
Constipation: Occasionally
Urinary leaks: Occasionally
Erection problems: Often
Current pain severity: 2
Aching pain: Occasionally, mild
Allodynia: None
Burning pain: None
Lancinating pain: None
Numbness: Often, mild
Prickling sensation: Often, mild

AUTONOMIC TESTING INTERPRETATION

- Severe generalized autonomic failure, most likely of central nervous system origin (preganglionic).

COMMENT

Autonomic testing showed a pattern strongly suggestive of MSA, including severe sympathetic adrenergic (Figure 48.1) and mild parasympathetic failure. A combination of supine hypertension and orthostatic hypotension is seen in advanced adrenergic sympathetic failure. The absence of postganglionic abnormalities (QSART, small fiber densities

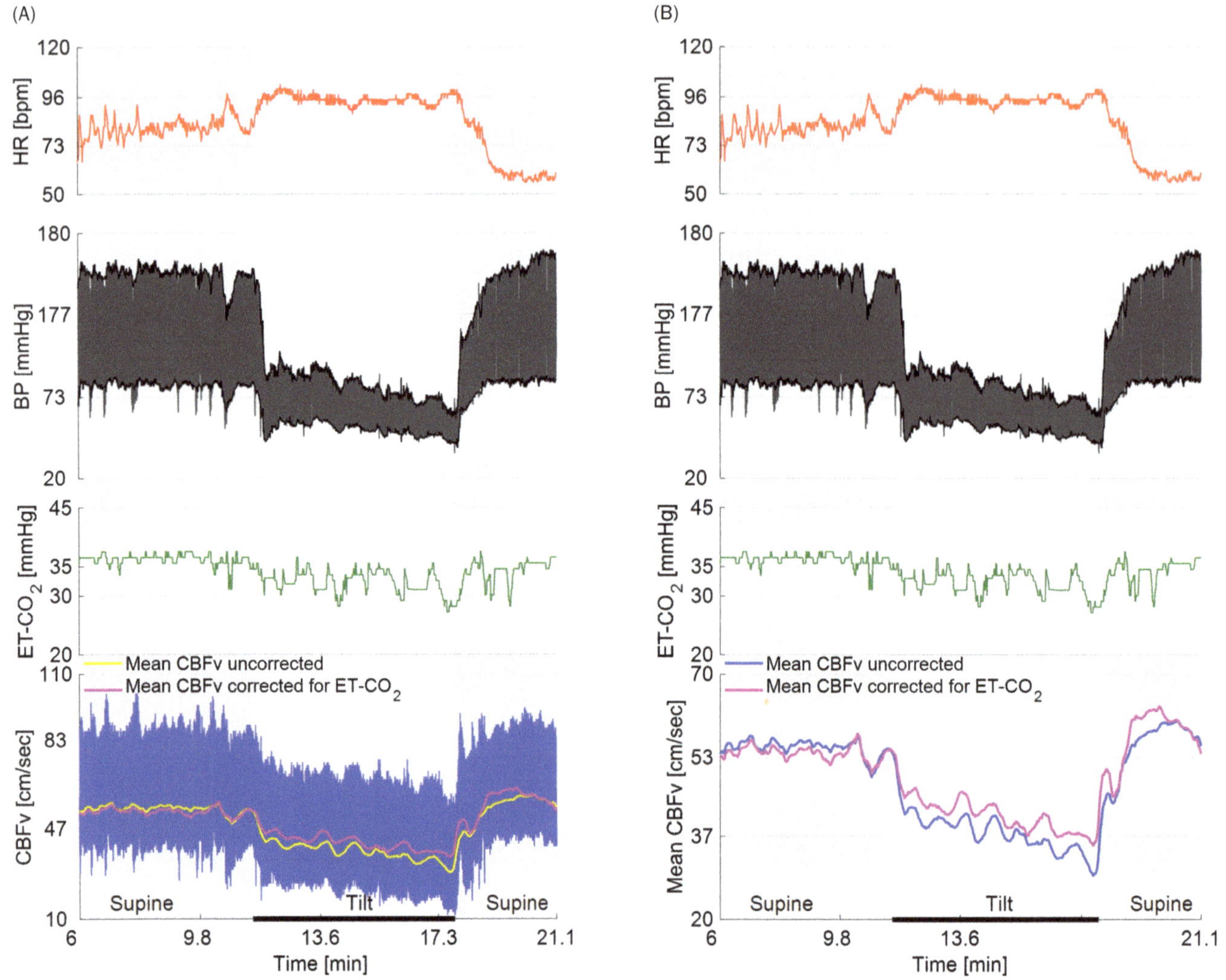

Figure 48.1 The tilt test showed severe abnormality. There was a progressive and severe orthostatic hypotension associated with a decline in cerebral blood flow velocity (CBFv) (A, B). The decline in CBFv was mainly due to orthostatic hypotension. There was mild hypocapnic hyperventilation during the tilt that further reduced CBFv (B). However, the hypocapnia was mild and hence the decline in CBFv due to vasoconstrictive effect of hypocapnia was minor as well. Heart rate response to tilt were also reduced but not absent. The patient became dizzy at the beginning of the tilt, then he became progressively confused and encephalopathic. The tilt was aborted at the sixth minute of the tilt because of severe acute encephalopathy. Note also lack of widening in the transcranial Doppler signal which indicate cerebral autoregulatory failure.

on skin biopsy) indicates that the lesion is located in the central nervous system (preganglionic). Dysautonomia of central nervous system origin is typically seen in MSA.

TREATMENT AND FOLLOW-UP

- Follow-up with the MSA clinic.

CAVEATS

- MSA is associated with severe generalized autonomic failure of central nervous system origin.[1]
- MSA diagnosis cannot be made solely based on autonomic testing, but autonomic testing may provide evidence of autonomic failure, which is one of the diagnostic criterion for MSA in addition to cerebellar syndrome and parkinsonism.

REFERENCE

1. Iodice V, Low DA, Vichayanrat E, Mathias CJ. Cardiovascular autonomic dysfunction in MSA and Parkinson's disease: similarities and differences. *J Neurol Sci*. 2011;310(1-2):133–138. doi:10.1016/j.jns.2011.07.014.

49.

CASE 43: MULTIPLE SYSTEM ATROPHY AND VITAMIN B_{12} DEFICIENCY

Chief complaint: Progressive imbalance and incontinence.

Case presentation: A 61-year-old man presented with prominent sphincter and balance problems. Five years ago, he experienced reduced urinary flow, which transiently improved after transurethral resection of the prostate. A year later, he noted erectile dysfunction and urinary incontinence. About 5 years ago, he experienced hoarse voice, numbness and tingling in the legs, and feeling of imbalance while walking. Within 2 years, he was unable to walk and had to use a motorized scooter. Other more recent symptoms include fatigue, incoordination of the upper limbs, loss of dexterity, slurred speech, nocturnal jerking of the limbs, and twitching of the muscles of his right leg upon standing. Patient was seen by multiple neurologists. MRIs of the brain and spine were normal. Electromyogram and nerve conduction studies 4 years ago were normal. Ataxia panel, including evaluation for hereditary spastic paraplegia, was normal. He has a history of B_{12} deficiency, treated with oral replacement. More recent neurological evaluation was consistent with prominent cerebellar syndrome and mild parkinsonism. Since the emergence of autonomic failure (as evidenced by urinary incontinence and erectile dysfunction), multiple system atrophy (MSA) has been suspected. (MSA is characterized by a combination of cerebellar syndrome, parkinsonism, and dysautonomia in variable proportion.) Patient was referred for formal evaluation of autonomic functions.

Past medical history: Dyslipidemia, vitamin B_{12} deficiency.

Current medication: Modafinil, oxybutynin, stool softeners, aspirin, vitamins D and B_{12}, probiotic, calcium.

Assessment plan: Functional autonomic tests and skin biopsy.

AUTONOMIC TESTING EVALUATION

See Table 49.1.

Heart rate: Supine heart rate was normal. Heart rate responses to deep breathing were reduced to 77.4% of normal value. Heart rate increment during the tilt (13 BPM) was normal.

Blood pressure:

Valsalva maneuver: Mean blood pressure failed to return to baseline at the end of Phase 2 by 33 mm Hg (i.e., 67.2% of baseline).

Tilt: Supine blood pressure was elevated. Blood pressure responses to tilt were abnormal and consistent with marked orthostatic hypotension.

Sudomotor evaluation: Electrochemical skin conductance was abnormal (reduced to 13.6% of normal limit) at hands and abnormal (reduced to 7% of normal limit) at feet. Sweat output was abnormal (reduced to 10% of

TABLE 49.1 **RESULTS OF AUTONOMIC TESTING**

Blood pressure evaluation					
Test: Valsalva maneuver					
Pressure [mmHg]	Baseline	Phase 2			Phase 4
		Early	End		
Systolic	142	81	81		
Mean	100.7	67.7	67.7	n/a	
Diastolic	80	61	61	n/a	

Heart rate evaluation	
Test: Deep breathing	
Results	Norm*
5.42	≥7
Test: Valsalva ratio	
1.22	≥1.29
* adjusted for a gender and age	

(continued)

TABLE 49.1 **CONTINUED**

Test: Tilt test										
Position		HR [BPM]	Blood pressure [mmHg]		MCA Blood flow velocity [cm/s]				Respiratory frequency [breaths/min]	End tidal CO_2 [mmHg]
			Systolic	Diastolic	Systolic	Mean	Mean drop [%]	Diastolic		
Supine		63	152	89	66	38.7		25	13	38
Tilt [min]	1	66	138	83	65	38.3	1	25	14	38
	2	66	128	83						
	3	68	118	79						
	4	71	118	78						
	5	70	117	78	63	34.5	10.9	20.2	20	33
	6	71	115	78						
	7	76	108	73						
	8	73	109	73						
	9	75	111	76						
	10	75	104	69	62	34	12.1	20	17	37
	15									
	20									
	30									
	40									

Sudomotor evaluation - functional

Test: Quantitative sudomotor axon reflex test (QSART)				
Location	Site (l/r)	Latency [min]	Volume [µl]	Norm [µl]*
Forearm	l	3.09	0.03	≥0.3
Prox. leg				≥0.23
Distal leg	l	1.12	0.995	≥0.23
Foot	l	3.49	0.104	≥0.27

* Normative data are adjusted for gender and age of patient.

Test: Electrochemical skin conductance (ESC)				
Location	Left [µS]	Right [µS]	Average [µS/k]	Norm [µS/kg]
Hand	12	16	0.14	≥1.03
Feet	9	8	0.08	≥1.14
Forehead				

For grading uses ESC [µS] adjusted for weight [µS/k].

TABLE 49.1 CONTINUED

Small fiber (sensory + sudomotor) evaluation - morphological					
Test: Skin biopsy					
Location	Site (l/r)	Nerve fibers			
		Epidermal*		Sweat glands	
		Density	Norm	Density	Norm
Proximal leg – thigh	Right	7.66	≥8.3	27.9	≥37.8
Distal leg - calf	Right	3.86	≥4.7	34.3	≥36.5
Foot	Right		≥3.11		≥34.8

*Normative data for distal leg are adjusted for gender and age of patient.

QASAT*										
Heart rate		BP		CBFv		ET-CO2		Sudomotor		Total QASAT score
S. bradycardia	0	Low supine	0	Low supine	1	Low supine	0	QSART	2	
S. tachycardia	0	High supine	1	High supine	0	High supine	0	ESC	4	
Increase tilt	0	OH	8	Tilt response	0	Tilt low	0			
Decrease tilt	0	OHTN	0	CA	0	Tilt high	0	**Skin biopsy**		25
Deep breathing	1	VM	2	CVR	0			Epidermal	2	
VR	1			VM	0			Sweat gland	3	
Total	2	Total	11	Total	1	Total	0			

*QASAT. See Novak. Quantitative Scale for Grading of Cardiovascular Autonomic Reflex Tests and Small Fibers from Skin Biopsies. *J Neurol Disord* 2015;3:2.

S, supine; Increase tilt, increased response to tilt; Decrease tilt, decreased response to tilt; BP, blood pressure; VM, Valsalva maneuver; CBFv, cerebral blood flow velocity; CA, cerebral autoregulation; MCA, middle cerebral artery; VR, Valsalva ratio; CVR, cerebral vasoreactivity.

lower limit) at forearm, normal at distal leg, and abnormal (reduced to 38.5% of lower limit) at foot.

Respiratory system: Respiratory frequency and end tidal CO_2 were normal in supine position and during the tilt.

Cerebral blood flow velocity (CBFv): CBFv in middle cerebral artery was reduced in supine position (38.7 cm/s, normal ≥ 45.4 cm/s) but was stable during the tilt.

Skin biopsy (sensory-epidermal): Epidermal nerve fiber density was abnormal (reduced to 92.3% of normal limit) at proximal leg and abnormal (reduced to 82.1% of normal limit) at distal leg.

Skin biopsy (sweat glands): Sweat gland nerve fiber density was abnormal (reduced to 73.8% of normal limit) at proximal leg and abnormal (reduced to 94% of normal limit) at distal leg.

Patient-reported symptoms during testing: None during the tilt.

Patient-reported symptoms for past 2 weeks:

Lightheadedness or dizziness: Occasionally
Dry eyes or mouth: Yes, minor annoyance
Pale feet: None
Cold feet: Occasionally
Reduced sweating: Occasionally
Reduced sweating after exercise: None
Increased sweating: Yes, minor annoyance
Nausea: Yes, minor annoyance
Diarrhea: None
Constipation: Occasionally
Urinary leaks: Often
Erection problems: Often
Aching pain: None
Allodynia: None
Burning pain: None
Lancinating pain: None
Numbness: Often, moderate
Prickling sensation: Often, mild

AUTONOMIC TESTING INTERPRETATION

- Severe generalized autonomic failure associated with compensated orthostatic hypotension.
- Cerebral vasoconstriction, associated with low supine CBFv.

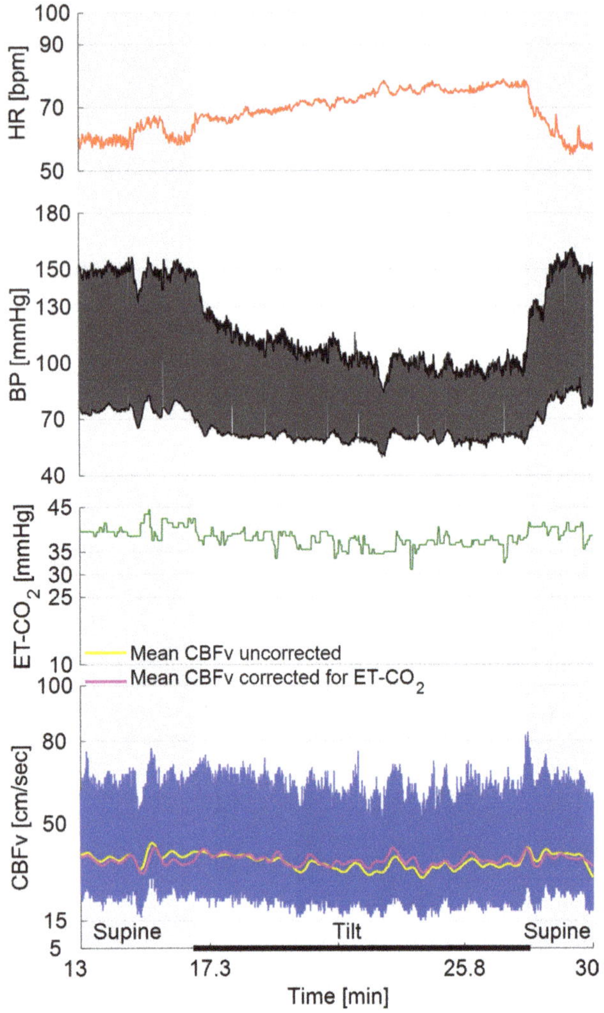

Figure 49.1 Tilt test showed a progressive orthostatic hypotension with normal heart rate increment. Cerebral blood flow velocity (CBFv) was stable.

- Small fiber neuropathy, biopsy-proven, mixed, affecting both sensory and autonomic fibers.

COMMENT

Autonomic testing showed generalized autonomic failure (Figure 49.1), which is consistent with MSA.[1,2] However, MSA affects predominantly the central nervous system and testing showed also evidence of involvement of the peripheral nervous system, as implicated by abnormal skin biopsy and abnormal sudomotor function. Patient has history of B_{12} deficiency that can explain the peripheral nerve lesion.

The autonomic failure was associated with compensated orthostatic CBFv, which means orthostatic CBFv was stable.

Nevertheless, the supine CBFv was reduced. In the context of elevated supine blood pressure and absent hypocapnia, low supine CBFv is due to cerebral vasoconstriction. This pattern is seen in hypertension and small vessel disease. Cerebral vasoconstriction can result in cerebral hypoperfusion. Since orthostatic CBFv was stable, the compensatory orthostatic vasodilation was preserved in this patient.

TREATMENT AND FOLLOW-UP

- Referral to MSA clinic.
- Consider calcium channel blockers that are cerebral vasodilators and may improve cerebral perfusion.

CAVEATS

- MSA is associated with widespread autonomic failure.
- Coexisting peripheral nerve damage may indicate an additional process, as in this case the B_{12} deficiency.

REFERENCES

1. Iodice V, Low DA, Vichayanrat E, Mathias CJ. Cardiovascular autonomic dysfunction in MSA and Parkinson's disease: similarities and differences. *J Neurol Sci.* 2011;310(1–2):133–138. doi:10.1016/j.jns.2011.07.014.
2. Novak V, Novak P, Spies JM, Low PA. Autoregulation of cerebral blood flow in orthostatic hypotension. *Stroke.* 1998;29(1):104–111.

50.

CASE 45: MULTIPLE SYSTEM ATROPHY?

Chief complaint: Dizziness.

Case presentation: A 47-year-old man presents with dizziness. Initially, he experienced left-sided weakness and balance problems with falls at age 35. Two years ago, his physician detected very mild rigidity and bradykinesia consistent with parkinsonian syndrome. At this time, he has limited strength, and he can walk intermittently for short distances. He gets dizzy and his arms frequently become numb. He has lost muscle bulk at the forearms. His vision has declined, and he noted droopy eyelids. He has also dry eyes, dry mouth, diarrhea, and memory and vision problems. High humidity and hot weather exacerbate symptoms, particularly the pain.

A positron emission tomography (PET) scan of the brain showed normal metabolism. MRI of the brain and the cervical spine were normal. Electromyogram and nerve conduction studies were normal. Patient was referred for evaluation of suspected autonomic failure as a part of multiple system atrophy (MSA).

Past medical history: Dyslipidemia, MSA?

Current medication: Simvastatin, Levodopa (on hold), Proamatine (on hold).

Assessment plan: Functional autonomic tests and skin biopsy.

AUTONOMIC TESTING EVALUATION

See Table 50.1.

Heart rate: Supine heart rate was normal. Heart rate responses to deep breathing were normal. Heart rate increment during the tilt (29 BPM) was normal.

Blood pressure:

Valsalva maneuver: Mean blood pressure failed to return to baseline at the end of Phase 2 by 2.7 mm Hg (i.e., 97% of baseline).

Tilt: Supine blood pressure was normal. Blood pressure responses to tilt were normal.

Sudomotor evaluation: Patient could not tolerate quantitative sudomotor axon reflex test (QSART).

Respiratory system: Respiratory frequency was normal in supine position and during the tilt. End tidal CO_2 was normal in supine position but was moderately reduced during the tilt.

Cerebral blood flow velocity (CBFv): CBFv in middle cerebral artery was normal in supine position but was severely reduced during the tilt.

Skin biopsy (sensory-epidermal): Epidermal nerve fiber density was abnormal (reduced to 65.7% of normal limit) at proximal leg and abnormal (reduced to 89% of normal limit) at distal leg.

TABLE 50.1 **RESULTS OF AUTONOMIC TESTING**

Blood pressure evaluation					
Test: Valsalva maneuver					
Pressure [mmHg]	Baseline	Phase 2			Phase 4
		Early	End		
Systolic	129	85	107		
Mean	89	71	86.3	n/a	
Diastolic	69	64	76	n/a	

Heart rate evaluation	
Test: Deep breathing	
Results	Norm*
22.8	≥10
Test: Valsalva ratio	
1.79	≥1.44
* adjusted for a gender and age	

(continued)

Test: Tilt test										
Position		HR [BPM]	Blood pressure [mmHg]		MCA Blood flow velocity [cm/s]				Respiratory frequency [breaths/min]	End tidal CO2 [mmHg]
			Systolic	Diastolic	Systolic	Mean	Mean drop [%]	Diastolic		
Supine		81	118	81	104	74.7		60	11	35
Tilt [min]	1	94	119	88	95	64.3	13.9	49	13	33
	2	98	114	81						
	3	90	118	84						
	4	89	123	86						
	5	95	126	84	68	45.3	39.4	34	12	26
	6	96	113	79						
	7	100	122	83						
	8	103	115	82						
	9	104	106	76						
	10	110	112	76	66	40	46.5	27	8	22
	15									
	20									
	30									
	40									

Sudomotor evaluation - functional

Test: Quantitative sudomotor axon reflex test (QSART)				
Location	Site (l/r)	Latency [min]	Volume [μl]	Norm [μl]*
Forearm				≥0.3
Prox. leg				≥0.37
Distal leg				≥0.38
Foot				≥0.31

* Normative data are adjusted for gender and age of patient.

Test: Electrochemical skin conductance (ESC)				
Location	Left [μS]	Right [μS]	Average [μS/k]	Norm [μS/kg]
Hand				≥1.03
Feet				≥1.14
Forehead				

For grading uses ESC [μS] adjusted for weight [μS/k].

TABLE 50.1 CONTINUED

Small fiber (sensory + sudomotor) evaluation - morphological					
Test: Skin biopsy					
Location	Site (l/r)	Nerve fibers			
		Epidermal*		Sweat glands	
		Density	Norm	Density	Norm
Proximal leg – thigh	Right	5.45	≥8.3		≥37.8
Distal leg - calf	Right	5.32	≥5.975	9.9	≥36.5
Foot	Right		≥3.11		≥34.8

*Normative data for distal leg are adjusted for gender and age of patient.

QASAT*

Heart rate		BP		CBFv		ET CO2		Sudomotor			Total QASAT score
S. bradycardia		Low sup.	0	Low sup.	0	Low sup.	0	QSART			
S. tachycardia	0	High sup.	0	High sup.	0	High sup.	0	ESC			
Increase. tilt	0	OH	0	Tilt resp.	7	Tilt low	4				
Decreas. tilt	0	OHTN	0	CA	0	Tilt high	0	**Skin biopsy**			19
Deep breath	0	VM	1	CVR	0			Epidermal	3		
VR	0			VM	0			Sweat gland	4		
Total	0	Total	1	Total	7	Total	4				

*QASAT. See Novak. Quantitative Scale for Grading of Cardiovascular Autonomic Reflex Tests and Small Fibers from Skin Biopsies. *J Neurol Disord* 2015;3:2.

S, supine; Increase tilt, increased response to tilt; Decrease tilt, decreased response to tilt; BP, blood pressure; VM, Valsalva maneuver; CBFv, cerebral blood flow velocity; CA, cerebral autoregulation; MCA, middle cerebral artery; VR, Valsalva ratio; CVR, cerebral vasoreactivity.

Skin biopsy (sweat glands): Sweat gland nerve fiber density was abnormal (reduced to 27.1% of normal limit) at distal leg.

Patient-reported symptoms during testing: Dizziness during the tilt.

Patient-reported symptoms for past 2 weeks:

Lightheadedness or dizziness: Often
Dry eyes or mouth: Often
Pale feet: Occasionally
Cold feet: Often
Reduced sweating: Occasionally
Reduced sweating after exercise: Occasionally
Increased sweating: Occasionally
Nausea: Occasionally
Diarrhea: Often
Constipation: None
Urinary leaks: Occasionally
Erection problems: Occasionally
Aching pain: None
Allodynia: None
Burning pain: None
Lancinating pain: None
Numbness: None
Prickling sensation: None

AUTONOMIC TESTING INTERPRETATION

- Small fiber neuropathy, mixed, severe, length-dependent, affecting sensory and autonomic fibers, biopsy-proven.
- Autonomic dysfunction, mild, affecting adrenergic system. There was no evidence of orthostatic hypotension.
- Hypocapnic cerebral hypoperfusion (HYCH), severe.
- Hypocapnic hyperventilation during the tilt.

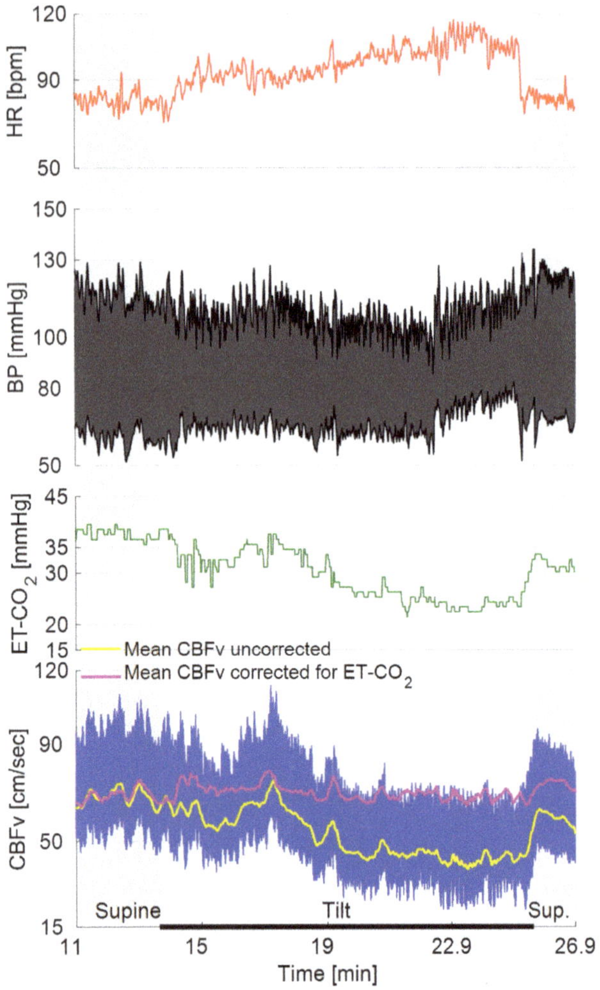

Figure 50.1 The tilt test showed severe reduction in end tidal CO_2 and cerebral blood flow velocity (CBFv). Heart rate and blood pressure responses were normal.

COMMENT

The tilt test showed marked reduction in CBFv (46.5%, Figure 50.1), which was associated with hypocapnia without orthostatic hypotension. The decline in CBFv was due to hypocapnia-induced cerebral vasoconstriction since corrected CBFv was stable.

There are several facts in this study that speak against the diagnosis of MSA. First, the dysautonomia detected in this study is much milder than seen in typical MSA. Typical MSA is associated with generalized autonomic failure with orthostatic hypotension.[1,2] Second, the study detected small fiber neuropathy that is not part of MSA. Third, the duration of symptoms is much longer than in typical MSA.

This study was not only useful to rule out MSA, but it also provides some explanation for the patient's symptoms. In particular, small fiber neuropathy can be responsible for some of the sensory complaints and HYCH[3] for orthostatic intolerance.

TREATMENT AND FOLLOW-UP

- Clinical workup for neuropathy and HYCH.

CAVEATS

- Autonomic testing can be useful in evaluation of suspected MSA.

REFERENCES

1. Gilman S, Wenning GK, Low PA, et al. Second consensus statement on the diagnosis of multiple system atrophy. *Neurology*. 2008;71(9):670–676. doi:10.1212/01.wnl.0000324625.00404.15.
2. Iodice V, Low DA, Vichayanrat E, Mathias CJ. Cardiovascular autonomic dysfunction in MSA and Parkinson's disease: similarities and differences. *J Neurol Sci*. 2011;310(1-2):133–138. doi:10.1016/j.jns.2011.07.014.
3. Novak P. Hypocapnic cerebral hypoperfusion: A biomarker of orthostatic intolerance. *PloS One*. 2018;13(9):e0204419. doi:10.1371/journal.pone.0204419

51.

CASE 46: AMYOTROPHIC LATERAL SCLEROSIS

Chief complaint: Dizziness and exertional dyspnea.

Case presentation: A 61-year-old man presents with a progressive exertional dyspnea, fatigue, orthostatic intolerance, and weakness for 4 years. He was admitted to the hospital for severe dyspnea. Neurological examination showed signs of upper and lower motor neuron damage with normal sensory functions. Electromyogram and nerve conduction studies (EMG/NCS) showed widespread denervation with sparing of sensory conductions. The office evaluation also showed severe symptomatic orthostatic hypotension. Although clinical examination and EMG/NCS was suggestive of a motor neuron disease, neurogenic orthostatic hypotension and associated autonomic failure are usually not part of amyotrophic lateral sclerosis (ALS). Typically, mild dysautonomia can be seen in ALS.[1] The patient was referred for autonomic testing to determine if dysautonomia can be responsible for some of his symptoms.

Past medical history: Lyme disease.

Current medication: None.

Assessment plan: Functional autonomic tests and skin biopsy.

AUTONOMIC TESTING EVALUATION

See Table 51.1.

Heart rate: Supine heart rate was normal. Heart rate responses to deep breathing were normal. Heart rate increment during the tilt (13 BPM) was normal.

Blood pressure:

Valsalva maneuver: Blood pressure responses were normal.

Tilt: Supine blood pressure was normal. Blood pressure responses to tilt were normal.

Sudomotor evaluation: Electrochemical skin conductance was normal at hands and normal at feet.

Respiratory system: Respiratory frequency was increased in supine position and during the tilt. End tidal CO_2 was reduced in supine position and was further reduced during the tilt.

Cerebral blood flow velocity (CBFv): CBFv in middle cerebral artery was normal in supine position. CBFv in middle cerebral artery was reduced during the tilt.

Skin biopsy (sensory-epidermal): Epidermal nerve fiber density was normal at proximal leg and normal at distal leg.

Skin biopsy (sweat glands): Sweat gland nerve fiber density was abnormal (reduced to 57.5% of normal limit) at distal leg.

Patient-reported symptoms during testing: Shortness of breath during the tilt.

Patient-reported symptoms for past 2 weeks:

Lightheadedness or dizziness: Occasionally
Dry eyes or mouth: Often
Pale feet: None
Cold feet: Often

TABLE 51.1 RESULTS OF AUTONOMIC TESTING

Blood pressure evaluation					
Test: Valsalva maneuver					
Pressure [mmHg]	Baseline	Phase 2			Phase 4
		Early	End		
Systolic	138	120	152		
Mean	100	90.7	108.7	n/a	
Diastolic	81	76	87	n/a	

Heart rate evaluation	
Test: Deep breathing	
Results	Norm*
7.1	≥7
Test: Valsalva ratio	
1	≥1.29
* adjusted for a gender and age	

(continued)

TABLE 51.1 **CONTINUED**

Test: Tilt test											
Position		HR [BPM]	Blood pressure [mmHg]		MCA Blood flow velocity [cm/s]				Respiratory frequency [breaths/min]	End tidal CO_2 [mmHg]
			Systolic	Diastolic	Systolic	Mean	Mean drop [%]	Diastolic		
Supine		91	131	80	75	45.7		31	30	32
Tilt [min]	1	98	127	85	68	41.3	9.6	28	32	33
	2	96	128	86						
	3	96	128	87						
	4	96	132	85						
	5	95	134	90	64	38.7	15.3	26	34	26
	6	94	137	91						
	7	96	136	87						
	8	104	114	84						
	9	102	121	85						
	10	97	142	91	63	37.7	17.5	25	29	22
	15									
	20									
	30									
	40									

Sudomotor evaluation - functional

Test: Quantitative sudomotor axon reflex test (QSART)				
Location	Site (l/r)	Latency [min]	Volume [μl]	Norm [μl]*
Forearm				≥0.3
Prox. leg				≥0.23
Distal leg				≥0.23
Foot				≥0.27

* Normative data are adjusted for gender and age of patient.

Test: Electrochemical skin conductance (ESC)				
Location	Left [μS]	Right [μS]	Average [μS/k]	Norm [μS/kg]
Hand	80	73	1.34	≥1.03
Feet	81	82	1.45	≥1.14
Forehead				

For grading uses ESC [μS] adjusted for weight [μS/k].

TABLE 51.1 CONTINUED

Small fiber (sensory + sudomotor) evaluation - morphological					
Test: Skin biopsy					
Location	Site (l/r)	Nerve fibers			
		Epidermal*		Sweat glands	
		Density	Norm	Density	Norm
Proximal leg – thigh	Right	11.66	≥8.3		≥37.8
Distal leg - calf	Right	7.37	≥4.93	21	≥36.5
Foot	Right		≥3.11		≥34.8

*Normative data for distal leg are adjusted for gender and age of patient.

QASAT*										
Heart rate		BP		CBFv		ET-CO2		Sudomotor		Total QASAT score
S. bradycardia	0	Low supine	0	Low supine	0	Low supine	1	QSART		
S. tachycardia	0	High supine	0	High supine	0	High supine	0	ESC	0	
Increase tilt	0	OH	0	Tilt response	2	Tilt low	4			
Decrease tilt	0	OHTN	0	CA	0	Tilt high	0	**Skin biopsy**		11
Deep breathing	0	VM	0	CVR	0			Epidermal	0	
VR	1			VM	0			Sweat gland	3	
Total	1	Total	0	Total	2	Total	5			

*QASAT. See Novak. Quantitative Scale for Grading of Cardiovascular Autonomic Reflex Tests and Small Fibers from Skin Biopsies. *J Neurol Disord* 2015;3:2.

S, supine; Increase tilt, increased response to tilt; Decrease tilt, decreased response to tilt; BP, blood pressure; VM, Valsalva maneuver; CBFv, cerebral blood flow velocity; CA, cerebral autoregulation; MCA, middle cerebral artery; VR, Valsalva ratio; CVR, cerebral vasoreactivity; RR, respiratory rate.

Reduced sweating: None
Reduced sweating after exercise: None
Increased sweating: None
Nausea: None
Diarrhea: None
Constipation: None
Urinary leaks: Occasionally
Erection problems: None
Current pain severity: 2
Aching pain: Occasionally, severe
Allodynia: None
Burning pain: None
Lancinating pain: Occasional, severe
Numbness: None
Prickling sensation: None

AUTONOMIC TESTING INTERPRETATION

- Small fiber neuropathy, affecting predominantly autonomic fibers.
- Autonomic functions were normal.
- Hypocapnic cerebral hypoperfusion.
- Respiratory failure associated with hypocapnic hyperventilation and tachypnea.

COMMENT

Autonomic testing showed normal autonomic functions. However, there was evidence of respiratory failure associated with tachypnea and hypocapnia (Figure 51.1). The decline in the orthostatic CBFv was because of hypocapnia.

TREATMENT AND FOLLOW-UP

- Referral to ALS clinic.
- Continue adequate hydration.

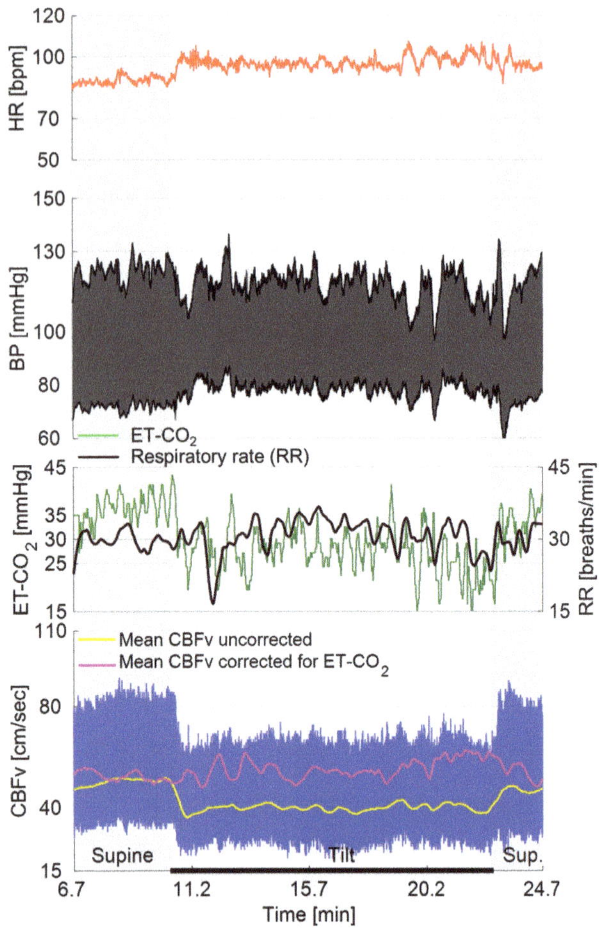

Figure 51.1 Patient was dyspneic both in supine position and during the tilt, which was associated with tachypnea (respiratory frequency >20 breath/minute) and hypocapnia (end tidal CO_2 <35 mm Hg). Heart rate responses to tilt were normal, and orthostatic blood pressure was stable. The decline in cerebral blood flow velocity (CBFv) was entirely due to hypocapnia-induced cerebral vasoconstriction because the CBFv adjusted for end tidal CO_2 was stable during the tilt. The oxygen saturation at the middle finger was ~93% throughout the testing.

CAVEATS

- Respiratory failure is characteristically seen in ALS. Normal oxygen saturation as measured by pulse oximetry is more than 95% on room air. Although in acute respiratory failure the oxygen saturation is less than 90%,[2] this patient was hyperventilating, as evidenced by tachypnea with hypocapnia.
- Previous orthostatic hypotension detected in the office was probably due to dehydration. Indeed, a review of the hospital chart showed patient was extensively hydrated for the past few days.

REFERENCES

1. Baltadzhieva R, Gurevich T, Korczyn AD. Autonomic impairment in amyotrophic lateral sclerosis. *Curr Opin Neurol.* 2005;18(5):487–493.
2. Lam T, Nagappa M, Wong J, Singh M, Wong D, Chung F. Continuous pulse oximetry and capnography monitoring for postoperative respiratory depression and adverse events: a systematic review and meta-analysis. *Anesth Analg.* 2017;125(6):2019–2029. doi:10.1213/ANE.0000000000002557.

PART VIII

MULTIPLE SCLEROSIS

52.

CASE 47: MOEBIUS SYNDROME

Chief complaint: Dizziness.

Case presentation: A 34-year-old man with Moebius syndrome and multiple sclerosis (MS) presents with intermittent dizziness. According to his mother, his heart rate was widely fluctuating after he was born. He had multiple resuscitations before age 6 since his "heart would spontaneously stop or he would not breath." For example, he would scream, exhale, and then stop breathing. At one point, he was intubated for respiratory failure. Nevertheless, he was doing relatively well until age 21, when he began to experience dizziness and passing-out episodes. He was then diagnosed with MS. He was stable again until the past 6 months. He began to have episodes in which he suddenly feels sick, his whole body becomes red, and his blood pressure becomes elevated. The spells happen several times per month with durations of less than 10 minutes. Electroencephalogram was normal. Multiple MRIs of the brain showed periventricular lesions consistent with MS, with the impression that they are not likely associated with a seizure disorder. He was referred for autonomic testing because, for past 2 years, he had several syncopal episodes and he was found to have orthostatic hypotension.

Past medical history: Moebius syndrome, MS.

Current medication: Tecfidera, gabapentin, citalopram, solifenacin.

Assessment plan: Functional autonomic tests and skin biopsy.

AUTONOMIC TESTING EVALUATION

See Table 52.1.

Heart rate: Supine heart rate was normal. Heart rate responses to deep breathing were reduced to 36.1% of normal value. Heart rate increment during the tilt (5 BPM) was reduced (Figure 52.1).

Blood pressure:

Valsalva maneuver: Blood pressure responses were normal.

Tilt: Supine blood pressure was normal. Blood pressure responses to tilt were abnormal and consistent with transient orthostatic hypotensions and presyncope.

Sudomotor evaluation: Electrochemical skin conductance was abnormal (reduced to 44.4% of normal limit) at hands and abnormal (reduced to 55.4% of normal limit) at feet.

Respiratory system: Respiratory frequency was elevated in supine position and during the tilt. End tidal CO_2 was normal in supine position and during the tilt.

Cerebral blood flow velocity (CBFv): CBFv in middle cerebral artery was normal in supine position but was moderately reduced during the tilt.

Skin biopsy (sensory-epidermal): Epidermal nerve fiber density was abnormal (reduced to 71.4% of normal limit) at proximal leg and normal at distal leg.

TABLE 52.1 RESULTS OF AUTONOMIC TESTING

Blood pressure evaluation					
Test: Valsalva maneuver					
Pressure [mmHg]	Baseline	Phase 2			Phase 4
		Early	End		
Systolic	118.2	119.3	129		
Mean	85.4	78.6	94.1	n/a	
Diastolic	69	58.3	76.7	n/a	

Heart rate evaluation	
Test: Deep breathing	
Results	Norm*
4.33	≥12
Test: Valsalva ratio	
1.1	≥1.52
* adjusted for a gender and age	

(continued)

TABLE 52.1 **CONTINUED**

Test: Tilt test										
Position		HR [BPM]	Blood pressure [mmHg]		MCA Blood flow velocity [cm/s]				Respiratory frequency [breaths/min]	End tidal CO_2 [mmHg]
			Systolic	Diastolic	Systolic	Mean	Mean drop [%]	Diastolic		
Supine		82	130	87	88	55.3		39	23	37
Tilt [min]	1	85	106	74	81	45.7	17.4	28	28	35
	2	87	102	70						
	3	86	94	69						
	4	87	106	74						
	5	86	114	79	83	47.7	13.7	30	29	37
	6	85	117	82						
	7	86	108	76						
	8	87	113	79						
	9	82	123	88						
	10	87	115	81	77	43	22.2	26	25	38
	15									
	20									
	30									
	40									

Sudomotor evaluation - functional

Test: Quantitative sudomotor axon reflex test (QSART)				
Location	Site (l/r)	Latency [min]	Volume [µl]	Norm [µl]*
Forearm				≥0.3
Prox. leg				≥0.37
Distal leg				≥0.38
Foot				≥0.31

* Normative data are adjusted for gender and age of patient.

Test: Electrochemical skin conductance (ESC)				
Location	Left [µS]	Right [µS]	Average [µS/k]	Norm [µS/kg]
Hand	48	52	0.46	≥1.03
Feet	71	67	0.61	≥1.14
Forehead				

For grading uses ESC [µS] adjusted for weight [µS/k].

TABLE 52.1 **CONTINUED**

Small fiber (sensory + sudomotor) evaluation - morphological					
Test: Skin biopsy					
Location	Site (l/r)	Nerve fibers			
		Epidermal*		Sweat glands	
		Density	Norm	Density	Norm
Proximal leg – thigh	Right	5.93	≥8.3	23.1	≥37.8
Distal leg - calf	Right	9.27	≥6.95	20.6	≥36.5
Foot	Right		≥3.11		≥34.8

*Normative data for distal leg are adjusted for gender and age of patient.

QASAT*										
Heart rate		**BP**		**CBFv**		**ET-CO2**		**Sudomotor**		**Total QASAT score**
S. bradycardia	0	Low supine	0	Low supine	0	Low supine	0	QSART		
S. tachycardia	0	High supine	0	High supine	0	High supine	0	ESC	3	
Increase tilt	0	OH	4	Tilt response	3	Tilt low	0			
Decrease tilt	1	OHTN	0	CA	0	Tilt high	0	**Skin biopsy**		19
Deep breathing	2	VM	0	CVR	0			Epidermal	1	
VR	1			VM	0			Sweat gland	4	
Total	4	Total	4	Total	3	Total	0			

*QASAT. See Novak. Quantitative Scale for Grading of Cardiovascular Autonomic Reflex Tests and Small Fibers from Skin Biopsies. *J Neurol Disord* 2015;3:2.

S, supine; Increase tilt, increased response to tilt; Decrease tilt, decreased response to tilt; BP, blood pressure; VM, Valsalva maneuver; CBFv, cerebral blood flow velocity; CA, cerebral autoregulation; MCA, middle cerebral artery; VR, Valsalva ratio; CVR, cerebral vasoreactivity.

Skin biopsy (sweat glands): Sweat gland nerve fiber density was abnormal (reduced to 61.1% of normal limit) at proximal leg and abnormal (reduced to 56.4% of normal limit) at distal leg.

Patient-reported symptoms during testing: Dizziness during the tilt.

Patient-reported symptoms for past 2 weeks:

Lightheadedness or dizziness: Occasionally
Dry eyes or mouth: Occasionally
Pale feet: None
Cold feet: None
Reduced sweating: None
Reduced sweating after exercise: None
Increased sweating: None
Nausea: None
Diarrhea: None
Constipation: None
Urinary leaks: None
Erection problems: None
Current pain severity: 0
Aching pain: Occasionally, mild
Allodynia: None
Burning pain: None
Lancinating pain: None
Numbness: Occasionally, mild
Prickling sensation: None

AUTONOMIC TESTING INTERPRETATION

- Small fiber neuropathy, mixed, length-dependent, affecting sensory and autonomic fibers.
- Cardiovagal failure.
- Orthostatic cerebral hypoperfusion syndrome (OCHOS).

COMMENT

Autonomic testing showed small fiber neuropathy, OCHOS and presyncope (Figure 52.1). Paroxysmal hypertension (not seen in this case), orthostatic hypotension, and autonomic symptoms were described in Moebius syndrome.[1] Although this patient was also diagnosed with MS, he experienced autonomic symptoms since birth. Therefore,

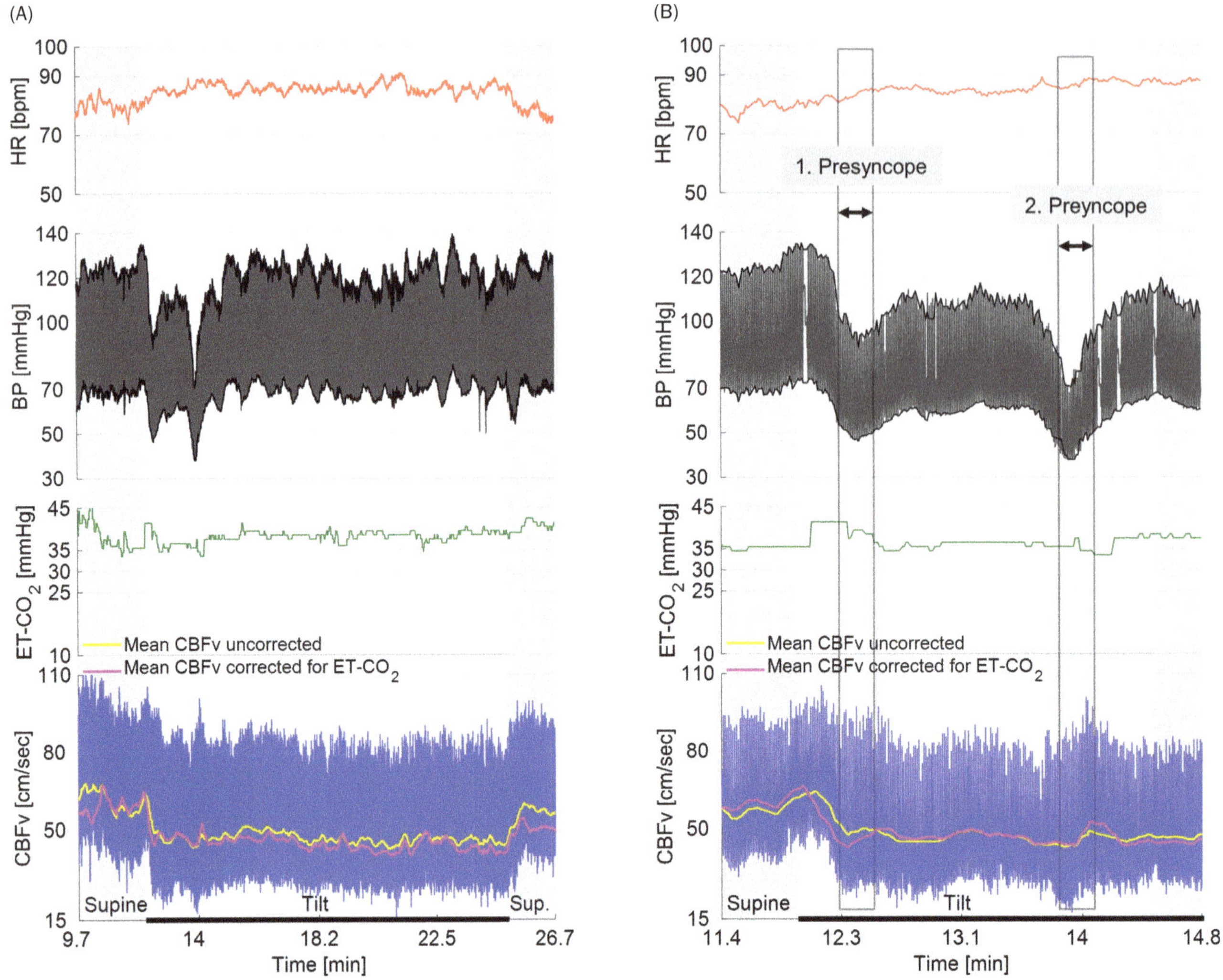

Figure 52.1 The tilt provoked transient orthostatic hypotension twice at the beginning of the tilt. On both occasions, blood pressure recovered but there was no compensatory tachycardia during the hypotensive episodes. The spells were associated with a cerebral vasodilation pattern in cerebral blood flow velocity (CBFv) with widening of the transcranial Doppler signal (increase in systolic and decrease in diastolic CBFv). In addition, CBFv was reduced during the tilt.

it is more likely that Moebius syndrome is responsible for dysautonomia. Also, MRI of the brain showed typical MS periventricular white matter lesions without any lesions in the brainstem that can potentially explain dysautonomia.

Small fiber neuropathy is likely associated with MS,[2,3] although usually skin biopsy and autonomic testing cannot differentiate between causes of neuropathies.

TREATMENT AND FOLLOW-UP

- Continuous monitoring of respiratory status.

CAVEATS

- Presyncope does not necessary lead to syncope, recovery is possible.
- Cardiovagal failure and OCHOS can be associated with Moebius syndrome.

REFERENCES

1. Bowers M, Simson GG. Moebius syndrome with baroreflex failure in an adolescent female. *J Pediatr Genet*. 2012;1(3):199–203. doi:10.3233/PGE-2012-031.
2. Khan A, Kamran S, Ponirakis G, et al. Peripheral neuropathy in patients with multiple sclerosis. *PloS One*. 2018;13(3):e0193270. doi:10.1371/journal.pone.0193270.
3. Habek M, Crnošija L, Lovrić M, Junaković A, Krbot Skorić M, Adamec I. Sympathetic cardiovascular and sudomotor functions are frequently affected in early multiple sclerosis. *Clin Auton Res Off J Clin Auton Res Soc*. 2016;26(6):385–393. doi:10.1007/s10286-016-0370-x.

53.

CASE 48: DYSPNEA

Chief complaint: Dyspnea and labile blood pressure.

Case presentation: A 62-year-old man, a life-long nonsmoker without known chronic pulmonary disease, presented with slowly progressive chronic exertional dyspnea. Dyspnea began after severe community-acquired pneumonia 4 years ago complicated by slow clinical and radiographic improvement with hypoxemia. Pulmonary evaluations showed normal pulmonary functions, including resting and peak exercise oximetry. Chest imaging has been normal; pulmonary function tests were essentially normal except for a mild decline in diffusing capacity. Methacholine challenge has demonstrated moderate airway reactivity. A ventilation perfusion (V/Q) scan was without perfusion defects. Echocardiogram has demonstrated a mild increase in right ventricular systolic pressure. Noninvasive cardiopulmonary exercise testing demonstrated a decrease in maximum aerobic capacity and marked increase in VE/VCO_2 slope (50, normal <30). Exercise tolerance test with a radioactive tracer (ETT-MIBI) was unrevealing for ischemia.

Other causes of dyspnea such as anemia, renal dysfunction, and thyroid disease were ruled out.

Empiric therapy for asthma with inhaled corticosteroid, long-acting β-agonists, and reconditioning exercise with a graded aerobic training regimen did not improve dyspnea.

Patient has relapsing and remitting multiple sclerosis (MS), stable on natalizumab.

Past medical history: Relapsing and remitting MS.

Current medication: Natalizumab, venlafaxine, gabapentin.

Assessment plan: Functional autonomic test and skin biopsy.

AUTONOMIC TESTING EVALUATION

See Table 53.1.

Heart rate: Supine heart rate was normal. Heart rate responses to deep breathing were reduced to 35.7% of normal value. Heart rate increment during the tilt (19 BPM) was normal.

Blood pressure:

Valsalva maneuver: Blood pressure responses were normal.

Tilt: Supine blood pressure was normal. Blood pressure responses to tilt were abnormal and consistent with marked orthostatic hypotension.

Sudomotor evaluation: Electrochemical skin conductance was abnormal (reduced to 34.4% of normal limit) at hands and abnormal (reduced to 50.9% of normal limit) at feet.

Respiratory system: Respiratory frequency was normal in supine position and during the tilt. End tidal CO_2 was reduced in supine position and was further severely reduced during the tilt.

TABLE 53.1 **RESULTS OF AUTONOMIC TESTING**

Blood pressure evaluation					
Test: Valsalva maneuver					
Pressure [mmHg]	Baseline	Phase 2			Phase 4
		Early	End		
Systolic	83	74	74		
Mean	65	68.7	68.7	n/a	
Diastolic	56	66	66	n/a	

Heart rate evaluation	
Test: Deep breathing	
Results	Norm*
2.5	≥7
Test: Valsalva ratio	
1.069	≥1.29
* adjusted for a gender and age	

(continued)

TABLE 53.1 CONTINUED

Test: Tilt test											
Position		HR [BPM]	Blood pressure [mmHg]		MCA Blood flow velocity [cm/s]				Respiratory frequency [breaths/min]	End tidal CO_2 [mmHg]
			Systolic	Diastolic	Systolic	Mean	Mean drop [%]	Diastolic		
Supine		94	107	74	65	42.7		31.5	12	28
Tilt [min]	1	110	70	40	54	30.7	28.1	19	9	24
	2	110	70	40						
	3	113	74	52						
	4	101	80	56						
	5	100	84	58	50	28.7	32.8	18	6	25
	6	100	67	50						
	7	101	85	60						
	8	100	80	56						
	9	98	73	52						
	10	100	76	54	53	30.3	29	19	8	26
	15									
	20									
	30									
	40									

Sudomotor evaluation - functional

Test: Quantitative sudomotor axon reflex test (QSART)				
Location	Site (l/r)	Latency [min]	Volume [µl]	Norm [µl]*
Forearm				≥0.3
Prox. leg				≥0.23
Distal leg				≥0.23
Foot				≥0.27

* Normative data are adjusted for gender and age of patient.

Test: Electrochemical skin conductance (ESC)				
Location	Left [µS]	Right [µS]	Average [µS/k]	Norm [µS/kg]
Hand	40	39	0.35	≥1.03
Feet	73	56	0.51	≥1.14
Forehead				

For grading uses ESC [µS] adjusted for weight [µS/k].

TABLE 53.1 **CONTINUED**

Small fiber (sensory + sudomotor) evaluation - morphological					
Test: Skin biopsy					
Location	Site (l/r)	Nerve fibers			
		Epidermal*		Sweat glands	
		Density	Norm	Density	Norm
Proximal leg – thigh	Right		≥8.3		≥37.8
Distal leg - calf	Right	2.67	≥4.85	20.6	≥36.5
Foot	Right		≥3.11		≥34.8

*Normative data for distal leg are adjusted for gender and age of patient.

QASAT*											
Heart rate		BP		CBFv		ET-CO2		Sudomotor		Total QASAT score	
S. bradycardia	0	Low supine	0	Low supine	1	Low supine	1	QSART			
S. tachycardia	0	High supine	0	High supine	0	High supine	0	ESC	3		
Increase tilt	0	OH	10	Tilt response	7	Tilt low	6				
Decrease tilt	0	OHTN	0	CA	0	Tilt high	0	**Skin biopsy**		37	
Deep breathing	2	VM	0	CVR	0			Epidermal	3		
VR	1			VM	0			Sweat gland	3		
Total	3	Total	10	Total	8	Total	7				

*QASAT. See Novak. Quantitative Scale for Grading of Cardiovascular Autonomic Reflex Tests and Small Fibers from Skin Biopsies. *J Neurol Disord* 2015;3:2.

S, supine; Increase tilt, increased response to tilt; Decrease tilt, decreased response to tilt; BP, blood pressure; VM, Valsalva maneuver; CBFv, cerebral blood flow velocity; CA, cerebral autoregulation; MCA, middle cerebral artery; VR, Valsalva ratio; CVR, cerebral vasoreactivity.

Cerebral blood flow velocity (CBFv): CBFv in middle cerebral artery was reduced in supine position and was further severely reduced during the tilt.

Skin biopsy (sensory-epidermal): Epidermal nerve fiber density was abnormal (reduced to 55.1% of normal limit) at distal leg.

Skin biopsy (sweat glands): Sweat gland nerve fiber density was abnormal (reduced to 56.4% of normal limit) at distal leg.

Patient-reported symptoms during testing: Dizziness, floating, shortness of breath during the tilt.

Patient-reported symptoms for past 2 weeks:

Lightheadedness or dizziness: Occasionally
Dry eyes or mouth: Often
Pale feet: None
Cold feet: None
Reduced sweating: None
Reduced sweating after exercise: None
Increased sweating: None
Nausea: None
Diarrhea: Occasionally
Constipation: Occasionally
Urinary leaks: Occasionally
Erection problems: Often
Current pain severity: 0
Aching pain: Often, moderate
Allodynia: None
Burning pain: None
Lancinating pain: Occasionally, mild
Numbness: Often, moderate
Prickling sensation: Often, severe

AUTONOMIC TESTING INTERPRETATION

- Severe autonomic failure.
- Small fiber neuropathy, mixed, severe.
- Hypocapnic cerebral hypoperfusion.
- Hypocapnic hyperventilation.

COMMENT

The testing showed severe abnormality in several domains, with a total QASAT score of 37 (Figure 53.1). There was evidence of severe autonomic failure likely due to small fiber neuropathy. CBFv was abnormally low even at supine position (42.5 cm/s, normal ≥45.4 cm/s), which is likely due to hypocapnia. CBFv further declined during the tilt, which was driven by worsening of hypocapnia (Figure 53.1). The oxygen saturation measured from the finger was around 96% throughout the testing. The cause of severe dyspnea may include chronic cerebral hypoperfusion.

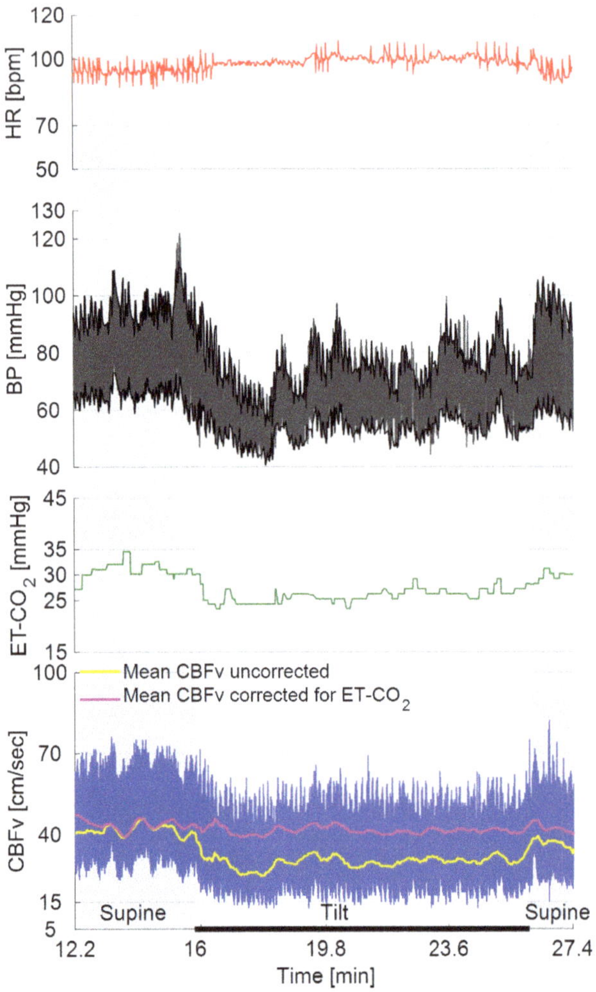

Figure 53.1 The tilt test showed supine tachycardia with normal heart rate response to the tilt, orthostatic hypotension, reduced end tidal CO_2, and reduced cerebral blood flow velocity.

Cardiopulmonary exercise testing showed an elevated VE/VCO_2, which can be seen in congestive heart failure (CHF) or pulmonary hypertension.[1] While CHF has been already ruled out in this patient, an evaluation for pulmonary hypertension is still needed since it may be related to dysautonomia.[2]

Small fiber neuropathy can be associated with MS.[3,4]

TREATMENT AND FOLLOW-UP

- For autonomic failure, consider volume expansion through high fluid and high salt intake.
- Consider pressor medication (pyridostigmine, proamatine, fludrocortisone, or droxidopa)[5] that may improve cerebral perfusion and reduce dyspnea.

CAVEATS

- Severe dyspnea can be associated with autonomic failure.

REFERENCES

1. Adachi H. Cardiopulmonary exercise test. *Int Heart J.* 2017;58(5):654–665. doi:10.1536/ihj.17-264.
2. Vaillancourt M, Chia P, Sarji S, et al. Autonomic nervous system involvement in pulmonary arterial hypertension. *Respir Res.* 2017;18(1):201. doi:10.1186/s12931-017-0679-6.
3. Khan A, Kamran S, Ponirakis G, et al. Peripheral neuropathy in patients with multiple sclerosis. *PloS One.* 2018;13(3):e0193270. doi:10.1371/journal.pone.0193270.
4. Habek M, Crnošija L, Lovrić M, Junaković A, Krbot Skorić M, Adamec I. Sympathetic cardiovascular and sudomotor functions are frequently affected in early multiple sclerosis. *Clin Auton Res Off J Clin Auton Res Soc.* 2016;26(6):385–393. doi:10.1007/s10286-016-0370-x.
5. Hale GM, Valdes J, Brenner M. The treatment of primary orthostatic hypotension. *Ann Pharmacother.* 2017;51(5):417–428. doi:10.1177/1060028016689264.

54.

CASE 49: DIZZINESS DUE TO MULTIPLE SCLEROSIS OR DUE TO DYSAUTONOMIA?

Chief complaint: Dizziness.

Case presentation: A 25-year-old woman with a past medical history of multiple sclerosis (MS) since age 13 years presents with dizziness. She became dizzy and noted being off balance for several weeks. More recently, she had two episodes of severe lightheadedness and feeling of disorientation for 2 hours. Evaluation by her MS specialist was negative for relapse. Patient was referred for evaluation of dysautonomia to determine if dysautonomia can be responsible for her orthostatic complaints.

Past medical history: MS, relapsing-remitting, associated with mainly visual symptoms.

Current medication: Natalizumab.

Assessment plan: Functional autonomic tests and skin biopsy.

AUTONOMIC TESTING EVALUATION

See Table 54.1.

Heart rate: Supine heart rate was normal. Heart rate responses to deep breathing were normal. Heart rate increment during the tilt (23 BPM) was normal (Figure 54.1).

Blood pressure:

Valsalva maneuver: Blood pressure responses were normal.

Tilt: Supine blood pressure was normal. The tilt provoked syncope at minute 6, then the tilt was terminated.

Sudomotor evaluation: Electrochemical skin conductance was abnormal (reduced to 89.4% of normal limit) at hands and normal at feet.

Respiratory system: Respiratory frequency was normal in supine position and during the tilt. End tidal CO_2 was reduced in supine position and declined further during the tilt.

Cerebral blood flow velocity (CBFv): CBFv in middle cerebral artery was normal in supine position but was severely reduced during the tilt.

Skin biopsy (sensory-epidermal): Epidermal nerve fiber density was normal at proximal leg and abnormal (reduced to 90.4% of normal limit) at distal leg.

Skin biopsy (sweat glands): Sweat gland nerve fiber density was abnormal (reduced to 73.2% of normal limit) at distal leg.

Patient-reported symptoms during testing: Syncope, dizziness, and nausea during the tilt.

Patient-reported symptoms for past 2 weeks:

Lightheadedness or dizziness: Occasionally
Dry eyes or mouth: None
Pale feet: None

TABLE 54.1 **RESULTS OF AUTONOMIC TESTING**

Blood pressure evaluation					
Test: Valsalva maneuver					
Pressure [mmHg]	Baseline	Phase 2			Phase 4
		Early	End		
Systolic	96	56	66		
Mean	68.7	70.7	79.3	n/a	
Diastolic	55	78	86	n/a	

Heart rate evaluation	
Test: Deep breathing	
Results	Norm*
24.2	≥14
Test: Valsalva ratio	
2.3	≥1.46
* adjusted for a gender and age	

(continued)

TABLE 54.1 **CONTINUED**

Test: Tilt test										
Position		HR [BPM]	Blood pressure [mmHg]		MCA Blood flow velocity [cm/s]				Respiratory frequency [breaths/min]	End tidal CO_2 [mmHg]
			Systolic	Diastolic	Systolic	Mean	Mean drop [%]	Diastolic		
Supine		80	116	82	116	78.7		60	5	33
Tilt [min]	1	94	105	73	117	77	2.2	57	9	33
	2	86	102	71						
	3	101	96	67						
	4	103	106	73						
	5	85	89	60	112	45.3	42.4	12	13	30
	6	69	64	44	101	41.7	47	12	15	25
	7									
	8									
	9									
	10									
	15									
	20									
	30									
	40									

Sudomotor evaluation - functional

Test: Quantitative sudomotor axon reflex test (QSART)				
Location	Site (l/r)	Latency [min]	Volume [µl]	Norm [µl]*
Forearm				≥0.08
Prox. leg				≥0.14
Distal leg				≥0.24
Foot				≥0.09

* Normative data are adjusted for gender and age of patient.

Test: Electrochemical skin conductance (ESC)				
Location	Left [µS]	Right [µS]	Average [µS/k]	Norm [µS/kg]
Hand	58	65	0.92	≥1.03
Feet	87	70	1.06	≥1.14
Forehead				

For grading uses ESC [µS] adjusted for weight [µS/k].

TABLE 54.1 CONTINUED

Small fiber (sensory + sudomotor) evaluation - morphological					
Test: Skin biopsy					
Location	Site (l/r)	Nerve fibers			
		Epidermal*		Sweat glands	
		Density	Norm	Density	Norm
Proximal leg – thigh	Right	8.85	≥8.3		≥37.8
Distal leg - calf	Right	8.23	≥9.1	26.7	≥36.5
Foot	Right		≥3.11		≥34.8

*Normative data for distal leg are adjusted for gender and age of patient.

QASAT*										
Heart rate		**BP**		**CBFv**		**ET-CO2**		**Sudomotor**		**Total QASAT score**
S. bradycardia	0	Low supine	0	Low supine	0	Low supine	1	QSART		
S. tachycardia	0	High supine	0	High supine	0	High supine	0	ESC	1	
Increase tilt		OH		Tilt response		Tilt low				
Decrease tilt		OHTN		CA	0	Tilt high		**Skin biopsy**		16
Deep breathing	0	VM	0	CVR	0			Epidermal	1	
VR	0			VM	0			Sweat gland	3	
Total	0	Total	0	Total	0	Total	1			

*QASAT. See Novak. Quantitative Scale for Grading of Cardiovascular Autonomic Reflex Tests and Small Fibers from Skin Biopsies. *J Neurol Disord* 2015;3:2. Orthostatic (tilt) responses were not graded since QASAT requires the duration of the tilt at least 10 minutes.

S, supine; Increase tilt, increased response to tilt; Decrease tilt, decreased response to tilt; BP, blood pressure; VM, Valsalva maneuver; CBFv, cerebral blood flow velocity; CA, cerebral autoregulation; MCA, middle cerebral artery; VR, Valsalva ratio; CVR, cerebral vasoreactivity.

Cold feet: None
Reduced sweating: None
Reduced sweating after exercise: None
Increased sweating: None
Nausea: None
Diarrhea: None
Constipation: None
Urinary leaks: None
Current pain severity: 0
Aching pain: None
Allodynia: None
Burning pain: None
Lancinating pain: None
Numbness: None
Prickling sensation: Occasionally, mild

AUTONOMIC TESTING INTERPRETATION

- Syncope, mixed, neutrally mediated.
- Small fiber neuropathy, mixed, affecting sensory and autonomic fibers.
- No evidence of autonomic failure.

COMMENT

The tilt provoked syncope (Figure 54.1). Patient confirmed that the symptoms during the tilt test were very similar to those she was referred for. Small fiber neuropathy can be associated with multiple sclerosis.[1,2]

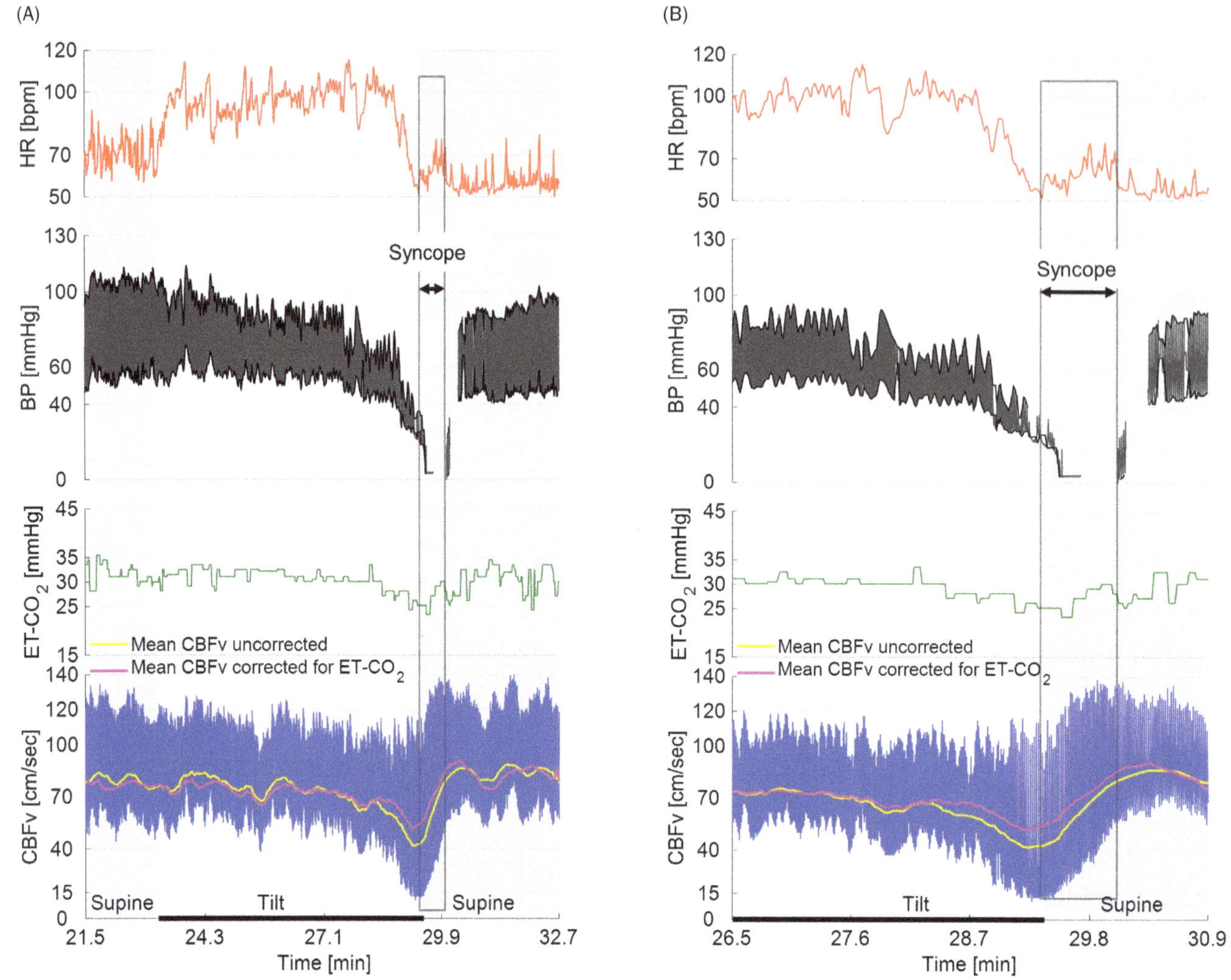

Figure 54.1 The initial responses to tilt were normal, then the patient experienced mixed neurally mediated syncope at minute 6 (A–F). The finger cuff device amplifies blood pressure decline. Blood pressure is spuriously almost zero but cerebral blood flow is well preserved during syncope. E shows details of signals during supine baseline and F shows the signals during syncope.

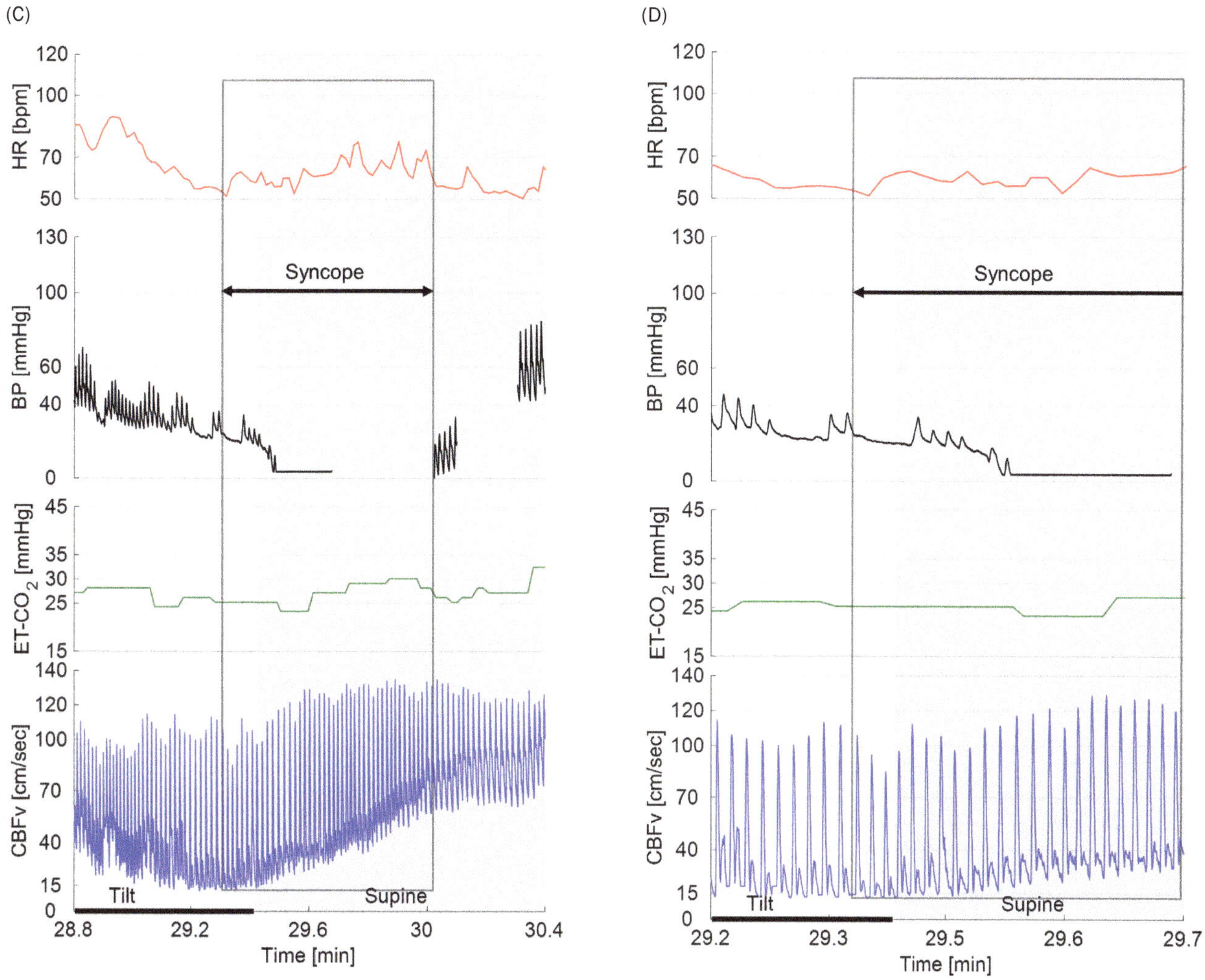

Figure 54.1 Continued

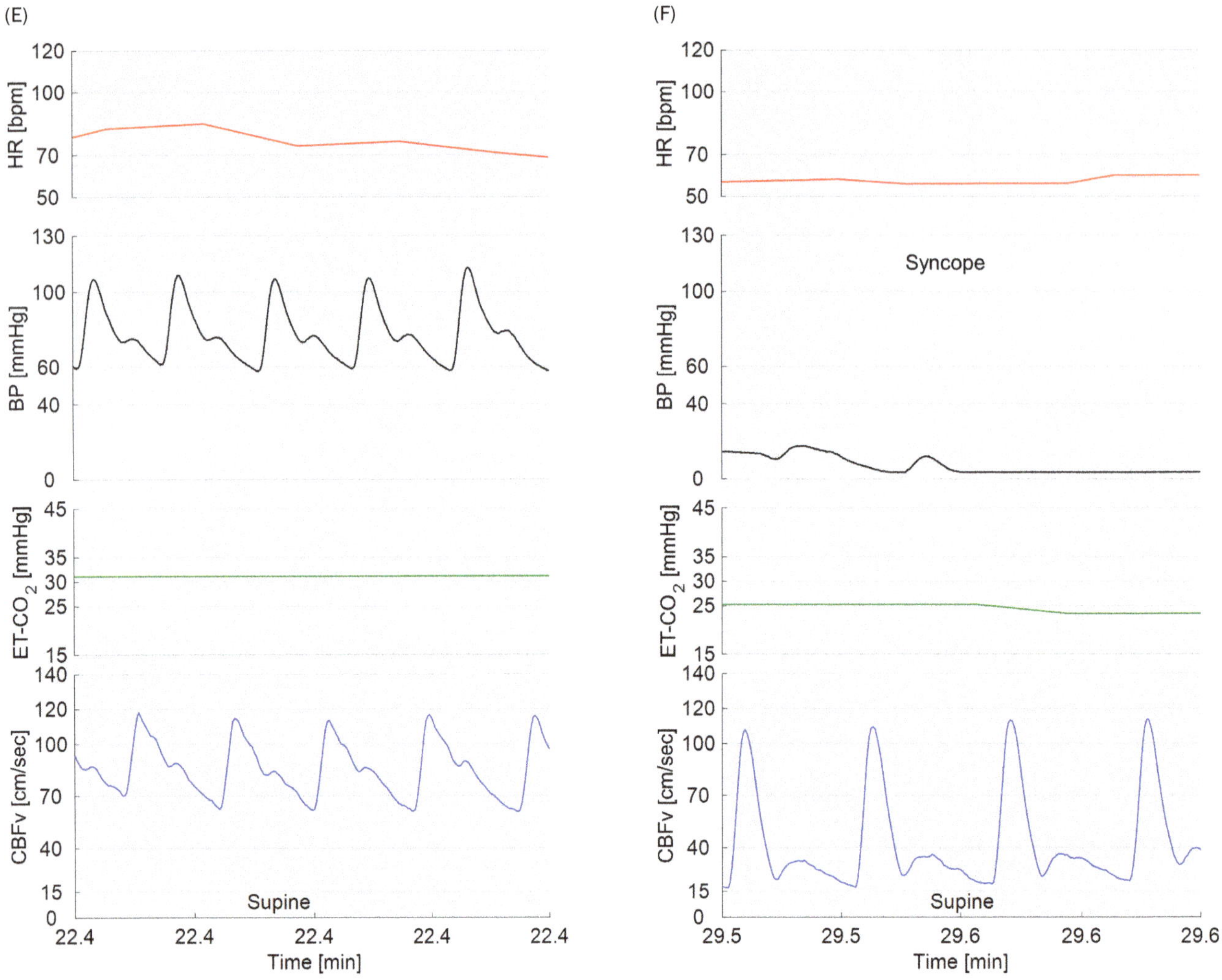

Figure 54.1 Continued

TREATMENT AND FOLLOW-UP

- Recommended nonpharmacological and pharmacological treatment of syncope.[3]

CAVEATS

- The tilt test can be diagnostic for syncope.
- Syncope and small fiber neuropathy are associated with MS.

REFERENCES

1. Khan A, Kamran S, Ponirakis G, et al. Peripheral neuropathy in patients with multiple sclerosis. *PloS One*. 2018;13(3):e0193270. doi:10.1371/journal.pone.0193270.
2. Habek M, Crnošija L, Lovrić M, Junaković A, Krbot Skorić M, Adamec I. Sympathetic cardiovascular and sudomotor functions are frequently affected in early multiple sclerosis. *Clin Auton Res Off J Clin Auton Res Soc*. 2016;26(6):385–393. doi:10.1007/s10286-016-0370-x.
3. Task Force for the Diagnosis and Management of Syncope, European Society of Cardiology (ESC), European Heart Rhythm Association (EHRA), et al. Guidelines for the diagnosis and management of syncope (version 2009). *Eur Heart J*. 2009;30(21):2631–2671. doi:10.1093/eurheartj/ehp298.

PART IX

SMALL FIBER NEUROPATHY

55.

CASE 50: SMALL FIBER NEUROPATHY AND SEVERE AUTONOMIC FAILURE IN DIABETES

Chief complaint: Dizziness.

Case presentation: A 59-year-old woman with past medical history of insulin-dependent diabetes mellitus presents with postural dizziness. She noted the sudden onset of dizziness on standing for past 3 months. She has a history of coronary artery disease treated with drug-eluting stents also 3 months ago. Repeated cardiac catheterization showed patent coronary arteries. MRI and magnetic resonance angiography (MRA) of the brain was unremarkable. She was referred for evaluation of suspected diabetic autonomic failure.

Past medical history: Diabetes mellitus, insulin-dependent for 30 years, pericardial effusion, orthostatic hypotension, hypothyroidism, headaches, coronary artery disease, status post drug-eluting stent placements.

Current medication: Insulin pump, levothyroxine, clopidogrel, duloxetine, atorvastatin.

Assessment plan: Functional autonomic tests and skin biopsy.

AUTONOMIC TESTING EVALUATION

See Table 55.1.

Heart rate: Supine heart rate was normal. Heart rate responses to deep breathing were reduced to 11.1% of normal value. Heart rate increment during the tilt (11 BPM) was normal.

Blood pressure:

Valsalva maneuver: Mean blood pressure failed to return to baseline at the end of Phase 2 by 19.7 mm Hg (i.e., 77% of baseline).

Tilt: Supine blood pressure was elevated. Blood pressure responses to tilt were abnormal and consistent with marked orthostatic hypotension.

Sudomotor evaluation: Sweat output was normal at forearm, normal at proximal leg, normal at distal leg, and normal at foot.

Respiratory system: Respiratory frequency and end tidal CO_2 were normal during in supine position and during the tilt.

Cerebral blood flow velocity (CBFv): CBFv in middle cerebral artery was increased in supine position. CBFv in middle cerebral artery was intermittently reduced during the tilt.

Skin biopsy (sensory-epidermal): Epidermal nerve fiber density was abnormal (reduced to 19.9% of normal limit) at proximal leg and abnormal (reduced to 0% of normal limit) at distal leg.

Skin biopsy (sweat glands): Sweat gland nerve fiber density was abnormal (reduced to 60.3% of normal limit)

TABLE 55.1 RESULTS OF AUTONOMIC TESTING

Blood pressure evaluation					
Test: Valsalva maneuver					
Pressure [mmHg]	Baseline	Phase 2			Phase 4
		Early	End		
Systolic	131	82	82		
Mean	85.7	66	66	n/a	
Diastolic	63	58	58	n/a	

Heart rate evaluation	
Test: Deep breathing	
Results	Norm*
1	≥9
Test: Valsalva ratio	
1.14	≥1.47
* adjusted for a gender and age	

(continued)

TABLE 55.1 **CONTINUED**

Test: Tilt test											
Position		HR [BPM]	Blood pressure [mmHg]		MCA Blood flow velocity [cm/s]				Respiratory frequency [breaths/min]	End tidal CO_2 [mmHg]
			Systolic	Diastolic	Systolic	Mean	Mean drop [%]	Diastolic		
Supine		88	175	90	144	86		57	17	42
Tilt [min]	1	92	127	78	150	88	-2.3	57	13	41
	2	93	121	76						
	3	94	121	77						
	4	95	125	79						
	5	95	123	77	160	92	-7	58	18	41
	6	99	122	78						
	7	94	106	69						
	8	95	95	64						
	9	94	91	62						
	10	94	91	61	166	96	-11.6	61	16	39
	15									
	20									
	30									
	40									

Sudomotor evaluation - functional

Test: Quantitative sudomotor axon reflex test (QSART)				
Location	Site (l/r)	Latency [min]	Volume [µl]	Norm [µl]*
Forearm	l	1.15	0.45	≥0.08
Prox. leg	l	1.14	0.763	≥0.14
Distal leg	l	1.11	0.197	≥0.07
Foot	l	1.14	0.16	≥0.05

* Normative data are adjusted for gender and age of patient.

Test: Electrochemical skin conductance (ESC)				
Location	Left [µS]	Right [µS]	Average [µS/k]	Norm [µS/kg]
Hand				≥
Feet				≥
Forehead				

For grading uses ESC [µS] adjusted for weight [µS/k].

TABLE 55.1 **CONTINUED**

Small fiber (sensory + sudomotor) evaluation - morphological					
Test: Skin biopsy					
Location	Site (l/r)	Nerve fibers			
		Epidermal*		Sweat glands	
		Density	Norm	Density	Norm
Proximal leg – thigh	Right	1.65	≥8.3	22.8	≥37.8
Distal leg - calf	Right	0	≥6.38	33.5	≥36.5
Foot	Right		≥3.11		≥34.8

*Normative data for distal leg are adjusted for gender and age of patient.

QASAT*										
Heart rate		**BP**		**CBFv**		**ET-CO2**		**Sudomotor**		**Total QASAT score**
S. bradycardia	0	Low supine	0	Low supine	0	Low supine	0	QSART	1	
S. tachycardia	0	High supine	2	High supine	1	High supine	0	ESC		
Increase tilt	0	OH	10	Tilt response	0	Tilt low	0			
Decrease tilt	0	OHTN	0	CA	0	Tilt high	0	**Skin biopsy**		27
Deep breathing	3	VM	2	CVR	0			Epidermal	4	
VR	1			VM	0			Sweat gland	3	
Total	4	Total	14	Total	1	Total	0			

*QASAT. See Novak. Quantitative Scale for Grading of Cardiovascular Autonomic Reflex Tests and Small Fibers from Skin Biopsies. *J Neurol Disord* 2015;3:2.

S, supine; Increase tilt, increased response to tilt; Decrease tilt, decreased response to tilt; BP, blood pressure; VM, Valsalva maneuver; CBFv, cerebral blood flow velocity; CA, cerebral autoregulation; MCA, middle cerebral artery; VR, Valsalva ratio; CVR, cerebral vasoreactivity.

at proximal leg and abnormal (reduced to 91.8% of normal limit) at distal leg.

Patient-reported symptoms during testing: Dizziness during the tilt.

Patient-reported symptoms for past 2 weeks:

Lightheadedness or dizziness: Occasionally
Dry eyes or mouth: Occasionally
Pale feet: Yes, minor annoyance
Cold feet: Yes, minor annoyance
Reduced sweating: Yes, minor annoyance
Reduced sweating after exercise: Yes, minor annoyance
Increased sweating: None
Nausea: Yes, minor annoyance
Diarrhea: None
Constipation: Occasionally
Urinary leaks: Occasionally
Current pain severity: 0
Aching pain: Occasionally, mild
Allodynia: None
Burning pain: Occasionally, mild
Lancinating pain: Occasionally, moderate
Numbness: Occasionally, mild
Prickling sensation: Occasionally, mild

AUTONOMIC TESTING INTERPRETATION

- Small fiber neuropathy, severe, mixed, affecting both sensory and autonomic fibers.
- Generalized autonomic failure, severe, due to small fiber neuropathy.

COMMENT

This is an example of a typical autonomic failure associated with diabetes (Figure 55.1).

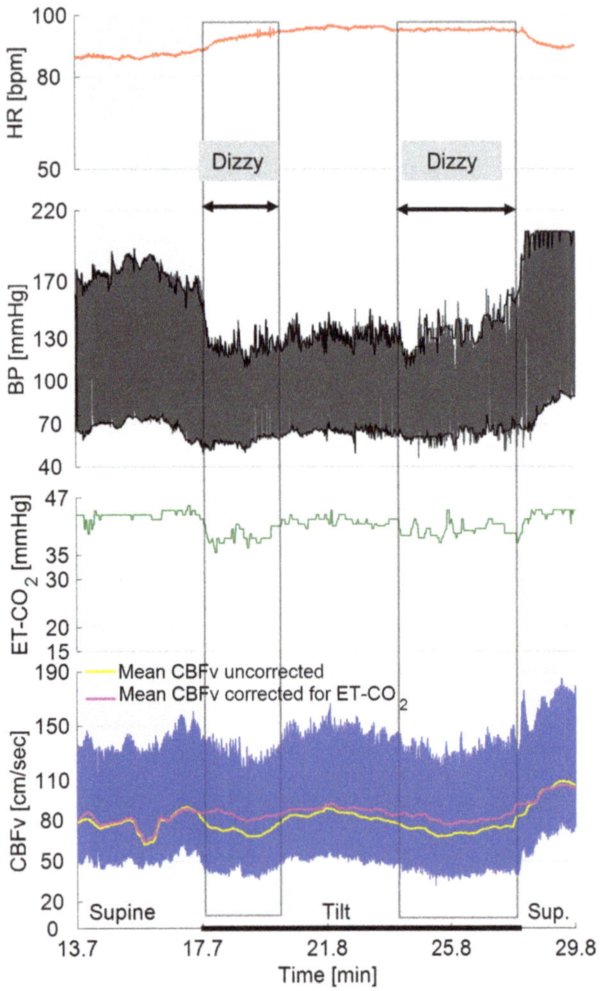

Figure 55.1 The tilt showed orthostatic hypotension. The patient became transiently dizzy twice during the tilt; on both occasions, the dizziness coincided with the decline in cerebral blood flow velocity even as blood pressure was reduced throughout the tilt.

TREATMENT AND FOLLOW-UP

- Compression stockings and pressor medication (pyridostigmine and/or proamatine) during daytime.
- Avoid daytime supine position.
- At night, sleep with elevated head.
- May use angiotensin-receptor antagonists for supine hypertension.

CAVEATS

- Diabetes is associated with small fiber neuropathy affecting sensory and autonomic fibers.[1,2]
- Damage of sensory fibers results in distal numbness and pain.
- Damage to autonomic fibers is associated with autonomic failure including orthostatic hypotension.
- During the day, avoiding the supine position is often effective in avoiding supine hypertension.[3] At night, the patient should sleep with the head elevated and use short-acting angiotensin-receptor antagonists for supine hypertension.[4]

REFERENCES

1. Fisher VL, Tahrani AA. Cardiac autonomic neuropathy in patients with diabetes mellitus: current perspectives. *Diabetes Metab Syndr Obes Targets Ther*. 2017;10:419–434. doi:10.2147/DMSO.S129797.
2. Russell JW, Zilliox LA. Diabetic neuropathies. *Contin Minneap Minn*. 2014;20(5 Peripheral Nervous System Disorders):1226–1240. doi:10.1212/01.CON.0000455884.29545.d2.
3. Jordan J, Biaggioni I. Diagnosis and treatment of supine hypertension in autonomic failure patients with orthostatic hypotension. *J Clin Hypertens Greenwich Conn*. 2002;4(2):139–145.
4. Naschitz JE, Slobodin G, Elias N, Rosner I. The patient with supine hypertension and orthostatic hypotension: a clinical dilemma. *Postgrad Med J*. 2006;82(966):246–253. doi:10.1136/pgmj.2005.037457.

56.

CASE 51: SMALL FIBER NEUROPATHY AND TRANSIENT ORTHOSTATIC HYPOTENSION IN DIABETES

Chief complaint: Dizziness.

Case presentation: A 45-year-old woman presents with dizziness. She has had type 1 diabetes for 30 years and is on an insulin pump. She has a history of chronic fatigue, shortness of breath, excessive sweating, nausea, vomiting, insomnia, and orthostatic dizziness associated with blurred vision for 1 year. She had multiple presyncopal episodes. She also experienced distal burning pain and joint pain. She had several hypertensive emergencies last year. Cardiac evaluation, including Holter monitoring and 2D echocardiogram was normal. She was referred for evaluation of suspected diabetic autonomic failure.

Past medical history: Type 1 diabetes mellitus for 30 years, dyslipidemia.

Current medication: Insulin pump, levothyroxine, sertraline, gabapentin, atorvastatin, omeprazole, ondansetron, vitamin D, loratadine, ipratropium, albuterol, fluticasone, metoclopramide.

Assessment plan: Functional autonomic tests and skin biopsy.

AUTONOMIC TESTING EVALUATION

See Table 56.1.

Heart rate: Supine heart rate was normal. Heart rate responses to deep breathing were reduced to 36% of normal value. Heart rate increment during the tilt (24 BPM) was normal.

Blood pressure:

Valsalva maneuver: Blood pressure responses were normal.

Tilt: Supine blood pressure was elevated. Blood pressure responses to tilt were abnormal and consistent with moderate orthostatic hypotension.

Sudomotor evaluation: Electrochemical skin conductance was abnormal (reduced to 79.5% of normal limit) at hands and abnormal (reduced to 62.6% of normal limit) at feet.

Respiratory system: Respiratory frequency was normal in supine position and during the tilt. End tidal CO_2 was normal in supine position but was severely reduced during the tilt.

Cerebral blood flow velocity (CBFv): CBFv in middle cerebral artery was normal in supine position but was severely reduced during the tilt test.

Skin biopsy (sensory-epidermal): Epidermal nerve fiber density was abnormal (reduced to 5.3% of normal limit) at proximal leg and abnormal (reduced to 3.6% of normal limit) at distal leg.

Skin biopsy (sweat glands): Sweat gland nerve fiber density was abnormal (reduced to 30.7% of normal limit) at proximal leg and abnormal (reduced to 31.2% of normal limit) at distal leg.

TABLE 56.1 **RESULTS OF AUTONOMIC TESTING**

Blood pressure evaluation					
Test: Valsalva maneuver					
Pressure [mmHg]	Baseline	Phase 2			Phase 4
		Early	End		
Systolic	154	102	130		
Mean	102.7	90.7	109.3	n/a	
Diastolic	77	85	99	n/a	

Heart rate evaluation	
Test: Deep breathing	
Results	Norm*
3.6	≥10
Test: Valsalva ratio	
1.23	≥1.51
* adjusted for a gender and age	

(continued)

TABLE 56.1 CONTINUED

Test: Tilt test										
Position		HR [BPM]	Blood pressure [mmHg]		MCA Blood flow velocity [cm/s]				Respiratory frequency [breaths/min]	End tidal CO_2 [mmHg]
			Systolic	Diastolic	Systolic	Mean	Mean drop [%]	Diastolic		
Supine		85	160	89	114	63.3		38	16	36
Tilt [min]	1	102	136	78	101	55.7	12	33	10	30
	2	106	127	74						
	3	106	111	73						
	4	107	125	82						
	5	109	145	80	88	46	27.3	25	17	25
	6	105	157	88						
	7	106	132	78						
	8	105	150	80						
	9	104	134	74						
	10	104	122	78	87	49.7	21.5	31	18	23
	15									
	20									
	30									
	40									

Sudomotor evaluation - functional

Test: Quantitative sudomotor axon reflex test (QSART)				
Location	Site (l/r)	Latency [min]	Volume [μl]	Norm [μl]*
Forearm				≥0.08
Prox. leg				≥0.14
Distal leg				≥0.15
Foot				≥0.07

* Normative data are adjusted for gender and age of patient.

Test: Electrochemical skin conductance (ESC)				
Location	Left [μS]	Right [μS]	Average [μS/k]	Norm [μS/kg]
Hand	35	43	0.82	≥1.03
Feet	27	42	0.88	≥1.14
Forehead				

For grading uses ESC [μS] adjusted for weight [μS/k].

TABLE 56.1 CONTINUED

Small fiber (sensory + sudomotor) evaluation - morphological					
Test: Skin biopsy					
Location	Site (l/r)	Nerve fibers			
		Epidermal*		Sweeat glands	
		Density	Norm	Density	Norm
Proximal leg – thigh	Right	0.44	≥8.3	11.6	≥37.8
Distal leg - calf	Right	0.27	≥7.5	11.4	≥36.5
Foot	Right		≥3.11		≥34.8

*Normative data for distal leg are adjusted for gender and age of patient.

QASAT*											
Heart rate		BP		CBFv		ET-CO2		Sudomotor			Total QASAT score
S. bradycardia	0	Low supine	0	Low supine	0	Low supine	0	QSART			
S. tachycardia	0	High supine	2	High supine	0	High supine	0	ESC	2		
Increase tilt	0	OH	4	Tilt response	4	Tilt low	5				
Decrease tilt	0	OHTN	0	CA	0	Tilt high	0	**Skin biopsy**			28
Deep breathing	2	VM	0	CVR	0			Epidermal	4		
VR	1			VM	0			Sweat gland	4		
Total	3	Total	6	Total	4	Total	5				

*QASAT. See Novak. Quantitative Scale for Grading of Cardiovascular Autonomic Reflex Tests and Small Fibers from Skin Biopsies. *J Neurol Disord* 2015;3:2.

S, supine; Increase tilt, increased response to tilt; Decrease tilt, decreased response to tilt; BP, blood pressure; VM, Valsalva maneuver; CBFv, cerebral blood flow velocity; CA, cerebral autoregulation; MCA, middle cerebral artery; VR, Valsalva ratio; CVR, cerebral vasoreactivity.

Patient-reported symptoms during testing: Dizziness, shortness of breath, tremor during the tilt test.

Patient-reported symptoms for past 2 weeks:

Lightheadedness or dizziness: Often
Dry eyes or mouth: Occasionally
Pale feet: Occasionally
Cold feet: Occasionally
Reduced sweating: Occasionally
Reduced sweating after exercise: Occasionally
Increased sweating: Yes, minor annoyance
Nausea: Often
Diarrhea: Occasionally
Constipation: Occasionally
Urinary leaks: Occasionally
Current pain severity: 0
Aching pain: Continuous, severe
Allodynia: Often, mild
Burning pain: Continuous, moderate
Lancinating pain: Often, severe
Numbness: Often, mild
Prickling sensation: Often, moderate

AUTONOMIC TESTING INTERPRETATION

- Small fiber neuropathy, mixed, severe, non–length-dependent, affecting sensory and autonomic fibers.
- Generalized autonomic failure associated with transient orthostatic hypotension.
- Reduced CBFv due to orthostatic hypotension and hypocapnia. Hypocapnia induces cerebral vasoconstriction and reduces CBFv.
- Hypocapnic hyperventilation during the supine position and during the tilt.

COMMENT

Autonomic neuropathy is common in diabetes.[1] Although the autonomic testing showed autonomic failure (Figure 56.1), the orthostatic hypotension was moderate (QASAT score for orthostatic hypotension during tilt was 4) and not responsible for all orthostatic symptoms. The primary cause of orthostatic

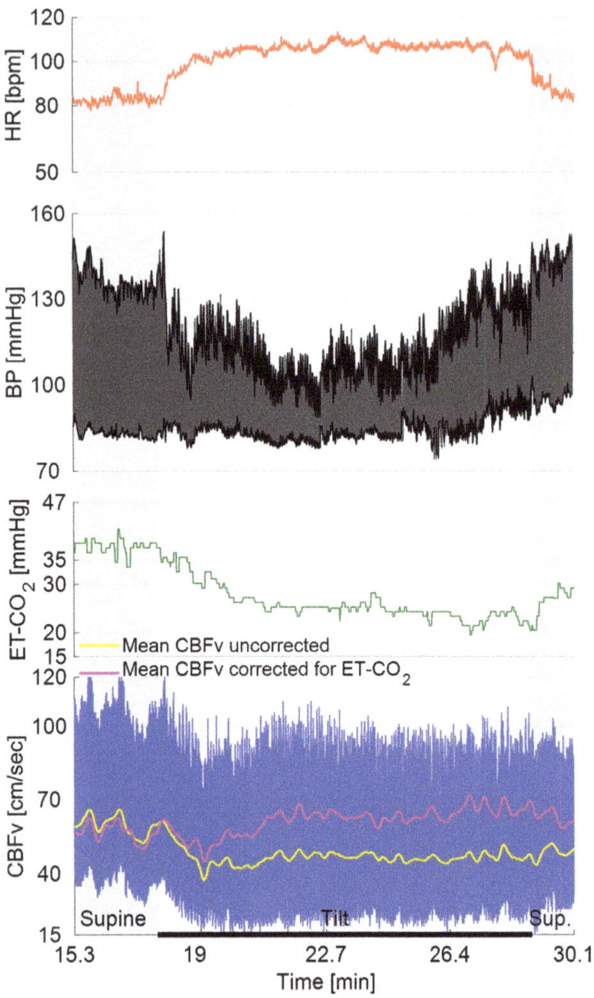

Figure 56.1 The tilt test provoked initial orthostatic hypotension (IOH) associated with decline in blood pressure and cerebral blood flow velocity when the patient became dizzy. IOH partially corrected later but then worsened again at around minute 22.7. Finally, blood pressure recovered 3 minutes before the tilt end.

dizziness in this patient was the effect of hypocapnia on the CBFv (Figure 56.1). CBFv was reduced due to orthostatic hypotension only at the beginning and in the middle of the tilt; later the reduced CBFv was due to reduced end tidal CO_2.

The testing also showed non–length-dependent small fiber neuropathy. In a typical diabetes, the small fiber neuropathy is distal (e.g., length-dependent),[2] therefore this patient also needs evaluation for non–length-dependent neuropathy.[3]

TREATMENT AND FOLLOW-UP

- Clinical workup for non–length-dependent neuropathy.
- Volume expansion through high fluid and high salt intake.
- Pulmonary evaluation for orthostatic hypocapnia.

CAVEATS

- Quantitative autonomic testing is useful to assess severity of dysautonomia and small fiber neuropathy, which can be helpful in clinical management.
- Hypocapnia may play an important role in orthostatic intolerance in diabetes.

REFERENCES

1. Fisher VL, Tahrani AA. Cardiac autonomic neuropathy in patients with diabetes mellitus: current perspectives. *Diabetes Metab Syndr Obes Targets Ther*. 2017;10:419–434. doi:10.2147/DMSO.S129797.
2. Said G. Diabetic neuropathy: a review. *Nat Clin Pract Neurol*. 2007;3(6):331–340. doi:10.1038/ncpneuro0504.
3. Terkelsen AJ, Karlsson P, Lauria G, Freeman R, Finnerup NB, Jensen TS. The diagnostic challenge of small fibre neuropathy: clinical presentations, evaluations, and causes. *Lancet Neurol*. 2017;16(11):934–944. doi:10.1016/S1474-4422(17)30329-0.

57.

CASE 52: PAINFUL SMALL FIBER NEUROPATHY

Chief complaint: Burning pain in the feet.

Case presentation: A 56-year-old man presents with disabling severe pain in the feet. The pain started at the first toe and within 1 year spread to the whole foot. The patient saw several podiatrists and neurologists without establishing a diagnosis. Nerve conduction study was normal.

Neurological examination showed normal reflexes, muscle strength, and large fibers examination (soft touch, vibration, and proprioception sensation) but abnormal small fiber examination (pin-prick and temperature sensation at distal legs). The skin at the bottom of the feet was red and thin. Even a soft touch to the bottom of the feet was painful. Patient was referred for evaluation of suspected painful small fiber neuropathy.

Past medical history: None.

Current medication: None.

Assessment plan: Functional autonomic tests and skin biopsy.

AUTONOMIC TESTING EVALUATION

See Table 57.1.

Heart rate: Supine heart rate was normal. Heart rate responses to deep breathing were reduced to 65.6% of normal value. Heart rate increment during the tilt (20 BPM) was normal.

Blood pressure:

Valsalva maneuver: Blood pressure responses were normal.

Tilt: Supine blood pressure was normal. Blood pressure was elevated during the tilt.

Sudomotor evaluation: Sweat output was normal at forearm, normal at proximal leg, normal at distal leg, and normal at foot.

Respiratory system: N/A

Cerebral blood flow velocity (CBFv): N/A

Skin biopsy (sensory-epidermal): Epidermal nerve fiber density was abnormal (reduced to 86.9% of normal limit) at proximal leg and abnormal (reduced to 2.5% of normal limit) at distal leg.

Skin biopsy (sweat glands): Sweat gland nerve fiber density was abnormal (reduced to 60.8% of normal limit) at distal leg.

Patient-reported symptoms during testing: None during the tilt.

Patient-reported symptoms for past 2 weeks:

Lightheadedness or dizziness: Occasionally
Dry eyes or mouth: Occasionally
Pale feet: Occasionally
Cold feet: Occasionally
Reduced sweating: Occasionally
Reduced sweating after exercise: Occasionally
Increased sweating: Yes, minor annoyance
Nausea: Yes, minor annoyance
Diarrhea: Occasionally
Constipation: Yes, minor annoyance
Urinary leaks: Occasionally

TABLE 57.1 RESULTS OF AUTONOMIC TESTING

Blood pressure evaluation					
Test: Valsalva maneuver					
Pressure [mmHg]	Baseline	Phase 2			Phase 4
		Early	End		
Systolic	108	115	141		
Mean	74.7	86.3	109.7	n/a	
Diastolic	58	72	94	n/a	

Heart rate evaluation	
Test: Deep breathing	
Results	Norm*
5.9	≥9
Test: Valsalva ratio	
1.51	≥1.36

* adjusted for a gender and age

(continued)

TABLE 57.1 CONTINUED

Test: Tilt test											
Position		HR [BPM]	Blood pressure [mmHg]		MCA Blood flow velocity [cm/s]				Respiratory frequency [breaths/min]	End tidal CO_2 [mmHg]
			Systolic	Diastolic	Systolic	Mean	Mean drop [%]	Diastolic		
Supine		60	120	79						
Tilt [min]	1	80	122	88						
	2	75	145	90						
	3	73	124	84						
	4	80	149	97						
	5	80	149	94						
	6	76	141	97						
	7	80	147	98						
	8	75	139	91						
	9	72	139	96						
	10	66	144	100						
	15									
	20									
	30									
	40									

Sudomotor evaluation - functional

Test: Quantitative sudomotor axon reflex test (QSART)				
Location	Site (l/r)	Latency [min]	Volume [µl]	Norm [µl]*
Forearm	l	0.58	1.013	≥0.3
Prox. leg	l	1.35	0.84	≥0.23
Distal leg	l	0.39	0.701	≥0.23
Foot	l	0.49	1.563	≥0.27

* Normative data are adjusted for gender and age of patient.

Test: Electrochemical skin conductance (ESC)				
Location	Left [µS]	Right [µS]	Average [µS/k]	Norm [µS/kg]
Hand				≥
Feet				≥
Forehead				

For grading uses ESC [µS] adjusted for weight [µS/k].

TABLE 57.1 **CONTINUED**

Small fiber (sensory + sudomotor) evaluation - morphological					
Test: Skin biopsy					
Location	Site (l/r)	Nerve fibers			
		Epidermal*		Sweat glands	
		Density	Norm	Density	Norm
Proximal leg – thigh	Right	7.21	≥8.3		≥37.8
Distal leg - calf	Right	0.13	≥5.3	22.2	≥36.5
Foot	Right	0.08	≥3.11	35.1	≥34.8

*Normative data for distal leg are adjusted for gender and age of patient.

QASAT*												
Heart rate		BP		CBFv		ET-CO2		Sudomotor			Total QASAT score
S. bradycardia	0	Low supine	0	Low supine		Low supine		QSART	0		
S. tachycardia	0	High supine	0	High supine		High supine		ESC			
Increase tilt	0	OH	0	Tilt response		Tilt low					
Decrease tilt	0	OHTN	6	CA		Tilt high		**Skin biopsy**			14
Deep breathing	1	VM	0	CVR				Epidermal	4		
VR	0			VM				Sweat gland	3		
Total	1	Total	6	Total		Total					

*QASAT. See Novak. Quantitative Scale for Grading of Cardiovascular Autonomic Reflex Tests and Small Fibers from Skin Biopsies. *J Neurol Disord* 2015;3:2.

S, supine; Increase tilt, increased response to tilt; Decrease tilt, decreased response to tilt; BP, blood pressure; VM, Valsalva maneuver; CBFv, cerebral blood flow velocity; CA, cerebral autoregulation; MCA, middle cerebral artery; VR, Valsalva ratio; CVR, cerebral vasoreactivity.

Erection problems: Yes, minor annoyance
Aching pain: Continuous, severe
Allodynia: Occasionally, moderate
Burning pain: Often, moderate
Lancinating pain: Continuous, moderate
Numbness: Continuous, moderate
Prickling sensation: Continuous, moderate
Current pain severity: 7

AUTONOMIC TESTING INTERPRETATION

- Small fiber neuropathy.

COMMENT

This patient exhibited characteristic symptoms of painful small fiber neuropathy which was confirmed by abnormal skin biopsy.[1] The pain was disabling, causing considerable discomfort. Clinical workup for neuropathy was positive for neuronal voltage-gated potassium antibody (titer 0.09, normal ≤0.02 nmol/L). The patient has been treated with intravenous immunoglobulins (IVIG), at a dose of 2 g/kg, monthly, for a presumed autoimmune process.[2] Within a year, the pain improved by at least 60%.

TREATMENT AND FOLLOW-UP

- Intravenous immunoglobulin.
- Gabapentin for the pain.

CAVEAT

- Painful small fiber neuropathy can have an autoimmune cause and may respond to IVIG.

REFERENCES

1. Novak V, Freimer ML, Kissel JT, et al. Autonomic impairment in painful neuropathy. *Neurology*. 2001;56(7):861–868.
2. Oaklander AL. Immunotherapy prospects for painful small-fiber sensory neuropathies and ganglionopathies. *Neurotherapeutics*. 2016;13(1):108–117. doi:10.1007/s13311-015-0395-1.

58.

CASE 53: SMALL FIBER NEUROPATHY WITH STRIATIONAL ANTIBODIES

Chief complaint: Dizziness.

Case presentation: A 32-year-old woman presents with orthostatic intolerance. She experienced a viral illness 2 months ago. Since then, her blood pressure is low and heart rate elevated. She was admitted, diagnosed with postural tachycardia syndrome (POTS), and placed on proamatine and fludrocortisone. She experienced some improvement but she still gets dizzy when standing up or when she moves; her whole body shakes and she also stutters. She also experienced numbness and a burning sensation in her arms and chest, usually on the right, sometimes on the left. She became disabled, able to stand only for minutes before becoming short of breath and dizzy. MRI of the brain was normal. Usual workup for neuropathy (vitamin B_{12} level, thyroid stimulation test, rapid plasma reagin, protein electrophoresis) was normal.

Past medical history: Asthma, depression.

Current medication: Nortriptyline, cetirizine.

Assessment plan: Functional autonomic tests and skin biopsy.

AUTONOMIC TESTING EVALUATION

See Table 58.1.

Heart rate: Supine heart rate was normal. Heart rate responses to deep breathing were reduced to 65.6% of normal value. Heart rate increment during the tilt (56 BPM) was exaggerated and exceeded 130 BPM.

Blood pressure:

Valsalva maneuver: Mean blood pressure failed to return to baseline at the end of Phase 2 by 37.6 mm Hg (i.e., 61.3% of baseline).

Tilt: Supine blood pressure was normal. Blood pressure responses to tilt were normal.

Sudomotor evaluation: Patient did not tolerate quantitative sudomotor axon reflex test (QSART).

Respiratory system: Respiratory frequency was normal in supine position and during the tilt. End tidal CO_2 was normal in supine position and was reduced during the tilt.

Cerebral blood flow velocity (CBFv): CBFv in middle cerebral artery was normal in supine position. CBFv in middle cerebral artery was severely reduced during the tilt.

Skin biopsy (sensory-epidermal): Epidermal nerve fiber density was normal at proximal leg and abnormal (reduced to 29.9% of normal limit) at distal leg.

Skin biopsy (sweat glands): Sweat gland nerve fiber density was normal at proximal leg.

Patient-reported symptoms during testing: Chest pressure and dizziness during the tilt.

Patient-reported symptoms for past 2 weeks:

Lightheadedness or dizziness: Occasionally
Dry eyes or mouth: Occasionally
Pale feet: Yes, minor annoyance

TABLE 58.1 **RESULTS OF AUTONOMIC TESTING**

Blood pressure evaluation					
Test: Valsalva maneuver					
Pressure [mmHg]	Baseline	Phase 2			Phase 4
		Early	End		
Systolic	131.1	63.1	63.1		
Mean	97.2	59.6	59.6	n/a	
Diastolic	80.3	57.8	57.8	n/a	

Heart rate evaluation	
Test: Deep breathing	
Results	Norm*
21	≥12
Test: Valsalva ratio	
2.1	≥1.5
* adjusted for a gender and age	

TABLE 58.1 **CONTINUED**

Test: Tilt test										
Position		HR [BPM]	Blood pressure [mmHg]		MCA Blood flow velocity [cm/s]				Respiratory frequency [breaths/min]	End tidal CO_2 [mmHg]
			Systolic	Diastolic	Systolic	Mean	Mean drop [%]	Diastolic		
Supine		76	114	74	96	58		39	16	41
Tilt [min]	1	99	111	77	63	41	29.3	30	16	28
	2	120	117	77						
	3	127	104	74						
	4	118	115	80						
	5	120	111	79	76	52.7	9.1	41	15	29
	6	125	111	78						
	7	129	117	82						
	8	123	115	81						
	9	132	115	83						
	10	122	116	83	63	42.3	27.1	32	15	27
	15									
	20									
	30									
	40									

Sudomotor evaluation - functional

Test: Quantitative sudomotor axon reflex test (QSART)				
Location	Site (l/r)	Latency [min]	Volume [µl]	Norm [µl]*
Forearm				≥0.08
Prox. leg				≥0.14
Distal leg				≥0.15
Foot				≥0.07

* Normative data are adjusted for gender and age of patient.

Test: Electrochemical skin conductance (ESC)				
Location	Left [µS]	Right [µS]	Average [µS/k]	Norm [µS/kg]
Hand				≥1.03
Feet				≥1.14
Forehead				

For grading uses ESC [µS] adjusted for weight [µS/k].

(continued)

TABLE 58.1 **CONTINUED**

Small fiber (sensory + sudomotor) evaluation - morphological					
Test: Skin biopsy					
Location	Site (l/r)	Nerve fibers			
		Epidermal*		Sweat glands	
		Density	Norm	Density	Norm
Proximal leg – thigh	Right	17.79	≥8.3	50.7	≥37.8
Distal leg - calf	Right	2.55	≥8.54		≥36.5
Foot	Right		≥3.11		≥34.8

*Normative data for distal leg are adjusted for gender and age of patient.

QASAT*												
Heart rate		BP		CBFv		ET-CO2		Sudomotor			Total QASAT score
S. bradycardia	0	Low supine	0	Low supine	0	Low supine	0	QSART			
S. tachycardia	0	High supine	0	High supine	0	High supine	0	ESC			
Increase tilt	8	OH	0	Tilt response	4	Tilt low	2				
Decrease tilt	0	OHTN	0	CA	0	Tilt high	0	**Skin biopsy**			19
Deep breathing	0	VM	2	CVR	0			Epidermal	3		
VR	0			VM	0			Sweat gland	0		
Total	8	Total	2	Total	4	Total	2				

*QASAT. See Novak. Quantitative Scale for Grading of Cardiovascular Autonomic Reflex Tests and Small Fibers from Skin Biopsies. *J Neurol Disord* 2015;3:2.

S, supine; Increase tilt, increased response to tilt; Decrease tilt, decreased response to tilt; BP, blood pressure; VM, Valsalva maneuver; CBFv, cerebral blood flow velocity; CA, cerebral autoregulation; MCA, middle cerebral artery; VR, Valsalva ratio; CVR, cerebral vasoreactivity.

Cold feet: Occasionally
Reduced sweating: None
Reduced sweating after exercise: Yes, minor annoyance
Increased sweating: Occasionally
Nausea: Occasionally
Diarrhea: None
Constipation: Occasionally
Urinary leaks: Yes, minor annoyance
Aching pain: Occasionally, mild
Allodynia: Occasionally, mild
Burning pain: Occasionally, moderate
Lancinating pain: None
Numbness: Often, mild
Prickling sensation: None

AUTONOMIC TESTING INTERPRETATION

- Small fiber neuropathy affecting sensory fibers.
- POTS, neuropathic form.

TREATMENT AND FOLLOW-UP

- Clinical workup for neuropathy.

COMMENT

Further evaluation showed elevated striational antibody (titer 1: 240, normal <1:120). Cancer screen was negative. Patient did not benefit from β-blockers, proamatine, or fludrocortisone. She did benefit modestly from physical therapy. Since failure of conservative therapy and because of the presumed autoimmune cause of her neuropathy, a therapy with IVIG at a dose of 2 g/kg/month has been initiated. After 8 months, she noted significant improvement of orthostatic tolerance, up to the point where she was able to walk 50 meters or more.

Striational autoantibodies bind to skeletal and heart muscle.[1,2] They are found in 30% of adult patients with myasthenia gravis and in 80% of those with thymoma. They also may be detected in patients with Lambert-Eaton myasthenic syndrome, small-cell lung carcinoma, breast carcinoma, patients treated with D-penicillamine, and bone marrow transplant recipients having graft-versus-host disease.

The case presented here suggests that striational antibodies can be associated with small fiber neuropathy or POTS and can respond to IVIG.

CAVEATS

- POTS, neuropathic form with positive striational antibodies, may respond to IVIG.

REFERENCES

1. Cikes N, Momoi MY, Williams CL, et al. Striational autoantibodies: quantitative detection by enzyme immunoassay in myasthenia gravis, thymoma, and recipients of D-penicillamine or allogeneic bone marrow. *Mayo Clin Proc* 1988;63:474–481.
2. McKeon A, Lennon VA, LaChance DH, et al. Striational antibodies in a paraneoplastic context. *Muscle and Nerve*. 2013;47: 585–587.

59.

CASE 54: POLYNEUROPATHY AFFECTING LARGE AND SMALL FIBERS IN MULTIPLE AUTOIMMUNE DISORDERS

Chief complaint: Orthostatic intolerance and pain.

Case presentation: A 38-year-old woman has a history of multiple autoimmune disorders. She has history of juvenile rheumatoid arthritis at age 7, systemic lupus erythematosus at age 15, and Sjögren syndrome at age 18. She was also diagnosed with psoriasis, fibromyalgia, and Graves disease with hypothyroidism. Her clinical course is associated with flaring symptoms including severe joint pain, deep muscle pain, distal superficial burning pain, weakness, vision loss, loss of teeth, chronic diarrhea, orthostatic intolerance, excessive sweating, fatigue, and multiple gastrointestinal symptoms. She can ambulate for several minutes, but uses a wheelchair most of the times. She has been treated with prednisone, hydroxychloroquine, pilocarpine, pregabalin, duloxetine, gabapentin, naproxen, celecoxib, and tramadol. She developed allergies to essentially all medications. Neurological examination showed red and dystrophic skin at distal legs with mild distal muscle wasting. Motor examination revealed 4/5 strength in proximal and distal muscles at both legs. There was diffuse areflexia. Vibration sensation was absent at ankles, temperature was reduced at knees and elbows. Nerve conduction study showed a generalized, symmetric sensory neuropathy. She was referred for evaluation of orthostatic intolerance.

Past medical history: Systemic lupus erythematosus, Sjögren syndrome, psoriasis, juvenile rheumatoid arthritis, fibromyalgia, hypothyroidism, vitamin D deficiency, depression.

Current medication: Liothyronine, hydroxyzine, alprazolam, oxycodone, ibuprofen.

Assessment plan: Functional autonomic tests and skin biopsy.

AUTONOMIC TESTING EVALUATION

See Table 59.1.

Heart rate: Supine tachycardia. Heart rate increment during the tilt (23 BPM) was normal.

Blood pressure:

Valsalva maneuver: Mean blood pressure failed to return to baseline at the end of Phase 2 by 25.4 mm Hg (i.e., 73.7% of baseline).

Tilt: Supine blood pressure was normal. Blood pressure responses to tilt were normal.

Sudomotor evaluation: Sweat output was normal at forearm, abnormal (reduced to 65% of lower limit) at proximal leg, normal at distal leg, and normal at foot.

Respiratory system: Respiratory frequency was normal in supine position and during the tilt. End tidal

TABLE 59.1 **RESULTS OF AUTONOMIC TESTING**

Blood pressure evaluation					
Test: Valsalva maneuver					
Pressure [mmHg]	Baseline	Phase 2			Phase 4
		Early	End		
Systolic	132	80	80		
Mean	96.7	71.3	71.3	n/a	
Diastolic	79	67	67	n/a	

Heart rate evaluation	
Test: Deep breathing	
Results	Norm*
10.4	≥12
Test: Valsalva ratio	
1.63	≥1.5
* adjusted for a gender and age	

TABLE 59.1 **CONTINUED**

Test: Tilt test										
Position		HR [BPM]	Blood pressure [mmHg]		MCA Blood flow velocity [cm/s]				Respiratory frequency [breaths/min]	End tidal CO_2 [mmHg]
			Systolic	Diastolic	Systolic	Mean	Mean drop [%]	Diastolic		
Supine		118	130	84	70	38.7		23	12	34
Tilt [min]	1	140	130	82	64	36.7	5.2	23	13	32
	2	140	121	87						
	3	132	113	74						
	4	132	118	77						
	5	133	120	86	57	33	14.7	21	13	34
	6	131	115	83						
	7	129	115	88						
	8	132	120	82						
	9	131	119	76						
	10	141	119	79	62	35.3	8.8	22	9	33
	15									
	20									
	30									
	40									

Sudomotor evaluation - functional

Test: Quantitative sudomotor axon reflex test (QSART)				
Location	Site (l/r)	Latency [min]	Volume [μl]	Norm [μl]*
Forearm	l	1.29	0.09	≥0.08
Prox. leg	l	0.57	0.091	≥0.14
Distal leg	l	0.43	0.257	≥0.15
Foot	l	0.43	0.09	≥0.07

* Normative data are adjusted for gender and age of patient.

Test: Electrochemical skin conductance (ESC)				
Location	Left [μS]	Right [μS]	Average [μS/k]	Norm [μS/kg]
Hand				≥
Feet				≥
Forehead				

For grading uses ESC [μS] adjusted for weight [μS/k].

(continued)

TABLE 59.1 CONTINUED

Small fiber (sensory + sudomotor) evaluation - morphological					
Test: Skin biopsy					
Location	Site (l/r)	Nerve fibers			
		Epidermal*		Sweat glands	
		Density	Norm	Density	Norm
Proximal leg – thigh	Right	11.53	≥8.3		≥37.8
Distal leg - calf	Right	3.63	≥8.06		≥36.5
Foot	Right		≥3.11		≥34.8

*Normative data for distal leg are adjusted for gender and age of patient.

QASAT*											
Heart rate		BP		CBFv		ET-CO2		Sudomotor			Total QASAT score
S. bradycardia	0	Low supine	0	Low supine	1	Low supine	1	QSART	2		
S. tachycardia	1	High supine	0	High supine	0	High supine	0	ESC			
Increase tilt	0	OH	0	Tilt response	1	Tilt low	0				
Decrease tilt	0	OHTN	0	CA	0	Tilt high	0	**Skin biopsy**			12
Deep breathing	1	VM	2	CVR	0			Epidermal	3		
VR	0			VM	0			Sweat gland			
Total	2	Total	2	Total	2	Total	1				

*QASAT. See Novak. Quantitative Scale for Grading of Cardiovascular Autonomic Reflex Tests and Small Fibers from Skin Biopsies. *J Neurol Disord* 2015;3:2.

S, supine; Increase tilt, increased response to tilt; Decrease tilt, decreased response to tilt; BP, blood pressure; VM, Valsalva maneuver; CBFv, cerebral blood flow velocity; CA, cerebral autoregulation; MCA, middle cerebral artery; VR, Valsalva ratio; CVR, cerebral vasoreactivity.

CO_2 was minimally reduced in supine position but was normal during the tilt test.

Cerebral blood flow velocity (CBFv): CBFv in middle cerebral artery was reduced in supine position and was further reduced during the tilt.

Skin biopsy (sensory-epidermal): Epidermal nerve fiber density was normal at proximal leg and abnormal (reduced to 45% of normal limit) at distal leg.

Skin biopsy (sweat glands): No sweat glands found in the specimen.

Patient-reported symptoms during testing: Dizziness during the tilt test.

Patient-reported symptoms for past 2 weeks:

Lightheadedness or dizziness: Occasionally
Dry eyes or mouth: Yes, minor annoyance
Pale feet: Occasionally
Cold feet: Yes, minor annoyance
Reduced sweating: Occasionally
Reduced sweating after exercise: Occasionally
Increased sweating: None
Nausea: Occasionally
Diarrhea: None
Constipation: Occasionally
Urinary leaks: Yes, minor annoyance
Current pain severity: 8
Aching pain: Continuous, severe
Allodynia: Continuous, severe
Burning pain: Continuous, severe
Lancinating pain: Continuous, severe
Numbness: Continuous, severe
Prickling sensation: Continuous, moderate

AUTONOMIC TESTING INTERPRETATION

- Small fiber neuropathy, severe, length-dependent.
- Cerebral autoregulatory failure with reduced CBFv.
- Mild autonomic failure.

COMMENT

This patient has diagnoses of multiple autoimmune disorders including Sjögren syndrome, rheumatoid arthritis,

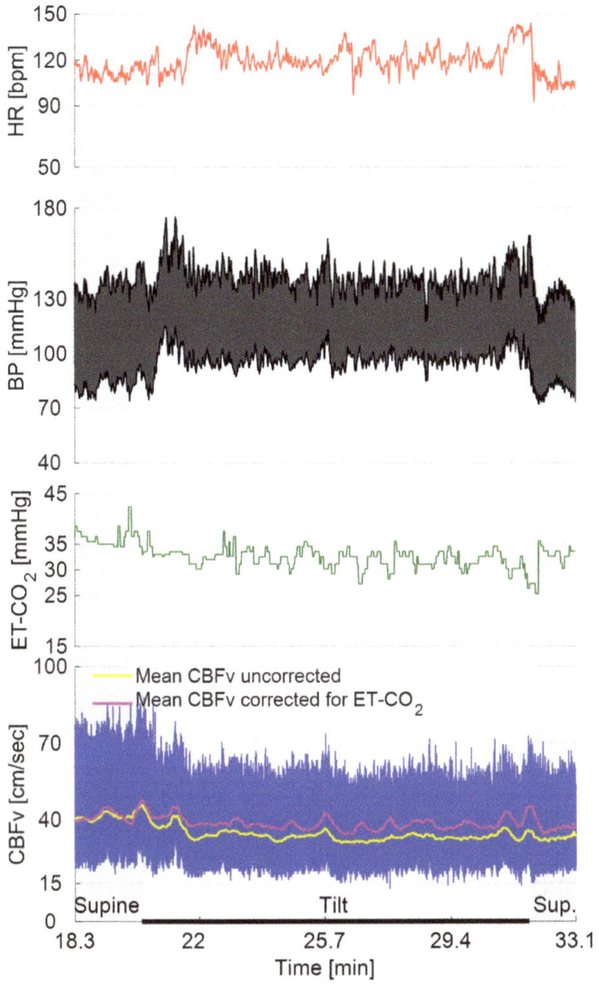

Figure 59.1 The tilt test showed supine tachycardia that was further worsened during the tilt but did not reach criteria for postural tachycardia syndrome (heart rate increment ≥ 30 BPM). Blood pressure was stable. Cerebral blood flow was reduced in supine position and was further reduced during the tilt.

and systemic lupus erythematosus. These disorders, particularly Sjögren syndrome, can be associated with variable dysautonomia[1] and sensory neuropathy.[2] The skin biopsy showed small fiber sensory neuropathy, with the length-dependent pattern. In this patient, small fiber neuropathy is part of a generalized neuropathy affecting both small and large fibers since her nerve conduction study was consistent with large fiber neuropathy.

The main reason for referral was unexplained orthostatic intolerance and chronic fatigue. Autonomic testing showed only mild dysautonomia (Figure 59.1), which is unlikely responsible for orthostatic intolerance. There was resting tachycardia, which can be related to chronic pain and/or volume depletion. Heart rate increment during the tilt was normal. Nevertheless, the main finding on the autonomic testing was low CBFv in both supine position and during the tilt. Low CBFv is likely due to cerebral autoregulatory failure with abnormal cerebral vasoconstriction. Low cardiac output may play a role. Low CBFv may results in cerebral hypoperfusion including orthostatic intolerance.

The testing was also positive for small fiber neuropathy and mild autonomic failure. Patient has a history of several disorders that are associated with neuropathy or dysautonomia including Sjögren syndrome,[1] rheumatoid arthiritis,[3] systemic lupus erythematosus,[4] and psoriasis.[5] Autonomic testing and skin biopsies are sensitive to detect abnormal findings, however in general they cannot differentiate between causes of abnormalities, which is one of the major limitation of the testing.

TREATMENT AND FOLLOW-UP

- Consider immunomodulatory treatment.

CAVEATS

- Orthostatic intolerance can be due to cerebral autoregulatory failure.
- Although autonomic testing and skin biopsies are in general sensitive to detect abnormal findings, they cannot differentiate between causes of abnormalities.

REFERENCES

1. Goodman BP, Crepeau A, Dhawan PS, Khoury JA, Harris LA. Spectrum of autonomic nervous system impairment in Sjögren syndrome. *The Neurologist.* 2017;22(4):127–130. doi:10.1097/NRL.0000000000000134.
2. Pereira PR, Viala K, Maisonobe T, et al. Sjögren sensory neuronopathy (Sjögren Ganglionopathy): long-term outcome and treatment response in a series of 13 cases. *Medicine (Baltimore).* 2016;95(19):e3632. doi:10.1097/MD.0000000000003632.
3. Syngle V, Syngle A, Garg N, Krishan P, Verma I. Predictors of autonomic neuropathy in rheumatoid arthritis. *Auton Neurosci Basic Clin.* 2016;201:54–59. doi:10.1016/j.autneu.2016.07.008.
4. Florica B, Aghdassi E, Su J, Gladman DD, Urowitz MB, Fortin PR. Peripheral neuropathy in patients with systemic lupus erythematosus. *Semin Arthritis Rheum.* 2011;41(2):203–211. doi:10.1016/j.semarthrit.2011.04.001.
5. Halıgür BD, Cicek D, Bulut S, Berilgen MS. The investigation of autonomic functions in patients with psoriasis. *Int J Dermatol.* 2012;51(5):557–563. doi:10.1111/j.1365-4632.2011.05111.x.

60.

CASE 55: SMALL FIBER NEUROPATHY WITH AUTONOMIC FAILURE

Chief complaint: Dizziness.

Case presentation: A 56-year-old woman presents with unexplained orthostatic dizziness, weakness, chronic pain at distal legs, numbness, and fatigue for several years. She passed out several times. She had normal neurological examination. Electromyogram and nerve conductions studies, EEG, and MRI of the brain were all normal. Patient was referred for evaluation of suspected autonomic failure.

Past medical history: Wolff-Parkinson-White syndrome, status post ablation 11 years ago, dyslipidemia.

Current medication: Atorvastatin.

Assessment plan: Functional autonomic tests and skin biopsy.

AUTONOMIC TESTING EVALUATION

See Table 60.1.

Heart rate: Supine heart rate was normal. Heart rate responses to deep breathing were reduced to 71.4% of normal value. Heart rate increment during the tilt (11 BPM) was normal (Figure 60.1).

Blood pressure:

Valsalva maneuver: Mean blood pressure failed to return to baseline at the end of Phase 2 by 30.7 mm Hg (i.e., 68% of baseline).

Tilt: Supine blood pressure was normal. Blood pressure responses to tilt were abnormal and consistent with severe orthostatic hypotension.

Sudomotor evaluation: Sweat output was normal at forearm, normal at proximal leg, normal at distal leg, and normal at foot.

Respiratory system: Respiratory frequency was normal in supine position. Respiratory frequency was normal during the tilt. End tidal CO_2 was normal in supine position. End tidal CO_2 was normal during the tilt.

Cerebral blood flow velocity (CBFv): CBFv in middle cerebral artery was normal in supine position but was moderately reduced during the tilt.

Skin biopsy (sensory-epidermal): Epidermal nerve fiber density was abnormal (reduced to 44.1% of normal limit) at proximal leg and abnormal (reduced to 89.1% of normal limit) at distal leg.

Skin biopsy (sweat glands): Sweat gland nerve fiber density was abnormal (reduced to 43.7% of normal limit) at proximal leg.

Patient-reported symptoms during testing: Weakness during the tilt.

Patient-reported symptoms for past 2 weeks:

Lightheadedness or dizziness: Occasionally
Dry eyes or mouth: Occasionally
Pale feet: None

TABLE 60.1 RESULTS OF AUTONOMIC TESTING

Blood pressure evaluation						Heart rate evaluation	
Test: Valsalva maneuver						Test: Deep breathing	
Pressure [mmHg]	Baseline	Phase 2			Phase 4	Results	Norm*
		Early	End			6.43	≥9
Systolic	140	82	82			Test: Valsalva ratio	
Mean	96	65.3	65.3	n/a		1.24	≥1.47
Diastolic	74	57	57	n/a		* adjusted for a gender and age	

TABLE 60.1 CONTINUED

Test: Tilt test										
Position		HR [BPM]	Blood pressure [mmHg]		MCA Blood flow velocity [cm/s]				Respiratory frequency [breaths/min]	End tidal CO_2 [mmHg]
			Systolic	Diastolic	Systolic	Mean	Mean drop [%]	Diastolic		
Supine		61	128	84	82	54		40	16	42
Tilt [min]	1	72	86	60	80	48.7	9.8	33	11	40
	2	69	88	59						
	3	68	84	57						
	4	67	105	66						
	5	67	89	60	68	42	22.2	29	10	40
	6	69	91	61						
	7	68	96	65						
	8	70	96	65						
	9	66	94	64						
	10	69	108	72	68	44	18.5	32	14	37
	15									
	20									
	30									
	40									

Sudomotor evaluation - functional

Test: Quantitative sudomotor axon reflex test (QSART)				
Location	Site (l/r)	Latency [min]	Volume [μl]	Norm [μl]*
Forearm	l	0.46	1.282	≥0.08
Prox. leg	l	1.35	0.657	≥0.14
Distal leg	l	1.36	0.45	≥0.07
Foot	l	2.07	0.671	≥0.05

* Normative data are adjusted for gender and age of patient.

Test: Electrochemical skin conductance (ESC)				
Location	Left [μS]	Right [μS]	Average [μS/k]	Norm [μS/kg]
Hand				≥
Feet				≥
Forehead				

For grading uses ESC [μS] adjusted for weight [μS/k].

(continued)

TABLE 60.1 CONTINUED

Small fiber (sensory + sudomotor) evaluation - morphological					
Test: Skin biopsy					
Location	Site (l/r)	Nerve fibers			
		Epidermal*		Sweat glands	
		Density	Norm	Density	Norm
Proximal leg – thigh	Right	3.66	≥8.3	16.5	≥37.8
Distal leg - calf	Right	5.9	≥6.62		≥36.5
Foot	Right		≥3.11		≥34.8

*Normative data for distal leg are adjusted for gender and age of patient.

QASAT*										
Heart rate		**BP**		**CBFv**		**ET-CO2**		**Sudomotor**		**Total QASAT score**
S. bradycardia	0	Low supine	0	Low supine	0	Low supine	0	QSART	0	
S. tachycardia	0	High supine	0	High supine	0	High supine	0	ESC		
Increase tilt	0	OH	9	Tilt response	3	Tilt low	0			
Decrease tilt	0	OHTN	0	CA	0	Tilt high	0	**Skin biopsy**		23
Deep breathing	1	VM	2	CVR	0			Epidermal	3	
VR	1			VM	0			Sweat gland	4	
Total	2	Total	11	Total	3	Total	0			

*QASAT. See Novak. Quantitative Scale for Grading of Cardiovascular Autonomic Reflex Tests and Small Fibers from Skin Biopsies. *J Neurol Disord* 2015;3:2.

S, supine; Increase tilt, increased response to tilt; Decrease tilt, decreased response to tilt; BP, blood pressure; VM, Valsalva maneuver; CBFv, cerebral blood flow velocity; CA, cerebral autoregulation; MCA, middle cerebral artery; VR, Valsalva ratio; CVR, cerebral vasoreactivity.

Cold feet: Occasionally
Reduced sweating: Often
Reduced sweating after exercise: Occasionally
Increased sweating: Occasionally
Nausea: Occasionally
Diarrhea: None
Constipation: Occasionally
Urinary leaks: Occasionally
Current pain severity: 5
Aching pain: Often, moderate
Allodynia: None
Burning pain: Often, moderate
Lancinating pain: None
Numbness: Often, moderate
Prickling sensation: Occasionally, moderate

AUTONOMIC TESTING INTERPRETATION

- Small fiber neuropathy, severe, mixed, affecting sensory and autonomic fibers, non–length-dependent.
- Autonomic failure, affecting cardiovagal and sympathetic adrenergic fibers, associated with small fiber neuropathy.
- Neurogenic orthostatic hypotension, symptomatic, due autonomic adrenergic failure.
- Reduced orthostatic CBFv throughout the tilt.

COMMENT

This patient has a typical symptomatic neurogenic orthostatic hypotension due to autonomic sympathetic failure (Figure 60.1). The orthostatic symptoms reflect cerebral hypoperfusion with reduced orthostatic CBFv. Abnormal skin biopsy confirmed that autonomic failure is due to mixed small fiber neuropathy. Non–length-dependent small fiber neuropathy is less common than length-dependent neuropathy, and it can be seen in a variety of conditions including abnormal glucose metabolism, Sjögren syndrome, and paraproteinemia.[1]

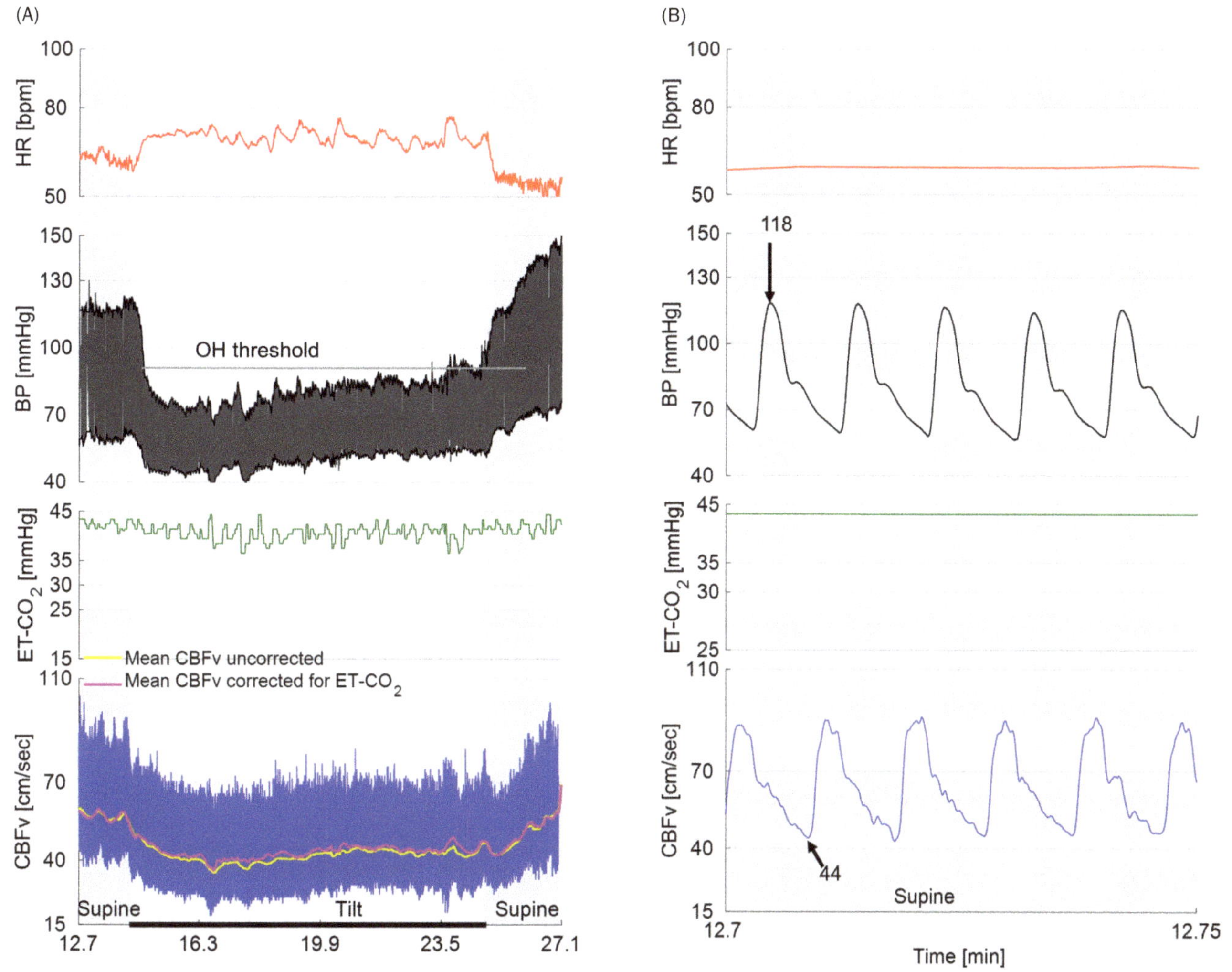

Figure 60.1 Tilt test induced symptomatic orthostatic hypotension (A). The patient complained of dizziness and weakness throughout the tilt, which was accompanied by a decline in blood pressure and cerebral blood flow velocity. The lowest blood pressure (systolic/diastolic 64/39.5 mm Hg) occurred at the first minute of the tilt, then blood pressure slowly recovered, and, at minute 10 of the tilt, orthostatic hypotension was no longer present.
(B) Details of signals during supine and tilt (B, C).

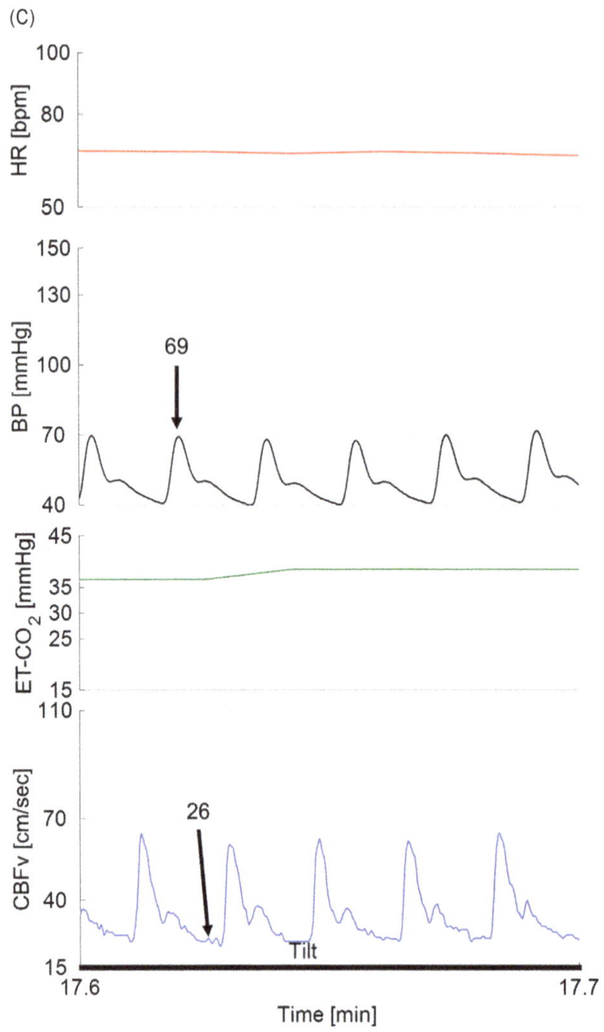

Figure 60.1 Continued

TREATMENT AND FOLLOW-UP

- Workup for non–length-dependent small fiber neuropathy.[1]
- Volume expansion through high fluid intake and high-salt diet.
- The use of compression stockings is recommended.
- Start fludrocortisone 0.1 mg/day orally.

CAVEATS

- Symptomatic neurogenic orthostatic hypotension is due to cerebral hypoperfusion when the decline in orthostatic blood pressure is out of autoregulatory range.[2]
- Reduced heart rate increment during the tilt and orthostatic hypotension are markers of autonomic failure.
- Skin biopsy is useful to localize the lesion. This patient had both abnormal sensory and autonomic fiber density, suggesting that mixed (sensory and autonomic) small fiber neuropathy underlies both sensory symptoms (pain, numbness) and autonomic failure.

REFERENCES

1. Gorson KC, Herrmann DN, Thiagarajan R, et al. Non-length dependent small fibre neuropathy/ganglionopathy. *J Neurol Neurosurg Psychiatry*. 2008;79(2):163–169. doi:10.1136/jnnp.2007.128801.
2. Novak P. Cerebral blood flow, heart rate, and blood pressure patterns during the tilt test in common orthostatic syndromes. *Neurosci J*. 2016;2016:6127340. doi:10.1155/2016/6127340.

61.

CASE 56: AUTOIMMUNE SMALL FIBER NEUROPATHY WITH POSITIVE GANGLIONIC ACETYLCHOLINE RECEPTOR ANTIBODY

Chief complaint: Dizziness.

Case presentation: A 48-year-old woman presents with disabling abdominal pain after each meal, weight loss, fatigue, and postural dizziness for several years. Neurologic examination showed a frail patient (body mass index of 17), but otherwise was unrevealing. She has been seen by multiple specialties without finding a cause. She was referred for evaluation of small fiber neuropathy and autonomic failure.

Past medical history: Migraine, gastritis.

Current medication: Rizatriptan, linaclotide.

Assessment plan: Functional autonomic tests and skin biopsy.

AUTONOMIC TESTING EVALUATION

See Table 61.1.

Heart rate: Supine tachycardia. Heart rate increment during the tilt (17 BPM) was normal (Figure 61.1).

Blood pressure:

Valsalva maneuver: Mean blood pressure failed to return to baseline at the end of Phase 2 by 22.4 mm Hg (i.e., 66.9% of baseline).

Tilt: Supine blood pressure was normal. Blood pressure responses to tilt were normal.

Sudomotor evaluation: Sweat output was abnormal (reduced to 30% of lower limit) at forearm, abnormal (reduced to 57.1% of lower limit) at proximal leg, normal at distal leg, and abnormal (reduced to 44.3% of lower limit) at foot.

Respiratory system: Respiratory frequency was normal in supine position and during the tilt. End tidal CO_2 was reduced in supine position and was further reduced during the tilt.

Cerebral blood flow velocity (CBFv): CBFv in middle cerebral artery was normal in supine position but was reduced during the tilt.

Skin biopsy (sensory-epidermal): Epidermal nerve fiber density was normal at proximal leg and abnormal (reduced to 88% of normal limit) at distal leg.

Skin biopsy (sweat glands): Sweat gland nerve fiber density was normal at proximal leg and normal at distal leg.

Patient-reported symptoms during testing: Dizziness during the tilt.

Patient-reported symptoms for past 2 weeks:

Lightheadedness or dizziness: Often
Dry eyes or mouth: Often
Pale feet: Occasionally
Cold feet: Often

TABLE 61.1 **RESULTS OF AUTONOMIC TESTING**

Blood pressure evaluation					
Test: Valsalva maneuver					
Pressure [mmHg]	Baseline	Phase 2			Phase 4
		Early	End		
Systolic	93	52	52		
Mean	67.7	45.3	45.3	n/a	
Diastolic	55	42	42	n/a	

Heart rate evaluation	
Test: Deep breathing	
Results	Norm*
6.5	≥10
Test: Valsalva ratio	
1.73	≥1.51
* adjusted for a gender and age	

(continued)

TABLE 61.1 **CONTINUED**

Test: Tilt test										
Position		HR [BPM]	Blood pressure [mmHg]		MCA Blood flow velocity [cm/s]				Respiratory frequency [breaths/min]	End tidal CO_2 [mmHg]
			Systolic	Diastolic	Systolic	Mean	Mean drop [%]	Diastolic		
Supine		105	96	64	93	65.7		52	19	23
Tilt [min]	1	115	106	72	82	60	8.7	49	20	31
	2	116	106	71						
	3	115	109	73						
	4	118	99	73						
	5	118	105	71	77	55.7	15.2	45	17	30
	6	119	106	73						
	7	120	107	69						
	8	120	107	73						
	9	121	106	76						
	10	122	113	77	79	57	13.2	46	16	23
	15									
	20									
	30									
	40									

Sudomotor evaluation - functional

Test: Quantitative sudomotor axon reflex test (QSART)				
Location	Site (l/r)	Latency [min]	Volume [µl]	Norm [µl]*
Forearm	l	2.27	0.024	≥0.08
Prox. leg	l	1.54	0.08	≥0.14
Distal leg	l	1.12	0.343	≥0.15
Foot	l	3.49	0.031	≥0.07

* Normative data are adjusted for gender and age of patient.

Test: Electrochemical skin conductance (ESC)				
Location	Left [µS]	Right [µS]	Average [µS/k]	Norm [µS/kg]
Hand				≥1.03
Feet				≥1.14
Forehead				

For grading uses ESC [µS] adjusted for weight [µS/k].

TABLE 61.1 CONTINUED

Small fiber (sensory + sudomotor) evaluation - morphological					
Test: Skin biopsy					
Location	Site (l/r)	Nerve fibers			
		Epidermal*		Sweat glands	
		Density	Norm	Density	Norm
Proximal leg – thigh	Right	12.34	≥8.3	54.2	≥37.8
Distal leg - calf	Right	6.39	≥7.26	43.6	≥36.5
Foot	Right		≥3.11		≥34.8

*Normative data for distal leg are adjusted for gender and age of patient.

QASAT*										
Heart rate		**BP**		**CBFv**		**ET-CO2**		**Sudomotor**		**Total QASAT score**
S. bradycardia	0	Low supine	0	Low supine	0	Low supine	1	QSART	2	
S. tachycardia	1	High supine	0	High supine	0	High supine	0	ESC		
Increase tilt	0	OH	0	Tilt response	1	Tilt low	4			
Decrease tilt	0	OHTN	0	CA	0	Tilt high	0	**Skin biopsy**		13
Deep breathing	1	VM	2	CVR	0			Epidermal	1	
VR	0			VM	0			Sweat gland	0	
Total	2	Total	2	Total	1	Total	5			

*QASAT. See Novak. Quantitative Scale for Grading of Cardiovascular Autonomic Reflex Tests and Small Fibers from Skin Biopsies. *J Neurol Disord* 2015;3:2.

S, supine; Increase tilt, increased response to tilt; Decrease tilt, decreased response to tilt; BP, blood pressure; VM, Valsalva maneuver; CBFv, cerebral blood flow velocity; CA, cerebral autoregulation; MCA, middle cerebral artery; VR, Valsalva ratio; CVR, cerebral vasoreactivity.

Reduced sweating: None
Reduced sweating after exercise: None
Increased sweating: None
Nausea: Often
Diarrhea: Occasionally
Constipation: Often
Urinary leaks: Occasionally
Current pain severity: 4
Aching pain: Often, moderate
Allodynia: None
Burning pain: Occasionally, moderate
Lancinating pain: Often, severe
Numbness: Occasionally, moderate
Prickling sensation: Often, moderate

AUTONOMIC TESTING INTERPRETATION

- Small fiber neuropathy, mixed, length-dependent.
- Autonomic failure due to small fiber neuropathy.
- Syncope induced by the Valsalva maneuver.
- Volume depletion.

COMMENT

The testing showed mixed small fiber neuropathy affecting sensory (detected by skin biopsy) and cholinergic autonomic (detected by QSART) fibers. There was also evidence of autonomic failure (Figure 61.1). Patient's gastrointestinal symptoms are likely due to enteric cholinergic neuropathy that is part of small fiber neuropathy. Clinical workup for neuropathy revealed elevated ganglionic acetylcholine receptor (AChR) antibody (0.14 nmol/L, normal ≤0.02 nmol/L). She was started on intravenous immune globulin (IVIG), at a dose of 2 g/kg/month. The gastrointestinal problems improved after about 8 months

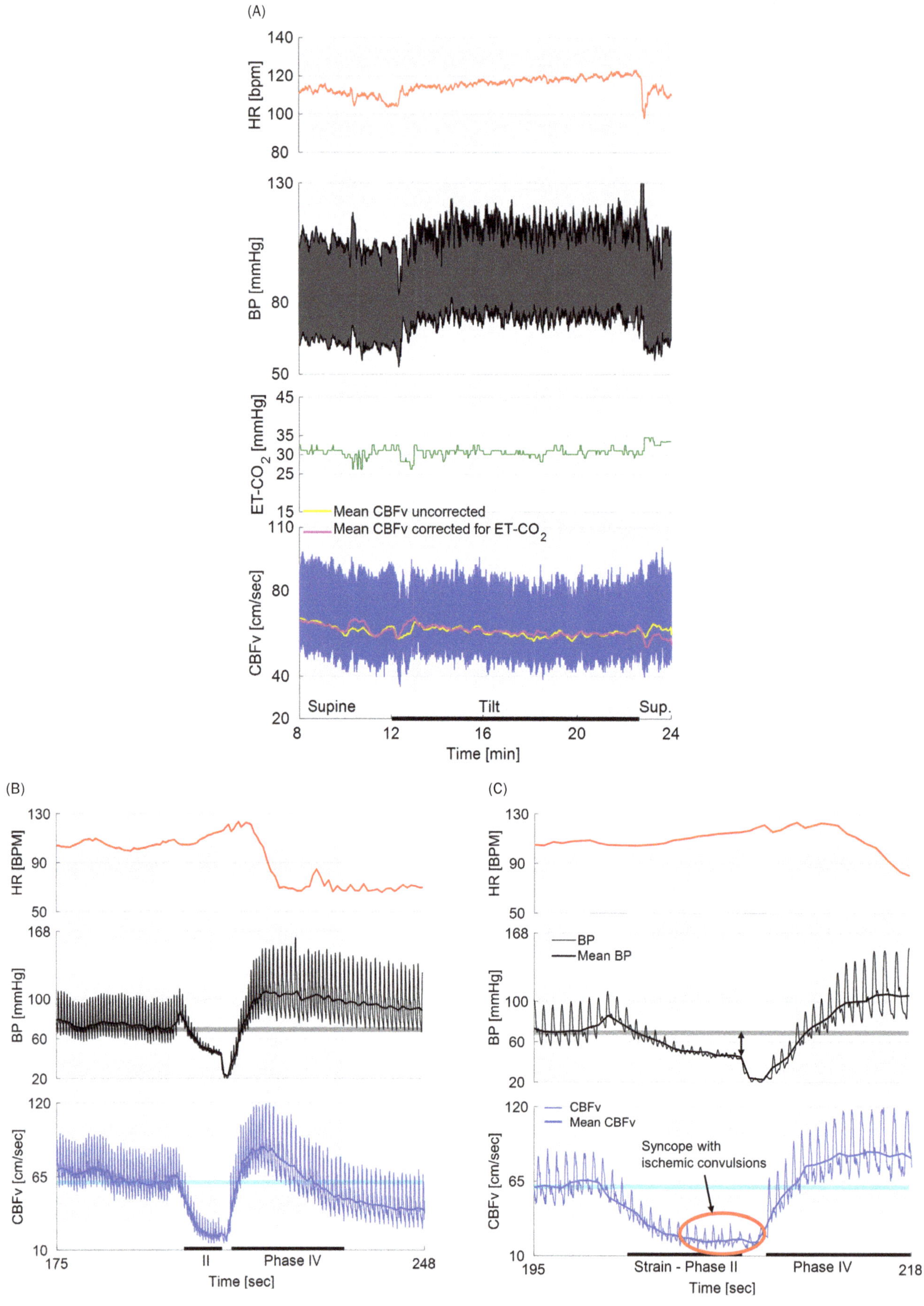

Figure 61.1 The tilt test showed supine tachycardia with preserved orthostatic heart rate acceleration (A). Blood pressure and cerebral blood flow velocity responses to tilt were normal. The Valsalva maneuver showed abnormality in both blood pressure and cerebral blood flow velocity (CBFv, B, C). There was a pulse pressure collapse (difference between systolic and diastolic blood pressure) during the phase II and absent recovery in blood pressure at the end of phase II. CBFv was markedly reduced during the phase II. The diastolic CBFv was close to 10 cm/s and the CBFv railed to return to baseline at the end of phase II. Patient passed out during the Valsalva maneuver when the diastolic CBFv was at its lowest level (B,C).

of IVIG therapy, and she was able to gain weight. Repeat titer of ganglionic AChR antibody obtained 1 year after onset of the immunomodudulatory therapy was within normal range.

The ganglionic AChR modulates synaptic activity in sympathetic, parasympathetic and enteric autonomic ganglia.[1] AChR antibody may impair synaptic transmission in autonomic ganglia. AChR antibodies are positive in 50% of subjects with subacute autonomic autoimmune ganglionopathy,[1–3] and immunotherapy with IVIG may be effective.[4]

TREATMENT AND FOLLOW-UP

- Continue therapy with IVIG.

CAVEATS

- Small fiber neuropathy with elevated ganglionic AChR antibody may respond to immunotherapy with IVIG.

REFERENCES

1. Vernino S. Antibody testing as a diagnostic tool in autonomic disorders. *Clin Auton Res Off J Clin Auton Res Soc*. 2009;19(1):13–19. doi:10.1007/s10286-008-0488-6.
2. Li Y, Jammoul A, Mente K, et al. Clinical experience of seropositive ganglionic acetylcholine receptor antibody in a tertiary neurology referral center. *Muscle Nerve*. 2015;52(3):386–391. doi:10.1002/mus.24559.
3. Koike H, Sobue G. [Autoimmune autonomic ganglionopathy and acute autonomic and sensory neuropathy]. *Rinsho Shinkeigaku*. 2013;53(11):1326–1329.
4. Iodice V, Kimpinski K, Vernino S, Sandroni P, Fealey RD, Low PA. Efficacy of immunotherapy in seropositive and seronegative putative autoimmune autonomic ganglionopathy. *Neurology*. 2009;72(23):2002–2008. doi:10.1212/WNL.0b013e3181a92b52.

62.

CASE 57: SMALL FIBER NEUROPATHY AND HYPOCAPNIC CEREBRAL HYPOPERFUSION WITH ELEVATED ANTIBODIES TO N-TYPE CALCIUM CHANNEL

Chief complaint: Dizziness.

Case presentation: A 38-year-old woman experienced headaches associated with facial numbness 3 years ago. At that time, she tested positive for Lyme disease. She completed therapy with doxycycline, minocycline, trimethoprim, and sulfamethoxazole. She improved temporarily but for the past few months she has experienced fluctuating numbness of the whole body and intermittent weakness of her legs. Feet and hands are cold and painful. She is very sensitive to light. The most disabling problem is chronic fatigue. She was referred for evaluation of autonomic failure and small fiber neuropathy.

Past medical history: Lyme disease, dyslipidemia.

Current medication: None.

Assessment plan: Functional autonomic tests and skin biopsy.

AUTONOMIC TESTING EVALUATION

See Table 62.1.

Heart rate: Supine heart rate was normal. Heart rate responses to deep breathing were reduced to 79.2% of normal value. Heart rate increment during the tilt (19 BPM) was normal.

Blood pressure:

Valsalva maneuver: Blood pressure responses were normal.

Tilt: Supine blood pressure was normal. Blood pressure responses to tilt were normal.

Sudomotor evaluation: Electrochemical skin conductance was abnormal (reduced to 64.9% of normal limit) at hands and abnormal (reduced to 99.9% of normal limit) at feet.

Respiratory system: Respiratory frequency was normal in supine position and during the tilt. End tidal CO_2 was normal in supine position but was moderately reduced during the tilt.

Cerebral blood flow velocity (CBFv): CBFv in middle cerebral artery was normal in supine position but was reduced during the tilt.

Skin biopsy (sensory-epidermal): Epidermal nerve fiber density was abnormal (reduced to 67.3% of normal limit) at proximal leg and abnormal (reduced to 5.8% of normal limit) at distal leg.

Skin biopsy (sweat glands): Sweat gland nerve fiber density was abnormal (reduced to 40.7% of normal limit) at proximal leg and abnormal (reduced to 28.2% of normal limit) at distal leg.

Patient-reported symptoms during testing: Dizziness during the tilt.

TABLE 62.1 RESULTS OF AUTONOMIC TESTING

Blood pressure evaluation

Test: Valsalva maneuver

Pressure [mmHg]	Baseline	Phase 2			Phase 4
		Early	End		
Systolic	101	86	95		
Mean	73	68.7	80.3	n/a	
Diastolic	59	60	73	n/a	

Heart rate evaluation

Test: Deep breathing	
Results	Norm*
9.5	≥12
Test: Valsalva ratio	
1.45	≥1.5

* adjusted for a gender and age

TABLE 62.1 **CONTINUED**

Test: Tilt test										
Position		HR [BPM]	Blood pressure [mmHg]		MCA Blood flow velocity [cm/s]				Respiratory frequency [breaths/min]	End tidal CO_2 [mmHg]
			Systolic	Diastolic	Systolic	Mean	Mean drop [%]	Diastolic		
Supine		71	96	64	107	68.3		49	10	36
Tilt [min]	1	71	88	62	83	54.3	20.5	40	15	30
	2	75	95	60						
	3	90	101	65						
	4	80	101	65						
	5	73	121	67	87	55	19.5	39	11	32
	6	81	91	63						
	7	79	90	61						
	8	82	91	63						
	9	85	90	62						
	10	84	91	62	86	54	20.9	38	9	24
	15									
	20									
	30									
	40									

Sudomotor evaluation - functional

Test: Quantitative sudomotor axon reflex test (QSART)				
Location	Site (l/r)	Latency [min]	Volume [μl]	Norm [μl]*
Forearm				≥0.08
Prox. leg				≥0.14
Distal leg				≥0.15
Foot				≥0.07

* Normative data are adjusted for gender and age of patient.

Test: Electrochemical skin conductance (ESC)				
Location	Left [μS]	Right [μS]	Average [μS/k]	Norm [μS/kg]
Hand	32	43	0.67	≥1.03
Feet	64	63	1.14	≥1.14
Forehead				

For grading uses ESC [μS] adjusted for weight [μS/k].

(continued)

TABLE 62.1 CONTINUED

Small fiber (sensory + sudomotor) evaluation - morphological					
Test: Skin biopsy					
Location	Site (l/r)	Nerve fibers			
		Epidermal*		Sweat glands	
		Density	Norm	Density	Norm
Proximal leg – thigh	Right	5.59	≥8.3	15.4	≥37.8
Distal leg - calf	Right	0.47	≥8.06	10.3	≥36.5
Foot	Right		≥3.11		≥34.8

*Normative data for distal leg are adjusted for gender and age of patient.

QASAT*											
Heart rate		BP		CBFv		ET-CO2		Sudomotor		Total QASAT score
S. bradycardia	0	Low supine	0	Low supine	0	Low supine	0	QSART		
S. tachycardia	0	High supine	0	High supine	0	High supine	0	ESC	2	
Increase tilt	0	OH	0	Tilt response	4	Tilt low	3			
Decrease tilt	0	OHTN	0	CA	0	Tilt high	0	**Skin biopsy**		19
Deep breathing	1	VM	0	CVR	0			Epidermal	4	
VR	1			VM	0			Sweat gland	4	
Total	2	Total	0	Total	4	Total	3			

*QASAT. See Novak. Quantitative Scale for Grading of Cardiovascular Autonomic Reflex Tests and Small Fibers from Skin Biopsies. *J Neurol Disord* 2015;3:2.

S, supine; Increase tilt, increased response to tilt; Decrease tilt, decreased response to tilt; BP, blood pressure; VM, Valsalva maneuver; CBFv, cerebral blood flow velocity; CA, cerebral autoregulation; MCA, middle cerebral artery; VR, Valsalva ratio; CVR, cerebral vasoreactivity.

Patient-reported symptoms for past 2 weeks:

Lightheadedness or dizziness: Occasionally
Dry eyes or mouth: Occasionally
Pale feet: Yes, minor annoyance
Cold feet: Occasionally
Reduced sweating: Occasionally
Reduced sweating after exercise: Occasionally
Increased sweating: Occasionally
Nausea: Occasionally
Diarrhea: Yes, minor annoyance
Constipation: Yes, minor annoyance
Urinary leaks: Yes, minor annoyance
Current pain severity: 7
Aching pain: often, moderate
Allodynia: Occasionally, moderate
Burning pain: None
Lancinating pain: Occasionally, moderate
Numbness: Often, moderate
Prickling sensation: Often, moderate

AUTONOMIC TESTING INTERPRETATION

- Small fiber neuropathy, mixed, severe, length-dependent.
- Hypocapnic cerebral hypoperfusion (HYCH).
- Mild autonomic dysfunction.

COMMENT

The testing showed severe small fiber neuropathy and HYCH (Figure 62.1). Both findings are relevant to patient symptoms. Small fiber neuropathy can be responsible for pain and numbness. HYCH may be associated with cognitive deficit. The dysautonomia was mild and of questionable clinical significance.

Further evaluation showed elevated calcium binding antibody, N type (titer 0.05, normal ≤0.03 nmol/L). Cancer screening was negative.

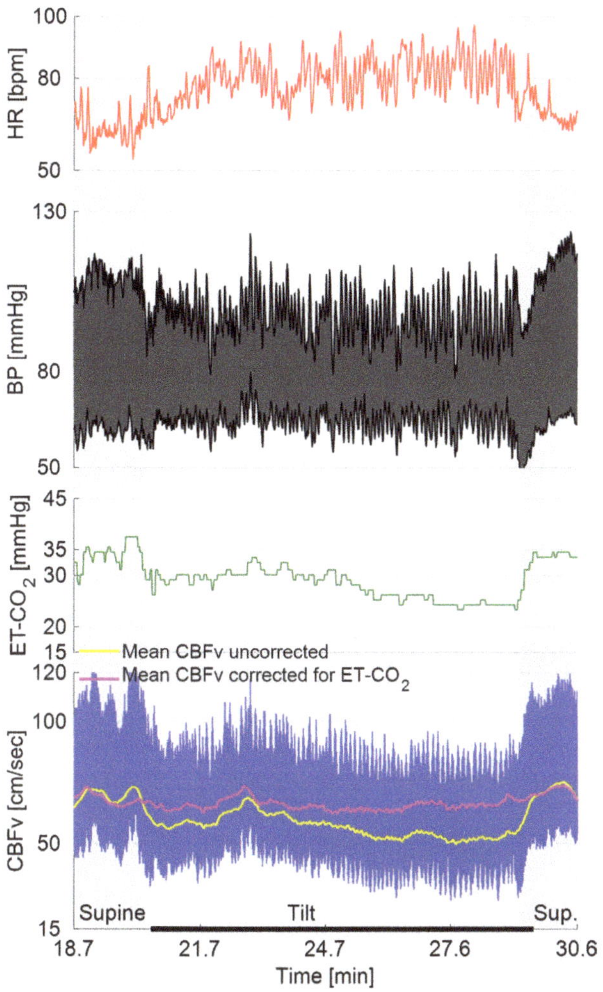

Figure 62.1 The tilt showed normal heart rate and blood pressure responses. The end tidal CO_2 and cerebral blood flow velocity were reduced during the tilt.

Antibodies against the N-type calcium channel are detectable in about 30% of patients with Lambert Eaton myasthenic syndrome. These antibodies are occasionally found in autoimmune gastrointestinal dysmotility, which is a form autoimmune dysautonomia.[1] Patients with dysmotility problems may respond to immunotherapy.

TREATMENT AND FOLLOW-UP

- Trial with immunotherapy.

CAVEATS

- Small fiber neuropathy is associated with antibodies against the N-type calcium channel.

REFERENCE

1. Dhamija R, Tan KM, Pittock SJ, Foxx-Orenstein A, Benarroch E, Lennon VA. Serological profiles aiding the diagnosis of autoimmune gastrointestinal dysmotility. *Clin Gastroenterol Hepatol Off Clin Pract J Am Gastroenterol Assoc.* 2008;6(9):988–992. doi:10.1016/j.cgh.2008.04.009.

63.

CASE 58: SMALL FIBER NEUROPATHY AND ORTHOSTATIC CEREBRAL HYPOPERFUSION SYNDROME WITH POSITIVE AUTOANTIBODIES TO N-TYPE CALCIUM CHANNEL

Chief complaint: Chronic pain and dizziness.

Case presentation: A 58-year-old woman presents with fatigue, joint pain, shortness of breath, memory problems, brain fog, and orthostatic dizziness probably of subacute onset 16 years ago. For the past few months, she complains of severe shooting nerve pain at her distal arms and legs.

Past medical history: Obesity (body mass index of 48), hypertension, dyslipidemia, osteoarthritis, chronic pain, depression, fibromyalgia, Lyme disease.

Current medication: Gabapentin, diphenhydramine, baclofen, losartan (on hold), hydrochlorothiazide (on hold), atenolol (on hold).

Assessment plan: Functional autonomic tests and skin biopsy.

AUTONOMIC TESTING EVALUATION

See Table 63.1.

Heart rate: Supine heart rate was normal. Heart rate responses to deep breathing were normal. Heart rate increment during the tilt (14 BPM) was normal.

Blood pressure:

Valsalva maneuver: Blood pressure responses were normal.

Tilt: Supine blood pressure was elevated. Blood pressure responses to tilt were normal.

Sudomotor evaluation: Electrochemical skin conductance was abnormal (reduced to 45.4% of normal limit) at hands and abnormal (reduced to 53.2% of normal limit) at feet.

Respiratory system: Respiratory frequency and end tidal CO_2 were normal in supine position and during the tilt.

Cerebral blood flow velocity (CBFv): CBFv in middle cerebral artery was normal in supine position but was severely reduced during the tilt.

Skin biopsy (sensory-epidermal): Epidermal nerve fiber density was abnormal (reduced to 32.8% of normal limit) at proximal leg and abnormal (reduced to 76.3% of normal limit) at distal leg.

Skin biopsy (sweat glands): Sweat gland nerve fiber density was normal at distal leg.

Patient-reported symptoms during testing: Dizziness, chest pain, and shortness of breath during the tilt.

Patient-reported symptoms for past 2 weeks:

Lightheadedness or dizziness: Occasionally
Dry eyes or mouth: Occasionally
Pale feet: None
Cold feet: Occasionally
Reduced sweating: None
Reduced sweating after exercise: None
Increased sweating: None

TABLE 63.1 **RESULTS OF AUTONOMIC TESTING**

Blood pressure evaluation					
Test: Valsalva maneuver					
Pressure [mmHg]	Baseline	Phase 2			Phase 4
		Early	End		
Systolic	143	112	140		
Mean	95.7	84	108.7	n/a	
Diastolic	72	70	93	n/a	

Heart rate evaluation	
Test: Deep breathing	
Results	Norm*
9.2	≥9
Test: Valsalva ratio	
1.18	≥1.47

* adjusted for a gender and age

TABLE 63.1 CONTINUED

Test: Tilt test										
Position		HR [BPM]	Blood pressure [mmHg]		MCA Blood flow velocity [cm/s]				Respiratory frequency [breaths/min]	End tidal CO_2 [mmHg]
			Systolic	Diastolic	Systolic	Mean	Mean drop [%]	Diastolic		
Supine		65	159	100	94	53.3		33	15	36
Tilt [min]	1	71	137	86	74	44	17.4	29	12	35
	2	79	142	104						
	3	78	141	88						
	4	73	148	97						
	5	76	149	89	69	39.7	25.5	25	17	36
	6	76	143	89						
	7	79	146	86						
	8	79	146	86						
	9	78	146	86						
	10	78	146	89	69	39.7	25.5	25	15	38
	15									
	20									
	30									
	40									

Sudomotor evaluation - functional

Test: Quantitative sudomotor axon reflex test (QSART)				
Location	Site (l/r)	Latency [min]	Volume [µl]	Norm [µl]*
Forearm				≥0.08
Prox. leg				≥0.14
Distal leg				≥0.07
Foot				≥0.05

* Normative data are adjusted for gender and age of patient.

Test: Electrochemical skin conductance (ESC)				
Location	Left [µS]	Right [µS]	Average [µS/k]	Norm [µS/kg]
Hand	65	69	0.47	≥1.03
Feet	87	88	0.61	≥1.14
Forehead				

For grading uses ESC [µS] adjusted for weight [µS/k].

(continued)

TABLE 63.1 **CONTINUED**

Small fiber (sensory + sudomotor) evaluation - morphological

Test: Skin biopsy

Location	Site (l/r)	Nerve fibers			
		Epidermal*		Sweat glands	
		Density	Norm	Density	Norm
Proximal leg – thigh	Right	2.72	≥8.3		≥37.8
Distal leg - calf	Right	4.93	≥6.46	36.5	≥36.5
Foot	Right		≥3.11		≥34.8

*Normative data for distal leg are adjusted for gender and age of patient.

QASAT*

Heart rate		**BP**		**CBFv**		**ET-CO2**		**Sudomotor**			**Total QASAT score**
S. bradycardia	0	Low supine	0	Low supine	0	Low supine	0	QSART			
S. tachycardia	0	High supine	2	High supine	0	High supine	0	ESC	3		
Increase tilt	0	OH	0	Tilt response	5	Tilt low	0				
Decrease tilt	0	OHTN	0	CA	0	Tilt high	0	**Skin biopsy**			14
Deep breathing	0	VM	0	CVR	0			Epidermal	3		
VR	1			VM	0			Sweat gland	0		
Total	1	Total	2	Total	5	Total	0				

*QASAT. See Novak. Quantitative Scale for Grading of Cardiovascular Autonomic Reflex Tests and Small Fibers from Skin Biopsies. *J Neurol Disord* 2015;3:2.

S, supine; Increase tilt, increased response to tilt; Decrease tilt, decreased response to tilt; BP, blood pressure; VM, Valsalva maneuver; CBFv, cerebral blood flow velocity; CA, cerebral autoregulation; MCA, middle cerebral artery; VR, Valsalva ratio; CVR, cerebral vasoreactivity.

Nausea: None
Diarrhea: None
Constipation: None
Urinary leaks: Occasionally
Current pain severity: 7
Aching pain: Often, moderate
Allodynia: Occasionally, mild
Burning pain: Occasionally, severe
Lancinating pain: Occasionally, severe
Numbness: Occasionally, moderate
Prickling sensation: Occasionally, moderate

AUTONOMIC TESTING INTERPRETATION

- Small fiber neuropathy, mixed, length-dependent.
- Orthostatic cerebral hypoperfusion syndrome (OCHOS).
- No evidence of autonomic failure.

COMMENT

The testing showed small fiber neuropathy and OCHOS (Figure 63.1).[1] Further evaluation showed elevated antibodies against the N-type calcium channel (titer 0.15, normal ≤0.03 nmL/L). Cancer screening was negative.

Antibodies against the N-type calcium channel can be occasionally found in autoimmune dysautonomia.[2] Patients with dysmotility problems may respond to immunotherapy.

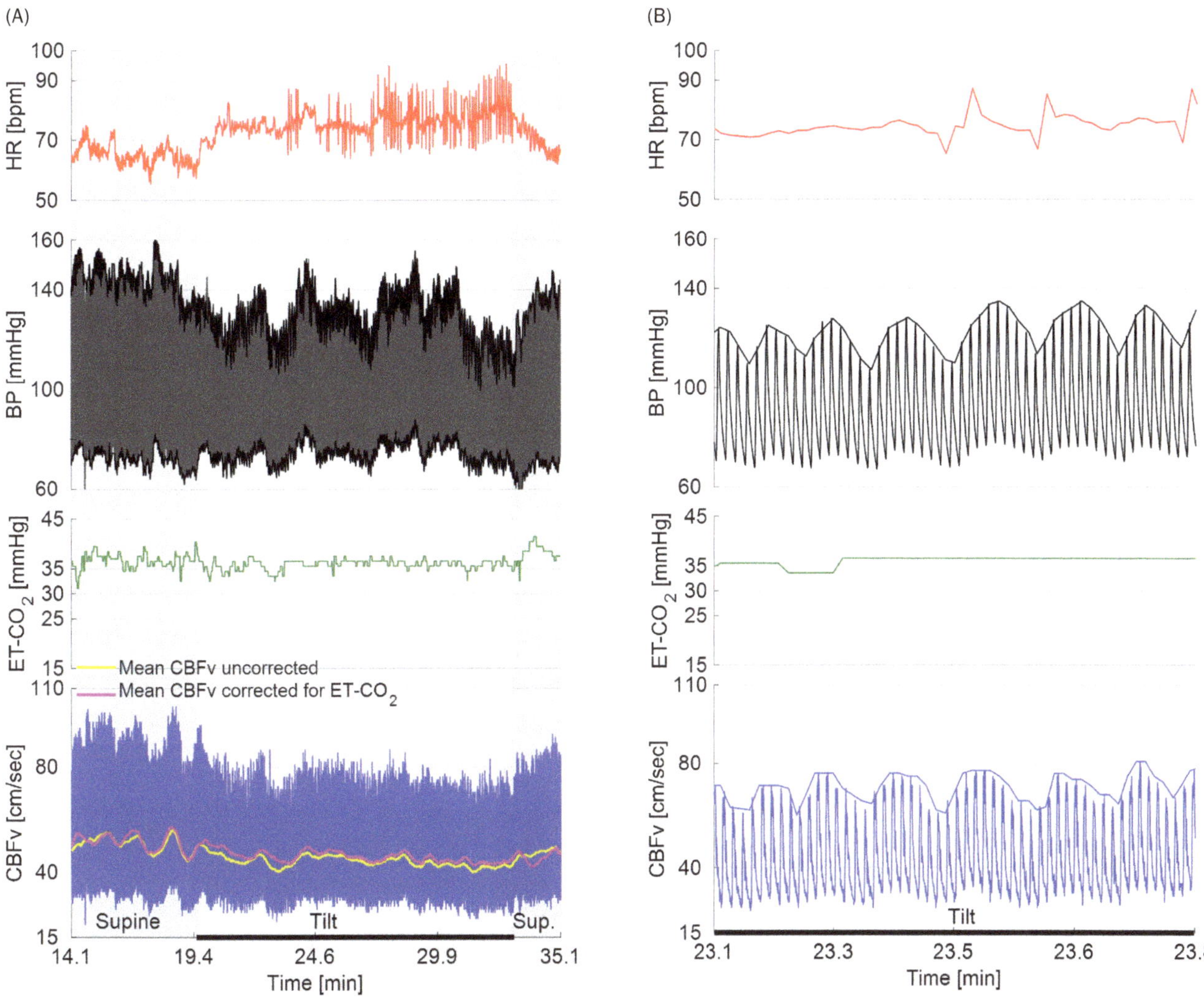

Figure 63.1 Heart rate, blood pressure, and end tidal CO_2 responses to tilt were normal (A). Cerebral blood flow velocity (CBFv) was reduced during the tilt. CBFv and blood pressure started to oscillate during the tilt (B), which usually indicates sympathetic excitation and is probably a compensatory response to reduced cerebral perfusion.

TREATMENT AND FOLLOW-UP

- Trial with immunotherapy.

CAVEATS

- Small fiber neuropathy and OCHOS are associated with antibodies against the N-type calcium channel.

REFERENCES

1. Novak P. Orthostatic cerebral hypoperfusion syndrome. *Front Aging Neurosci*. 2016;8:22. doi:10.3389/fnagi.2016.00022.
2. Dhamija R, Tan KM, Pittock SJ, Foxx-Orenstein A, Benarroch E, Lennon VA. Serological profiles aiding the diagnosis of autoimmune gastrointestinal dysmotility. *Clin Gastroenterol Hepatol Off Clin Pract J Am Gastroenterol Assoc*. 2008;6(9):988–992. doi:10.1016/j.cgh.2008.04.009.

64.

CASE 59: SMALL FIBER NEUROPATHY AND AUTONOMIC FAILURE WITH ELEVATED VOLTAGE-GATED POTASSIUM CHANNEL ANTIBODIES

Chief complaint: Dizziness.

Case presentation: A 48-year-old woman was in good health until 2 years ago, when she suddenly experienced postural palpitations, shortness of breath, and chest pains. Within the next 2 weeks, she noted nausea, fluctuating numbness affecting different parts of her body, insomnia, severe daily and night sweats, blurred vision, muscle twitches, postural dizziness, diffuse pain, and loss of appetite. At one point, she was disabled, could barely walk, and became very anxious. Extensive evaluations including multiple emergency visits and admissions with consults by cardiology, rheumatology, and neurology were unrevealing. She tested initially negative for Lyme disease, then positive for infections with *Bartonella, Ehrlichia,* and *Babesia* as well as for Lyme disease. She was treated with multiple antibiotics by infectious disease specialists for suspected Lyme disease and other tick-borne infections. She improved only marginally on antibiotics; therefore, she was referred for evaluation of autonomic functions and small fiber neuropathy.

Past medical history: Lyme disease, tested also positive for *Bartonella, Ehrlichia,* and *Babesia.*

Current medication: Gabapentin, citalopram.

Assessment plan: Functional autonomic tests and skin biopsy.

AUTONOMIC TESTING EVALUATION

See Table 64.1.

Heart rate: Supine heart rate was normal. Heart rate responses to deep breathing were normal. Heart rate increment during the tilt (14 BPM) was normal.

Blood pressure:

Valsalva maneuver: Mean blood pressure failed to return to baseline at the end of Phase 2 by 11.7 mm Hg (i.e., 83.5% of baseline).

Tilt: Supine blood pressure was normal. Blood pressure responses to tilt were abnormal and consistent with severe orthostatic hypotension.

Sudomotor evaluation: Sweat output was normal at forearm, normal at proximal leg, normal at distal leg, and normal at foot.

Respiratory system: Respiratory frequency and end tidal CO_2 were normal in supine position and during the tilt.

Cerebral blood flow velocity (CBFv): CBFv in middle cerebral artery was normal in supine position but was mildly reduced during the tilt.

Skin biopsy (sensory-epidermal): Epidermal nerve fiber density was normal at proximal leg and abnormal (reduced to 76.9% of normal limit) at distal leg.

TABLE 64.1 **RESULTS OF AUTONOMIC TESTING**

Blood pressure evaluation					
Test: Valsalva maneuver					
Pressure [mmHg]	Baseline	Phase 2			Phase 4
		Early	End		
Systolic	97	68	76		
Mean	71	55.3	59.3	n/a	
Diastolic	58	49	51	n/a	

Heart rate evaluation	
Test: Deep breathing	
Results	Norm*
10.4	≥10
Test: Valsalva ratio	
1.37	≥1.51
* adjusted for a gender and age	

TABLE 64.1 **CONTINUED**

Test: Tilt test										
Position		HR [BPM]	Blood pressure [mmHg]		MCA Blood flow velocity [cm/s]				Respiratory frequency [breaths/min]	End tidal CO_2 [mmHg]
			Systolic	Diastolic	Systolic	Mean	Mean drop [%]	Diastolic		
Supine		80	122	80	91	61		46	18	40
Tilt [min]	1	91	104	72	80	54.7	10.3	42	15	40
	2	88	105	74						
	3	87	103	71						
	4	90	101	70						
	5	92	94	69	79	53.7	12	41	11	40
	6	92	93	67						
	7	91	99	68						
	8	94	95	67						
	9	94	91	67						
	10	90	90	65	79	53	13.1	40	16	40
	15									
	20									
	30									
	40									

Sudomotor evaluation - functional

Test: Quantitative sudomotor axon reflex test (QSART)				
Location	Site (l/r)	Latency [min]	Volume [µl]	Norm [µl]*
Forearm	l	1.47	0.391	≥0.08
Prox. leg	l	0.38	0.413	≥0.14
Distal leg	l	1.5	0.471	≥0.15
Foot	l	1.55	0.318	≥0.07

* Normative data are adjusted for gender and age of patient.

Test: Electrochemical skin conductance (ESC)				
Location	Left [µS]	Right [µS]	Average [µS/k]	Norm [µS/kg]
Hand				≥1.03
Feet				≥1.14
Forehead				

For grading uses ESC [µS] adjusted for weight [µS/k].

(continued)

TABLE 64.1 CONTINUED

Small fiber (sensory + sudomotor) evaluation - morphological					
Test: Skin biopsy					
Location	Site (l/r)	Nerve fibers			
		Epidermal*		Sweat glands	
		Density	Norm	Density	Norm
Proximal leg – thigh	Right	11.05	≥8.3		≥37.8
Distal leg - calf	Right	5.58	≥7.26	36.8	≥36.5
Foot	Right		≥3.11		≥34.8

*Normative data for distal leg are adjusted for gender and age of patient.

QASAT*										
Heart rate		BP		CBFv		ET-CO2		Sudomotor		Total QASAT score
S. bradycardia	0	Low supine	0	Low supine	0	Low supine	0	QSART	0	
S. tachycardia	0	High supine	0	High supine	0	High supine	0	ESC		12
Increase tilt	0	OH	6	Tilt response	2	Tilt low	0			
Decrease tilt	0	OHTN	0	CA	0	Tilt high	0	**Skin biopsy**		
Deep breathing	0	VM	2	CVR	0			Epidermal	1	
VR	1			VM	0			Sweat gland	0	
Total	1	Total	8	Total	2	Total	0			

*QASAT. See Novak. Quantitative Scale for Grading of Cardiovascular Autonomic Reflex Tests and Small Fibers from Skin Biopsies. *J Neurol Disord* 2015;3:2.

S, supine; Increase tilt, increased response to tilt; Decrease tilt, decreased response to tilt; BP, blood pressure; VM, Valsalva maneuver; CBFv, cerebral blood flow velocity; CA, cerebral autoregulation; MCA, middle cerebral artery; VR, Valsalva ratio; CVR, cerebral vasoreactivity.

Skin biopsy (sweat glands): Sweat gland nerve fiber density was normal at distal leg.

Patient-reported symptoms during testing: Dizziness during the tilt.

Patient-reported symptoms for past 2 weeks:

Lightheadedness or dizziness: Occasionally
Dry eyes or mouth: Occasionally
Pale feet: Occasionally
Cold feet: Occasionally
Reduced sweating: Yes, minor annoyance
Reduced sweating after exercise: Yes, minor annoyance
Increased sweating: Occasionally
Nausea: Occasionally
Diarrhea: Yes, minor annoyance
Constipation: Yes, minor annoyance
Urinary leaks: Occasionally
Current pain severity: 4
Aching pain: Occasionally, mild
Allodynia: Continuous, moderate
Burning pain: Often, moderate
Lancinating pain: Occasionally, mild
Numbness: Often, moderate
Prickling sensation: Often, moderate

AUTONOMIC TESTING INTERPRETATION

- Abnormal study. The results are consistent with small fiber neuropathy, length-dependent, affecting predominantly sensory fibers.
- Adrenergic autonomic failure associated with orthostatic hypotension.

TREATMENT AND FOLLOW-UP

- Immunotherapy with the intravenous immunoglobulins.

COMMENT

The testing showed small fiber neuropathy and severe autonomic failure (Figure 64.1). Clinical course is consistent

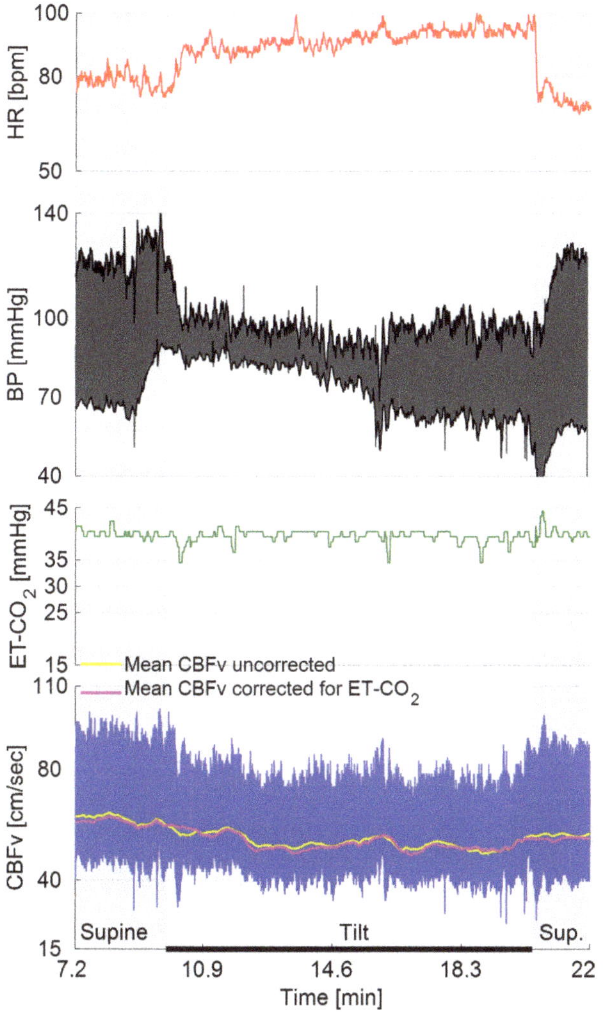

Figure 64.1 The tilt provoked symptomatic orthostatic hypotension and a decline in cerebral blood flow velocity. Heart rate responses and end tidal CO_2 were normal.

with an autoimmune process. Further evaluation was positive for elevated voltage-gated potassium channel (VGKC) antibodies with a titer of 0.12 (normal ≤0.02 nmol/L). The LGI1 and Caspr2 antibodies were absent. Cancer screening was negative. Patient was recommended to start immunotherapy with intravenous immunoglobulins.

Chronic pain is linked to VKGC antibodies (VKGC syndrome), and it is present in 50% of seropositive patients.[1–3] The clinical spectrum of VGKC-positive patients is heterogeneous and includes epilepsy, pain syndromes, cognitive decline, polyneuropathy, and cramp fasciculation syndrome.[3] There is a report describing a positive VKGC antibody in a child with painful small fiber neuropathy.[4] VGKC-positive patients should be further stratified based on the presence of LGI1 and Caspr2 antibodies. The immunotherapy can be of benefit if either LGI1 and Caspr2 antibodies are present. There are limited data regarding the effects of immunotherapy in VGKC-positive and LGI1/Caspr2 negative antibodies as have been found in this patient.

CAVEATS

- Hyperhidrosis and muscle twitches can be seen in small fiber neuropathy associated with elevated VGKC antibodies.[1,2]

REFERENCES

1. Irani SR, Vincent A. Voltage-gated potassium channel-complex autoimmunity and associated clinical syndromes. *Handb Clin Neurol.* 2016;133:185–197. doi:10.1016/B978-0-444-63432-0.00011-6.
2. Lahoria R, Pittock SJ, Gadoth A, Engelstad JK, Lennon VA, Klein CJ. Clinical-pathologic correlations in voltage-gated Kv1 potassium channel complex-subtyped autoimmune painful polyneuropathy. *Muscle Nerve.* August 2016. doi:10.1002/mus.25371.
3. van Sonderen A, Schreurs MWJ, Wirtz PW, Sillevis Smitt P a. E, Titulaer MJ. From VGKC to LGI1 and Caspr2 encephalitis: the evolution of a disease entity over time. *Autoimmun Rev.* 2016;15(10):970–974. doi:10.1016/j.autrev.2016.07.018.
4. Oaklander AL, Klein MM. Evidence of small-fiber polyneuropathy in unexplained, juvenile-onset, widespread pain syndromes. *Pediatrics.* 2013;131(4):e1091–e1100. doi:10.1542/peds.2012-2597.

65.

CASE 60: SMALL FIBER NEUROPATHY, SERONEGATIVE, TREATED WITH IMMUNE GLOBULINS

Chief complaint: Numbness.

Case presentation: A 59-year-old woman presents with a progressive numbness at the distal legs for 2 years of subacute onset. She also has experienced intermittent diarrhea for 6 years, excessive sweating with hot flashes, fatigue, exertional dyspnea, and exercise intolerance. Sometimes she has to sit down when doing the dishes. She may wake up several times during the night due to excessive sweating spells, and in the morning she does not feel refreshed but she denies depression. She denies cough or sputum production, hemoptysis, or pleuritic pain. Sometimes she notes chest flutter but denies chest pain. She gets dizzy and tired when standing or going upstairs but denies syncope.

Cardiac evaluation including Holter monitoring and echocardiogram was normal. She was seen by endocrine specialists, but except for an elevated antinuclear antibody level, her evaluation was unrevealing. She had normal results of tests of thyroid functions, 24-hour urine cortisol, serum metanephrine, normetanephrine, vasoactive intestinal peptide, chromogranin A, and 24-hour urinary N-methylhistamine.

Her nerve conduction study was normal. She was referred for evaluation of suspected small fiber neuropathy.

Past medical history: Small fiber neuropathy?

Current medication: None.

Assessment plan: Functional autonomic tests and skin biopsy.

AUTONOMIC TESTING EVALUATION

See Table 65.1.

Heart rate: Supine heart rate was normal. Heart rate responses to deep breathing were normal. Heart rate increment during the tilt (16 BPM) was normal.

Blood pressure:

Valsalva maneuver: Blood pressure responses were normal.

Tilt: Supine blood pressure was normal. Blood pressure responses to tilt were normal.

Sudomotor evaluation: Electrochemical skin conductance was abnormal (reduced to 98.3% of normal limit) at hands and normal at feet.

Respiratory system: Respiratory frequency and end tidal CO_2 were normal in supine position and during the tilt.

Cerebral blood flow velocity (CBFv): CBFv in middle cerebral artery was normal in supine position and was stable during the tilt.

Skin biopsy (sensory-epidermal): Epidermal nerve fiber density was normal at proximal leg and abnormal (reduced to 57.7% of normal limit) at distal leg.

Skin biopsy (sweat glands): Sweat gland nerve fiber density was abnormal (reduced to 87.6% of normal limit) at proximal leg and abnormal (reduced to 77.3% of normal limit) at distal leg.

TABLE 65.1 **RESULTS OF AUTONOMIC TESTING**

Blood pressure evaluation					
Test: Valsalva maneuver					
Pressure [mmHg]	Baseline	Phase 2			Phase 4
		Early	End		
Systolic	135	109	123		
Mean	91.7	93.7	107	n/a	
Diastolic	70	86	99	n/a	

Heart rate evaluation	
Test: Deep breathing	
Results	Norm*
14.71	≥9
Test: Valsalva ratio	
1.57	≥1.47
* adjusted for a gender and age	

TABLE 65.1 **CONTINUED**

Test: Tilt test										
Position		HR [BPM]	Blood pressure [mmHg]		MCA Blood flow velocity [cm/s]				Respiratory frequency [breaths/min]	End tidal CO_2 [mmHg]
			Systolic	Diastolic	Systolic	Mean	Mean drop [%]	Diastolic		
Supine		52	121	80	97	59		40	13	35
Tilt [min]	1	65	134	86	89	56.3	4.6	40	17	34
	2	68	127	83						
	3	65	128	85						
	4	66	127	85						
	5	65	134	82	84	53.3	9.7	38	14	34
	6	59	124	81						
	7	59	123	81						
	8	64	123	85						
	9	65	119	79						
	10	67	111	77	83	51.7	12.4	36	16	35
	15									
	20									
	30									
	40									

Sudomotor evaluation - functional

Test: Quantitative sudomotor axon reflex test (QSART)				
Location	Site (l/r)	Latency [min]	Volume [μl]	Norm [μl]*
Forearm				≥0.08
Prox. leg				≥0.14
Distal leg				≥0.07
Foot				≥0.05

* Normative data are adjusted for gender and age of patient.

Test: Electrochemical skin conductance (ESC)				
Location	Left [μS]	Right [μS]	Average [μS/k]	Norm [μS/kg]
Hand	59	65	1.01	≥1.03
Feet	91	92	1.5	≥1.14
Forehead				

For grading uses ESC [μS] adjusted for weight [μS/k].

(continued)

TABLE 65.1 **CONTINUED**

Small fiber (sensory + sudomotor) evaluation - morphological					
Test: Skin biopsy					
Location	Site (l/r)	Nerve fibers			
		Epidermal*		Sweat glands	
		Density	Norm	Density	Norm
Proximal leg – thigh	Right	10.07	≥8.3	33.1	≥37.8
Distal leg - calf	Right	3.68	≥6.38	28.2	≥36.5
Foot	Right		≥3.11		≥34.8

*Normative data for distal leg are adjusted for gender and age of patient.

QASAT*										
Heart rate		BP		CBFv		ET-CO2		Sudomotor		Total QASAT score
S. bradycardia	0	Low supine	0	Low supine	0	Low supine	0	QSART		
S. tachycardia	0	High supine	0	High supine	0	High supine	0	ESC	1	
Increase tilt	0	OH	0	Tilt response	0	Tilt low	0			
Decrease tilt	0	OHTN	0	CA	0	Tilt high	0	**Skin biopsy**		7
Deep breathing	0	VM	0	CVR	0			Epidermal	3	
VR	0			VM	0			Sweat gland	3	
Total	0	Total	0	Total	0	Total	0			

*QASAT. See Novak. Quantitative Scale for Grading of Cardiovascular Autonomic Reflex Tests and Small Fibers from Skin Biopsies. *J Neurol Disord* 2015;3:2.

S, supine; Increase tilt, increased response to tilt; Decrease tilt, decreased response to tilt; BP, blood pressure; VM, Valsalva maneuver; CBFv, cerebral blood flow velocity; CA, cerebral autoregulation; MCA, middle cerebral artery; VR, Valsalva ratio; CVR, cerebral vasoreactivity.

Patient-reported symptoms during testing: None during the tilt.

Patient-reported symptoms for past 2 weeks:

Lightheadedness or dizziness: Occasionally
Dry eyes or mouth: Often
Pale feet: None
Cold feet: Occasionally
Reduced sweating: Occasionally
Reduced sweating after exercise: Occasionally
Increased sweating: Occasionally
Nausea: Occasionally
Diarrhea: Often
Constipation: Yes, minor annoyance
Urinary leaks: Occasionally
Current pain severity: 0
Aching pain: Often, moderate
Allodynia: None
Burning pain: Often, severe
Lancinating pain: Occasionally, moderate
Numbness: Often, moderate
Prickling sensation: Often, moderate

AUTONOMIC TESTING INTERPRETATION

- Small fiber neuropathy, mixed, length-dependent.
- No evidence of autonomic failure.

COMMENT

This patient has small fiber neuropathy. Further evaluation for autoimmunity was negative. History, including subacute onset and relative broad range of autonomic symptoms with negative clinical workup, is suggestive of an autoimmune cause.[1] Indeed, patient responded well to intravenous immunoglobulin (IVIG) therapy, 2 g/kg/month. Sensory symptoms resolved; fatigue and dyspnea improved at least 50% within a year of therapy.

TREATMENT AND FOLLOW-UP

- Continue IVIG.

CAVEATS

- Small fiber neuropathy with a suspected autoimmune cause and with negative neuronal antibodies may respond to IVIG.

REFERENCE

1. Oaklander AL. Immunotherapy prospects for painful small-fiber sensory neuropathies and ganglionopathies. *Neurotherapeutics*. 2016;13(1):108–117. doi:10.1007/s13311-015-0395-1.

66.

CASE 61: SMALL FIBER NEUROPATHY, PATCHY, WITH ELEVATED VOLTAGE-GATED POTASSIUM CHANNEL ANTIBODIES

Chief complaint: Pain.

Case presentation: A 34-year-old woman presents with disabling pain in the feet for several years. She was bit by a tick at age 10 but she did not recollect having a skin rash. Subsequently, she became depressed, noted back pain, later diffuse pain. For past 2 years, she experienced chronic fatigue, cold legs, and weakness. She was diagnosed with Lyme disease 2 years ago but did not respond to multiple trials of antibiotics. She had detailed neurologic evaluations including MRI of the brain, nerve conduction studies, and spinal taps that were all within normal limits. The patient was referred for evaluation of painful small fiber neuropathy.

Past medical history: Headaches, Lyme disease.

Current medication: Oxycodone, gabapentin, lamotrigine.

Assessment plan: Functional autonomic tests and skin biopsy. Since the most severe pain was just below the knees, two additional skin biopsies were taken about 10 cm below the knee, bilaterally.

AUTONOMIC TESTING EVALUATION

See Table 66.1.

Heart rate: Heart rate was within the normal range in supine position. Heart rate responses to deep breathing and to tilt were normal.

Blood pressure:

Valsalva maneuver: Mean blood pressure failed to return to baseline at the end of Phase 2 by 40.3 mm Hg (i.e., 59.3% of baseline).

Tilt: Supine blood pressure was within normal range. Blood pressure responses to tilt were normal.

Sudomotor evaluation: Electrochemical skin conductance was normal at hands and normal at feet.

Respiratory system: Respiratory frequency was normal in supine position and during the tilt. End tidal CO_2 was reduced in supine position and during the tilt. Oxygen saturation was 99% throughout the testing.

Cerebral blood flow velocity (CBFv): CBFv in middle cerebral artery was reduced in supine position and was reduced further during the tilt.

Skin biopsy (sensory-epidermal): Epidermal nerve fiber density was normal at proximal leg and normal at distal leg. Additional skin biopsy below the knee showed 1.56/3.16 fibers/mm (left/right) epidermal nerve fiber density.

Skin biopsy (sweat glands): Sweat gland nerve fiber density was normal at proximal leg and normal at distal leg. Additional skin biopsy below the knee showed 20.6/16.3 fibers/mm (left/right) sweat gland nerve fiber density.

Patient-reported symptoms during testing: Dizziness, shortness of breath during the tilt.

TABLE 66.1 RESULTS OF AUTONOMIC TESTING

Blood pressure evaluation					
Test: Valsalva maneuver					
Pressure [mmHg]	Baseline	Phase 2			Phase 4
		Early	End		
Systolic	117	64	64		
Mean	99	58.7	58.7	n/a	
Diastolic	90	56	56	n/a	

Heart rate evaluation	
Test: Deep breathing	
Results	Norm*
14.2	≥12
Test: Valsalva ratio	
1.9	≥1.5
* adjusted for a gender and age	

TABLE 66.1 CONTINUED

Test: Tilt test										
Position		HR [BPM]	Blood pressure [mmHg]		MCA Blood flow velocity [cm/s]				Respiratory frequency [breaths/min]	End tidal CO_2 [mmHg]
			Systolic	Diastolic	Systolic	Mean	Mean drop [%]	Diastolic		
Supine		86	129	82	77	45		29	10	24
Tilt [min]	1	93	124	81	71	41	8.9	26	11	20
	2	87	118	73						
	3	92	134	85						
	4	95	135	84						
	5	97	119	82	74	46	-2.2	32	8	20
	6	96	118	81						
	7	94	130	84						
	8	95	123	79						
	9	101	126	84						
	10	96	108	73	62	35.3	21.6	22	10	20
	15									
	20									
	30									
	40									

Sudomotor evaluation - functional

Test: Quantitative sudomotor axon reflex test (QSART)				
Location	Site (l/r)	Latency [min]	Volume [µl]	Norm [µl]*
Forearm				≥0.08
Prox. leg				≥0.14
Distal leg				≥0.15
Foot				≥0.07

* Normative data are adjusted for gender and age of patient.

Test: Electrochemical skin conductance (ESC)				
Location	Left [µS]	Right [µS]	Average [µS/k]	Norm [µS/kg]
Hand	86	84	1.33	≥1.03
Feet	79	84	1.31	≥1.14
Forehead				

For grading uses ESC [µS] adjusted for weight [µS/k].

(continued)

Small fiber (sensory + sudomotor) evaluation - morphological					
Test: Skin biopsy					
Location	Site (l/r)	Nerve fibers			
		Epidermal*		Sweat glands	
		Density	Norm	Density	Norm
Proximal leg – thigh	Right	15.82	≥8.3		≥37.8
Distal leg - calf	Right	9.34	≥8.38	53.1	≥36.5
Foot	Right		≥3.11		≥34.8

*Normative data for distal leg are adjusted for gender and age of patient.

QASAT*											
Heart rate		BP		CBFv		ET-CO2		Sudomotor			Total QASAT score
S. bradycardia	0	Low supine	0	Low supine	1	Low supine	1	QSART			
S. tachycardia	0	High supine	0	High supine	0	High supine	0	ESC	0		
Increase tilt	0	OH	0	Tilt response	1	Tilt low	9				
Decrease tilt	0	OHTN	0	CA	0	Tilt high	0	**Skin biopsy**			15
Deep breathing	0	VM	3	CVR	0			Epidermal	0**		
VR	0			VM	0			Sweat gland	0**		
Total	0	Total	3	Total	2	Total	10				

*QASAT. See Novak. Quantitative Scale for Grading of Cardiovascular Autonomic Reflex Tests and Small Fibers from Skin Biopsies. *J Neurol Disord* 2015;3:2.

** The skin biopsy scores reflect results from standardized biopsy locations.

S, supine; Increase tilt, increased response to tilt; Decrease tilt, decreased response to tilt; BP, blood pressure; VM, Valsalva maneuver; CBFv, cerebral blood flow velocity; CA, cerebral autoregulation; MCA, middle cerebral artery; VR, Valsalva ratio; CVR, cerebral vasoreactivity.

Patient-reported symptoms for past 2 weeks:

Lightheadedness or dizziness: Occasionally
Dry eyes or mouth: Often
Pale feet: Occasionally
Cold feet: Often
Reduced sweating: Occasionally
Reduced sweating after exercise: None
Increased sweating: Occasionally
Nausea: Occasionally
Diarrhea: None
Constipation: Occasionally
Urinary leaks: None
Current pain severity: 5
Aching pain: Continuous, severe
Allodynia: Continuous, moderate
Burning pain: Often, moderate
Lancinating pain: Occasionally, severe
Numbness: Continuous, mild
Prickling sensation: Often, moderate

AUTONOMIC TESTING INTERPRETATION

- Small fiber neuropathy, severe, mixed, affecting sensory and autonomic sudomotor fibers, with a patchy distribution pattern.
- Mild autonomic adrenergic failure (Figure 66.1).
- Severe hypocapnic hyperventilation.
- Low CBFv and hypocapnic cerebral hypoperfusion (HYCH).

TREATMENT AND FOLLOW-UP

- Clinical workup for neuropathy showed elevated voltage-gated potassium channel (VGKC) antibodies with titer 0.21 (normal ≤0.02 nmol/L). LGI1 and Caspr2 antibodies were absent.
- Cancer screening was negative. Patient was recommended to start immunotherapy with the intravenous immunoglobulins.

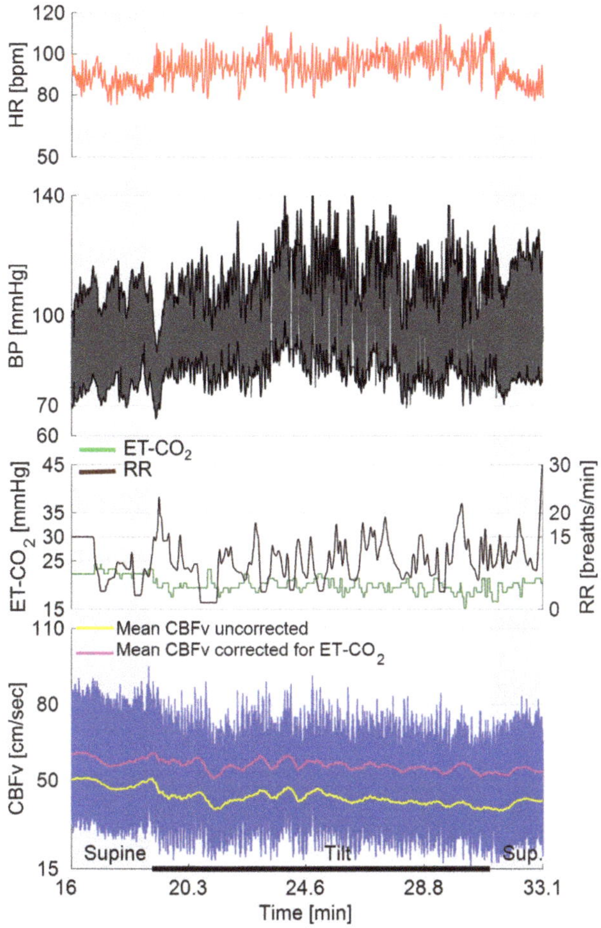

Figure 66.1 Patient complained of severe shortness of breath, weakness, dizziness, and fatigue during the tilt test. The heart rate and blood pressure response to tilt were normal. However, there was severe hypocapnic hyperventilation in supine position and during the tilt. The respiratory rate (RR) was erratic. Cerebral blood flow velocity (CBFv) was reduced both in supine and during the tilt. Velocity corrected for the effect of end tidal CO_2 was normal indicating that the reduction in CBFv was entirely due to hypocapnia.

- Respiratory and behavior therapy for hypocapnic hyperventilation.

COMMENT

This example shows small fiber neuropathy associated with VGKC antibodies and HYCH (Figure 66.1). The small fiber neuropathy is likely autoimmune, considering the clinical course (subacute onset) and the presence of VGKC antibodies. VGKCs modulate the nociceptive sensory threshold.[1–4]

CAVEATS

- Small fiber neuropathy with positive VGKC antibodies can have a patchy distribution. Standard biopsy sites would miss the diagnosis.
- Severe hypocapnic hyperventilation in this patient may be related to chronic pain and cerebral hypoperfusion.

REFERENCES

1. Irani SR, Vincent A. Voltage-gated potassium channel-complex autoimmunity and associated clinical syndromes. *Handb Clin Neurol.* 2016;133:185–197. doi:10.1016/B978-0-444-63432-0.00011-6.
2. Lahoria R, Pittock SJ, Gadoth A, Engelstad JK, Lennon VA, Klein CJ. Clinical-pathologic correlations in voltage-gated Kv1 potassium channel complex-subtyped autoimmune painful polyneuropathy. *Muscle Nerve.* August 2016. doi:10.1002/mus.25371.
3. van Sonderen A, Schreurs MWJ, Wirtz PW, Sillevis Smitt P a. E, Titulaer MJ. From VGKC to LGI1 and Caspr2 encephalitis: the evolution of a disease entity over time. *Autoimmun Rev.* 2016; 15(10):970–974. doi:10.1016/j.autrev.2016.07.018.
4. Oaklander AL, Klein MM. Evidence of small-fiber polyneuropathy in unexplained, juvenile-onset, widespread pain syndromes. *Pediatrics.* 2013;131(4):e1091–e1100. doi:10.1542/peds.2012-2597.

67.

CASE 62: SMALL FIBER NEUROPATHY WITH SYMPTOMATIC IMPROVEMENT ON IMMUNE GLOBULINS

Chief complaint: Fatigue.

Case presentation: A 65-year-old man presents with a chronic disabling fatigue. He suddenly experienced respiratory failure of unknown cause 12 years ago; a nonspecific connective tissue disorder has been suspected. Patient responded to steroids. Since then, he has experienced worsening of exertional intolerance, disabling shortness of breath, postural dizziness, brain fog, and diffuse aching pain, mainly affecting distal limbs. Autonomic testing confirmed small fiber neuropathy. Ganglionic acetylcholine receptor antibody was elevated at 0.04 nmol/L (normal ≤0.02 nmol/L). Patient was started on intravenous immune globulins (IVIG) at a dose of 2 g/kg/month for presumed autoimmune small fiber neuropathy.[1] The patient noted improvement of fatigue by at least 50% and improvement of shortness of breath by 70%. He still has days when he is tired. He was referred for repeated testing, including level of antibodies to assess interval changes.

Past medical history: Migraine, respiratory failure.

Current medication: None.

Assessment plan: Functional autonomic tests and skin biopsy.

AUTONOMIC TESTING EVALUATION

See Table 67.1.

Heart rate: Supine heart rate was normal. Heart rate responses to deep breathing were reduced to 42.9% of normal value. Heart rate increment during the tilt (11 BPM) was normal.

Blood pressure:

Valsalva maneuver: Blood pressure responses were normal.

Tilt: Supine blood pressure was normal. Blood pressure responses to tilt were normal.

Sudomotor evaluation: Electrochemical skin conductance was normal at hands and normal at feet.

Respiratory system: Respiratory frequency was normal in supine position and during the tilt. End tidal CO_2 was reduced in supine position and during the tilt.

Cerebral blood flow velocity (CBFv): CBFv in middle cerebral artery was normal in supine position but was mildly reduced during the tilt.

Skin biopsy (sensory-epidermal): Epidermal nerve fiber density was abnormal (reduced to 69.4% of normal

TABLE 67.1 RESULTS OF AUTONOMIC TESTING

Blood pressure evaluation					
Test: Valsalva maneuver					
Pressure [mmHg]	Baseline	Phase 2			Phase 4
		Early	End		
Systolic	82	66	66		
Mean	56.7	56.7	56.7	n/a	
Diastolic	44	52	52	n/a	

Heart rate evaluation	
Test: Deep breathing	
Results	Norm*
3	≥7
Test: Valsalva ratio	
1.69	≥1.29
* adjusted for a gender and age	

TABLE 67.1 CONTINUED

Test: Tilt test										
Position		HR [BPM]	Blood pressure [mmHg]		MCA Blood flow velocity [cm/s]				Respiratory frequency [breaths/min]	End tidal CO_2 [mmHg]
			Systolic	Diastolic	Systolic	Mean	Mean drop [%]	Diastolic		
Supine		68	135	76	99	53		30	13	30
Tilt [min]	1	70	122	73	103	53.7	-1.3	29	19	27
	2	73	121	69						
	3	71	132	73						
	4	76	121	72						
	5	74	123	77	104	54.7	-3.2	30	20	29
	6	75	126	74						
	7	73	131	80						
	8	79	129	74						
	9	68	138	72						
	10	74	138	79	103	40.3	24	9	19	27
	15									
	20									
	30									
	40									

Sudomotor evaluation - functional

Test: Quantitative sudomotor axon reflex test (QSART)				
Location	Site (l/r)	Latency [min]	Volume [µl]	Norm [µl]*
Forearm				≥0.3
Prox. leg				≥0.23
Distal leg				≥0.23
Foot				≥0.27

* Normative data are adjusted for gender and age of patient.

Test: Electrochemical skin conductance (ESC)				
Location	Left [µS]	Right [µS]	Average [µS/k]	Norm [µS/kg]
Hand	76	78	1.06	≥1.03
Feet	91	88	1.21	≥1.14
Forehead				

For grading uses ESC [µS] adjusted for weight [µS/k].

(continued)

TABLE 67.1 CONTINUED

Small fiber (sensory + sudomotor) evaluation - morphological					
Test: Skin biopsy					
Location	Site (l/r)	Nerve fibers			
		Epidermal*		Sweat glands	
		Density	Norm	Density	Norm
Proximal leg – thigh	Right	5.76	≥8.3		≥37.8
Distal leg - calf	Right	1.61	≥4.48		≥36.5
Foot	Right		≥3.11		≥34.8

*Normative data for distal leg are adjusted for gender and age of patient.

QASAT*											
Heart rate		BP		CBFv		ET-CO2		Sudomotor			Total QASAT score
S. bradycardia	0	Low supine	0	Low supine	0	Low supine	1	QSART			
S. tachycardia	0	High supine	0	High supine	0	High supine	0	ESC	0		
Increase tilt	0	OH	0	Tilt response	2	Tilt low	2				
Decrease tilt	0	OHTN	0	CA	0	Tilt high	0	**Skin biopsy**			10
Deep breathing	2	VM	0	CVR	0			Epidermal	3		
VR	0			VM	0			Sweat gland			
Total	2	Total	0	Total	2	Total	3				

*QASAT. See Novak. Quantitative Scale for Grading of Cardiovascular Autonomic Reflex Tests and Small Fibers from Skin Biopsies. *J Neurol Disord* 2015;3:2.

S, supine; Increase tilt, increased response to tilt; Decrease tilt, decreased response to tilt; BP, blood pressure; VM, Valsalva maneuver; CBFv, cerebral blood flow velocity; CA, cerebral autoregulation; MCA, middle cerebral artery; VR, Valsalva ratio; CVR, cerebral vasoreactivity.

limit) at proximal leg and abnormal (reduced to 36% of normal limit) at distal leg (Figure 67.1).

Skin biopsy (sweat glands): No sweat glands detected on the biopsy.

Patient-reported symptoms during testing: None.

Patient-reported symptoms for past 2 weeks:

Lightheadedness or dizziness: Often
Dry eyes or mouth: Yes, minor annoyance
Pale feet: Occasionally
Cold feet: Often
Reduced sweating: None
Reduced sweating after exercise: None
Increased sweating: Occasionally
Nausea: Occasionally
Diarrhea: Occasionally
Constipation: Occasionally
Urinary leaks: Occasionally
Erection problems: Yes, minor annoyance
Current pain severity: 0
Aching pain: Occasionally, mild
Allodynia: Occasionally, moderate
Burning pain: Occasionally, mild
Lancinating pain: Occasionally, moderate
Numbness: None
Prickling sensation: Often, moderate

AUTONOMIC TESTING INTERPRETATION

- Small fiber neuropathy affecting sensory fibers, length-dependent.
- No evidence of autonomic failure.
- Orthostatic cerebral hypoperfusion syndrome (OCHOS)

COMMENT

The autonomic testing was consistent with small fiber neuropathy associated with OCHOS (Figure 67.1).

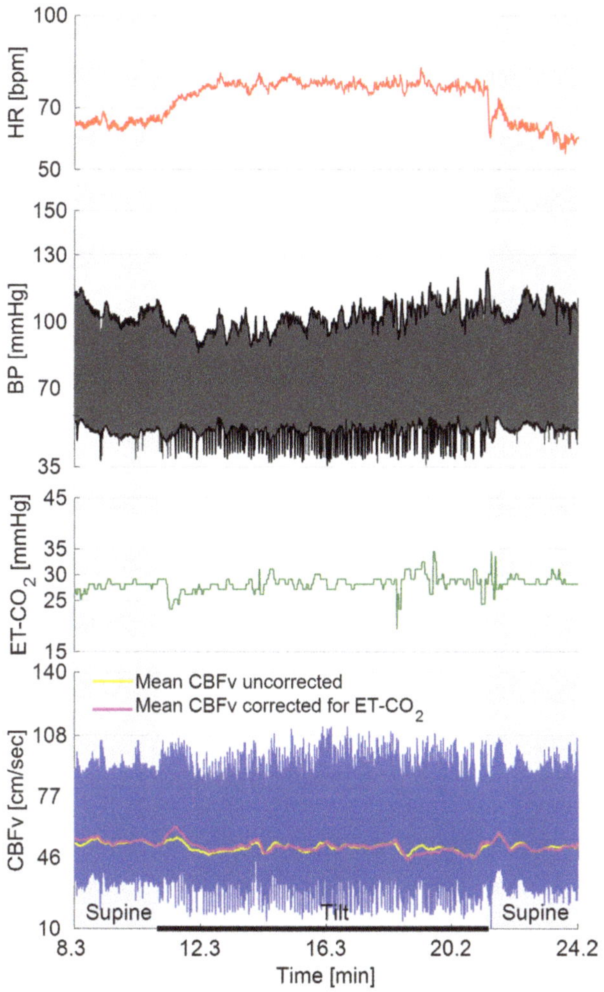

Figure 67.1 Tilt test showed mild hypocapnia in the supine position and during the tilt and a decline in orthostatic cerebral blood flow velocity. Heart rate and blood pressure responses to tilt were normal.

Repeated titer of ganglionic receptor acetylcholine antibody was zero, but the repeated epidermal nerve fiber density deteriorated to 1.61 fibers/mm (previously 4.34 fibers/mm). Autonomic scores were similar (e.g., initial QASAT- autonomic failure score = 3, repeat score = 2. QASAT- autonomic failure score is defined as sum of deep breathing score [cardiovagal index], blood pressure score [adrenergic index] and sudomotor score.

TREATMENT AND FOLLOW-UP

- Continue therapy with IVIG since symptomatic improvement was noted.

CAVEATS

- IVIG may improve symptoms even if small fiber neuropathy deteriorates, as determined by the skin biopsy.

REFERENCE

1. Oaklander AL. Immunotherapy prospects for painful small-fiber sensory neuropathies and ganglionopathies. *Neurotherapeutics*. 2016;13(1):108–117. doi:10.1007/s13311-015-0395-1.

68.

CASE 63: SMALL FIBER SENSORY NEUROPATHY WITH ELEVATED GANGLIONIC ACETYLCHOLINE RECEPTOR ANTIBODY RESPONDING TO IMMUNOGLOBULINS

Chief complaint: Dizziness.

Case presentation: A 43-year-old woman has a history of multiple tick bites associated with skin rash for the past 5 years. She was treated for about a year with multiple antibiotics for suspected Lyme disease. In spite of treatment, she experienced postural and nonpostural dizziness, lack of energy, weakness, cold intolerance, and fatigue. Most of complaints had a fluctuating character. She was again treated with multiple courses of antibiotics for Lyme disease including doxycycline, erythromycin, amoxicillin, rifampin, and ceftriaxone. Latest Western blot testing for Lyme disease showed four positive IgG bands, which is boderline. CDC Lyme criteria require the presence 5 bands or more. She was referred for evaluation of posttreatment Lyme disease syndrome.

Past medical history: Lyme disease.

Current medication: Lexapro, thyroid replacement.

Assessment plan: Functional autonomic tests and skin biopsy.

AUTONOMIC TESTING EVALUATION

See Table 68.1.

Heart rate: Supine heart rate was normal. Heart rate responses to deep breathing were normal. Heart rate increment during the tilt (25 BPM) was normal.

Blood pressure:

Valsalva maneuver: Blood pressure responses were normal.

Tilt: Supine blood pressure was normal. Blood pressure responses to tilt were normal.

Sudomotor evaluation: Sweat output was normal at forearm, normal at proximal leg, normal at distal leg, and normal at foot. Quantitative sudomotor axon reflex test (QSART) showed length-dependent pattern with a decrease of sweat output distally of at least 33%.

Respiratory system: Respiratory frequency and end tidal CO_2 were normal in supine position and during the tilt.

Cerebral blood flow velocity (CBFv): CBFv in middle cerebral artery was normal in supine position and was stable during the tilt.

Skin biopsy (sensory-epidermal): Epidermal nerve fiber density was abnormal (reduced to 82.4% of normal limit) at proximal leg and abnormal (reduced to 32.3% of normal limit) at distal leg.

Skin biopsy (sweat glands): Sweat gland nerve fiber density was normal at proximal leg and normal at distal leg.

Patient-reported symptoms during testing: None during the tilt.

TABLE 68.1 RESULTS OF AUTONOMIC TESTING

Blood pressure evaluation					
Test: Valsalva maneuver					
Pressure [mmHg]	Baseline	Phase 2			Phase 4
		Early	End		
Systolic	107	79	100		
Mean	81.7	69	87.3	n/a	
Diastolic	69	64	81	n/a	

Heart rate evaluation	
Test: Deep breathing	
Results	Norm*
20.3	≥10
Test: Valsalva ratio	
2.32	≥1.51

* adjusted for a gender and age

TABLE 68.1 CONTINUED

Test: Tilt test										
Position		HR [BPM]	Blood pressure [mmHg]		MCA Blood flow velocity [cm/s]				Respiratory frequency [breaths/min]	End tidal CO_2 [mmHg]
			Systolic	Diastolic	Systolic	Mean	Mean drop [%]	Diastolic		
Supine		81	110	73	110	70		50	13	38
Tilt [min]	1	105	114	79	109	69	1.4	49	11	36
	2	106	110	76						
	3	95	111	77						
	4	95	109	75						
	5	105	111	75	106	68.7	1.9	50	21	37
	6	90	112	76						
	7	95	116	78						
	8	91	116	81						
	9	92	114	78						
	10	95	113	80	99	64.3	8.1	47	19	38
	15									
	20									
	30									
	40									

Sudomotor evaluation - functional

Test: Quantitative sudomotor axon reflex test (QSART)				
Location	Site (l/r)	Latency [min]	Volume [µl]	Norm [µl]*
Forearm	l	1.34	1.37	≥0.08
Prox. leg	l	1.08	1.325	≥0.14
Distal leg	l	1.38	0.816	≥0.15
Foot	l	2.05	0.455	≥0.07

* Normative data are adjusted for gender and age of patient.

Test: Electrochemical skin conductance (ESC)				
Location	Left [µS]	Right [µS]	Average [µS/k]	Norm [µS/kg]
Hand				≥
Feet				≥
Forehead				

For grading uses ESC [µS] adjusted for weight [µS/k].

(continued)

TABLE 68.1 CONTINUED

Small fiber (sensory + sudomotor) evaluation - morphological					
Test: Skin biopsy					
Location	Site (l/r)	Nerve fibers			
		Epidermal*		Sweat glands	
		Density	Norm	Density	Norm
Proximal leg – thigh	Right	6.84	≥8.3	48.4	≥37.8
Distal leg - calf	Right	2.5	≥7.74	51.8	≥36.5
Foot	Right		≥3.11		≥34.8

*Normative data for distal leg are adjusted for gender and age of patient.

QASAT*											
Heart rate		BP		CBFv		ET-CO2		Sudomotor			Total QASAT score
S. bradycardia	0	Low supine	0	Low supine	0	Low supine	0	QSART	1		
S. tachycardia	0	High supine	0	High supine	0	High supine	0	ESC			
Increase tilt	0	OH	0	Tilt response	0	Tilt low	0				
Decrease tilt	0	OHTN	0	CA	0	Tilt high	0	**Skin biopsy**			4
Deep breathing	0	VM	0	CVR	0			Epidermal	3		
VR	0			VM	0			Sweat gland	0		
Total	0	Total	0	Total	0	Total	0				

*QASAT. See Novak. Quantitative Scale for Grading of Cardiovascular Autonomic Reflex Tests and Small Fibers from Skin Biopsies. *J Neurol Disord* 2015;3:2.

S, supine; Increase tilt, increased response to tilt; Decrease tilt, decreased response to tilt; BP, blood pressure; VM, Valsalva maneuver; CBFv, cerebral blood flow velocity; CA, cerebral autoregulation; MCA, middle cerebral artery; VR, Valsalva ratio; CVR, cerebral vasoreactivity.

Patient-reported symptoms for past 2 weeks:

Lightheadedness or dizziness: Yes, minor annoyance
Dry eyes or mouth: Occasionally
Pale feet: Occasionally
Cold feet: Often
Reduced sweating: None
Reduced sweating after exercise: None
Increased sweating: None
Nausea: Yes, minor annoyance
Diarrhea: Yes, minor annoyance
Constipation: Yes, minor annoyance
Urinary leaks: Occasionally
Current pain severity: 0
Aching pain: Occasionally, mild
Allodynia: None
Burning pain: Often, mild
Lancinating pain: Occasionally, moderate
Numbness: Often, mild
Prickling sensation: Often, mild

AUTONOMIC TESTING INTERPRETATION

- Small fiber neuropathy, sensory, length-dependent.
- Autonomic functions were essentially normal; there was no evidence of autonomic failure or orthostatic intolerance.

COMMENT

Patient tested positive for ganglionic acetylcholine receptor antibody (0.04 nmol/L, normal ≤0.02 nmol/L). She was started on intravenous immune globulins (IVIG) at a dose of 2 g/kg/month. After 6 months, she noted improvement of pain and energy by 70%. After 1 year of IVIG therapy, she further improved although she appeared to reach a plateau and opted to discontinue the treatment. Repeated skin biopsy a year after initiation of the IVIG therapy showed 10.5 epidermal fibers/mm as compared to 2.5 fibers/mm at the beginning of the treatment.

TREATMENT AND FOLLOW-UP

- Patient improved on IVIG therapy.

CAVEATS

- IVIG therapy may be effective for inflammatory small fiber neuropathy.[1,2]

REFERENCES

1. Oaklander AL. Immunotherapy prospects for painful small-fiber sensory neuropathies and ganglionopathies. *Neurotherapeutics*. 2016;13(1):108–117. doi:10.1007/s13311-015-0395-1.
2. Liu X, Treister R, Lang M, Oaklander AL. IVIg for apparently autoimmune small-fiber polyneuropathy: first analysis of efficacy and safety. *Ther Adv Neurol Disord*. 2018;11:1756285617744484. doi:10.1177/1756285617744484.

69.

CASE 64: EHLERS-DANLOS SYNDROME AND SMALL FIBER NEUROPATHY

Chief complaint: Palpitations and chest pain

Case presentation: A 42-year-old woman presents with intermittent chest pain, dizziness, and anxiety. She was doing well until age 14, when she began to experience recurrent fevers of unknown origin. She was extensively investigated without a clear cause. The fevers generally occurred around January, and she recollects having to miss multiple weeks of school during the winter. She otherwise was fully functional until age 24, when she had prolonged severe exhaustion and fatigue following childbirth. Over the next few years, she developed new symptoms of dizziness and near syncope. Autonomic testing was positive for postural orthostatic tachycardia syndrome (POTS). Insidiously, she started to have numbness in her feet that has gradually ascended and now involves her hands. She cut herself several times without feeling it. She has toothache-like pain in the lower back and into the buttocks. She has urinary as well as episodes of stool incontinence. She has significant hypermobility and multiple joint subluxations, and she was diagnosed hypermobile Ehlers-Danlos syndrome. She experiences intermittent palpitations and chest pain. Cardiology evaluation including a 2D echocardiogram of the aorta was unrevealing. She was referred for autonomic testing to assess palpitations and to evaluate for small fiber neuropathy.

Past medical history: Ehlers-Danlos syndrome hypermobility type, POTS, migraine.

Current medication: None.

Assessment plan: Functional autonomic tests and skin biopsy.

AUTONOMIC TESTING EVALUATION

See Table 69.1.

Heart rate: Supine heart rate was normal. Heart rate responses to deep breathing were normal. Heart rate increment during the tilt (32 BPM) was exaggerated.

Blood pressure:

Valsalva maneuver: Blood pressure responses were normal. Supine blood pressure was normal.

Tilt: Blood pressure was elevated during the tilt. Blood pressure responses to tilt were normal.

Sudomotor evaluation: Electrochemical skin conductance was abnormal (reduced to 80.9% of normal limit) at hands and abnormal (reduced to 91.3% of normal limit) at feet.

Respiratory system: Respiratory frequency was normal in supine position. Respiratory frequency was normal during the tilt. End tidal CO_2 was normal in supine position. End tidal CO_2 was moderately reduced during the tilt.

Cerebral blood flow velocity (CBFv): CBFv in middle cerebral artery was normal in supine position. CBFv in middle cerebral artery was severely reduced during the tilt.

Skin biopsy (sensory-epidermal): Epidermal nerve fiber density was abnormal (reduced to 5.1% of normal limit) at proximal leg and abnormal (reduced to 1.7% of normal limit) at distal leg.

Skin biopsy (sweat glands): Sweat gland nerve fiber density was abnormal (reduced to 6.6% of normal limit) at proximal leg and abnormal (reduced to 13.7% of normal limit) at distal leg.

TABLE 69.1 RESULTS OF AUTONOMIC TESTING

Blood pressure evaluation					
Test: Valsalva maneuver					
Pressure [mmHg]	Baseline	Phase 2			Phase 4
		Early	End		
Systolic	147	116	132		
Mean	111	100	115.3	n/a	
Diastolic	93	92	107	n/a	

Heart rate evaluation	
Test: Deep breathing	
Results	Norm*
26	≥10
Test: Valsalva ratio	
1.98	≥1.51

* adjusted for a gender and age

TABLE 69.1 **CONTINUED**

Test: Tilt test										
Position		HR [BPM]	Blood pressure [mmHg]		MCA Blood flow velocity [cm/s]				Respiratory frequency [breaths/min]	End tidal CO_2 [mmHg]
			Systolic	Diastolic	Systolic	Mean	Mean drop [%]	Diastolic		
Supine		76	130	84	132	85.3		62	10	37
Tilt [min]	1	100	131	96	78	49.3	42.2	35	15	25
	2	106	122	86						
	3	104	120	82						
	4	97	142	90						
	5	97	135	97	88	58	32	43	15	31
	6	89	125	93						
	7	97	135	95						
	8	108	135	89						
	9	95	133	94						
	10	94	133	95	80	54.7	35.9	42	18	28
	15									
	20									
	30									
	40									

Sudomotor evaluation - functional

Test: Quantitative sudomotor axon reflex test (QSART)				
Location	Site (l/r)	Latency [min]	Volume [μl]	Norm [μl]*
Forearm				≥0.08
Prox. leg				≥0.14
Distal leg				≥0.15
Foot				≥0.07

* Normative data are adjusted for gender and age of patient.

Test: Electrochemical skin conductance (ESC)				
Location	Left [μS]	Right [μS]	Average [μS/k]	Norm [μS/kg]
Hand	70	66	0.83	≥1.03
Feet	85	86	1.05	≥1.14
Forehead				

For grading uses ESC [μS] adjusted for weight [μS/k].

(continued)

Small fiber (sensory + sudomotor) evaluation - morphological					
Test: Skin biopsy					
Location	Site (l/r)	Nerve fibers			
		Epidermal*		Sweat glands	
		Density	Norm	Density	Norm
Proximal leg – thigh	Right	0.42	≥8.3	2.5	≥37.8
Distal leg - calf	Right	0.13	≥7.74	5	≥36.5
Foot	Right		≥3.11		≥34.8

*Normative data for distal leg are adjusted for gender and age of patient.

QASAT*										
Heart rate		BP		CBFv		ET-CO2		Sudomotor		Total QASAT score
S. bradycardia	0	Low supine	0	Low supine	0	Low supine	0	QSART		
S. tachycardia	0	High supine	0	High supine	0	High supine	0	ESC	2	
Increase tilt	1	OH	0	Tilt response	9	Tilt low	3			
Decrease tilt	0	OHTN	0	CA	0	Tilt high	0	**Skin biopsy**		23
Deep breathing	0	VM	0	CVR	0			Epidermal	4	
VR	0			VM	0			Sweat gland	4	
Total	1	Total	0	Total	9	Total	3			

*QASAT. See Novak. Quantitative Scale for Grading of Cardiovascular Autonomic Reflex Tests and Small Fibers from Skin Biopsies. *J Neurol Disord* 2015;3:2.

S, supine; Increase tilt, increased response to tilt; Decrease tilt, decreased response to tilt; BP, blood pressure; VM, Valsalva maneuver; CBFv, cerebral blood flow velocity; CA, cerebral autoregulation; MCA, middle cerebral artery; VR, Valsalva ratio; CVR, cerebral vasoreactivity.

Patient-reported symptoms during testing: Dizziness, shortness of breath during the tilt.

Patient-reported symptoms for past 2 weeks:

Lightheadedness or dizziness: Occasionally
Dry eyes or mouth: Occasionally
Pale feet: None
Cold feet: Occasionally
Reduced sweating: Yes, minor annoyance
Reduced sweating after exercise: Yes, minor annoyance
Increased sweating: None
Nausea: Often
Diarrhea: Occasionally
Constipation: Occasionally
Urinary leaks: Often
Current pain severity: 3
Aching pain: Often, moderate
Allodynia: None
Burning pain: Often, moderate
Lancinating pain: Often, moderate
Numbness: continuous, severe
Prickling sensation: Often, moderate

AUTONOMIC TESTING INTERPRETATION

- Anxiety reaction during the tilt.
- Small fiber neuropathy, mixed, severe, non–length-dependent.
- No evidence of autonomic failure or POTS.
- Hypocapnic hyperventilation.
- Hypocapnic cerebral hypoperfusion (HYCH).

COMMENT

Ehlers-Danlos syndrome is a heterogeneous group of inherited connective tissue disorders characterized by joint hypermobility, skin hyperextensibility, and tissue fragility.[1] Hypermobile Ehlers-Danlos syndrome (formerly called type III), as seen in this patient, is, in addition to joint hypermobility and skin problems, also associated with sleep disturbance, fatigue, POTS, functional gastrointestinal disorders, dysautonomia, anxiety, depression, and small fiber neuropathy.[1,2] This patient had severe small fiber

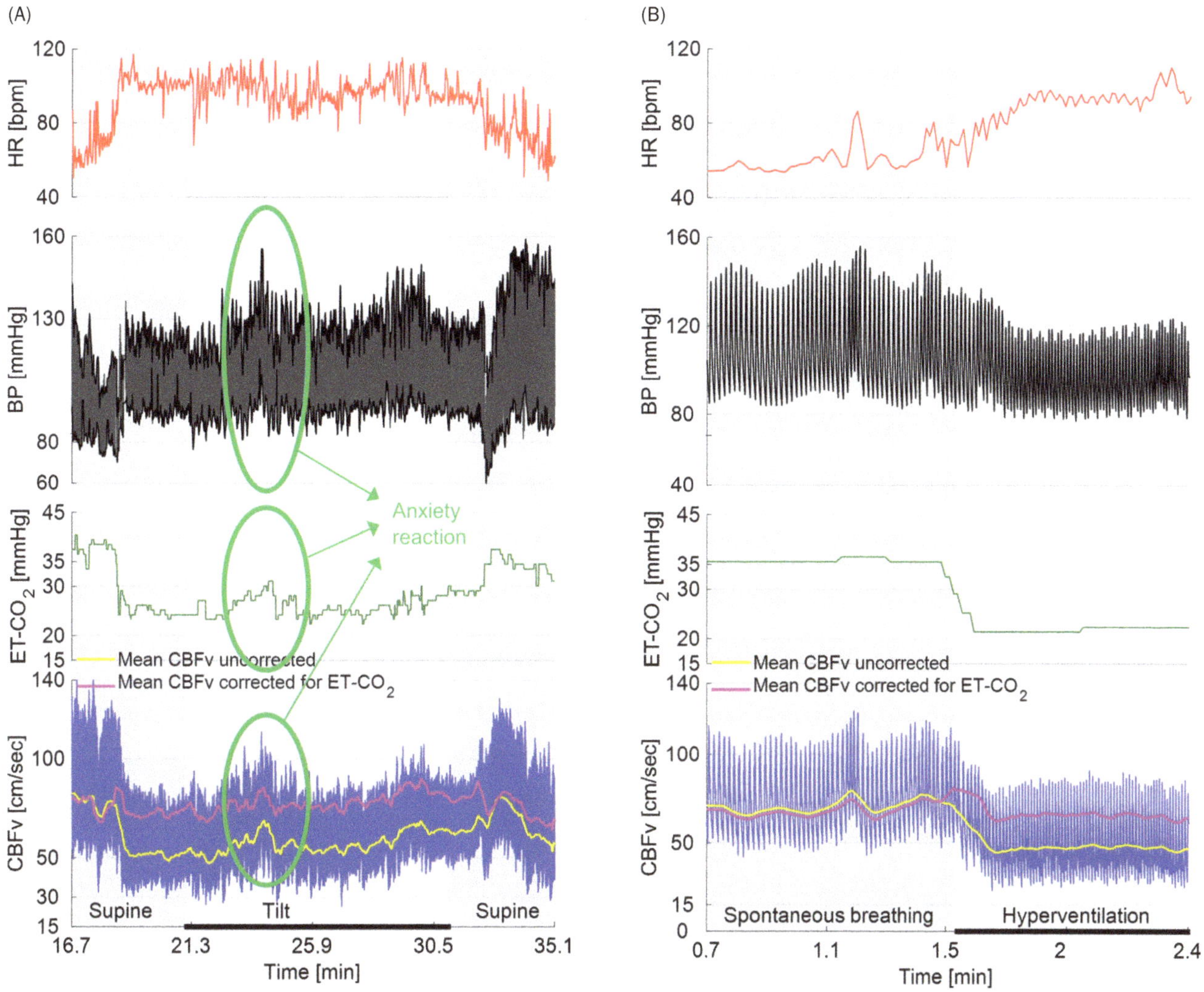

Figure 69.1 The tilt provoked the patient's typical chest pain and palpitations that occurred about 3 minutes after tilt onset. The spell's duration was about a minute and was associated with transient increase in blood pressure, heart rate, and cerebral blood flow (*green oval*). Patient was dizzy and short of breath throughout the tilt. Hyperventilation in supine position (B) did not reproduce the palpitations but induced a similar decline in CBFv and dizziness as seen during the tilt associated with dizziness (A).

neuropathy that can underlie some pain complaints. Tilt test showed that an anxiety reaction and not dysautonomia is related to the patient's palpitations (Figure 69.1). The tilt test also revealed HYCH that is associated with orthostatic intolerance.

TREATMENT AND FOLLOW-UP

- Treatment of anxiety and hypocapnic hyperventilation by respiratory and behavioral therapy.
- Pain control
- Imaging of the lower spine and lumbar-sacral roots to rule out compression since history of incontinence and autonomic testing was negative for autonomic failure.

CAVEATS

- Autonomic testing with skin biopsy can dissect the cause of symptoms and can help in planning effective therapy in hypermobile Ehlers-Danlos syndrome.

REFERENCES

1. Malfait F, Francomano C, Byers P, et al. The 2017 international classification of the Ehlers-Danlos syndromes. *Am J Med Genet C Semin Med Genet.* 2017;175(1):8–26. doi:10.1002/ajmg.c.31552.
2. Cazzato D, Castori M, Lombardi R, et al. Small fiber neuropathy is a common feature of Ehlers-Danlos syndromes. *Neurology.* 2016;87(2):155–159. doi:10.1212/WNL.0000000000002847.

70.

CASE 65: EHLERS-DANLOS SYNDROME WITH POSTURAL TACHYCARDIA SYNDROME, PRESYNCOPE, AND ANXIETY

Chief complaint: Dizziness.

Case presentation: A 32-year-old woman presents with orthostatic intolerance since age 7.

Previous tilt test was positive for postural tachycardia syndrome (POTS). Nevertheless, she responded only partially to proamatine. The dose higher than 2.5 mg and caused urinary retention and may even have exacerbated symptoms. She was reluctant to try other medications. She has good and bad days. When she is symptomatic, she experiences disabling tachycardia, is very anxious, noted blurred vision, but is rarely very dizzy. MRI of the brain, EEG, and nerve conduction study were all unrevealing.

Past medical history: POTS.

Current medication: None.

Assessment plan: Functional autonomic tests and skin biopsy.

AUTONOMIC TESTING EVALUATION

See Table 70.1.

Heart rate: Supine heart rate was normal. Heart rate responses to deep breathing were normal. Heart rate increment during the tilt (65 BPM) was exaggerated and exceeded 130 BPM.

Blood pressure:

Valsalva maneuver: Blood pressure responses were normal. Supine blood pressure was normal. Blood pressure was elevated during the tilt.

Tilt: Blood pressure responses to tilt were normal.

Sudomotor evaluation: Sweat output was normal at forearm, normal at proximal leg, normal at distal leg, and normal at foot. Quantitative sudomotor axon reflex test (QSART) showed length-dependent pattern with a decrease of sweat output distally of at least 33%.

Respiratory system: Respiratory frequency was normal in supine position and during the tilt. End tidal CO_2 was normal in supine position but was mildly reduced during the tilt.

Cerebral blood flow velocity (CBFv): CBFv in middle cerebral artery was normal in supine position but was mildly reduced during the tilt.

Skin biopsy (sensory-epidermal): Epidermal nerve fiber density was normal at proximal leg and normal at distal leg.

Skin biopsy (sweat glands): Sweat gland nerve fiber density was normal at proximal leg and normal at distal leg.

Patient-reported symptoms during testing: Dizziness, chest tightness, shaking, unclear vision during the tilt.

Patient-reported symptoms for past 2 weeks:

Lightheadedness or dizziness: Occasionally
Dry eyes or mouth: Occasionally

TABLE 70.1 **RESULTS OF AUTONOMIC TESTING**

Blood pressure evaluation					
Test: Valsalva maneuver					
Pressure [mmHg]	Baseline	Phase 2			Phase 4
		Early	End		
Systolic	128	114	125		
Mean	104	102.7	114.3	n/a	
Diastolic	92	97	109	n/a	

Heart rate evaluation	
Test: Deep breathing	
Results	Norm*
16.4	≥12
Test: Valsalva ratio	
1.97	≥1.5
* adjusted for a gender and age	

TABLE 70.1 **CONTINUED**

Test: Tilt test										
Position		HR [BPM]	Blood pressure [mmHg]		MCA Blood flow velocity [cm/s]				Respiratory frequency [breaths/min]	End tidal CO_2 [mmHg]
			Systolic	Diastolic	Systolic	Mean	Mean drop [%]	Diastolic		
Supine		91	111	72	107	79		65	15	37
Tilt [min]	1	156	135	87	104	70.7	10.5	54	16	29
	2	150	130	92						
	3	141	132	84						
	4	139	122	87						
	5	138	131	84	108	72	8.9	54	16	34
	6	121	113	82						
	7	132	114	83						
	8	128	107	75						
	9	129	118	86						
	10	128	115	83	98	66	16.5	50	17	33
	15									
	20									
	30									
	40									

Sudomotor evaluation - functional

Test: Quantitative sudomotor axon reflex test (QSART)				
Location	Site (l/r)	Latency [min]	Volume [μl]	Norm [μl]*
Forearm	l	1.19	0.161	≥0.08
Prox. leg	l	2.05	0.498	≥0.14
Distal leg	l	0.34	0.316	≥0.15
Foot	l	3.4	0.104	≥0.07

* Normative data are adjusted for gender and age of patient.

Test: Electrochemical skin conductance (ESC)				
Location	Left [μS]	Right [μS]	Average [μS/k]	Norm [μS/kg]
Hand				≥
Feet				≥
Forehead				

For grading uses ESC [μS] adjusted for weight [μS/k].

(continued)

TABLE 70.1 **CONTINUED**

Small fiber (sensory + sudomotor) evaluation - morphological					
Test: Skin biopsy					
Location	Site (l/r)	Nerve fibers			
		Epidermal*		Sweat glands	
		Density	Norm	Density	Norm
Proximal leg – thigh	Right	13.79	≥8.3	52.3	≥37.8
Distal leg - calf	Right	9.24	≥8.54	53.5	≥36.5
Foot	Right		≥3.11		≥34.8

*Normative data for distal leg are adjusted for gender and age of patient.

QASAT*												
Heart rate		**BP**		**CBFv**		**ET-CO2**		**Sudomotor**			**Total QASAT score**
S. bradycardia	0	Low supine	0	Low supine	0	Low supine	0	QSART	1		
S. tachycardia	0	High supine	0	High supine	0	High supine	0	ESC			
Increase tilt	10	OH	0	Tilt response	2	Tilt low	1				
Decrease tilt	0	OHTN	3	CA	0	Tilt high	0	**Skin biopsy**			17
Deep breathing	0	VM	0	CVR	0			Epidermal	0		
VR	0			VM	0			Sweat gland	0		
Total	10	Total	3	Total	2	Total	1				

*QASAT. See Novak. Quantitative Scale for Grading of Cardiovascular Autonomic Reflex Tests and Small Fibers from Skin Biopsies. *J Neurol Disord* 2015;3:2.

S, supine; Increase tilt, increased response to tilt; Decrease tilt, decreased response to tilt; BP, blood pressure; VM, Valsalva maneuver; CBFv, cerebral blood flow velocity; CA, cerebral autoregulation; MCA, middle cerebral artery; VR, Valsalva ratio; CVR, cerebral vasoreactivity.

Pale feet: Occasionally
Cold feet: Yes, minor annoyance
Reduced sweating: Occasionally
Reduced sweating after exercise: Occasionally
Increased sweating: Occasionally
Nausea: Occasionally
Diarrhea: Occasionally
Constipation: Yes, minor annoyance
Urinary leaks: Yes, minor annoyance
Current pain severity: 4
Aching pain: Often, moderate
Allodynia: None
Burning pain: Occasionally, mild
Lancinating pain: Occasionally, moderate
Numbness: Occasionally, moderate
Prickling sensation: Occasionally, mild

AUTONOMIC TESTING INTERPRETATION

- Anxiety.
- Presyncope, vasodepressor.
- POTS.

COMMENT

The tilt test showed a combination of anxiety, POTS, and presyncope (Figure 70.1). The POTS is mild, and anxiety may exacerbate symptoms; as such, both disorders have to be addressed.[1]

TREATMENT AND FOLLOW-UP

- Simultaneous therapy for anxiety and POTS.

CAVEATS

- POTS patients may recover from presyncope without terminating the tilt test.

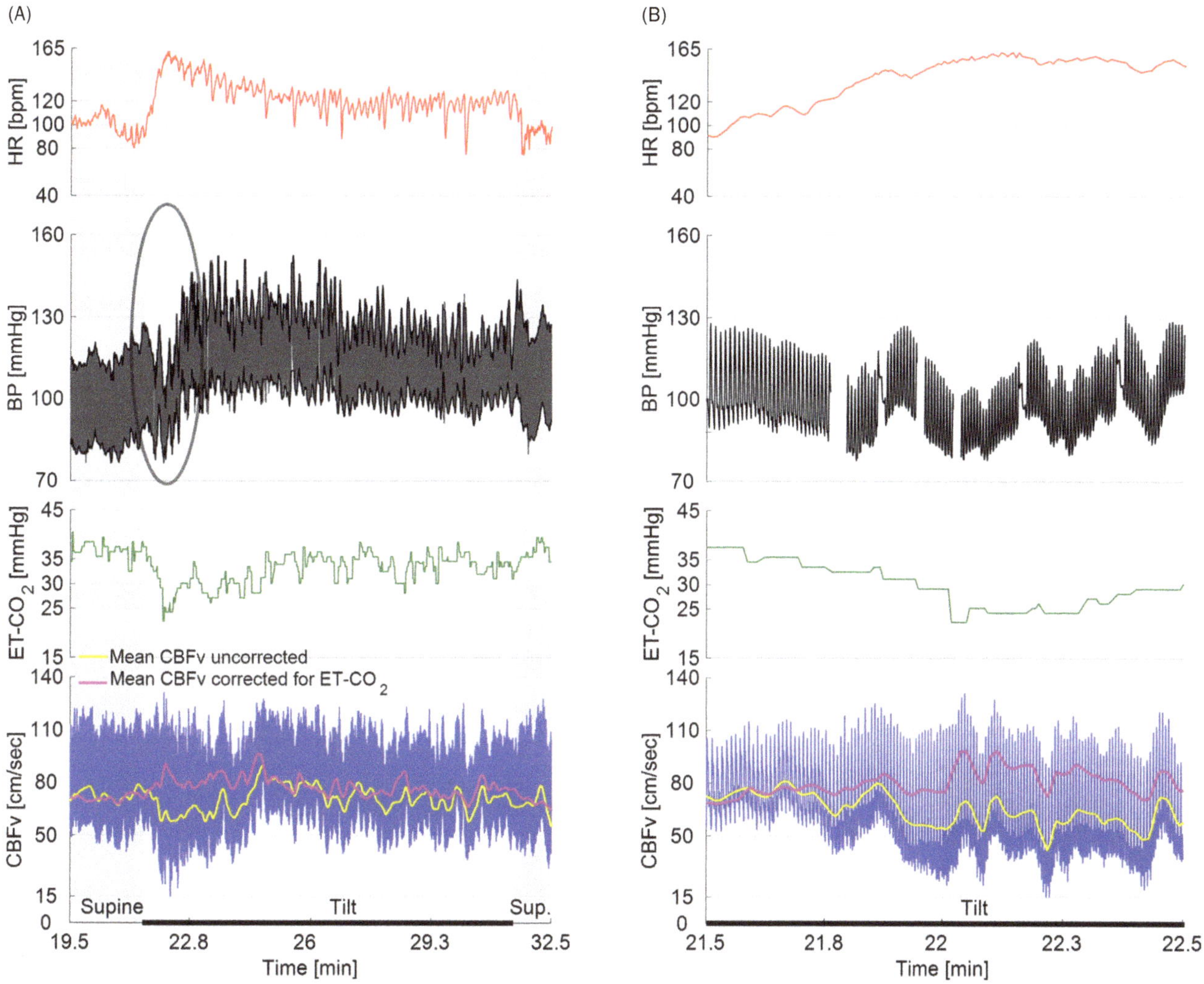

Figure 70.1 Tilt test (A–C) provoked severe tachycardia, decrease in blood pressure and end tidal CO_2, cerebral vasodilation pattern, e.g. widening of cerebral blood flow signal (decrease in diastolic cerebral blood flow velocity [CBFv], and an increase or no change in systolic CBFv. Patient was very anxious and dizzy throughout the tilt test. The initial responses to tilt is consistent with presyncope (decline in blood pressure and cerebral vasodilation). The patient recovered without terminating the tilt. Immediately after presyncope, patient experienced anxiety reaction (at around minute 22.3 (B) associated with severe tachycardia. Subsequently orthopstatic tachycardia improved but still remained at the POTS range (~120 BPM). B and C shows details of presyncope.

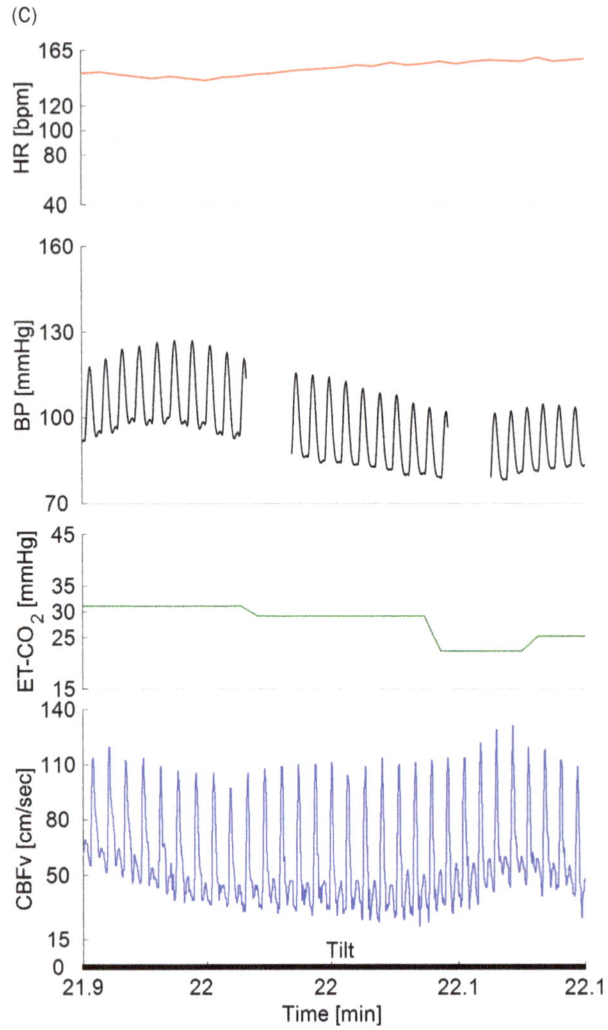

Figure 70.1 Continued

- Severe initial tachycardia during the tilt test most likely is due to the combined effect of anxiety and compensation of presyncopal reaction.

REFERENCE

1. Raj V, Opie M, Arnold AC. Cognitive and psychological issues in postural tachycardia syndrome. *Auton Neurosci Basic Clin*. March 2018. doi:10.1016/j.autneu.2018.03.004.

71.

CASE 66: HYPERVENTILATION SYNDROME, SMALL FIBER NEUROPATHY, AND POSTURAL TACHYCARDIA SYNDROME IN EHLERS-DANLOS SYNDROME

Chief complaint: Dizziness.

Case presentation: A 23-year-old woman presents with anxiety, brain fog, and unexplained fatigue and diffuse pain with numbness for 10 years. Additional present complaints are chronic diffuse pain, shortness of breath, brain fog, muscle spasms, hand tremor, postural dizziness, syncope, and anxiety. On some days, she is bedridden due extreme fatigue. She uses a cane occasionally due to unsteadiness. She was referred for autonomic testing to determine if dysautonomia can be responsible for her symptoms.

Past medical history: Chromosome 20 trisomy, obsessive compulsive disorder, Ehlers-Danlos syndrome hypermobility type, Lyme disease, migraine.

Current medication: None.

Assessment plan: Functional autonomic tests and skin biopsy.

AUTONOMIC TESTING EVALUATION

See Table 71.1.

Heart rate: Supine heart rate was normal. Heart rate responses to deep breathing were reduced to 44.1% of normal value. Heart rate increment during the tilt (39 BPM) was exaggerated.

Blood pressure:

Valsalva maneuver: Mean blood pressure failed to return to baseline at the end of Phase 2 by 22 mm Hg (i.e., 77.1% of baseline).

Tilt: Supine blood pressure was normal. Blood pressure responses to tilt were normal.

Sudomotor evaluation: Electrochemical skin conductance was abnormal (reduced to 77.4% of normal limit) at hands and normal at feet.

Respiratory system: Respiratory frequency was normal supine position and during the tilt. End tidal CO_2 was reduced in supine position and during the tilt.

Cerebral blood flow velocity (CBFv): CBFv in middle cerebral artery was normal in supine position. CBFv in middle cerebral artery was stable during the tilt.

Skin biopsy (sensory-epidermal): Epidermal nerve fiber density was normal at proximal leg and abnormal (reduced to 79.6% of normal limit) at distal leg.

Skin biopsy (sweat glands): Sweat gland nerve fiber density was normal at proximal leg and normal at distal leg.

TABLE 71.1 **RESULTS OF AUTONOMIC TESTING**

Blood pressure evaluation					
Test: Valsalva maneuver					
Pressure [mmHg]	Baseline	Phase 2			Phase 4
		Early	End		
Systolic	134	86	90		
Mean	96	68.7	74	n/a	
Diastolic	77	60	66	n/a	

Heart rate evaluation	
Test: Deep breathing	
Results	Norm*
6.17	≥14
Test: Valsalva ratio	
1.7	≥1.46
* adjusted for a gender and age	

(continued)

TABLE 71.1 CONTINUED

Test: Tilt test										
Position		HR [BPM]	Blood pressure [mmHg]		MCA Blood flow velocity [cm/s]				Respiratory frequency [breaths/min]	End tidal CO_2 [mmHg]
			Systolic	Diastolic	Systolic	Mean	Mean drop [%]	Diastolic		
Supine		81	121	79	102	71.3		56	12	28
Tilt [min]	1	111	121	84	97	68.3	4.2	54	13	28
	2	115	122	88						
	3	115	124	90						
	4	119	124	86						
	5	118	130	94	95	68.3	4.2	55	10	28
	6	119	129	87						
	7	117	124	88						
	8	118	126	87						
	9	120	117	86						
	10	120	119	86	94	67.3	5.6	54	11	30
	15									
	20									
	30									
	40									

Sudomotor evaluation - functional

Test: Quantitative sudomotor axon reflex test (QSART)				
Location	Site (l/r)	Latency [min]	Volume [µl]	Norm [µl]*
Forearm				≥0.08
Prox. leg				≥0.14
Distal leg				≥0.24
Foot				≥0.09

* Normative data are adjusted for gender and age of patient.

Test: Electrochemical skin conductance (ESC)				
Location	Left [µS]	Right [µS]	Average [µS/k]	Norm [µS/kg]
Hand	51	43	0.8	≥1.03
Feet	74	76	1.29	≥1.14
Forehead				

For grading uses ESC [µS] adjusted for weight [µS/k].

TABLE 71.1 CONTINUED

Small fiber (sensory + sudomotor) evaluation - morphological					
Test: Skin biopsy					
Location	Site (l/r)	Nerve fibers			
		Epidermal*		Sweat glands	
		Density	Norm	Density	Norm
Proximal leg – thigh	Right	14.69	≥8.3	38.8	≥37.8
Distal leg - calf	Right	7.37	≥9.26	36.5	≥36.5
Foot	Right		≥3.11		≥34.8

*Normative data for distal leg are adjusted for gender and age of patient.

QASAT*										
Heart rate		BP		CBFv		ET-CO2		Sudomotor		Total QASAT score
S. bradycardia	0	Low supine	0	Low supine	0	Low supine	1	QSART		
S. tachycardia	0	High supine	0	High supine	0	High supine	0	ESC	1	
Increase tilt	2	OH	0	Tilt response	0	Tilt low	2			
Decrease tilt	0	OHTN	0	CA	0	Tilt high	0	**Skin biopsy**		11
Deep breathing	2	VM	2	CVR	0			Epidermal	1	
VR	0			VM	0			Sweat gland	0	
Total	4	Total	2	Total	0	Total	3			

*QASAT. See Novak. Quantitative Scale for Grading of Cardiovascular Autonomic Reflex Tests and Small Fibers from Skin Biopsies. *J Neurol Disord* 2015;3:2.

S, supine; Increase tilt, increased response to tilt; Decrease tilt, decreased response to tilt; BP, blood pressure; VM, Valsalva maneuver; CBFv, cerebral blood flow velocity; CA, cerebral autoregulation; MCA, middle cerebral artery; VR, Valsalva ratio; CVR, cerebral vasoreactivity.

Patient-reported symptoms during testing: Dizziness during the tilt.

Patient-reported symptoms for past 2 weeks:

Lightheadedness or dizziness: Occasionally
Dry eyes or mouth: Occasionally
Pale feet: None
Cold feet: Occasionally
Reduced sweating: Occasionally
Reduced sweating after exercise: Occasionally
Increased sweating: Occasionally
Nausea: Often
Diarrhea: Often
Constipation: None
Urinary leaks: None
Current pain severity: 8
Aching pain: Occasionally, severe
Allodynia: None
Burning pain: None
Lancinating pain: Often, severe
Numbness: Occasionally, moderate
Prickling sensation: Often, moderate

AUTONOMIC TESTING INTERPRETATION

- Small fiber neuropathy, mild, length-dependent, affecting predominantly sensory fibers.
- Postural tachycardia syndrome (POTS), neuropathic form, mild.
- Hypocapnic hyperventilation, supine and orthostatic.

COMMENT

The testing showed supine and postural hypocapnia (Figure 71.1). Hypocapnia, particularly chronic, has multiple effects including reduction in cerebral blood flow ands changes in neuronal excitability. Hypocapnia can be physiologic or can be part of hyperventilation syndrome.[1–3] Postural hypocapnia is seen in POTS[4] or in hypocapnic cerebral hypoperfusion.

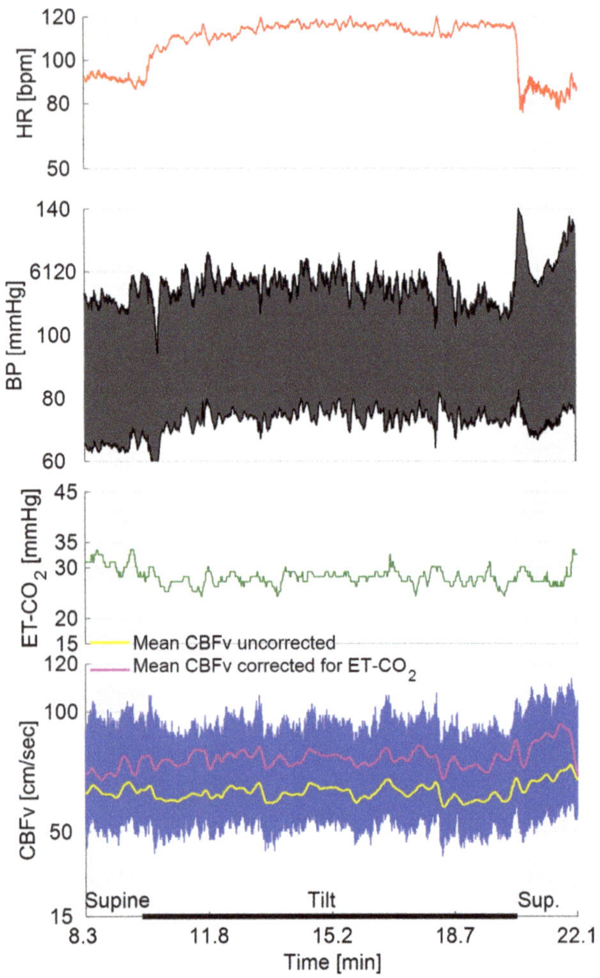

Figure 71.1 The tilt test showed mild orthostatic tachycardia with stable blood pressure and cerebral blood flow velocity. Patient was hyperventilating during both supine and tilt, as indicated by low end tidal CO_2.

The second finding of the study was mild POTS. Deconditioning also may play role in POTS.[5]

The third finding of the study was small fiber neuropathy, which is associated with hypermobile Ehlers-Danlos syndrome.[6] Combined effect of hypocapnia, POTS and small fiber neuropathy is probably responsible for patient's complaints.

TREATMENT AND FOLLOW-UP

- Evaluation of hypocapnia.
- Reconditioning program.

CAVEATS

- Hyperventilation syndrome can coexist with hypermobile Ehlers-Danlos syndrome and POTS.

REFERENCES

1. Hornsveld H, Garssen B. Hyperventilation syndrome: an elegant but scientifically untenable concept. *Neth J Med*. 1997;50(1):13–20.
2. Sikter A, Frecska E, Braun IM, Gonda X, Rihmer Z. The role of hyperventilation: hypocapnia in the pathomechanism of panic disorder. *Rev Bras Psiquiatr Sao Paulo Braz 1999*. 2007;29(4):375–379.
3. Pfortmueller CA, Pauchard-Neuwerth SE, Leichtle AB, Fiedler GM, Exadaktylos AK, Lindner G. Primary hyperventilation in the emergency department: a first overview. *PLoS ONE*. 2015;10(6). doi:10.1371/journal.pone.0129562
4. Novak V, Spies JM, Novak P, McPhee BR, Rummans TA, Low PA. Hypocapnia and cerebral hypoperfusion in orthostatic intolerance. *Stroke*. 1998;29(9):1876–1881.
5. Parsaik A, Allison TG, Singer W, et al. Deconditioning in patients with orthostatic intolerance. *Neurology*. 2012;79(14):1435–1439. doi:10.1212/WNL.0b013e31826d5f95.
6. Cazzato D, Castori M, Lombardi R, et al. Small fiber neuropathy is a common feature of Ehlers-Danlos syndromes. *Neurology*. 2016;87(2):155–159. doi:10.1212/WNL.0000000000002847.

72.

CASE 67: EHLERS-DANLOS SYNDROME WITH POSTURAL TACHYCARDIA SYNDROME AND PSYCHOGENIC PSEUDOSYNCOPE

Chief complaint: Dizziness.

Case presentation: A 19-year-old woman had variety of complaints since middle school. She was able to do only limited athletic activities in middle and high school since prolonged walking and running was associated with pain at joints or limbs. She was eventually diagnosed with hypermobile Ehlers-Danlos syndrome. She started to become dizzy on standing at age 14 and began to faint at age 16. She is using a wheelchair for 2 years, as a tool to prevent fainting. She faints daily if she tries to walk. In hot environments, she gets dizzy soon after standing up and may vomit. She also noted abdominal pain provoked by meals, and constipation. She responded only minimally to proamatine and propranolol for orthostatic intolerance. She was referred for suspected autonomic failure and small fiber neuropathy.

Past medical history: Ehlers-Danlos syndrome hypermobility type, attention deficit hyperactive disorder.

Current medication: Proamatine (on hold), propranolol (on hold), ondansetron, methylphenidate.

Assessment plan: Functional autonomic tests and skin biopsy.

AUTONOMIC TESTING EVALUATION

See Table 72.1.

Heart rate: Heart rate responses to deep breathing were normal. There was supine tachycardia. The heart rate increment during the tilt was exaggerated (45 BPM) and exceeded 163 BPM.

Blood pressure:

Valsalva maneuver: Mean blood pressure failed to return to baseline at the end of Phase 2 by 27.6 mm Hg (i.e., 62.9% of baseline).

Tilt: Supine blood pressure was within normal range. Patient became unresponsive at the first minute of the tilt, and tilt was aborted. At that time, the patient was tachycardic but blood pressure and cerebral blood flow were stable.

Sudomotor evaluation: Electrochemical skin conductance was abnormal (reduced to 94% of normal limit) at hands and normal at feet.

Respiratory system: The supine respiratory frequency and end tidal CO_2 were normal. There was tachypnea and hypocapnia during the tilt.

TABLE 72.1 **RESULTS OF AUTONOMIC TESTING**

Blood pressure evaluation					
Test: Valsalva maneuver					
Pressure [mmHg]	Baseline	Phase 2 Early	Phase 2 End		Phase 4
Systolic	103	52	52		
Mean	74.3	46.7	46.7	n/a	
Diastolic	60	44	44	n/a	

Heart rate evaluation	
Test: Deep breathing	
Results	Norm*
18.67	≥14
Test: Valsalva ratio	
2.3	≥1.46
* adjusted for a gender and age	

(continued)

TABLE 72.1 **CONTINUED**

Test: Tilt test											
Position		HR [BPM]	Blood pressure [mmHg]		MCA Blood flow velocity [cm/s]				Respiratory frequency [breaths/min]	End tidal CO_2 [mmHg]
			Systolic	Diastolic	Systolic	Mean	Mean drop [%]	Diastolic		
Supine		118	111	73	131	76.3		49	14	36
Tilt [min]	1	163	133	87	131	81		56	25	28
	2									
	3									
	4									
	5									
	6									
	7									
	8									
	9									
	10									
	15									
	20									
	30									
	40									

Sudomotor evaluation - functional

Test: Quantitative sudomotor axon reflex test (QSART)				
Location	Site (l/r)	Latency [min]	Volume [µl]	Norm [µl]*
Forearm				≥0.08
Prox. leg				≥0.14
Distal leg				≥0.24
Foot				≥0.09

* Normative data are adjusted for gender and age of patient.

Test: Electrochemical skin conductance (ESC)				
Location	Left [µS]	Right [µS]	Average [µS/k]	Norm [µS/kg]
Hand	53	55	0.97	≥1.03
Feet	88	88	1.58	≥1.14
Forehead				

For grading uses ESC [µS] adjusted for weight [µS/k].

TABLE 72.1 CONTINUED

Small fiber (sensory + sudomotor) evaluation - morphological					
Test: Skin biopsy					
Location	Site (l/r)	Nerve fibers			
		Epidermal*		Sweat glands	
		Density	Norm	Density	Norm
Proximal leg – thigh	Right	9.31	≥8.3		≥37.8
Distal leg - calf	Right	3.19	≥9.58		≥36.5
Foot	Right		≥3.11		≥34.8

*Normative data for distal leg are adjusted for gender and age of patient.

QASAT*											
Heart rate		**BP**		**CBFv**		**ET-CO2**		**Sudomotor**			**Total QASAT score**
S. bradycardia	0	Low supine	0	Low supine		Low supine		QSART			
S. tachycardia	0	High supine	0	High supine		High supine		ESC	1		
Increase tilt		OH		Tilt response		Tilt low					
Decrease tilt		OHTN		CA		Tilt high		**Skin biopsy**			6
Deep breathing	0	VM	2	CVR				Epidermal	3		
VR	0			VM				Sweat gland			
Total	0	Total	2	Total		Total					

*QASAT. See Novak. Quantitative Scale for Grading of Cardiovascular Autonomic Reflex Tests and Small Fibers from Skin Biopsies. *J Neurol Disord* 2015;3:2. Orthostatic (tilt) responses were not graded since QASAT requires the duration of the tilt at least 10 minutes.

S, supine; Increase tilt, increased response to tilt; Decrease tilt, decreased response to tilt; BP, blood pressure; VM, Valsalva maneuver; CBFv, cerebral blood flow velocity; CA, cerebral autoregulation; MCA, middle cerebral artery; VR, Valsalva ratio; CVR, cerebral vasoreactivity.

Cerebral blood flow velocity (CBFv): CBFv in middle cerebral artery was normal in supine position. CBFv in middle cerebral artery was stable during the tilt test.

Skin biopsy (sensory-epidermal): Epidermal nerve fiber density was normal at proximal leg and abnormal (reduced to 33.3% of normal limit) at distal leg.

Skin biopsy (sweat glands): No sweat glands found in the specimen.

Patient-reported symptoms during testing: Loss of consciousness.

Patient-reported symptoms for past 2 weeks:

Lightheadedness or dizziness: Often
Dry eyes or mouth: Occasionally
Pale feet: Often
Cold feet: Often
Reduced sweating: None
Reduced sweating after exercise: Occasionally
Increased sweating: Occasionally
Nausea: Often
Diarrhea: None
Constipation: Occasionally
Urinary leaks: Occasionally
Current pain severity: 4
Aching pain: Often, moderate
Allodynia: Occasionally, moderate
Burning pain: Occasionally, mild
Lancinating pain: Often, moderate
Numbness: Often, moderate
Prickling sensation: Occasionally, mild

AUTONOMIC TESTING INTERPRETATION

- Psychogenic pseudosyncope.
- Postural tachycardia syndrome (POTS), neuropathic form.
- Small fiber neuropathy, length-dependent, affecting predominantly sensory fibers.

COMMENT

Patient became unresponsive at the first minute of the tilt; she was tachycardic, but blood pressure and cerebral blood flow were stable, which is consistent with psychogenic pseudosyncope (Figure 72.1).

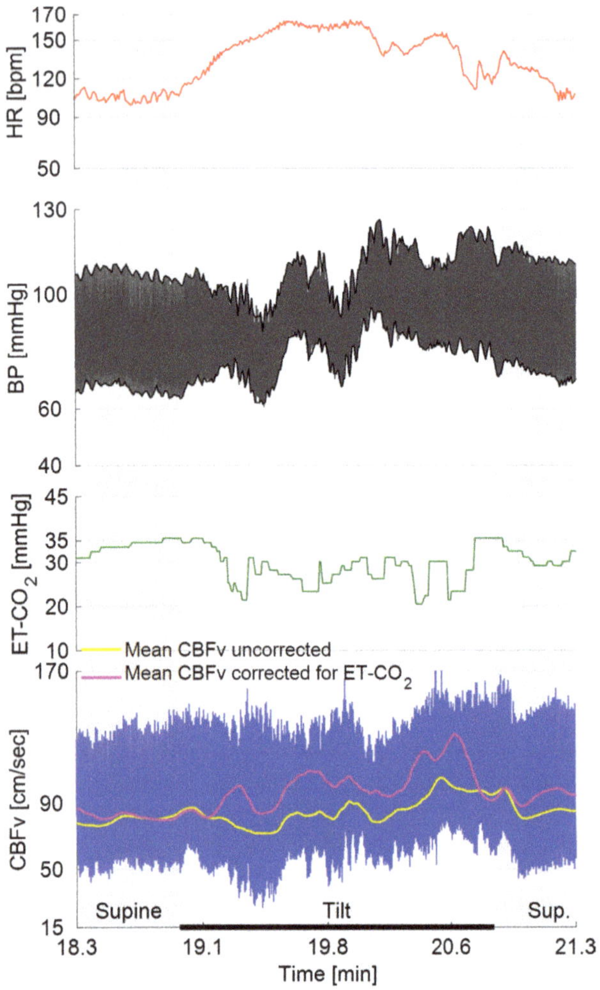

Figure 72.1 The tilt test provoked severe tachycardia almost immediately after tilting. Blood pressure and cerebral blood flow velocity (CBFv) were fluctuating, but respective means were stable. Patient was tilted for only 1 minute since she lost consciousness. Per request of her relative who was present during testing, the tilt was aborted.

It was concluded that the patient has POTS, even the POTS criteria require excessive tachycardia at the third minute of the tilt[1] and the tilt was terminated at the first minute. Nevertheless, the testing also showed orthostatic hypocapnia which is characteristic for POTS. It can be argued that the patient has inappropriate sinus tachycardia (IST) since the presence of supine tachycardia. However the supine tachycardia can be due to hypovolemia and/or deconditioning as suggests the collapse of the pulse pressure during the phase II of the Valsalva maneuver (Table 72.1).

Small fiber neuropathy is likely due to hypermobile Ehlers-Danlos syndrome.[2]

TREATMENT AND FOLLOW-UP

- Patient may need comprehensive care to address small fiber neuropathy, POTS, and psychogenic pseudosyncope.

CAVEATS

- Psychogenic pseudosyncope can be superimposed on POTS.
- Psychogenic pseudosyncope, small fiber neuropathy, and POTS are associated with hypermobile Ehlers-Danlos syndrome.

REFERENCES

1. Low PA, Sandroni P, Joyner M, Shen W-K. Postural tachycardia syndrome (POTS). *J Cardiovasc Electrophysiol.* 2009;20(3):352–358. doi:10.1111/j.1540-8167.2008.01407.x.
2. Cazzato D, Castori M, Lombardi R, et al. Small fiber neuropathy is a common feature of Ehlers-Danlos syndromes. *Neurology.* 2016;87(2):155–159. doi:10.1212/WNL.0000000000002847.

73.

CASE 68: UNKNOWN CONNECTIVE TISSUE DISORDER AND POSTURAL TACHYCARDIA SYNDROME

Chief complaint: Orthostatic intolerance.

Case presentation: A 33-year-old woman with marfanoid body habitus presents with chronic pain for most of her life. For the past 10 years, she also noted tremor of arms and legs, postural dizziness, abdominal pain, diarrhea, nosebleeds, vaginal bleeding, palpitations, and excessive sweating. There was no consensus if she satisfies the criteria for Ehlers-Danlos syndrome. Genetic testing was negative for the fibrillin-1 gene mutation but revealed variants of unknown significance in SKI and filamin A genes. Patient was referred for evaluation of orthostatic intolerance.

Past medical history: Marfanoid habitus.

Current medication: None.

Assessment plan: Functional autonomic tests and skin biopsy.

AUTONOMIC TESTING EVALUATION

See Table 73.1.

Heart rate: Supine heart rate was normal. Heart rate responses to deep breathing were reduced to 45.8% of normal value. Heart rate increment during the tilt (32 BPM) was exaggerated.

Blood pressure:

Valsalva maneuver: Mean blood pressure failed to return to baseline at the end of Phase 2 by 8.7 mm Hg (i.e., 90.6% of baseline).

Tilt: Supine blood pressure was normal. Blood pressure responses to tilt were normal.

Sudomotor evaluation: Electrochemical skin conductance was normal at hands and normal at feet.

Respiratory system: Respiratory frequency was normal in supine position but was increased during the tilt. End tidal CO_2 was normal in supine position but was reduced during the tilt.

Cerebral blood flow velocity (CBFv): CBFv in middle cerebral artery was normal in supine position.

Skin biopsy (sensory-epidermal): Epidermal nerve fiber density was normal at proximal leg and normal at distal leg.

Skin biopsy (sweat glands): Sweat gland nerve fiber density was normal at proximal leg and normal at distal leg.

Patient-reported symptoms during testing: Dizziness, shortness of breath during the tilt.

TABLE 73.1 **RESULTS OF AUTONOMIC TESTING**

Blood pressure evaluation

Test: Valsalva maneuver

Pressure [mmHg]	Baseline	Phase 2			Phase 4
		Early	End		
Systolic	117	81	97		
Mean	93	69	84.3	n/a	
Diastolic	81	63	78	n/a	

Heart rate evaluation

Test: Deep breathing	
Results	Norm*
5.5	≥12
Test: Valsalva ratio	
1.68	≥1.5

* adjusted for a gender and age

(continued)

TABLE 73.1 CONTINUED

Test: Tilt test										
Position		HR [BPM]	Blood pressure [mmHg]		MCA Blood flow velocity [cm/s]				Respiratory frequency [breaths/min]	End tidal CO_2 [mmHg]
			Systolic	Diastolic	Systolic	Mean	Mean drop [%]	Diastolic		
Supine		94	108	70	123	82.3		62	12	36
Tilt [min]	1	110	110	66	107	71.7	12.9	54	19	32
	2	122	113	81						
	3	118	116	77						
	4	118	115	81						
	5	119	114	79	111	73.7	10.4	55	23	31
	6	122	113	78						
	7	122	110	77						
	8	125	110	77						
	9	126	118	71						
	10	125	111	81	110	72.7	11.7	54	21	29
	15									
	20									
	30									
	40									

Sudomotor evaluation - functional

Test: Quantitative sudomotor axon reflex test (QSART)				
Location	Site (l/r)	Latency [min]	Volume [µl]	Norm [µl]*
Forearm				≥0.08
Prox. leg				≥0.14
Distal leg				≥0.15
Foot				≥0.07

* Normative data are adjusted for gender and age of patient.

Test: Electrochemical skin conductance (ESC)				
Location	Left [µS]	Right [µS]	Average [µS/k]	Norm [µS/kg]
Hand	87	86	1.76	≥1.03
Feet	88	94	1.92	≥1.14
Forehead				

For grading uses ESC [µS] adjusted for weight [µS/k].

TABLE 73.1 CONTINUED

Small fiber (sensory + sudomotor) evaluation - morphological					
Test: Skin biopsy					
Location	Site (l/r)	Nerve fibers			
		Epidermal*		Sweat glands	
		Density	Norm	Density	Norm
Proximal leg – thigh	Right	14.21	≥8.3	45.7	≥37.8
Distal leg - calf	Right	13.31	≥8.46	39.4	≥36.5
Foot	Right		≥3.11		≥34.8

*Normative data for distal leg are adjusted for gender and age of patient.

QASAT*												
Heart rate		**BP**		**CBFv**		**ET-CO2**		**Sudomotor**			**Total QASAT score**
S. bradycardia	0	Low supine	0	Low supine	0	Low supine	0	QSART			
S. tachycardia	0	High supine	0	High supine	0	High supine	0	ESC	0		
Increase tilt	3	OH	0	Tilt response	1	Tilt low	1				
Decrease tilt	0	OHTN	0	CA	0	Tilt high	0	**Skin biopsy**			8
Deep breathing	2	VM	1	CVR	0			Epidermal	0		
VR	0			VM	0			Sweat gland	0		
Total	5	Total	1	Total	1	Total	1				

*QASAT. See Novak. Quantitative Scale for Grading of Cardiovascular Autonomic Reflex Tests and Small Fibers from Skin Biopsies. *J Neurol Disord* 2015;3:2.

S, supine; Increase tilt, increased response to tilt; Decrease tilt, decreased response to tilt; BP, blood pressure; VM, Valsalva maneuver; CBFv, cerebral blood flow velocity; CA, cerebral autoregulation; MCA, middle cerebral artery; VR, Valsalva ratio; CVR, cerebral vasoreactivity.

Patient-reported symptoms for past 2 weeks:

Lightheadedness or dizziness: Often
Dry eyes or mouth: Occasionally
Pale feet: Yes, minor annoyance
Cold feet: Yes, minor annoyance
Reduced sweating: Yes, minor annoyance
Reduced sweating after exercise: None
Increased sweating: Occasionally
Nausea: Occasionally
Diarrhea: Often
Constipation: Yes, minor annoyance
Urinary leaks: None
Current pain severity: 4
Aching pain: Often, moderate
Allodynia: Occasionally, mild
Burning pain: Occasionally, moderate
Lancinating pain: Occasionally, severe
Numbness: Often, mild
Prickling sensation: Occasionally, mild

AUTONOMIC TEST INTERPRETATION

- Postural tachycardia syndrome (POTS), neuropathic form.
- There was no evidence of small fiber neuropathy on skin biopsy.

COMMENTS

The testing showed typical POTS, neuropathic form associated with autonomic adrenergic neuropathy as indicated by abnormal Valsalva maneuver (Figure 73.1). Although the patient has marfanoid habitus, she tested negative for the fibrillin-1 gene mutation which underlies the Marfan syndrome.[1] Genetic testing showed mutation in two genes: SKI and filamin A (FLNA): SKI (coding DNA c.1162G>A, variant p.Ala388Thr (A388T), heterozygous

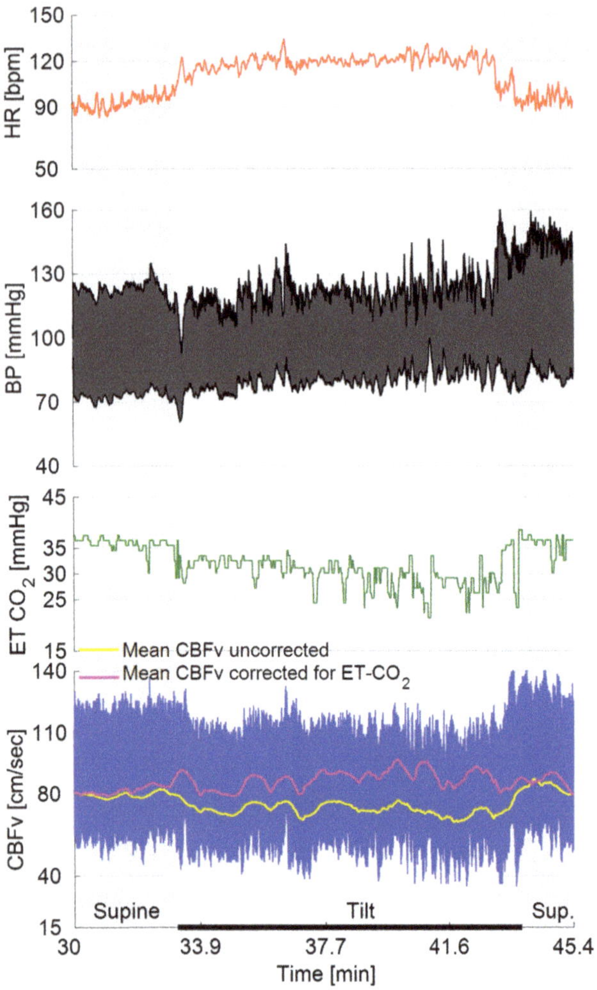

Figure 73.1 The tilt test was consistent with exaggerated heart rate responses but normal blood pressure. End tidal CO_2 and cerebral blood flow velocity were reduced during the tilt.

variant of uncertain significance and filamin A FLNA gene (coding DNA c.1411A>G, variant p.Thr471Ala (T471A), heterozygous, a novel variant of uncertain significance. Interestingly, FLNA plays a role in cytoskeleton and connective tissue development. A splice mutation results in Ehlers-Danlos syndrome.[2,3]

TREATMENT AND FOLLOW-UP

- Follow guidelines for therapy of Ehlers-Danlos syndrome and orthostatic intolerance.[4,5]

CAVEATS

- FLNA mutation can be associated with POTS.

REFERENCES

1. Rommel K, Karck M, Haverich A, et al. Identification of 29 novel and nine recurrent fibrillin-1 (FBN1) mutations and genotype-phenotype correlations in 76 patients with Marfan syndrome. *Hum Mutat*. 2005;26(6):529–539. doi:10.1002/humu.20239.
2. Ritelli M, Morlino S, Giacopuzzi E, et al. Ehlers-Danlos syndrome with lethal cardiac valvular dystrophy in males carrying a novel splice mutation in FLNA. *Am J Med Genet A*. 2017;173(1):169–176. doi:10.1002/ajmg.a.38004.
3. Sheen VL, Walsh CA. Periventricular heterotopia: new insights into Ehlers-Danlos syndrome. *Clin Med Res*. 2005;3(4):229–233.
4. Cazzato D, Castori M, Lombardi R, et al. Small fiber neuropathy is a common feature of Ehlers-Danlos syndromes. *Neurology*. 2016;87(2):155–159. doi:10.1212/WNL.0000000000002847.
5. Grigoriou E, Boris JR, Dormans JP. Postural orthostatic tachycardia syndrome (POTS): association with Ehlers-Danlos syndrome and orthopaedic considerations. *Clin Orthop*. 2015;473(2):722–728. doi:10.1007/s11999-014-3898-x.

74.

CASE 69: SMALL FIBER NEUROPATHY, HYPOCAPNIC CEREBRAL HYPOPERFUSION, AND GENERALIZED HYPERMOBILITY SPECTRUM DISORDER

Chief complaint: Dizziness.

Case presentation: A 34-year-old woman presents with a complex history. She has sinus infections every 3–4 months, starting at age 15. At about the same time, she noted purple feet and foot pain upon standing and walking. She also noted reduced sensation in her toes and numbness and tingling in her feet. Tingling occurs randomly in the legs; running may improve the numbness. She also has daily pain; her whole body aches, including joint pain and migraine. She has an electrical-like shock sensation at the neck when she bends her neck, radiating down to her legs. She has constant dry mouth and dry nose. She uses a saline spray for her nose and frequent eye drops. She has hives and sensitive skin and scarring on the sides of the neck from urticarial lesions. She has flushing and redness in the face, ears, and chest and feels like she is on fire. She has a history of elevated blood pressure since her 20s. She has a history of alternating constipation and diarrhea for many years. She has hypermobile joints, and her skin heals poorly. She has had normal chest computed tomography (CT). MRI of the brain and of the cervical spine was normal. Evaluations for Sjögren's syndrome, systemic lupus erythematosus, mast cell activation disorders, and Ehlers-Danlos syndrome were negative. She does, however, satisfy criteria for generalized hypermobility spectrum disorder. She was referred for evaluation of suspected small fiber neuropathy and/or autonomic failure.

Past medical history: Generalized hypermobility spectrum disorder, irritable bowel syndrome, migraine, insomnia.

Current medication: Topiramate.

Assessment plan: Functional autonomic tests and skin biopsy.

AUTONOMIC TESTING EVALUATION

See Table 74.1.

Heart rate: There was supine tachycardia. Heart rate increment during the tilt (27 BPM) was normal.

Blood pressure:

Valsalva maneuver: Mean blood pressure failed to return to baseline at the end of Phase 2 by 8 mm Hg (i.e., 92.1% of baseline). Supine blood pressure was normal.

Tilt: Blood pressure was elevated during the tilt.

Sudomotor evaluation: Sweat output was normal at forearm, normal at proximal leg, normal at distal leg, and normal at foot. Quantitative sudomotor axon reflex test

TABLE 74.1 **RESULTS OF AUTONOMIC TESTING**

Blood pressure evaluation					
Test: Valsalva maneuver					
Pressure [mmHg]	Baseline	Phase 2			Phase 4
		Early	End		
Systolic	138	90	108		
Mean	100.7	77.3	92.7	n/a	
Diastolic	82	71	85	n/a	

Heart rate evaluation	
Test: Deep breathing	
Results	Norm*
5	≥12
Test: Valsalva ratio	
2.27	≥1.5
* adjusted for a gender and age	

(continued)

TABLE 74.1 **CONTINUED**

Test: Tilt test											
Position		HR [BPM]	Blood pressure [mmHg]		MCA Blood flow velocity [cm/s]				Respiratory frequency [breaths/min]	End tidal CO_2 [mmHg]
			Systolic	Diastolic	Systolic	Mean	Mean drop [%]	Diastolic		
Supine		121	127	79	111	74.3		56	15	35
Tilt [min]	1	148	134	93	99	65.7	11.6	49	24	19
	2	145	131	92						
	3	140	142	92						
	4	148	132	95						
	5	145	128	87	83	52.3	29.6	37	13	21
	6	148	145	96						
	7	148	138	95						
	8	140	141	104						
	9	140	140	98						
	10	140	129	92	82	51.3	31	36	11	22
	15									
	20									
	30									
	40									

Sudomotor evaluation - functional

Test: Quantitative sudomotor axon reflex test (QSART)				
Location	Site (l/r)	Latency [min]	Volume [µl]	Norm [µl]*
Forearm	l	1.43	0.649	≥0.08
Prox. leg	l	1.2	0.986	≥0.14
Distal leg	l	0.58	1.177	≥0.15
Foot	l	3.51	0.204	≥0.07

* Normative data are adjusted for gender and age of patient.

Test: Electrochemical skin conductance (ESC)				
Location	Left [µS]	Right [µS]	Average [µS/k]	Norm [µS/kg]
Hand				≥1.03
Feet				≥1.14
Forehead				

For grading uses ESC [µS] adjusted for weight [µS/k].

TABLE 74.1 CONTINUED

Small fiber (sensory + sudomotor) evaluation - morphological					
Test: Skin biopsy					
Location	Site (l/r)	Nerve fibers			
		Epidermal*		Sweat glands	
		Density	Norm	Density	Norm
Proximal leg – thigh	Right	14.51	≥8.3		≥37.8
Distal leg - calf	Right	9.1	≥8.38	21.5	≥36.5
Foot	Right		≥3.11		≥34.8

*Normative data for distal leg are adjusted for gender and age of patient.

QASAT*										
Heart rate		BP		CBFv		ET-CO2		Sudomotor		Total QASAT score
S. bradycardia	0	Low supine	0	Low supine	0	Low supine	0	QSART	1	
S. tachycardia	1	High supine	0	High supine	0	High supine	0	ESC		
Increase tilt	0	OH	0	Tilt response	5	Tilt low	8			
Decrease tilt	0	OHTN	0	CA	0	Tilt high	0	**Skin biopsy**		22
Deep breathing	2	VM	1	CVR	0			Epidermal	0	
VR	1			VM	0			Sweat gland	3	
Total	4	Total	1	Total	5	Total	8			

*QASAT. See Novak. Quantitative Scale for Grading of Cardiovascular Autonomic Reflex Tests and Small Fibers from Skin Biopsies. *J Neurol Disord* 2015;3:2.

S, supine; Increase tilt, increased response to tilt; Decrease tilt, decreased response to tilt; BP, blood pressure; VM, Valsalva maneuver; CBFv, cerebral blood flow velocity; CA, cerebral autoregulation; MCA, middle cerebral artery; VR, Valsalva ratio; CVR, cerebral vasoreactivity.

(QSART) showed length-dependent pattern with a decrease of sweat output distally of at least 33%.

Respiratory system: Respiratory frequency was normal in supine position but was increased during the tilt. End tidal CO_2 was normal in supine position but was severely reduced during the tilt.

Cerebral blood flow velocity (CBFv): CBFv in middle cerebral artery was normal in supine position but was severely reduced during the tilt.

Skin biopsy (sensory-epidermal): Epidermal nerve fiber density was normal at proximal leg and normal at distal leg.

Skin biopsy (sweat glands): Sweat gland nerve fiber density was abnormal (reduced to 58.9% of normal limit) at distal leg.

Patient-reported symptoms during testing: Dizziness and shortness of breath during the tilt.

Patient-reported symptoms for past 2 weeks:

Lightheadedness or dizziness: Often
Dry eyes or mouth: Often
Pale feet: Often
Cold feet: Often
Reduced sweating: Occasionally
Reduced sweating after exercise: None
Increased sweating: Occasionally
Nausea: Often
Diarrhea: Occasionally
Constipation: Occasionally
Urinary leaks: Occasionally
Current pain severity: 7
Aching pain: Often, moderate
Allodynia: Often, moderate
Burning pain: Often, moderate
Lancinating pain: Often, severe
Numbness: Often, severe
Prickling sensation: Often, severe

AUTONOMIC TESTING INTERPRETATION

- Small fiber neuropathy, autonomic.
- Hypocapnic cerebral hypoperfusion (HYCH).
- Sinus tachycardia.

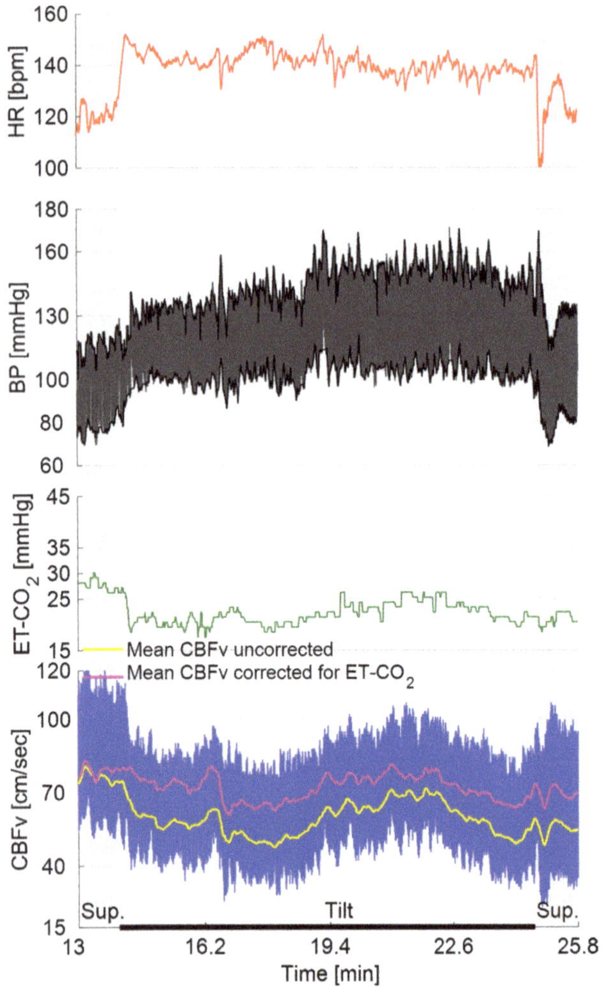

Figure 74.1 The tilt test showed severe tachycardia, both supine and orthostatic, with normal heart rate increment during the tilt. Orthostatic blood pressure was elevated. End tidal CO_2 and cerebral blood flow velocity (CBFv) were reduced during the tilt. CBFv adjusted for the end tidal CO_2 was normal.

COMMENT

Autonomic testing showed small fiber neuropathy affecting autonomic fibers. In addition, there was evidence of sinus tachycardia and HYCH, which may contribute to orthostatic intolerance (Figure 74.1).

This patient has joint hypermobility, and she was diagnosed with generalized hypermobility spectrum disorder (GHSD).[1] A GHSD has been defined recently as a diagnostic entity for patients with symptomatic joint hypermobility but who do not meet criteria for hypermobile Ehlers-Danlos syndrome or to any other syndromes with joint hypermobility.[1]

TREATMENT AND FOLLOW-UP

- β-Blockers for tachycardia.
- Pain control.

CAVEATS

- GHSD is associated with small fiber neuropathy and HYCH.

REFERENCE

1. Castori M, Tinkle B, Levy H, Grahame R, Malfait F, Hakim A. A framework for the classification of joint hypermobility and related conditions. *Am J Med Genet C Semin Med Genet.* 2017;175(1): 148–157. doi:10.1002/ajmg.c.31539.

75.

CASE 70: SMALL FIBER NEUROPATHY AND GENERALIZED HYPERMOBILITY SPECTRUM DISORDER

Chief complaint: Chronic pain.

Case presentation: A 26-year-old woman presents with chronic diffuse pain since age 11. The pain is of variable character, affecting joints, limbs, and muscles. Additional complains include dizziness on standing and balance problems with history of several falls per year, She has history of flexible joints. She was seen by a genetic specialist and diagnosed with generalized hypermobility spectrum disorder (GHSD). She was referred for evaluation of suspected small fiber neuropathy and/or autonomic failure.

Past medical history: GHSD, migraine, obstructive sleep apnea.

Current medication: Celecoxib, ranitidine.

Assessment plan: Functional autonomic tests and skin biopsy.

AUTONOMIC TESTING EVALUATION

See Table 75.1.

Heart rate: Supine heart rate was normal. Heart rate responses to deep breathing were reduced to 90% of normal value. Heart rate increment during the tilt (37 BPM) was exaggerated but did not reach 120 BPM.

Blood pressure:

Valsalva maneuver: Mean blood pressure failed to return to baseline at the end of Phase 2 by 5 mm Hg (i.e., 95.6% of baseline).

Tilt: Supine blood pressure was normal. Blood pressure was elevated during the tilt. Blood pressure responses to tilt were normal.

Sudomotor evaluation: Electrochemical skin conductance was abnormal (reduced to 72.3% of normal limit) at hands and abnormal (reduced to 77.4% of normal limit) at feet.

Respiratory system: Respiratory frequency was normal in supine position. Respiratory frequency was normal during the tilt. End tidal CO_2 was reduced in supine position. End tidal CO_2 was mildly reduced during the tilt.

Cerebral blood flow velocity (CBFv): CBFv in middle cerebral artery was normal in supine position. CBFv in middle cerebral artery was stable during the tilt.

Skin biopsy (sensory-epidermal): Epidermal nerve fiber density was normal at proximal leg and abnormal (reduced to 86% of normal limit) at distal leg.

Skin biopsy (sweat glands): Sweat gland nerve fiber density was normal at proximal leg and abnormal (reduced to 76.2% of normal limit) at distal leg.

TABLE 75.1 **RESULTS OF AUTONOMIC TESTING**

Blood pressure evaluation					
Test: Valsalva maneuver					
Pressure [mmHg]	Baseline	Phase 2			Phase 4
		Early	End		
Systolic	149	113	132		
Mean	114.3	90.3	109.3	n/a	
Diastolic	97	79	98	n/a	

Heart rate evaluation	
Test: Deep breathing	
Results	Norm*
12.6	≥14
Test: Valsalva ratio	
1.98	≥1.46
* adjusted for a gender and age	

(continued)

TABLE 75.1 CONTINUED

Test: Tilt test											
Position		HR [BPM]	Blood pressure [mmHg]		MCA Blood flow velocity [cm/s]				Respiratory frequency [breaths/min]	End tidal CO_2 [mmHg]
			Systolic	Diastolic	Systolic	Mean	Mean drop [%]	Diastolic		
Supine		75	128	85	94	62		46	17	31
Tilt [min]	1	99	130	91	91	61	1.6	46	18	31
	2	100	131	89						
	3	107	130	89						
	4	106	132	93						
	5	104	124	89	86	56.7	8.5	42	13	30
	6	112	123	91						
	7	103	125	88						
	8	103	129	86						
	9	109	127	89						
	10	111	126	86	88	56.7	8.5	41	14	30
	15									
	20									
	30									
	40									

Sudomotor evaluation - functional

Test: Quantitative sudomotor axon reflex test (QSART)				
Location	Site (l/r)	Latency [min]	Volume [µl]	Norm [µl]*
Forearm				≥0.08
Prox. leg				≥0.14
Distal leg				≥0.24
Foot				≥0.09

* Normative data are adjusted for gender and age of patient.

Test: Electrochemical skin conductance (ESC)				
Location	Left [µS]	Right [µS]	Average [µS/k]	Norm [µS/kg]
Hand	76	76	0.74	≥1.03
Feet	90	91	0.89	≥1.14
Forehead				

For grading uses ESC [µS] adjusted for weight [µS/k].

TABLE 75.1 CONTINUED

Small fiber (sensory + sudomotor) evaluation - morphological					
Test: Skin biopsy					
Location	Site (l/r)	Nerve fibers			
		Epidermal*		Sweat glands	
		Density	Norm	Density	Norm
Proximal leg – thigh	Right	9.99	≥8.3	43.3	≥37.8
Distal leg - calf	Right	7.76	≥9.02	27.8	≥36.5
Foot	Right		≥3.11		≥34.8

*Normative data for distal leg are adjusted for gender and age of patient.

QASAT*										
Heart rate		BP		CBFv		ET-CO2		Sudomotor		Total QASAT score
S. bradycardia	0	Low supine	0	Low supine	0	Low supine	1	QSART		
S. tachycardia	0	High supine	0	High supine	0	High supine	0	ESC	2	
Increase tilt	1	OH	0	Tilt response	0	Tilt low	2			
Decrease tilt	0	OHTN	0	CA	0	Tilt high	0	**Skin biopsy**		12
Deep breathing	1	VM	1	CVR	0			Epidermal	1	
VR	0			VM	0			Sweat gland	3	
Total	2	Total	1	Total	0	Total	3			

*QASAT. See Novak. Quantitative Scale for Grading of Cardiovascular Autonomic Reflex Tests and Small Fibers from Skin Biopsies. *J Neurol Disord* 2015;3:2.

S, supine; Increase tilt, increased response to tilt; Decrease tilt, decreased response to tilt; BP, blood pressure; VM, Valsalva maneuver; CBFv, cerebral blood flow velocity; CA, cerebral autoregulation; MCA, middle cerebral artery; VR, Valsalva ratio; CVR, cerebral vasoreactivity.

Patient-reported symptoms during testing: None during the tilt.

Patient-reported symptoms for past 2 weeks:

Lightheadedness or dizziness: Occasionally
Dry eyes or mouth: Occasionally
Pale feet: None
Cold feet: Occasionally
Reduced sweating: None
Reduced sweating after exercise: None
Increased sweating: None
Nausea: Occasionally
Diarrhea: Occasionally
Constipation: Occasionally
Urinary leaks: None
Current pain severity: 2
Aching pain: often, moderate
Allodynia: None
Burning pain: Occasionally, moderate
Lancinating pain: Occasionally, moderate
Numbness: Often, moderate
Prickling sensation: Often, moderate

AUTONOMIC TESTING INTERPRETATION

- Small fiber neuropathy, mixed, length-dependent, affecting sensory and autonomic fibers.
- Generalized autonomic failure, mild, affecting all major branches of autonomic nervous system (parasympathetic, adrenergic, and sudomotor). Orthostatic hypotension, a marker of more advanced adrenergic failure, was not seen in this study.
- CBFv was stable.
- Mild hypocapnic hyperventilation during the supine position and during the tilt.

COMMENT

The autonomic testing showed mixed small fiber neuropathy, which can be responsible for both sensory complaints and dysautonomia. The dysautonomia detected in the study was generalized but mild and was associated with mild

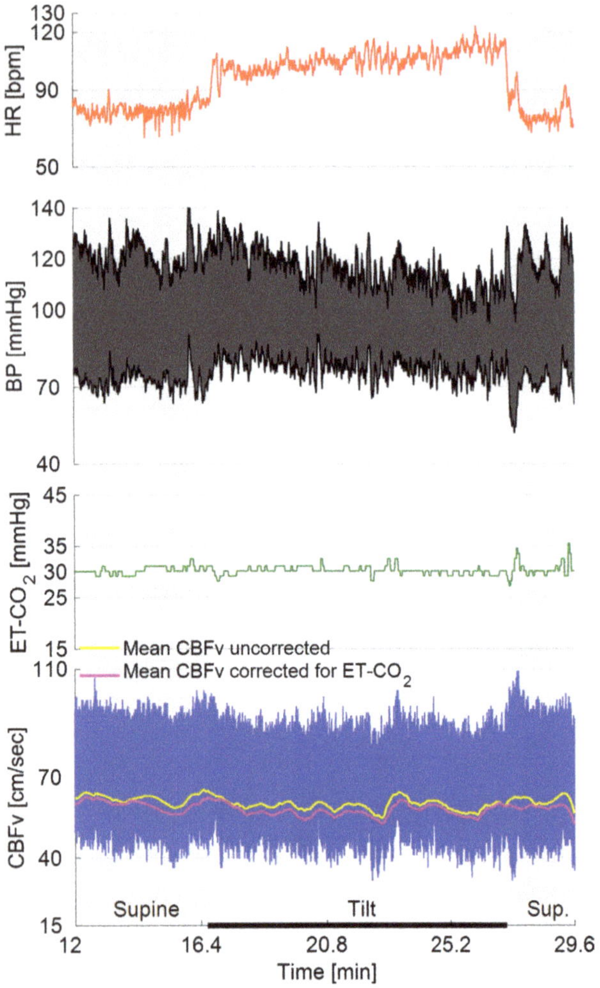

Figure 75.1 Tilt test showed mild orthostatic intolerance with stable cerebral blood flow velocity, end tidal CO_2, and blood pressure. Patient was asymptomatic.

orthostatic intolerance (Figure 75.1). Although the heart rate responses to tilt were exaggerated (BPM increment >30 BPM), the heart rate did not reach 120 BPM, which is also required in most definitions of postural tachycardia syndrome (POTS).[1] Furthermore, according to the POTS criteria, the patient should be symptomatic, which she was not during the tilt.

The patient has GHSD, which is related to hypermobile Ehlers-Danlos syndromes (h-EDS).[2] GHSD differs from h-EDS, although there is considerable overlap of symptoms while using stricter diagnostic criteria for h-EDS. In contrast to h-EDS, little is known about the involvement of small fibers and dysautonomia in GHSD. This study showed evidence of small fiber neuropathy and associated mild dysautonomia in this patient with GHSD.

TREATMENT AND FOLLOW-UP

- Volume expansion through high fluid and high salt intake.
- Physical therapy accommodated for hypermobility disorders.
- Pain control.

CAVEATS

- GHSD is associated with small fiber neuropathy and mild but generalized autonomic failure.

REFERENCES

1. Low PA, Sandroni P, Joyner M, Shen W-K. Postural tachycardia syndrome (POTS). *J Cardiovasc Electrophysiol*. 2009;20(3):352–358. doi:10.1111/j.1540-8167.2008.01407.x.
2. Castori M, Tinkle B, Levy H, Grahame R, Malfait F, Hakim A. A framework for the classification of joint hypermobility and related conditions. *Am J Med Genet C Semin Med Genet*. 2017;175(1): 148–157. doi:10.1002/ajmg.c.31539.

76.

CASE 71: SMALL FIBER NEUROPATHY, POSTURAL TACHYCARDIA, AND MAST CELL ACTIVATION SYNDROME

Chief complaint: Dizziness and fluctuating numbness.

Case presentation: A 49-year-old women presents with numbness, headaches, flushing, mental fog, abdominal pain, fatigue, dry skin, feeling cold, whole-body aches, postprandial hypotension, and intermittent lethargy with confusion for 12 years. She was diagnosed with mast cell activation syndrome (MCAS). She has a history of abdominal discomfort, bloating, and alternating diarrhea/constipation which was attributed to irritable bowel syndrome. An MRI of the brain was normal.

Past medical history: MCAS, hypothyroidism, interstitial cystitis, fibromyalgia, Barrett's esophagus, irritable bowel syndrome.

Current medication: Linaclotide, cromolyn, diphenhydramine, ketotifen.

Assessment plan: Functional autonomic tests and skin biopsy.

AUTONOMIC TESTING EVALUATION

See Table 76.1.

Heart rate: Supine heart rate was normal. Heart rate responses to deep breathing were normal. Heart rate increment during the tilt (46 BPM) was exaggerated and exceeded 120 BPM.

Blood pressure:

Valsalva maneuver: Blood pressure responses showed normal Phase 2 and exaggerated Phase 4.

Tilt: Supine blood pressure was normal. Blood pressure responses to tilt were normal.

Sudomotor evaluation: Electrochemical skin conductance was abnormal (reduced to 93.9% of normal limit) at hands and normal at feet.

Respiratory system: Respiratory frequency was normal in supine position and during the tilt. End tidal CO_2 was normal in supine position but was severely reduced during the tilt.

Cerebral blood flow velocity (CBFv): CBFv in middle cerebral artery was normal in supine position but was severely reduced during the tilt.

Skin biopsy (sensory-epidermal): Epidermal nerve fiber density was normal at proximal leg and abnormal (reduced to 92.1% of normal limit) at distal leg.

Skin biopsy (sweat glands): Sweat gland nerve fiber density was normal at proximal leg.

Patient-reported symptoms during testing: Dizziness during the tilt.

TABLE 76.1 **RESULTS OF AUTONOMIC TESTING**

Blood pressure evaluation					
Test: Valsalva maneuver					
Pressure [mmHg]	Baseline	Phase 2			Phase 4
		Early	End		
Systolic	122	98	119		
Mean	94.7	84.7	105.7	n/a	
Diastolic	81	78	99	n/a	

Heart rate evaluation	
Test: Deep breathing	
Results	Norm*
16.66	≥10
Test: Valsalva ratio	
2.2	≥1.51
* adjusted for a gender and age	

(continued)

TABLE 76.1 CONTINUED

Test: Tilt test										
Position		HR [BPM]	Blood pressure [mmHg]		MCA Blood flow velocity [cm/s]				Respiratory frequency [breaths/min]	End tidal CO_2 [mmHg]
			Systolic	Diastolic	Systolic	Mean	Mean drop [%]	Diastolic		
Supine		78	109	74	80	54.7		42	12	36
Tilt [min]	1	107	113	81	66	50.7	7.3	43	17	32
	2	115	120	88						
	3	120	115	77						
	4	124	113	87						
	5	121	114	82	53	31	43.3	20	13	21
	6	121	110	85						
	7	120	113	83						
	8	115	111	82						
	9	121	116	88						
	10	118	116	88	50	30	45.2	20	16	23
	15									
	20									
	30									
	40									

Sudomotor evaluation - functional

Test: Quantitative sudomotor axon reflex test (QSART)				
Location	Site (l/r)	Latency [min]	Volume [µl]	Norm [µl]*
Forearm				≥0.08
Prox. leg				≥0.14
Distal leg				≥0.15
Foot				≥0.07

* Normative data are adjusted for gender and age of patient.

Test: Electrochemical skin conductance (ESC)				
Location	Left [µS]	Right [µS]	Average [µS/k]	Norm [µS/kg]
Hand	66	71	0.97	≥1.03
Feet	84	85	1.21	≥1.14
Forehead				

For grading uses ESC [µS] adjusted for weight [µS/k].

TABLE 76.1 **CONTINUED**

Small fiber (sensory + sudomotor) evaluation - morphological					
Test: Skin biopsy					
Location	Site (l/r)	Nerve fibers			
		Epidermal*		Sweat glands	
		Density	Norm	Density	Norm
Proximal leg – thigh	Right	16.3	≥8.3	63.1	≥37.8
Distal leg - calf	Right	6.61	≥7.18		≥36.5
Foot	Right		≥3.11		≥34.8

*Normative data for distal leg are adjusted for gender and age of patient.

QASAT*										
Heart rate		**BP**		**CBFv**		**ET-CO2**		**Sudomotor**		**Total QASAT score**
S. bradycardia	0	Low supine	0	Low supine	0	Low supine	0	QSART		
S. tachycardia	0	High supine	0	High supine	0	High supine	0	ESC	1	
Increase tilt	6	OH	0	Tilt response	6	Tilt low	5			
Decrease tilt	0	OHTN	0	CA	0	Tilt high	0	**Skin biopsy**		19
Deep breathing	0	VM	0	CVR	0			Epidermal	1	
VR	0			VM	0			Sweat gland	0	
Total	6	Total	0	Total	6	Total	5			

*QASAT. See Novak. Quantitative Scale for Grading of Cardiovascular Autonomic Reflex Tests and Small Fibers from Skin Biopsies. *J Neurol Disord* 2015;3:2.

S, supine; Increase tilt, increased response to tilt; Decrease tilt, decreased response to tilt; BP, blood pressure; VM, Valsalva maneuver; CBFv, cerebral blood flow velocity; CA, cerebral autoregulation; MCA, middle cerebral artery; VR, Valsalva ratio; CVR, cerebral vasoreactivity.

Patient-reported symptoms for past 2 weeks:

Lightheadedness or dizziness: Occasionally
Dry eyes or mouth: Occasionally
Pale feet: Occasionally
Cold feet: Occasionally
Reduced sweating: None
Reduced sweating after exercise: None
Increased sweating: None
Nausea: Occasionally
Diarrhea: None
Constipation: Often
Urinary leaks: None
Current pain severity: 6
Aching pain: Often, moderate
Allodynia: None
Burning pain: Often, severe
Lancinating pain: Occasionally, severe
Numbness: Often, moderate
Prickling sensation: Often, moderate

AUTONOMIC TESTING INTERPRETATION

- Small fiber neuropathy, length-dependent, mild, affecting predominantly sensory fibers.
- Postural tachycardia syndrome (POTS).

COMMENT

The autonomic testing showed mild small fiber neuropathy and POTS (Figure 76.1). Patient was very dizzy during the tilt, and this was associated with severe decline in CBFv (by 45%). The decline was associated with hypocapnic hyperventilation. Hypocapnia induces cerebral vasoconstriction and reduces the CBFv. This finding is common in POTS.[1] Supine hyperventilation (Figure 76.1B) reproduced the CBFv decline and dizziness.

The patient has a history of MCAS, in which mast cells inappropriately release active substances including leukotriene and histamines.[2–4] Typical presentations include episodes of flushing, shortness of breath, headache, lightheadedness, excessive diuresis, and gastrointestinal symptoms such as diarrhea, nausea, and vomiting. The primary therapy of POTS associated with MCAS is the use of medications that stabilize the mast cells and prevent release of chemical mediators which may trigger POTS-like responses.

TREATMENT AND FOLLOW-UP

- Established treatment for MCAS and POTS.[3,5,6]

CAVEATS

- Small fiber neuropathy and POTS are associated with MCAS.

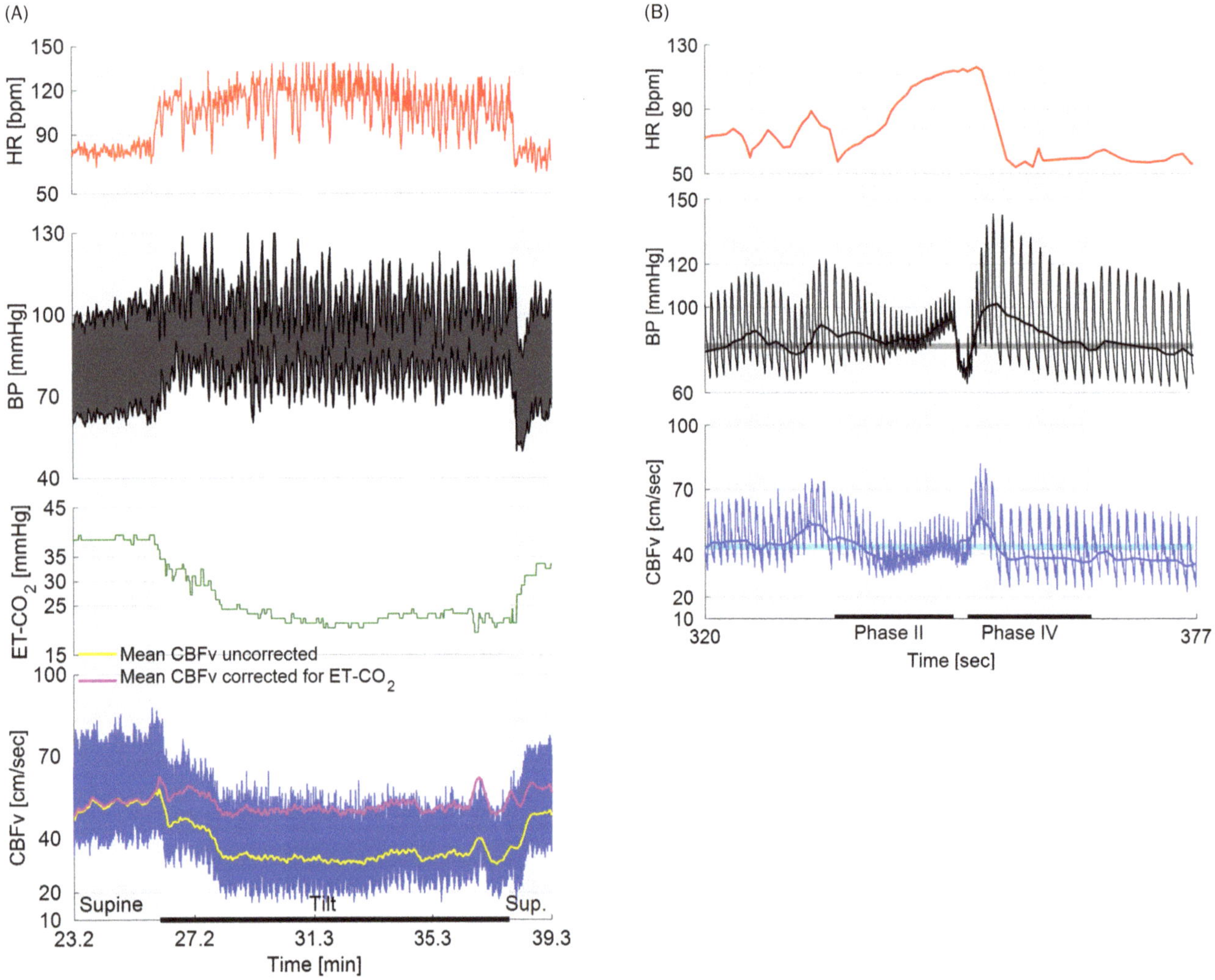

Figure 76.1 The tilt test showed exacerbated heart rate response to the tilt (A). Blood pressure was stable. End tidal CO_2 and cerebral blood flow velocity (CBFv) were reduced during the tilt. The Valsalva maneuver showed normal phase II and exaggerated phase IV which is characteristic for POTS (B). Hyperventilation in supine position reproduced major tilt findings including dizziness, decline in CBFv, elevation of blood pressure and tachycardia (C).

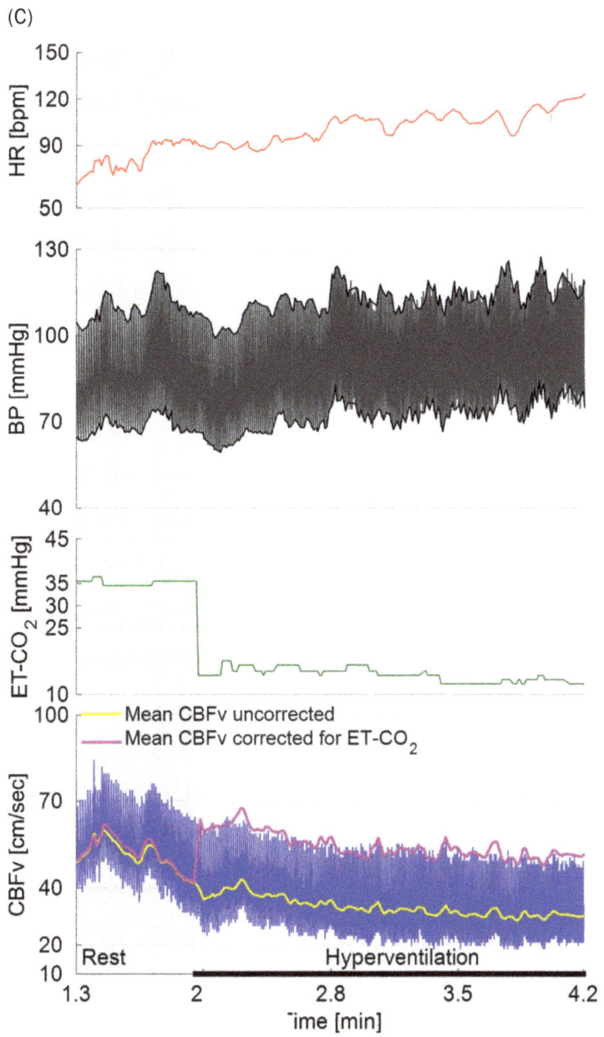

Figure 76.1 Continued

REFERENCES

1. Novak V, Spies JM, Novak P, McPhee BR, Rummans TA, Low PA. Hypocapnia and cerebral hypoperfusion in orthostatic intolerance. *Stroke*. 1998;29(9):1876–1881.
2. Shibao C, Arzubiaga C, Roberts LJ, et al. Hyperadrenergic postural tachycardia syndrome in mast cell activation disorders. *Hypertens Dallas Tex 1979*. 2005;45(3):385–390. doi:10.1161/01.HYP.0000158259.68614.40.
3. Seneviratne SL, Maitland A, Afrin L. Mast cell disorders in Ehlers-Danlos syndrome. *Am J Med Genet C Semin Med Genet*. 2017;175(1):226–236. doi:10.1002/ajmg.c.31555.
4. Frieri M, Patel R, Celestin J. Mast cell activation syndrome: a review. *Curr Allergy Asthma Rep*. 2013;13(1):27–32. doi:10.1007/s11882-012-0322-z.
5. Low PA, Sandroni P, Joyner M, Shen W-K. Postural tachycardia syndrome (POTS). *J Cardiovasc Electrophysiol*. 2009;20(3):352–358. doi:10.1111/j.1540-8167.2008.01407.x.
6. Benarroch EE. Postural tachycardia syndrome: a heterogeneous and multifactorial disorder. *Mayo Clin Proc*. 2012;87(12):1214–1225. doi:10.1016/j.mayocp.2012.08.013.

77.

CASE 72: POSTURAL TACHYCARDIA, MAST CELL ACTIVATION SYNDROME, AND EHLERS-DANLOS SYNDROME

Chief complaint: Orthostatic intolerance.

Case presentation: A 48-year-old woman presents with orthostatic intolerance. She has a history of urticaria, headaches, flushing, abdominal, and nausea for 8 years, all of intermittent character, associated with elevated urinary prostaglandin F. She was diagnosed with mast cell activation syndrome (MCAS) and was doing well on cromolyn, cetirizine, and montelukast. For the past 6 months, she has experienced several episodes of severe postural lightheadedness associated with palpitations, feeling hot, and exertional dyspnea. She was referred for autonomic testing to determine if her symptoms can be attributed to dysautonomia.

Past medical history: MCAS, hypermobile Ehlers-Danlos syndrome.

Current medication: Cromolyn, cetirizine, montelukast.

Assessment plan: Functional autonomic tests and skin biopsy.

AUTONOMIC TESTING EVALUATION

See Table 77.1.

Heart rate: Heart rate was within normal range in supine position. Heart rate responses to deep breathing were normal. Heart rate increment during the tilt (51 BPM) was exaggerated.

Blood pressure:

Valsalva maneuver: Blood pressure responses were normal.

Tilt: Supine blood pressure was elevated. Blood pressure was elevated during the tilt test. Patient experienced dizziness and shortness of breath during the tilt test.

Sudomotor evaluation: Electrochemical skin conductance was normal at hands and normal at feet.

Respiratory system: End tidal CO_2 was minimally reduced during supine and during the tilt.

Cerebral blood flow velocity (CBFv): CBFv in middle cerebral artery was normal in supine position. CBFv in middle cerebral artery was stable during the tilt test.

Skin biopsy (sensory-epidermal): Epidermal nerve fiber density was normal at proximal leg and normal at distal leg.

Skin biopsy (sweat glands): N/A

Patient-reported symptoms during testing: N/A

Patient-reported symptoms for past 2 weeks:

Lightheadedness or dizziness: Occasionally
Dry eyes or mouth: Occasionally
Pale feet: None
Cold feet: Occasionally
Reduced sweating: None

TABLE 77.1 RESULTS OF AUTONOMIC TESTING

Blood pressure evaluation

Test: Valsalva maneuver

Pressure [mmHg]	Baseline	Phase 2 Early	Phase 2 End		Phase 4
Systolic	150	122	135		
Mean	106	104	115	n/a	
Diastolic	84	95	105	n/a	

Heart rate evaluation

Test: Deep breathing	
Results	Norm*
14	≥10
Test: Valsalva ratio	
1.42	≥1.51

* adjusted for a gender and age

TABLE 77.1 CONTINUED

Test: Tilt test										
Position		HR [BPM]	Blood pressure [mmHg]		MCA Blood flow velocity [cm/s]				Respiratory frequency [breaths/min]	End tidal CO_2 [mmHg]
			Systolic	Diastolic	Systolic	Mean	Mean drop [%]	Diastolic		
Supine		69	143	94	98	60.7		42	12	34
Tilt [min]	1	97	167	100	98	61.3	-1	43	21	31
	2	99	159	114						
	3	104	174	121						
	4	101	164	123						
	5	101	171	115	84	56	7.7	42	17	32
	6	106	162	119						
	7	111	165	122						
	8	111	142	110						
	9	107	150	118						
	10	120	163	130	84	54.7	9.9	40	8	29
	15									
	20									
	30									
	40									

Sudomotor evaluation - functional

Test: Quantitative sudomotor axon reflex test (QSART)				
Location	Site (l/r)	Latency [min]	Volume [µl]	Norm [µl]*
Forearm				≥0.08
Prox. leg				≥0.14
Distal leg				≥0.15
Foot				≥0.07

* Normative data are adjusted for gender and age of patient.

Test: Electrochemical skin conductance (ESC)				
Location	Left [µS]	Right [µS]	Average [µS/k]	Norm [µS/kg]
Hand	83	81	1.21	≥1.03
Feet	92	90	1.33	≥1.14
Forehead				

For grading uses ESC [µS] adjusted for weight [µS/k].

(continued)

TABLE 77.1 **CONTINUED**

Small fiber (sensory + sudomotor) evaluation - morphological					
Test: Skin biopsy					
Location	Site (l/r)	Nerve fibers			
		Epidermal*		Sweat glands	
		Density	Norm	Density	Norm
Proximal leg – thigh	Right	16.09	≥8.3		≥37.8
Distal leg - calf	Right	9.67	≥7.26		≥36.5
Foot	Right		≥3.11		≥34.8

*Normative data for distal leg are adjusted for gender and age of patient.

QASAT*											
Heart rate		**BP**		**CBFv**		**ET-CO2**		**Sudomotor**			**Total QASAT score**
S. bradycardia	0	Low supine	0	Low supine	0	Low supine	1	QSART			
S. tachycardia	0	High supine	1	High supine	0	High supine	0	ESC	0		
Increase tilt	1	OH	0	Tilt response	0	Tilt low	2				
Decrease tilt	0	OHTN	6	CA	0	Tilt high	0	**Skin biopsy**			12
Deep breathing	0	VM	0	CVR	0			Epidermal	0		
VR	1			VM	0			Sweat gland			
Total	2	Total	7	Total	0	Total	3				

*QASAT. See Novak. Quantitative Scale for Grading of Cardiovascular Autonomic Reflex Tests and Small Fibers from Skin Biopsies. *J Neurol Disord* 2015;3:2.

S, supine; Increase tilt, increased response to tilt; Decrease tilt, decreased response to tilt; BP, blood pressure; VM, Valsalva maneuver; CBFv, cerebral blood flow velocity; CA, cerebral autoregulation; MCA, middle cerebral artery; VR, Valsalva ratio; CVR, cerebral vasoreactivity.

Reduced sweating after exercise: Occasionally
Increased sweating: Occasionally
Nausea: Often
Diarrhea: Occasionally
Constipation: Occasionally
Urinary leaks: Occasionally
Current pain severity: 4
Aching pain: Often, moderate
Allodynia: Often, mild
Burning pain: Occasionally, mild
Lancinating pain: Occasionally, mild
Numbness: Occasionally, mild
Prickling sensation: Occasionally, mild

AUTONOMIC TESTING INTERPRETATION

- Mild postural intolerance syndrome (POTS) associated with orthostatic hypertension.
- No evidence of autonomic failure.
- No evidence of small fiber neuropathy; skin biopsy and sudomotor testing were normal.

COMMENT

The study was consistent with POTS (Figure 77.1), probably of a hyperadrenergic variant because of orthostatic blood pressure was elevated. Hyperadrenergic POTS is associated with elevated orthostatic catecholamines.[1]

The patient has history of MCAS as well as hypermobile Ehlers-Danlos syndrome, and both syndromes are clustered with dysautonomia.[2]

TREATMENT AND FOLLOW-UP

- Catecholamines supine and standing to confirm hyperadrenergic variant of POTS.
- Treatment with mast cell stabilizers.[3,4]

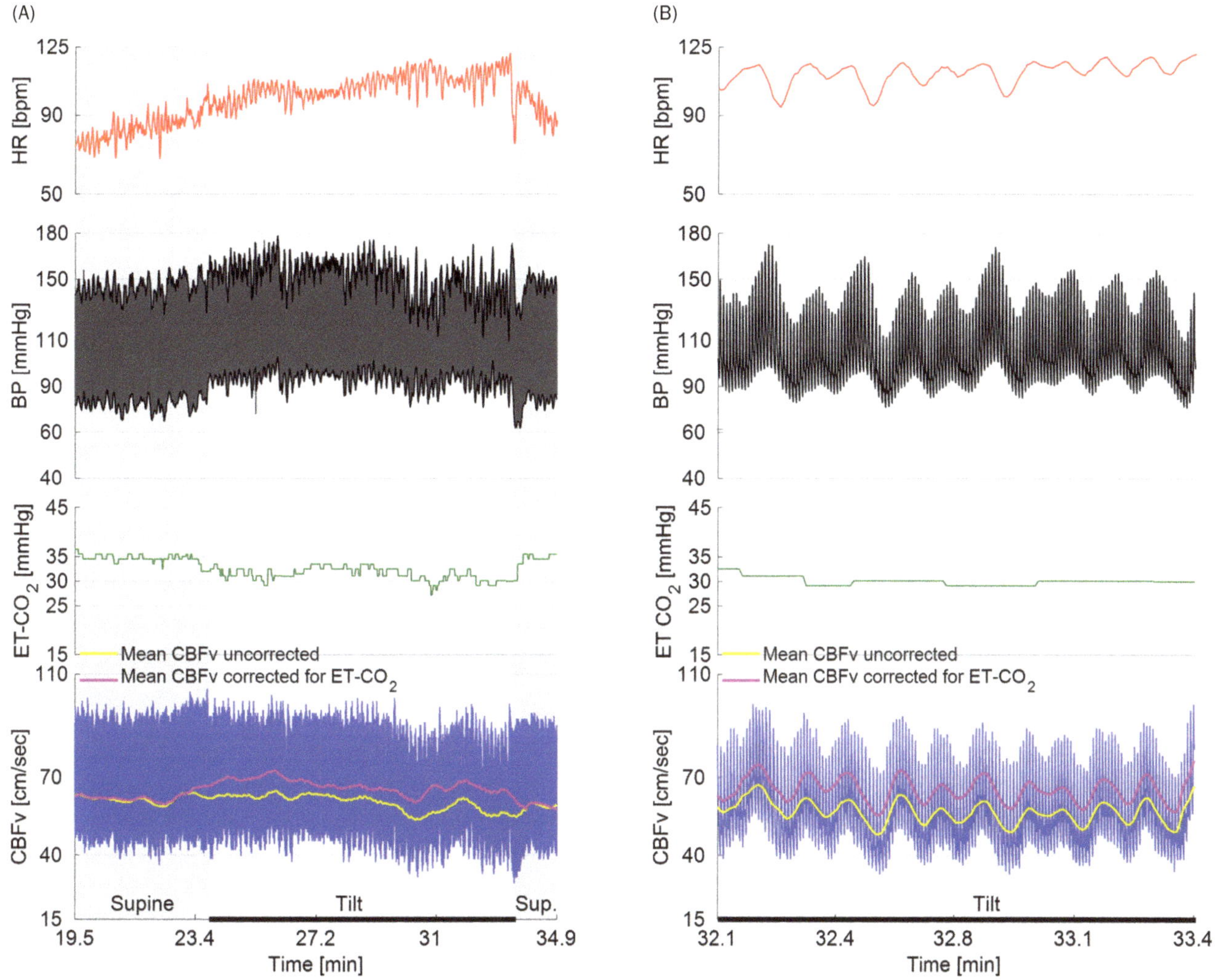

Figure 77.1 During the tilt, there was a progressive increase of the heart rate associated with orthostatic hypertension (A). The average blood flow velocity (CBFv) was minimally reduced but the reduction was within normal limits the tilt. Large fluctuations of the CBFv synchronous with blood pressure and respiratory sinus arrhythmia were seen at the second half of tilt (B) when the patient became dizzy and short of breath. Dizziness was likely caused by CBFv fluctuations since brain is very sensitive for even minor changes in blood flow.

CAVEATS

- POTS is associated with MCAS and hypermobile Ehlers-Danlos syndrome.

REFERENCES

1. Benarroch EE. Postural tachycardia syndrome: a heterogeneous and multifactorial disorder. *Mayo Clin Proc*. 2012;87(12):1214–1225. doi:10.1016/j.mayocp.2012.08.013.
2. Seneviratne SL, Maitland A, Afrin L. Mast cell disorders in Ehlers-Danlos syndrome. *Am J Med Genet C Semin Med Genet*. 2017;175(1):226–236. doi:10.1002/ajmg.c.31555.
3. Shibao C, Arzubiaga C, Roberts LJ, et al. Hyperadrenergic postural tachycardia syndrome in mast cell activation disorders. *Hypertens Dallas Tex 1979*. 2005;45(3):385–390. doi:10.1161/01.HYP.0000158259.68614.40.
4. Frieri M, Patel R, Celestin J. Mast cell activation syndrome: a review. *Curr Allergy Asthma Rep*. 2013;13(1):27–32. doi:10.1007/s11882-012-0322-z.

78.

CASE 73: DYSAUTONOMIA DUE TO MAST CELL ACTIVATION SYNDROME OR PSORIATIC ARTHRITIS?

Chief complaint: Fatigue.

Case presentation: A 39-year-old woman presents with fatigue. She was healthy a year ago, very active. She experienced severe postprandial diarrhea for 3 months, sometimes even after waking up or at night. She became nauseated after meals. She was found allergic to certain food, and also noted hives and itching. Evaluation for irritable bowel syndrome, including colonoscopy, was unrevealing. She was hospitalized recently due to abdominal pain, diarrhea, dyspnea, and orthostatic tachycardia. She was diagnosed with mast cell activation syndrome (MCAS). Cromolyn, ranitidine, diphenhydramine, and cetirizine help with the gastrointestinal problems. At the same time, she was also diagnosed with psoriatic arthritis (PA) and treated with prednisone. Patient failed pyridostigmine, fludrocortisone, and proamatine for suspected autonomic failure. She was referred for formal evaluation of autonomic functions and to determine if dysautonomia (if it exists) is due to PA or due to MCAS.

Past medical history: PA, MCAS.

Current medication: Cromolyn, lorazepam, ranitidine, diphenhydramine, cetirizine.

Assessment plan: Functional autonomic tests and skin biopsy.

AUTONOMIC TESTING EVALUATION

See Table 78.1.

Heart rate: Supine heart rate was normal. Heart rate responses to deep breathing were normal. Heart rate increment during the tilt (67 BPM) was exaggerated.

Blood pressure:

Valsalva maneuver: Mean blood pressure failed to return to baseline at the end of Phase 2 by 1.7 mm Hg (i.e., 98.5% of baseline).

Tilt: Supine blood pressure was normal. Blood pressure responses to tilt were normal.

Sudomotor evaluation: Electrochemical skin conductance was normal at hands and normal at feet.

Respiratory system: Respiratory frequency was normal in supine position but was increased during the tilt. End tidal CO_2 was reduced in supine position and declined further during the tilt.

Cerebral blood flow velocity (CBFv): CBFv in middle cerebral artery was normal in supine position but was severely reduced during the tilt.

Skin biopsy (sensory-epidermal): Epidermal nerve fiber density was abnormal (reduced to 99.8% of normal

TABLE 78.1 RESULTS OF AUTONOMIC TESTING

Blood pressure evaluation					
Test: Valsalva maneuver					
Pressure [mmHg]	Baseline	Phase 2			Phase 4
		Early	End		
Systolic	144	97	123		
Mean	114.7	89	113	n/a	
Diastolic	100	85	108	n/a	

Heart rate evaluation	
Test: Deep breathing	
Results	Norm*
16.25	≥12
Test: Valsalva ratio	
1.92	≥1.5
* adjusted for a gender and age	

TABLE 78.1 **CONTINUED**

Test: Tilt test											
Position		HR [BPM]	Blood pressure [mmHg]		MCA Blood flow velocity [cm/s]				Respiratory frequency [breaths/min]	End tidal CO_2 [mmHg]
			Systolic	Diastolic	Systolic	Mean	Mean drop [%]	Diastolic		
Supine		66	101	70	94	61.3		45	20	29
Tilt [min]	1	133	120	86	77	48.3	21.2	34	18	24
	2	108	114	84						
	3	106	113	84						
	4	105	114	82						
	5	106	106	79	79	45.7	25.4	29	27	21
	6	99	108	80						
	7	107	113	82						
	8	105	123	89						
	9	109	107	78						
	10	107	118	85	78	44.7	27.1	28	22	20
	15									
	20									
	30									
	40									

Sudomotor evaluation - functional

Test: Quantitative sudomotor axon reflex test (QSART)				
Location	Site (l/r)	Latency [min]	Volume [µl]	Norm [µl]*
Forearm				≥0.08
Prox. leg				≥0.14
Distal leg				≥0.15
Foot				≥0.07

* normative data are adjusted for a gender and age of a patient

Test: Electrochemical skin conductance (ESC)				
Location	Left [µS]	Right [µS]	Average [µS/k]	Norm [µS/kg]
Hand	74	63	1.34	≥1.03
Feet	83	83	1.63	≥1.14
Forehead				

For grading uses ESC [µS] adjusted for weight [µS/k].

(continued)

TABLE 78.1 CONTINUED

Small fiber (sensory + sudomotor) evaluation - morphological					
Test: Skin biopsy					
Location	Site (l/r)	Nerve fibers			
		Epidermal*		Sweat glands	
		Density	Norm	Density	Norm
Proximal leg – thigh	Right	8.28	≥8.3		≥37.8
Distal leg - calf	Right	5.26	≥8.06	21.4	≥36.5
Foot	Right		≥3.11		≥34.8

* normative data for distal leg are adjusted for a gender and age of a patient

QASAT*										
Heart rate		**BP**		**CBFv**		**ET-CO2**		**Sudomotor**		**Total QASAT score**
S. bradycardia	0	Low supine	0	Low supine	0	Low supine	1	QSART		
S. tachycardia	0	High supine	0	High supine	0	High supine	0	ESC	0	
Increase tilt	1	OH	0	Tilt response	6	Tilt low	8			
Decrease tilt	0	OHTN	0	CA	0	Tilt high	0	**Skin biopsy**		23
Deep breathing	0	VM	1	CVR	0			Epidermal	3	
VR	0			VM	0			Sweat gland	3	
Total	1	Total	1	Total	6	Total	9			

*QASAT = Quantitative Scale for Grading of Cardiovascular Autonomic Reflex Tests and Small Fibers from Skin Biopsies, Novak, J Neurol Disord 2015, 3:2, S. = supine, Increase tilt = increased response to tilt, Decrease tilt = decreased response to tilt, BP = blood pressure, VM = Valsalva maneuver, CBFv = cerebral blood flow velocity; CA = cerebral autoregulation, VR = Valsalva ratio, CVR = cerebral vasoreactivity.

limit) at proximal leg and abnormal (reduced to 65.3% of normal limit) at distal leg.

Skin biopsy (sweat glands): Sweat gland nerve fiber density was abnormal (reduced to 58.6% of normal limit) at distal leg.

Patient-reported symptoms during testing: Dizziness during the tilt.

Patient-reported symptoms for past 2 weeks:

Lightheadedness or dizziness: Often
Dry eyes or mouth: Occasionally
Pale feet: Occasionally
Cold feet: Often
Reduced sweating after exercise: Occasionally
Increased sweating: None
Nausea: Occasionally
Diarrhea: Occasionally
Constipation: Occasionally
Urinary leaks: None
Current pain severity: 0
Aching pain: Occasionally, mild
Allodynia: Occasionally, mild
Burning pain: Occasionally, mild
Lancinating pain: Occasionally, moderate
Numbness: Occasionally, mild
Prickling sensation: Occasionally, mild

AUTONOMIC TESTING INTERPRETATION

- Cerebral blood flow velocity was reduced during the tilt.
- Prominent anxiety and hyperventilation (Figure 78.1).

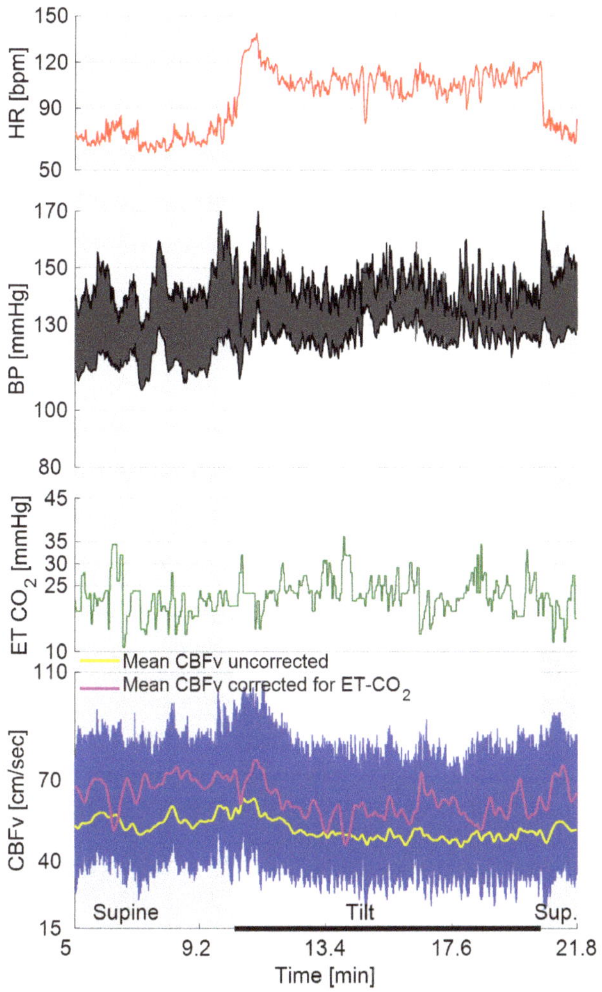

Figure 78.1 The tilt test showed initial tachycardia with a heart rate of almost 130 BPM within seconds of tilt onset. The tachycardia improved, but heart rate remained elevated during the tilt. Blood pressure was elevated but stable. End tidal CO_2 was very low throughout the testing.

- Small fiber neuropathy, mixed, length-dependent.
- Postural tachycardia syndrome (POTS), mild, neuropathic form.

COMMENT

The testing revealed anxiety with hyperventilation (Figure 78.1) and small fiber neuropathy. There was no evidence of severe autonomic failure, and this explains why pyridostigmine, fludrocortisone, and proamatine failed. The testing revealed mild POTS. Sympathetic dysfunction was reported in psoriasis,[1] while parasympathetic dysfunction was observed in PA.[2] Hyperadrenergic POTS was described in MCAS.[3]

TREATMENT AND FOLLOW-UP

- Clinical workup for neuropathy.
- Treatment of anxiety.
- Pulmonary evaluation of dyspnea and hyperventilation.

CAVEATS

- Both MCAS and PA can be associated with POTS and small fiber neuropathy.
- Severe anxiety with hyperventilation can be superimposed on POTS.

REFERENCES

1. Halıgür BD, Cicek D, Bulut S, Berilgen MS. The investigation of autonomic functions in patients with psoriasis. *Int J Dermatol.* 2012;51(5):557–563. doi:10.1111/j.1365-4632.2011.05111.x.
2. Syngle A, Verma I, Garg N, Krishan P. Autonomic dysfunction in psoriatic arthritis. *Clin Rheumatol.* 2013;32(7):1059–1064. doi:10.1007/s10067-013-2239-x.
3. Shibao C, Arzubiaga C, Roberts LJ, et al. Hyperadrenergic postural tachycardia syndrome in mast cell activation disorders. *Hypertens Dallas Tex 1979.* 2005;45(3):385–390. doi:10.1161/01.HYP.0000158259.68614.40.

79.

CASE 74: SMALL FIBER NEUROPATHY AND LYME DISEASE

Chief complaint: Dizziness.

Case presentation: A 62-year-old man presents with dizziness. He has worked all his life in the woods and has had many tick bites. Three years ago, after another bite, he experienced a number of symptoms including brain fog, intermittent confusion, sensitivity to light, numbness and pain in feet, anxiety, and weakness. Evaluations for neuropathy, including impaired glucose metabolism, monoclonal gammopathy, vitamin deficiencies, and Sjögren syndrome, have been negative or ruled out. MRI of the brain and nerve conduction studies were normal. He was treated with multiple oral and intravenous antibiotics for suspected Lyme disease. Patient was referred for evaluation of autonomic failure.

Past medical history: Lyme disease.

Current medication: None.

Assessment plan: Functional autonomic tests and skin biopsy.

AUTONOMIC TESTING EVALUATION

See Table 79.1.

Heart rate: Supine heart rate was normal. Heart rate responses to deep breathing were normal. Heart rate increment during the tilt (36 BPM) was exaggerated.

Blood pressure:

Valsalva maneuver: Mean blood pressure failed to return to baseline at the end of Phase 2 by 13 mm Hg (i.e., 86.1% of baseline).

Tilt: Supine blood pressure was normal. Blood pressure responses to tilt were normal.

Sudomotor evaluation: Electrochemical skin conductance was abnormal (reduced to 74.9% of normal limit) at hands and abnormal (reduced to 74.7% of normal limit) at feet.

Respiratory system: Respiratory frequency was normal in supine position but was reduced during the tilt. End tidal CO_2 was reduced in supine position and was declined further during the tilt.

Cerebral blood flow velocity (CBFv): CBFv in middle cerebral artery was reduced in supine position (mean 39 cm/s, normal ≥45.4 cm/s) but was stable during the tilt.

Skin biopsy (sensory-epidermal): Epidermal nerve fiber density was abnormal (reduced to 34.6% of normal limit) at distal leg.

Skin biopsy (sweat glands): Sweat gland nerve fiber density was abnormal (reduced to 22.7% of normal limit) at distal leg.

Patient-reported symptoms during testing: Dizziness during the tilt.

Patient-reported symptoms for past 2 weeks:

Lightheadedness or dizziness: Occasionally
Dry eyes or mouth: Occasionally
Pale feet: Occasionally
Cold feet: Often
Reduced sweating: Occasionally
Reduced sweating after exercise: Occasionally

TABLE 79.1 **RESULTS OF AUTONOMIC TESTING**

Blood pressure evaluation					
Test: Valsalva maneuver					
Pressure [mmHg]	Baseline	Phase 2			Phase 4
		Early	End		
Systolic	137	88	94		
Mean	93.7	76	80.7	n/a	
Diastolic	72	70	74	n/a	

Heart rate evaluation	
Test: Deep breathing	
Results	Norm*
11	≥7
Test: Valsalva ratio	
1.59	≥1.29
* adjusted for a gender and age	

TABLE 79.1 CONTINUED

Test: Tilt test										
Position		HR [BPM]	Blood pressure [mmHg]		MCA Blood flow velocity [cm/s]				Respiratory frequency [breaths/min]	End tidal CO_2 [mmHg]
			Systolic	Diastolic	Systolic	Mean	Mean drop [%]	Diastolic		
Supine		60	124	69	73	39		22	14	30
Tilt [min]	1	83	116	71	72	38	2.6	21	13	24
	2	91	118	81						
	3	86	128	72						
	4	91	129	79						
	5	90	123	77	77	39.7	-1.8	21	14	28
	6	82	127	78						
	7	87	123	76						
	8	93	122	79						
	9	96	129	80						
	10	86	129	80	78	38.7	0.8	19	18	25
	15									
	20									
	30									
	40									

Sudomotor evaluation - functional

Test: Quantitative sudomotor axon reflex test (QSART)				
Location	Site (l/r)	Latency [min]	Volume [μl]	Norm [μl]*
Forearm				≥0.3
Prox. leg				≥0.23
Distal leg				≥0.23
Foot				≥0.27

* Normative data are adjusted for gender and age of patient.

Test: Electrochemical skin conductance (ESC)				
Location	Left [μS]	Right [μS]	Average [μS/k]	Norm [μS/kg]
Hand	79	75	0.77	≥1.03
Feet	85	86	0.86	≥1.14
Forehead				

For grading uses ESC [μS] adjusted for weight [μS/k].

(continued)

TABLE 79.1 CONTINUED

Small fiber (sensory + sudomotor) evaluation - morphological					
Test: Skin biopsy					
Location	Site (l/r)	Nerve fibers			
		Epidermal*		Sweat glands	
		Density	Norm	Density	Norm
Proximal leg – thigh	Right		≥8.3		≥37.8
Distal leg - calf	Right	1.68	≥4.85	8.3	≥36.5
Foot	Right		≥3.11		≥34.8

*Normative data for distal leg are adjusted for gender and age of patient.

QASAT*											
Heart rate		BP		CBFv		ET-CO2		Sudomotor			Total QASAT score
S. bradycardia	0	Low supine	0	Low supine	1	Low supine	1	QSART			
S. tachycardia	0	High supine	0	High supine	0	High supine	0	ESC	2		
Increase tilt	1	OH	0	Tilt response	0	Tilt low	5				
Decrease tilt	0	OHTN	0	CA	0	Tilt high	0	**Skin biopsy**			19
Deep breathing	0	VM	2	CVR	0			Epidermal	3		
VR	0			VM	0			Sweat gland	4		
Total	1	Total	2	Total	1	Total	6				

*QASAT. See Novak. Quantitative Scale for Grading of Cardiovascular Autonomic Reflex Tests and Small Fibers from Skin Biopsies. *J Neurol Disord* 2015;3:2.

S, supine; Increase tilt, increased response to tilt; Decrease tilt, decreased response to tilt; BP, blood pressure; VM, Valsalva maneuver; CBFv, cerebral blood flow velocity; CA, cerebral autoregulation; MCA, middle cerebral artery; VR, Valsalva ratio; CVR, cerebral vasoreactivity.

Increased sweating: Occasionally
Nausea: Occasionally
Diarrhea: Occasionally
Constipation: Yes, minor annoyance
Urinary leaks: Yes, minor annoyance
Erection problems: Often
Current pain severity: 5
Aching pain: Often, moderate
Allodynia: None
Burning pain: Continuous, moderate
Lancinating pain: Occasionally, moderate
Numbness: Continuous, moderate
Prickling sensation: Often, moderate

AUTONOMIC TESTING INTERPRETATION

- Small fiber neuropathy, mixed, sever.
- Hypocapnic hyperventilation.
- Reduced CBFv was likely due to vasoconstrictive effect of hypocapnia.

COMMENT

The testing showed mild orthostatic intolerance without evidence of significant autonomic failure (Figure 79.1) but severe small fiber neuropathy affecting both sensory and autonomic fibers. Extensive clinical workup for neuropathy, including an autoimmune panel, has been negative; therefore the small fiber neuropathy has been attributed to Lyme disease.

Lyme disease is a transmitted tick-borne infection caused by the spirochete *Borrelia burgdorferi*[1] and can be associated with small fiber neuropathy.[2]

The testing also revealed reduced CBFv, which can be explained as due to the vasoconstrictive effect of hypocapnia. Hypocapnia induces cerebral arterioral vasoconstriction

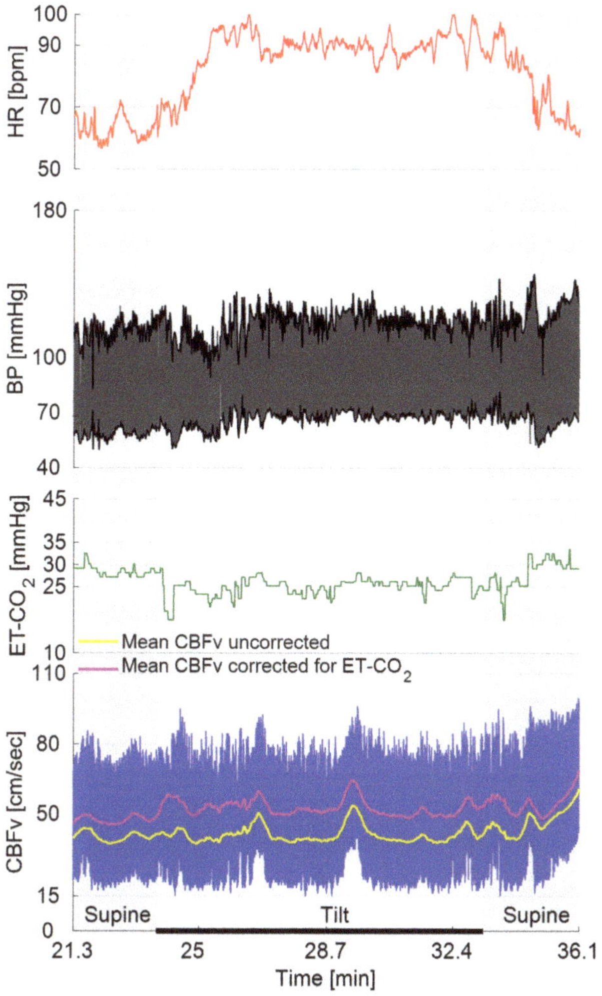

Figure 79.1 The tilt test showed increased orthostatic heart rate increment but it did not reach 120 BPM. Blood pressure was normal. Patient was hyperventilating throughout the test, including in supine position. Cerebral blood flow velocity was reduced throughout the tilt test.

and a decrease in the end tidal CO_2 such as a decrease in end tidal CO_2 by 1 mm Hg decreases CBFv by approximately 3%.[3] Reduced CBFv can be associated with cerebral hypoperfusion and patient's cognitive complaints. Why the patient was hyperventilating is unclear.

TREATMENT AND FOLLOW-UP

- Pulmonary consult for evaluation of hyperventilation.

CAVEATS

- Lyme disease can be associated with small fiber neuropathy and reduced cerebral blood flow velocity.

REFERENCES

1. Mead PS. Epidemiology of Lyme disease. *Infect Dis Clin North Am*. 2015;29(2):187–210. doi:10.1016/j.idc.2015.02.010.
2. Farhad K, Traub R, Ruzhansky KM, Brannagan TH. Causes of neuropathy in patients referred as "idiopathic neuropathy." *Muscle Nerve*. 2016;53(6):856–861. doi:10.1002/mus.24969.
3. Immink RV, Pott FC, Secher NH, van Lieshout JJ. Hyperventilation, cerebral perfusion, and syncope. *J Appl Physiol Bethesda Md 1985*. 2014;116(7):844–851. doi:10.1152/japplphysiol.00637.2013.

80.

CASE 75: SMALL FIBER NEUROPATHY, CEREBRAL AUTOREGULATORY FAILURE, AND POSTTREATMENT LYME DISEASE SYNDROME

Chief complaint: Dizziness.

Case presentation: A 65-year-old man with history of Lyme disease presents with diffuse pain, fatigue, orthostatic dizziness, and brain fog for about 2 years. Neurological examination showed reduction of small fiber modalities (temperature and soft touch at distal legs), but was otherwise normal. MRI of the brain showed nonspecific white matter changes related to small vessel disease. Nerve conduction studies were normal. The patient was referred for evaluation of small fiber neuropathy.

Past medical history: Lyme disease.

Current medication: Rifampicin.

Assessment plan: Functional autonomic tests and skin biopsy.

AUTONOMIC TESTING EVALUATION

See Table 80.1.

Heart rate: Supine heart rate was normal. Heart rate responses to deep breathing were reduced to 78.6% of normal value. Heart rate increment during the tilt (−3 BPM) was absent.

Blood pressure:

Valsalva maneuver: Mean blood pressure failed to return to baseline at the end of Phase 2 by 16 mm Hg (i.e., 78.9% of baseline).

Tilt: Supine blood pressure was normal. Blood pressure responses to tilt were normal.

Sudomotor evaluation: Electrochemical skin conductance was abnormal (reduced to 36.9% of normal limit) at hands and abnormal (reduced to 60.8% of normal limit) at feet.

Respiratory system: Respiratory frequency and end tidal CO_2 were normal in supine position and during the tilt.

Cerebral blood flow velocity (CBFv): CBFv in middle cerebral artery was reduced in supine position (mean 40.3 cm/s, normal ≥45.4 cm/s). CBFv in middle cerebral artery was stable during the tilt.

Skin biopsy (sensory-epidermal): Epidermal nerve fiber density was abnormal (reduced to 5.8% of normal limit) at distal leg.

Skin biopsy (sweat glands): Sweat gland nerve fiber density was abnormal (reduced to 51.2% of normal limit) at distal leg.

TABLE 80.1 RESULTS OF AUTONOMIC TESTING

Blood pressure evaluation					
Test: Valsalva maneuver					
Pressure [mmHg]	Baseline	Phase 2			Phase 4
		Early	End		
Systolic	96	68	68		
Mean	76	60	60	n/a	
Diastolic	66	56	56	n/a	

Heart rate evaluation	
Test: Deep breathing	
Results	Norm*
5.5	≥7
Test: Valsalva ratio	
1.1	≥1.29
* adjusted for a gender and age	

TABLE 80.1 **CONTINUED**

Test: Tilt test										
Position		HR [BPM]	Blood pressure [mmHg]		MCA Blood flow velocity [cm/s]				Respiratory frequency [breaths/min]	End tidal CO_2 [mmHg]
			Systolic	Diastolic	Systolic	Mean	Mean drop [%]	Diastolic		
Supine		65	104	61	77	40.3		22	12	40
Tilt [min]	1	62	113	76	69	37	8.2	21	13	40
	2	61	119	57						
	3	59	112	78						
	4	58	113	64						
	5	57	98	64	74	38.7	4	21	8	42
	6	57	118	80						
	7	58	111	58						
	8	54	110	58						
	9	59	100	52						
	10	60	116	59	72	36.7	8.9	19	14	36
	15									
	20									
	30									
	40									

Sudomotor evaluation - functional

Test: Quantitative sudomotor axon reflex test (QSART)				
Location	Site (l/r)	Latency [min]	Volume [μl]	Norm [μl]*
Forearm				≥0.3
Prox. leg				≥0.23
Distal leg				≥0.23
Foot				≥0.27

* Normative data are adjusted for gender and age of patient.

Test: Electrochemical skin conductance (ESC)				
Location	Left [μS]	Right [μS]	Average [μS/k]	Norm [μS/kg]
Hand	36	43	0.38	≥1.03
Feet	72	70	0.68	≥1.14
Forehead				

For grading uses ESC [μS] adjusted for weight [μS/k].

(continued)

TABLE 80.1 CONTINUED

Small fiber (sensory + sudomotor) evaluation - morphological					
Test: Skin biopsy					
Location	Site (l/r)	Nerve fibers			
		Epidermal*		Sweat glands	
		Density	Norm	Density	Norm
Proximal leg – thigh	Right		≥8.3		≥37.8
Distal leg - calf	Right	0.27	≥4.625	18.7	≥36.5
Foot	Right		≥3.11		≥34.8

*Normative data for distal leg are adjusted for gender and age of patient.

QASAT*										
Heart rate		BP		CBFv		ET-CO2		Sudomotor		Total QASAT score
S. bradycardia	0	Low supine	0	Low supine	1	Low supine	0	QSART		
S. tachycardia	0	High supine	0	High supine	0	High supine	0	ESC	3	
Increase tilt	0	OH	0	Tilt response	0	Tilt low	0			
Decrease tilt	1	OHTN	0	CA	0	Tilt high	0	**Skin biopsy**		16
Deep breathing	1	VM	2	CVR	0			Epidermal	4	
VR	1			VM	0			Sweat gland	3	
Total	3	Total	2	Total	1	Total	0			

*QASAT. See Novak. Quantitative Scale for Grading of Cardiovascular Autonomic Reflex Tests and Small Fibers from Skin Biopsies. *J Neurol Disord* 2015;3:2.

S, supine; Increase tilt, increased response to tilt; Decrease tilt, decreased response to tilt; BP, blood pressure; VM, Valsalva maneuver; CBFv, cerebral blood flow velocity; CA, cerebral autoregulation; MCA, middle cerebral artery; VR, Valsalva ratio; CVR, cerebral vasoreactivity.

Patient-reported symptoms during testing: Dizziness during the tilt.

Patient-reported symptoms for past 2 weeks:

Lightheadedness or dizziness: Yes, minor annoyance
Dry eyes or mouth: None
Pale feet: Often
Cold feet: Often
Reduced sweating: None
Reduced sweating after exercise: Occasionally
Increased sweating: None
Nausea: None
Diarrhea: None
Constipation: None
Urinary leaks: None
Erection problems: None
Current pain severity: 9
Aching pain: Continuous, severe
Allodynia: None
Burning pain: Occasionally, mild
Lancinating pain: Often, moderate
Numbness: Occasionally, moderate
Prickling sensation: Occasionally, moderate

AUTONOMIC TESTING INTERPRETATION

- Small fiber neuropathy, mixed, length-dependent (Figure 80.1).
- Low CBFv and cerebral autoregulatory failure (CAF).[1]

COMMENT

The autonomic testing showed small fiber neuropathy and CAF (Figure 80.1), the latter can be associated with cerebral small vessel disease. Very low diastolic CBFv may be seen in abnormal cerebral vasodilation. This patient has a history of Lyme disease with persistent cognitive and sensory symptoms, which is consistent with posttreatment Lyme disease syndrome (PLDS).

In between 10% and 45% of Lyme patients, symptoms associated with Lyme disease persist despite previous antibiotic therapy; these symptoms, referred as to as PLDS, include pain, fatigue, and cognitive complaints.[2,3] The origin of PLDS symptoms is unclear.[3]

The patient presented in this chapter has evidence of small fiber neuropathy and low CBFv. Small fiber neuropathy can

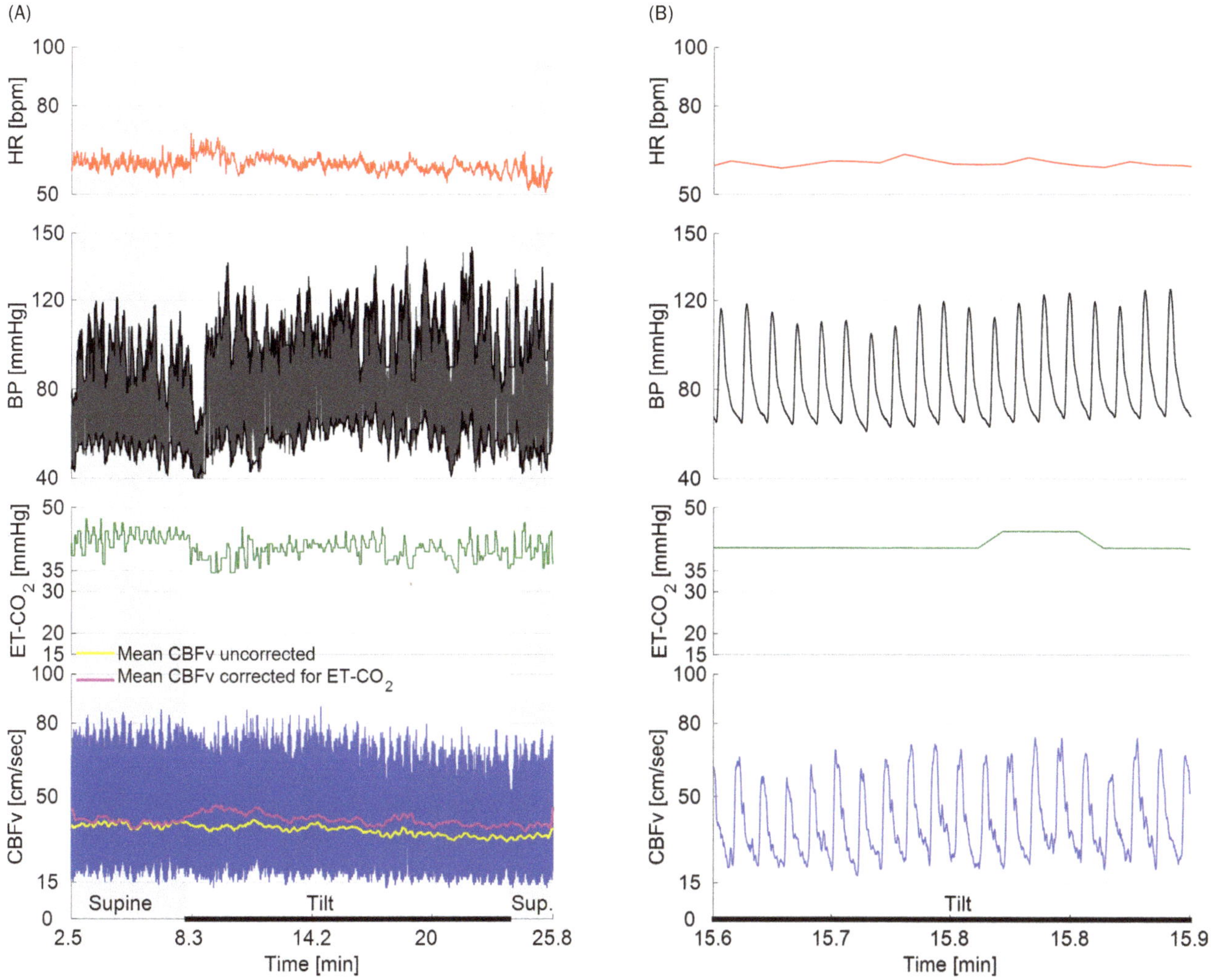

Figure 80.1 The tilt test showed reduced heart rate responses. The initial transient blood pressure decline to tilt is the movement-evoked artifact. Mean blood pressure was stable during the tilt. End tidal CO_2 was normal. Cerebral blood flow velocity was reduced in supine position and during the tilt (B).

explain the patient's sensory symptoms. Low CBFv can be linked to cerebral hypoperfusion and cognitive problems.

TREATMENT AND FOLLOW-UP

- Cerebral perfusion study.

CAVEATS

- PLDS can be associated with small fiber neuropathy and reduced CBFv.

REFERENCES

1. Novak P. Cerebral blood flow, heart rate, and blood pressure patterns during the tilt test in common orthostatic syndromes. *Neurosci J.* 2016;2016:6127340. doi:10.1155/2016/6127340.
2. Cairns V, Godwin J. Post-Lyme borreliosis syndrome: a meta-analysis of reported symptoms. *Int J Epidemiol.* 2005;34(6):1340–1345. doi:10.1093/ije/dyi129.
3. Aucott JN. Posttreatment Lyme disease syndrome. *Infect Dis Clin North Am.* 2015;29(2):309–323. doi:10.1016/j.idc.2015.02.012.

81.

CASE 76: SMALL FIBER NEUROPATHY, HYPOCAPNIC CEREBRAL HYPOPERFUSION, AND POSTTREATMENT LYME DISEASE SYNDROME

Chief complaint: Dizziness.

Case presentation: A 30-year-old woman presents with dizziness, blurred vision, gait problem, and joint and burning skin pain. She has a history of several tick bites at ages 12 and 28. She was empirically treated for Lyme disease with multiple antibiotics. For the past 2 years, she has experienced floaters, hot and cold flashes, orthostatic tremor, balance problems, chronic fatigue, abdominal pain, brain fog, and orthostatic dizziness. Patient was referred for autonomic testing to determine if autonomic failure can be responsible for her symptoms.

Past medical history: Posttreatment Lyme disease syndrome (PLDS).[1]

Current medication: None.

Assessment plan: Functional autonomic tests and skin biopsy.

AUTONOMIC TESTING EVALUATION

See Table 81.1.

Heart rate: Supine heart rate was normal. Heart rate responses to deep breathing were normal. Heart rate increment during the tilt (31 BPM) was exaggerated.

Blood pressure:

Valsalva maneuver: Mean blood pressure failed to return to baseline at the end of Phase 2 by 7 mm Hg (i.e., 92.4% of baseline).

Tilt: Supine blood pressure was normal. Blood pressure responses to tilt were normal.

Sudomotor evaluation: Sweat output was normal at forearm, normal at proximal leg, normal at distal leg, and normal at foot. Quantitative sudomotor axon reflex test (QSART) showed length-dependent pattern with a decrease of sweat output distally of at least 33%.

Respiratory system: Respiratory frequency was normal in supine position and during the tilt. End tidal CO_2 was normal in supine position but was moderately reduced during the tilt.

Cerebral blood flow velocity (CBFv): CBFv in middle cerebral artery was normal in supine position but was mildly reduced during the tilt.

Skin biopsy (sensory-epidermal): Epidermal nerve fiber density was normal at proximal leg and abnormal (reduced to 67.2% of normal limit) at distal leg.

Skin biopsy (sweat glands): Sweat gland nerve fiber density was normal at proximal leg and normal at distal leg.

TABLE 81.1 RESULTS OF AUTONOMIC TESTING

Blood pressure evaluation					
Test: Valsalva maneuver					
Pressure [mmHg]	Baseline	Phase 2			Phase 4
		Early	End		
Systolic	132	99	107		
Mean	92	79	85	n/a	
Diastolic	72	69	74	n/a	

Heart rate evaluation	
Test: Deep breathing	
Results	Norm*
12.16	≥12
Test: Valsalva ratio	
1.51	≥1.5

* adjusted for a gender and age

TABLE 81.1 **CONTINUED**

Test: Tilt test										
Position		HR [BPM]	Blood pressure [mmHg]		MCA Blood flow velocity [cm/s]				Respiratory frequency [breaths/min]	End tidal CO_2 [mmHg]
			Systolic	Diastolic	Systolic	Mean	Mean drop [%]	Diastolic		
Supine		66	107	70	103	67		49	15	35
Tilt [min]	1	84	106	74	107	69.7	-4	51	13	31
	2	97	120	82						
	3	80	106	74						
	4	82	104	72						
	5	93	107	72	96	57.3	14.5	38	15	27
	6	88	103	71						
	7	92	104	72						
	8	95	103	72						
	9	92	109	78						
	10	95	107	74	90	54.7	18.4	37	11	25
	15									
	20									
	30									
	40									

Sudomotor evaluation - functional

Test: Quantitative sudomotor axon reflex test (QSART)				
Location	Site (l/r)	Latency [min]	Volume [µl]	Norm [µl]*
Forearm	l	2.08	0.605	≥0.08
Prox. leg	l	2.05	0.829	≥0.14
Distal leg	l	1.37	0.638	≥0.15
Foot	l	2.37	0.186	≥0.07

* Normative data are adjusted for gender and age of patient.

Test: Electrochemical skin conductance (ESC)				
Location	Left [µS]	Right [µS]	Average [µS/k]	Norm [µS/kg]
Hand				≥
Feet				≥
Forehead				

For grading uses ESC [µS] adjusted for weight [µS/k].

(continued)

TABLE 81.1 CONTINUED

Small fiber (sensory + sudomotor) evaluation - morphological					
Test: Skin biopsy					
Location	Site (l/r)	Nerve fibers			
		Epidermal*		Sweat glands	
		Density	Norm	Density	Norm
Proximal leg – thigh	Right	16.41	≥8.3	48.5	≥37.8
Distal leg - calf	Right	5.85	≥8.7	69.3	≥36.5
Foot	Right		≥3.11		≥34.8

*Normative data for distal leg are adjusted for gender and age of patient.

QASAT*										
Heart rate		**BP**		**CBFv**		**ET-CO2**		**Sudomotor**		**Total QASAT score**
S. bradycardia	0	Low supine	0	Low supine	0	Low supine	0	QSART	1	
S. tachycardia	0	High supine	0	High supine	0	High supine	0	ESC		12
Increase tilt	1	OH	0	Tilt response	2	Tilt low	4			
Decrease tilt	0	OHTN	0	CA	0	Tilt high	0	**Skin biopsy**		
Deep breathing	0	VM	1	CVR	0			Epidermal	3	
VR	0			VM	0			Sweat gland	0	
Total	1	Total	1	Total	2	Total	4			

*QASAT. See Novak. Quantitative Scale for Grading of Cardiovascular Autonomic Reflex Tests and Small Fibers from Skin Biopsies. *J Neurol Disord* 2015;3:2.

S, supine; Increase tilt, increased response to tilt; Decrease tilt, decreased response to tilt; BP, blood pressure; VM, Valsalva maneuver; CBFv, cerebral blood flow velocity; CA, cerebral autoregulation; MCA, middle cerebral artery; VR, Valsalva ratio; CVR, cerebral vasoreactivity.

Patient-reported symptoms during testing: Dizziness during the tilt.

Patient-reported symptoms for past 2 weeks:

Lightheadedness or dizziness: Occasionally
Dry eyes or mouth: Occasionally
Pale feet: Yes, minor annoyance
Cold feet: Yes, minor annoyance
Reduced sweating: Occasionally
Reduced sweating after exercise: Yes, minor annoyance
Increased sweating: Yes, minor annoyance
Nausea: Occasionally
Diarrhea: None
Constipation: None
Urinary leaks: Yes, minor annoyance
Aching pain: Occasionally, mild
Allodynia: None
Burning pain: Occasionally, moderate
Lancinating pain: Occasionally, moderate
Numbness: Occasionally, moderate
Prickling sensation: Occasionally, mild

AUTONOMIC TESTING INTERPRETATION

- Small fiber neuropathy, sensory, length-dependent (Figure 81.1).
- Hypocapnic cerebral hypoperfusion (HYCH).
- Mild adrenergic failure.

COMMENT

The testing showed small fiber neuropathy and HYCH (Figure 81.1). Small fiber neuropathy can underlie some of the sensory complaints. HYCH can be linked to

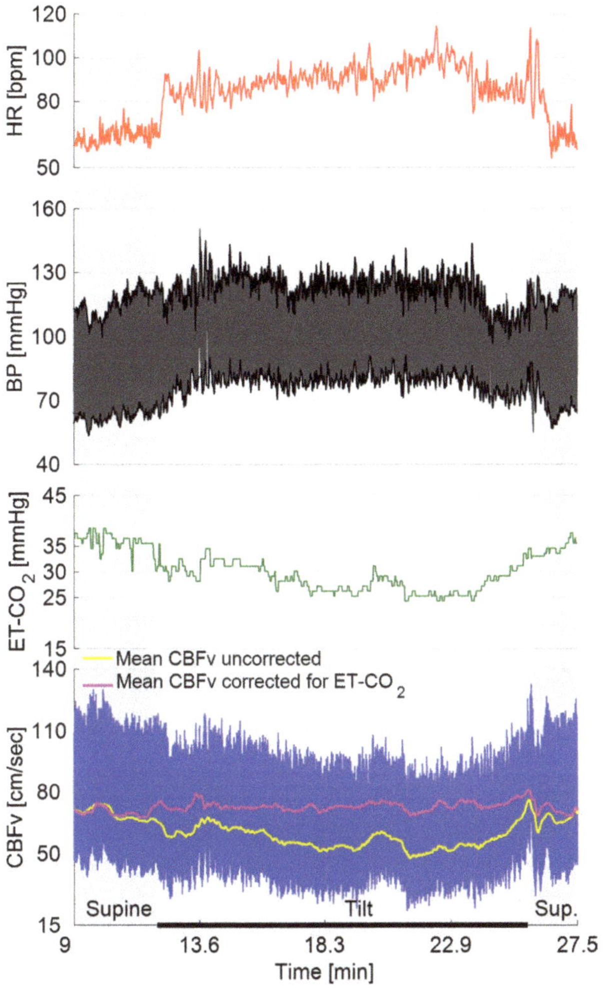

Figure 81.1 Heart rate responses to tilt were exaggerated but did not exceed 120 BPM which is typical for postural tachycardia syndrome. Blood pressure responses to tilt were normal. Orthostatic cerebral blood flow velocity declined due to hypocapnia-induced cerebral vasoconstriction.

cerebral hypoperfusion and thus be responsible for orthostatic intolerance and perhaps cognitive complaints. The dysautonomia was mild and cannot explain all symptoms.

TREATMENT AND FOLLOW-UP

- Pain control.
- Recommended management of orthostatic intolerance.[2–4]

CAVEATS

- PLDS can be associated with small fiber neuropathy and hypocapnic cerebral hypoperfusion.

REFERENCES

1. Aucott JN. Posttreatment Lyme disease syndrome. *Infect Dis Clin North Am*. 2015;29(2):309–323. doi:10.1016/j.idc.2015.02.012.
2. Low PA, Sandroni P, Joyner M, Shen W-K. Postural tachycardia syndrome (POTS). *J Cardiovasc Electrophysiol*. 2009;20(3):352–358. doi:10.1111/j.1540-8167.2008.01407.x.
3. Agarwal AK, Garg R, Ritch A, Sarkar P. Postural orthostatic tachycardia syndrome. *Postgrad Med J*. 2007;83(981):478–480. doi:10.1136/pgmj.2006.055046.
4. Garland EM, Celedonio JE, Raj SR. Postural Tachycardia Syndrome: Beyond Orthostatic Intolerance. *Curr Neurol Neurosci Rep*. 2015;15(9):60. doi:10.1007/s11910-015-0583-8.

82.

CASE 77: PAINFUL SMALL FIBER NEUROPATHY IN POSTTREATMENT LYME DISEASE SYNDROME

Chief complaint: Pain.

Case presentation: A 55-year-old woman presents with various pain syndromes for 12 years. The pain affects various part of her body at different time, including distal limbs. The pain is aching, stabbing, and associated with numbness. Patient tried multiple pain medications without any significant improvement although she noted some improvement on trigger point injections. She was diagnosed with Lyme disease 10 years ago and treated with multiple antibiotics. Previous electromyogram and nerve conduction studies were normal. Neurological examination showed normal reflexes and muscle strength, normal large fibers results (soft touch, vibration, and proprioception sensation), but abnormal small fiber results (pin-prick and temperature sensation at distal legs). Patient was referred for evaluation of suspected painful small fiber neuropathy.

Past medical history: Endometriosis, lumbar spine disk disease, Lyme disease, posttreatment Lyme disease syndrome (PLDS).

Current medication: Mirtazapine.

Assessment plan: Functional autonomic tests and skin biopsy.

AUTONOMIC TESTING EVALUATION

See Table 82.1.

Heart rate: Supine heart rate was normal. Heart rate responses to deep breathing were reduced to 80% of normal value. Heart rate increment during the tilt (18 BPM) was normal.

Blood pressure:

Valsalva maneuver: Mean blood pressure failed to return to baseline at the end of Phase 2 by 20 mm Hg (i.e., 82.5% of baseline).

Tilt: Supine blood pressure was elevated. Blood pressure responses to tilt were normal.

Sudomotor evaluation: Electrochemical skin conductance was normal at hands and normal at feet.

Respiratory system: Respiratory frequency was normal in supine position but was increased during the tilt. End tidal CO_2 was normal in supine position but was severely reduced during the tilt.

Cerebral blood flow velocity (CBFv): CBFv in middle cerebral artery was increased in supine position. CBFv in middle cerebral artery was reduced during the tilt.

Skin biopsy (sensory-epidermal): Epidermal nerve fiber density was abnormal (reduced to 87.6% of normal limit) at distal leg.

Skin biopsy (sweat glands): No sweat glands found in the specimen.

Patient-reported symptoms during testing: Dizziness and shortness of breath during the tilt.

TABLE 82.1 RESULTS OF AUTONOMIC TESTING

Blood pressure evaluation					
Test: Valsalva maneuver					
Pressure [mmHg]	Baseline	Phase 2			Phase 4
		Early	End		
Systolic	146	83	102		
Mean	114	77	94	n/a	
Diastolic	98	74	90	n/a	

Heart rate evaluation	
Test: Deep breathing	
Results	Norm*
7.2	≥9
Test: Valsalva ratio	
1.35	≥1.47

* adjusted for a gender and age

TABLE 82.1 **CONTINUED**

Test: Tilt test										
Position		HR [BPM]	Blood pressure [mmHg]		MCA Blood flow velocity [cm/s]				Respiratory frequency [breaths/min]	End tidal CO_2 [mmHg]
			Systolic	Diastolic	Systolic	Mean	Mean drop [%]	Diastolic		
Supine		90	154	90	167	103.7		72	17	36
Tilt [min]	1	97	133	87	126	80.7	22.2	58	24	25
	2	102	136	85						
	3	104	140	87						
	4	101	135	91						
	5	105	137	86	123	77	25.7	54	22	22
	6	108	131	85						
	7	107	133	87						
	8	107	132	82						
	9	108	130	92						
	10	108	133	88	140	88	15.1	62	20	22
	15									
	20									
	30									
	40									

Sudomotor evaluation - functional

Test: Quantitative sudomotor axon reflex test (QSART)				
Location	Site (l/r)	Latency [min]	Volume [μl]	Norm [μl]*
Forearm				≥0.08
Prox. leg				≥0.14
Distal leg				≥0.07
Foot				≥0.05

* Normative data are adjusted for gender and age of patient.

Test: Electrochemical skin conductance (ESC)				
Location	Left [μS]	Right [μS]	Average [μS/k]	Norm [μS/kg]
Hand	75	71	1.31	≥1.03
Feet	82	82	1.47	≥1.14
Forehead				

For grading uses ESC [μS] adjusted for weight [μS/k].

(continued)

TABLE 82.1 CONTINUED

Small fiber (sensory + sudomotor) evaluation - morphological					
Test: Skin biopsy					
Location	Site (l/r)	Nerve fibers			
		Epidermal*		Sweat glands	
		Density	Norm	Density	Norm
Proximal leg – thigh	Right		≥8.3		≥37.8
Distal leg - calf	Right	5.87	≥6.7		≥36.5
Foot	Right		≥3.11		≥34.8

*Normative data for distal leg are adjusted for gender and age of patient.

QASAT*												
Heart rate		BP		CBFv		ET-CO2		Sudomotor			Total QASAT score
S. bradycardia	0	Low supine	0	Low supine	0	Low supine	0	QSART			
S. tachycardia	0	High supine	1	High supine	1	High supine	0	ESC	0		
Increase tilt	0	OH	0	Tilt response	5	Tilt low	6				
Decrease tilt	0	OHTN	0	CA	0	Tilt high	0	**Skin biopsy**			18
Deep breathing	1	VM	2	CVR	0			Epidermal	1		
VR	1			VM	0			Sweat gland			
Total	2	Total	3	Total	6	Total	6				

*QASAT. See Novak. Quantitative Scale for Grading of Cardiovascular Autonomic Reflex Tests and Small Fibers from Skin Biopsies. *J Neurol Disord* 2015;3:2.

S, supine; Increase tilt, increased response to tilt; Decrease tilt, decreased response to tilt; BP, blood pressure; VM, Valsalva maneuver; CBFv, cerebral blood flow velocity; CA, cerebral autoregulation; MCA, middle cerebral artery; VR, Valsalva ratio; CVR, cerebral vasoreactivity.

Patient-reported symptoms for past 2 weeks:

Lightheadedness or dizziness: Yes, minor annoyance
Dry eyes or mouth: None
Pale feet: None
Cold feet: Occasionally
Reduced sweating: Occasionally
Reduced sweating after exercise: Occasionally
Increased sweating: Occasionally
Nausea: Yes, minor annoyance
Diarrhea: None
Constipation: Occasionally
Urinary leaks: Occasionally
Current pain severity: 10
Aching pain: Continuous, severe
Allodynia: Often, moderate
Burning pain: Continuous, severe
Lancinating pain: Continuous, severe
Numbness: Continuous, severe
Prickling sensation: Often, moderate

AUTONOMIC TESTING INTERPRETATION

1. Small fiber neuropathy, painful, affecting sensory fibers.
2. Hypocapnic cerebral hypoperfusion (HYCH).
3. Cerebral autoregulatory failure.

COMMENT

Patient reported severe shortness of breath, jerky movement, tremor, and worsening of the baselined chronic pain during the tilt (Figure 82.1). The symptoms were associated with reduced CBFv, and they may reflect cerebral hypoperfusion, which also can be associated with chronic pain, headaches, and fatigue.

High supine CBFv suggests impairment of cerebral autoregulation if other causes of high CBFV has been

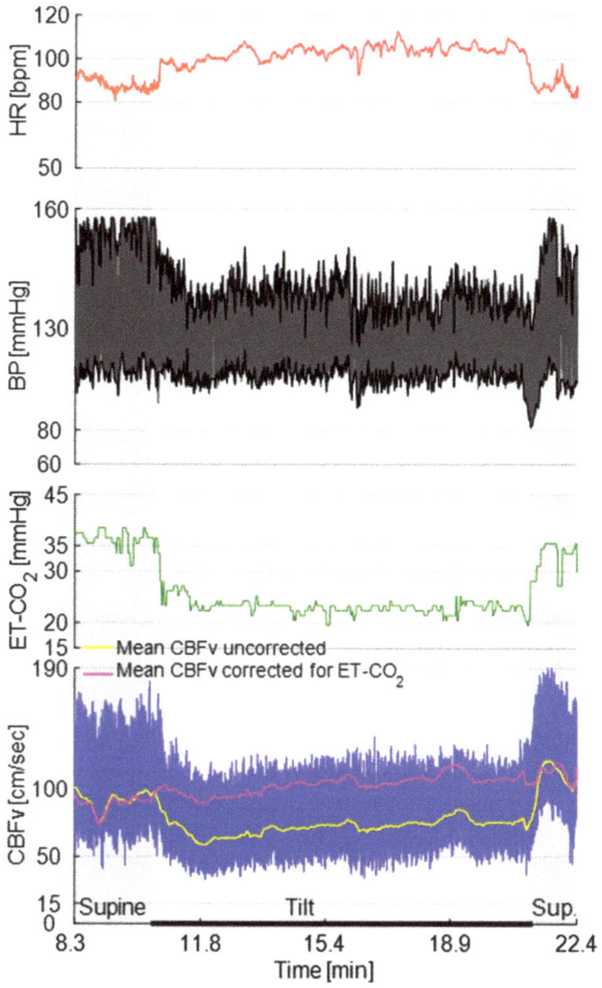

Figure 82.1 Cardiovascular responses to tilt showed supine hypertension and orthostatic decline in systolic blood pressure but it did not satisfy criteria for orthostatic hypotension. Cerebral blood flow velocity (CBFv) was elevated in supine position and declined significantly during the tilt due to hypocapnic vasoconstriction and not due to orthostatic decline in systolic blood pressure since CBFv adjusted for the effect of end tidal CO_2 was stable during the tilt.

ruled out such as anemia and middle cerebral artery stenosis.

CBFv responses in the Valsalva maneuver were also consistent with cerebral autoregulation failure (CAF) since the systolic CBFv exceeded 211 cm/s during Phase 4, which indicates a hyperemic response.[1]

Low orthostatic CBFv was not due to orthostatic hypotension but due to hypocapnic hyperventilation (Figure 82.1).

This patient has a history of Lyme disease, a tick-born infection[2–4] and PLDS since persistence of symptoms in spite of therapy with antibiotics.[5–7]

The patient presented in this chapter failed multiple pain medication. Since autoimmunity may play a role,[8] therapy with immune globulins (IVIG), 2 g/kg/month, was initiated. Patient noted improvement in her pain by about 40% after 12 months of the therapy.

TREATMENT AND FOLLOW-UP

- Trial of IVIG.

CAVEATS

- Chronic fatigue can be associated with cerebral hypoperfusion.
- IVIG can be effective in PLDS.

REFERENCES

1. Novak P. Quantitative scale for grading of cardiovascular autonomic reflex tests and small fibers from skin biopsies (QASAT). *J Neurol Disord*. April 2015. doi:10.4172/2329-6895.1000226.
2. Shapiro ED, Gerber MA. Lyme disease. *Clin Infect Dis Off Publ Infect Dis Soc Am*. 2000;31(2):533–542. doi:10.1086/313982.
3. Steere AC, Strle F, Wormser GP, et al. Lyme borreliosis. *Nat Rev Dis Primer*. 2016;2:16090. doi:10.1038/nrdp.2016.90.
4. Mead PS. Epidemiology of Lyme disease. *Infect Dis Clin North Am*. 2015;29(2):187–210. doi:10.1016/j.idc.2015.02.010.
5. Cairns V, Godwin J. Post-Lyme borreliosis syndrome: a meta-analysis of reported symptoms. *Int J Epidemiol*. 2005;34(6):1340–1345. doi:10.1093/ije/dyi129.
6. Aucott JN, Rebman AW, Crowder LA, Kortte KB. Post-treatment Lyme disease syndrome symptomatology and the impact on life functioning: is there something here? *Qual Life Res*. 2013;22(1):75–84. doi:10.1007/s11136-012-0126-6.
7. Aucott JN. Posttreatment Lyme disease syndrome. *Infect Dis Clin North Am*. 2015;29(2):309–323. doi:10.1016/j.idc.2015.02.012.
8. Maccallini P, Bonin S, Trevisan G. Autoimmunity against a glycolytic enzyme as a possible cause for persistent symptoms in Lyme disease. *Med Hypotheses*. 2018;110:1–8. doi:10.1016/j.mehy.2017.10.024.

83.

CASE 78: SMALL FIBER NEUROPATHY IN WILSON DISEASE

Chief complaint: Numbness.

Case presentation: A 45-year-old woman presented with bilateral hand pain and progressive loss of feeling in legs for 2 years. She has history of Wilson disease (proved mutation of ATP7B gene, associated with elevated urinary copper and low serum ceruloplasmin) treated with penicillamine for 36 years. Past medical history also includes Chiari malformation treated with occipital craniectomy. She also has a history of morbid obesity treated with bariatric surgery 3 years ago. Electromyogram (EMG) and nerve conduction studies (NCS) were normal. Repeat imaging of the upper cervical spine was without evidence of brainstem or spinal compression. Patient was referred for evaluation of sensory loss.

Past medical history: Wilson disease, Chiari malformation type I, obesity.

Current medication: Penicillamine, vitamin B_6, duloxetine, pregabalin.

Assessment plan: Functional autonomic tests and skin biopsy.

AUTONOMIC TESTING EVALUATION

See Table 83.1.

Heart rate: Supine heart rate was normal. Heart rate responses to deep breathing were reduced to 45.7% of normal value. Heart rate increment during the tilt (17 BPM) was normal.

Blood pressure:

Valsalva maneuver: Mean blood pressure failed to return to baseline at the end of Phase 2 by 6.4 mm Hg (i.e., 91.1% of baseline).

Tilt: Supine blood pressure was normal. Tilt provoked syncope at minute 6 and the tilt was aborted.

Sudomotor evaluation: Electrochemical skin conductance was abnormal (reduced to 70.7% of normal limit) at hands and abnormal (reduced to 70.1% of normal limit) at feet.

Respiratory system: Respiratory frequency was normal in supine position and during the tilt. End tidal CO_2 was minimally reduced in supine position and was further reduced during the tilt.

Cerebral blood flow velocity (CBFv): CBFv in middle cerebral artery was normal in supine position but was severely reduced during the tilt.

Skin biopsy (sensory-epidermal): Epidermal nerve fiber density was normal at proximal leg and abnormal (reduced to 53.6% of normal limit) at distal leg.

Skin biopsy (sweat glands): Sweat gland nerve fiber density was normal at proximal leg and abnormal (reduced to 26% of normal limit) at distal leg.

Patient-reported symptoms during testing: Syncope, dizziness, nausea during the tilt.

Patient-reported symptoms for past 2 weeks:

Lightheadedness or dizziness: Often
Dry eyes or mouth: Occasionally
Pale feet: Occasionally

TABLE 83.1 **RESULTS OF AUTONOMIC TESTING**

Blood pressure evaluation					
Test: Valsalva maneuver					
Pressure [mmHg]	Baseline	Phase 2			Phase 4
		Early	End		
Systolic	89	74	76		
Mean	71.7	63.3	65.3	n/a	
Diastolic	63	58	60	n/a	

Heart rate evaluation	
Test: Deep breathing	
Results	Norm*
4.57	≥10
Test: Valsalva ratio	
1.33	≥1.51
* adjusted for a gender and age	

TABLE 83.1 **CONTINUED**

Test: Tilt test											
Position		HR [BPM]	Blood pressure [mmHg]			MCA Blood flow velocity [cm/s]			Respiratory frequency [breaths/min]	End tidal CO_2 [mmHg]
			Systolic	Diastolic	Systolic	Mean	Mean drop [%]	Diastolic		
Supine		61	115	77	127	77		52	11	34
Tilt [min]	1	78	113	80	115	76.3	0.9	57	12	33
	2	78	111	77						
	3	76	112	77						
	4	78	102	70						
	5	60	76	52	108	68	11.7	48	11	28
	6	60	84	49	108	46	40.3	15	15	21
	7									
	8									
	9									
	10									
	15									
	20									
	30									
	40									

Sudomotor evaluation - functional

Test: Quantitative sudomotor axon reflex test (QSART)				
Location	Site (l/r)	Latency [min]	Volume [µl]	Norm [µl]*
Forearm				≥0.08
Prox. leg				≥0.14
Distal leg				≥0.15
Foot				≥0.07

* Normative data are adjusted for gender and age of patient.

Test: Electrochemical skin conductance (ESC)				
Location	Left [µS]	Right [µS]	Average [µS/k]	Norm [µS/kg]
Hand	73	72	0.73	≥1.03
Feet	81	78	0.79	≥1.14
Forehead				

For grading uses ESC [µS] adjusted for weight [µS/k].

(continued)

TABLE 83.1 CONTINUED

Small fiber (sensory + sudomotor) evaluation - morphological					
Test: Skin biopsy					
Location	Site (l/r)	Nerve fibers			
		Epidermal*		Sweat glands	
		Density	Norm	Density	Norm
Proximal leg – thigh	Right	10.42	≥8.3	38.5	≥37.8
Distal leg - calf	Right	4.02	≥7.5	9.5	≥36.5
Foot	Right		≥3.11		≥34.8

*Normative data for distal leg are adjusted for gender and age of patient.

QASAT*											
Heart rate		BP		CBFv		ET-CO2		Sudomotor			Total QASAT score
S. bradycardia	0	Low supine	0	Low supine	0	Low supine	1	QSART			
S. tachycardia	0	High supine	0	High supine	0	High supine	0	ESC	1		
Increase tilt		OH		Tilt response		Tilt low					
Decrease tilt		OHTN		CA		Tilt high		**Skin biopsy**			13
Deep breathing	2	VM	1	CVR	0			Epidermal	3		
VR	1			VM	0			Sweat gland	4		
Total	3	Total	1	Total	0	Total	1				

*QASAT. See Novak. Quantitative Scale for Grading of Cardiovascular Autonomic Reflex Tests and Small Fibers from Skin Biopsies. *J Neurol Disord* 2015;3:2. Orthostatic (tilt) responses were not graded since QASAT requires the duration of the tilt at least 10 minutes.

S, supine; Increase tilt, increased response to tilt; Decrease tilt, decreased response to tilt; BP, blood pressure; VM, Valsalva maneuver; CBFv, cerebral blood flow velocity; CA, cerebral autoregulation; MCA, middle cerebral artery; VR, Valsalva ratio; CVR, cerebral vasoreactivity.

Cold feet: Occasionally
Reduced sweating: None
Reduced sweating after exercise: None
Increased sweating: Occasionally
Nausea: Often
Diarrhea: Yes, minor annoyance
Constipation: None
Urinary leaks: None
Current pain severity: 4
Aching pain: Continuous, severe
Allodynia: Occasionally, mild
Burning pain: Occasionally, mild
Lancinating pain: None
Numbness: Continuous, severe
Prickling sensation: Occasionally, mild

AUTONOMIC TESTING INTERPRETATION

- Small fiber neuropathy, mixed, length-dependent.
- Syncope, neurally mediated, mixed.
- Autonomic failure due to small fiber neuropathy.

COMMENT

Autonomic testing showed severe, mixed, length-dependent small fiber neuropathy (Figure 83.1). Patient had several potential causes of small fiber neuropathy, including metabolic derangement after bariatric surgery, Wilson disease, and chronic therapy with penicillamine. In addition, patient had prominent bilateral hand pain, which can be seen in cervical cord compression. Further evaluations by imaging ruled out cervical cord compression and recurrence of Chiari malformation. Metabolic evaluation was negative for dyslipidemia, diabetes, nutritional deficiencies including vitamin B_{12}, and other disorders which were reported to be associated with small fiber neuropathy. Penicillamine may induce neuropathy,[1,2] and therefore penicillamine was replaced with triethylenetetramine. After a year of penicillamine replacement, patient still experienced progression of sensory symptoms.

Because discontinuation of penicillamine did not prevent progression of symptoms, Wilson disease is most likely the cause of small fiber neuropathy in this patient. Wilson disease is an autosomal recessive disorder of abnormal copper metabolism due to a mutations in the

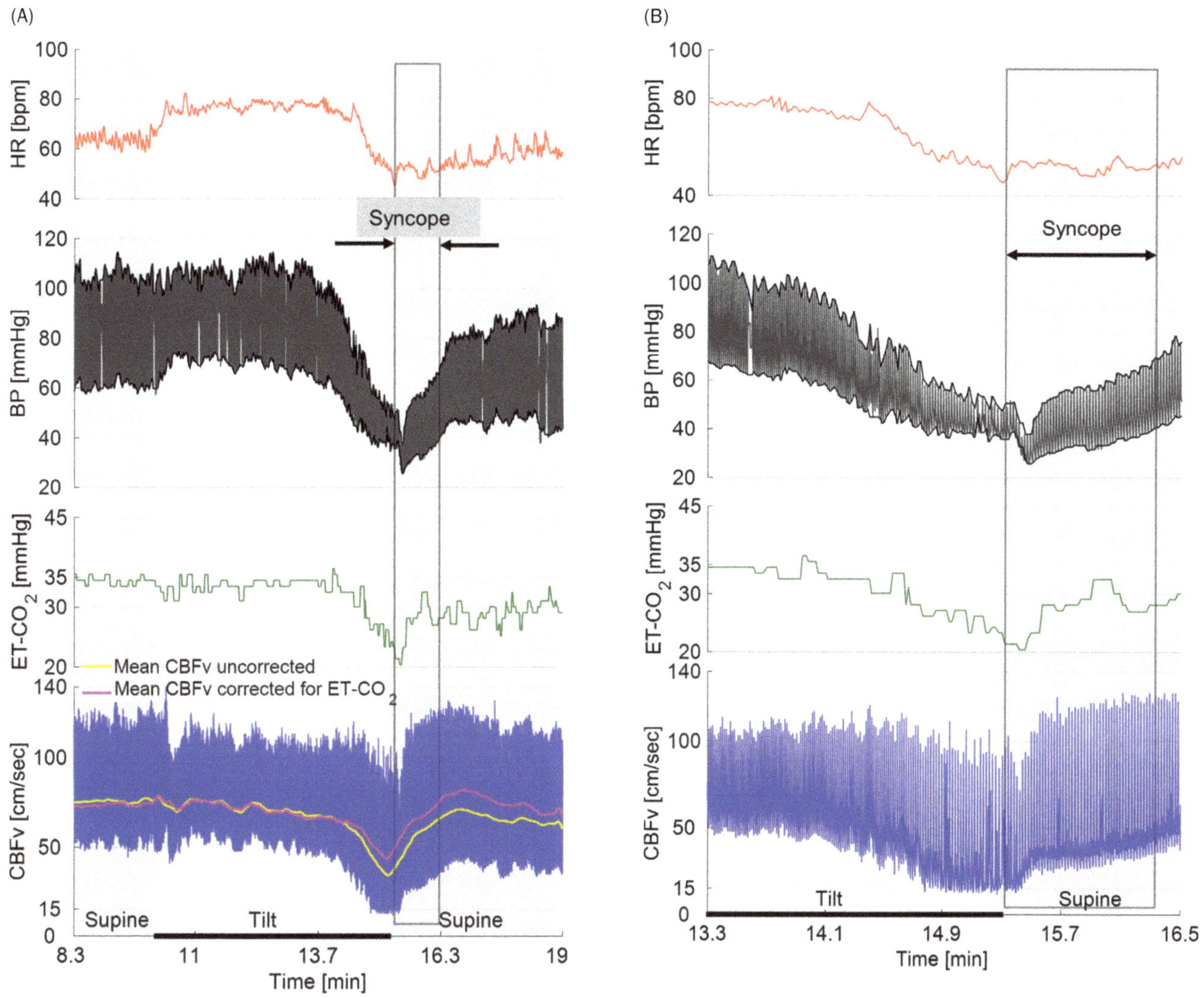

Figure 83.1 The tilt test provoked characteristic mixed syncope with a simultaneous decline in heart rate and blood pressure (A, B). Patient was hyperventilating (end tidal CO_2 <35 mm Hg) before and during the syncope. Cerebral blood flow velocity showed cerebral vasodilation pattern (widening of the signal), which is indicative of normal cerebral autoregulation.

ATP7B gene which codes for a copper-transporting P-type ATPase.[3] Wilson disease usually manifests with progressive liver cirrhosis, neurologic impairment, and renal malfunction.

Little is known about small fiber neuropathy in Wilson disease. Some Wilson disease patients were found to have changes in corneal subbasal nerve plexus on corneal confocal microscopy indicative of small fiber neuropathy.[4] Another study found abnormal skin wrinkling in Wilson disease consistent with small fiber neuropathy.[5] Two Wilson's disease patients had significant sensory and two had significant autonomic complaints, including syncopal spells.[5]

TREATMENT AND FOLLOW-UP

- Pain control.
- Continue chelating agents for Wilson disease.
- Start pyridostigmine for autonomic failure.

CAVEATS

- This patent has several potentials causes of small fiber neuropathy including Wilson disease, penicillamine toxicity, or sequela of bariatric surgery.
- Extensive evaluation of bariatric surgery–associated small fiber neuropathy (vitamin levels, metabolic derangement) has been unrevealing.
- Wilson disease is most likely the cause of small fiber neuropathy in this patient.
- This case provides an additional evidence of involvement of small fiber neuropathy in Wilson disease.

REFERENCES

1. Lee AH, Lawton NF. Penicillamine treatment of Wilson's disease and optic neuropathy. *J Neurol Neurosurg Psychiatry*. 1991;54(8):746.
2. Pedersen PB, Hogenhaven H. Penicillamin-induced neuropathy in rheumatoid arthritis. *Acta Neurol Scand*. 1990;81(2):188–190.
3. Bull PC, Thomas GR, Rommens JM, Forbes JR, Cox DW. The Wilson disease gene is a putative copper transporting P-type ATPase similar to the Menkes gene. *Nat Genet*. 1993;5(4):327–337. doi:10.1038/ng1293-327.
4. Sturniolo GC, Lazzarini D, Bartolo O, et al. Small fiber peripheral neuropathy in Wilson disease: an in vivo documentation by corneal confocal microscopy. *Invest Ophthalmol Vis Sci*. 2015;56(2): 1390–1395. doi:10.1167/iovs.14-15004.
5. Gondim F de AA, Gurgel Filha JH. Small fiber neuropathy and Wilson disease. *Invest Ophthalmol Vis Sci*. 2015;56(9):5330. doi:10.1167/iovs.15-17241.

84.

CASE 79: SMALL FIBER NEUROPATHY AND ABNORMAL CEREBRAL BLOOD FLOW

Chief complaint: Dizziness.

Case presentation: A 39-year-old woman presents with unexplained dizziness for 4 years. The dizziness is usually orthostatic and is associated with chest tightness or chest pain and shortness of breath. Patient also complains of numbness and pain at distal legs. Pulmonary and otorhinolaryngology evaluations were unrevealing. MRI of the brain, nerve conduction studies, and electroencephalogram were normal.

Past medical history: Allergic rhinitis, amenorrhea, anxiety disorder, asthma, herpes simplex, hypertension, hypothyroidism, lupus erythematosus, obstructive sleep apnea, osteoporosis.

Current medication: Duloxetine, diclofenac, fluticasone, hydroxychloroquine, vitamins B_{12} and D, coenzyme Q10, calcium.

Assessment Plan: Functional autonomic tests and skin biopsy.

AUTONOMIC TESTING EVALUATION

See Table 84.1.

Heart rate: Supine heart rate was normal. Heart rate responses to deep breathing were reduced to 16.7% of normal value. Heart rate increment during the tilt (36 BPM) was exaggerated.

Blood pressure:

Valsalva maneuver: Mean blood pressure failed to return to baseline at the end of Phase 2 by 46.4 mm Hg (i.e., 57.3% of baseline).

Tilt: Supine blood pressure was normal. Blood pressure responses to tilt were normal.

Sudomotor evaluation: Electrochemical skin conductance was normal at hands and abnormal (reduced to 76.2% of normal limit) at feet.

Respiratory system: Respiratory frequency was normal in supine and during the tilt. End tidal CO_2 was reduced in supine position and during the tilt.

Cerebral blood flow velocity (CBFv): CBFv in middle cerebral artery was minimally increased in supine position. CBFv in middle cerebral artery was severely reduced during the tilt.

Skin biopsy (sensory-epidermal): Epidermal nerve fiber density was abnormal (reduced to 44.3% of normal limit) at proximal leg and abnormal (reduced to 28.9% of normal limit) at distal leg.

Skin biopsy (sweat glands): Sweat gland nerve fiber density was abnormal (reduced to 92.9% of normal limit) at distal leg.

TABLE 84.1 RESULTS OF AUTONOMIC TESTING

Blood pressure evaluation					
Test: Valsalva maneuver					
Pressure [mmHg]	Baseline	Phase 2			Phase 4
		Early	End		
Systolic	140	61	71		
Mean	108.7	53	62.3	n/a	
Diastolic	93	49	58	n/a	

Heart rate evaluation	
Test: Deep breathing	
Results	Norm*
2	≥12
Test: Valsalva ratio	
1.1	≥1.5
* adjusted for a gender and age	

(continued)

TABLE 84.1 **CONTINUED**

Test: Tilt test											
Position		HR [BPM]	Blood pressure [mmHg]		MCA Blood flow velocity [cm/s]				Respiratory frequency [breaths/min]	End tidal CO_2 [mmHg]
			Systolic	Diastolic	Systolic	Mean	Mean drop [%]	Diastolic		
Supine		65	134	83	122	90.7		75	20	32
Tilt [min]	1	73	128	86	100	70.7	22.1	56	10	33
	2	78	145	95						
	3	76	138	91						
	4	76	136	94						
	5	83	144	93	100	73.3	19.2	60	12	32
	6	82	135	93						
	7	83	138	98						
	8	90	143	95						
	9	98	136	92						
	10	101	125	99	84	58	36.1	45	11	27
	15									
	20									
	30									
	40									

Sudomotor evaluation - functional

Test: Quantitative sudomotor axon reflex test (QSART)				
Location	Site (l/r)	Latency [min]	Volume [μl]	Norm [μl]*
Forearm				≥0.08
Prox. leg				≥0.14
Distal leg				≥0.15
Foot				≥0.07

* Normative data are adjusted for gender and age of patient.

Test: Electrochemical skin conductance (ESC)				
Location	Left [μS]	Right [μS]	Average [μS/k]	Norm [μS/kg]
Hand	82	77	1.06	≥1.03
Feet	67	63	0.84	≥1.14
Forehead				

For grading uses ESC [μS] adjusted for weight [μS/k].

TABLE 84.1 CONTINUED

Small fiber (sensory + sudomotor) evaluation - morphological					
Test: Skin biopsy					
Location	Site (l/r)	Nerve fibers			
		Epidermal*		Sweat glands	
		Density	Norm	Density	Norm
Proximal leg – thigh	Right	3.68	≥8.3		≥37.8
Distal leg - calf	Right	2.31	≥7.98	33.9	≥36.5
Foot	Right		≥3.11		≥34.8

*Normative data for distal leg are adjusted for gender and age of patient.

QASAT*											
Heart rate		BP		CBFv		ET-CO2		Sudomotor			Total QASAT score
S. bradycardia	0	Low supine	0	Low supine	0	Low supine	1	QSART			
S. tachycardia	0	High supine	0	High supine	1	High supine	0	ESC	2		
Increase tilt	1	OH	0	Tilt response	6	Tilt low	1				
Decrease tilt	0	OHTN	0	CA	0	Tilt high	0	**Skin biopsy**			23
Deep breathing	3	VM	3	CVR	0			Epidermal	3		
VR	1			VM	0			Sweat gland	1		
Total	5	Total	3	Total	7	Total	2				

*QASAT. See Novak. Quantitative Scale for Grading of Cardiovascular Autonomic Reflex Tests and Small Fibers from Skin Biopsies. *J Neurol Disord* 2015;3:2.

S, supine; Increase tilt, increased response to tilt; Decrease tilt, decreased response to tilt; BP, blood pressure; VM, Valsalva maneuver; CBFv, cerebral blood flow velocity; CA, cerebral autoregulation; MCA, middle cerebral artery; VR, Valsalva ratio; CVR, cerebral vasoreactivity.

Patient-reported symptoms during testing: Dizziness during the tilt.

Patient-reported symptoms for past 2 weeks:

Lightheadedness or dizziness: Occasionally
Dry eyes or mouth: Occasionally
Pale feet: Yes, minor annoyance
Cold feet: Occasionally
Reduced sweating: Occasionally
Reduced sweating after exercise: Yes, minor annoyance
Increased sweating: Occasionally
Nausea: Occasionally
Diarrhea: None
Constipation: Occasionally
Urinary leaks: Yes, minor annoyance
Current pain severity: 3
Aching pain: Often, moderate
Allodynia: Occasionally, mild
Burning pain: Occasionally, moderate
Lancinating pain: Occasionally
Numbness: Occasionally, mild
Prickling sensation: Occasionally, mild

AUTONOMIC TESTING INTERPRETATION

- Hypocapnic cerebral hypoperfusion (HYCH).
- Initial orthostatic hypotension.
- Small fiber neuropathy, mixed.

COMMENT

The tilt test showed initial orthostatic hypotension with recovery within the first minute (Figure 84.1A). However, the main finding was a progressive decline in CBFv during the tilt. Correction of CBFv by the end tidal CO_2 reduced the decline but did not normalize the orthostatic CBFv (Figure 84.1B). In another words, orthostatic CBFv declined more that can be attributed to the effect of end tidal CO_2. Therefore an exaggerated CO_2 induced vasoconstriction may play a role. This can be assessed by cerebral vasoreactivity study.[1]

The tilt test reproduced the patient's typical symptoms. She became dizzy immediately at the onset of the tilt, but symptoms resolved within a minute. She became again

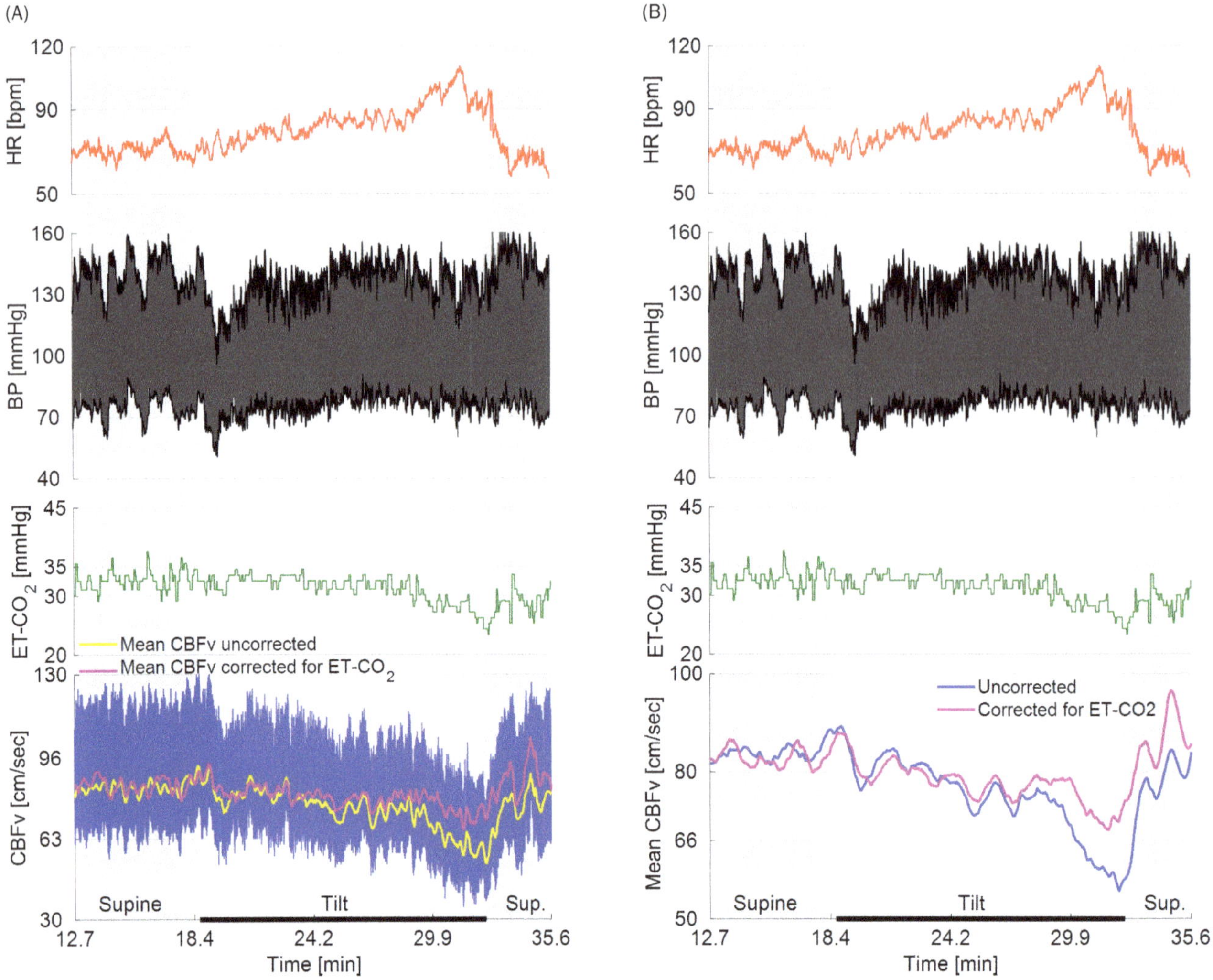

Figure 84.1 The tilt provoked immediate symptomatic decline in systolic blood pressure by 41 mm Hg and cerebral blood flow velocity (CBFv) by 18%, consistent with initial orthostatic hypotension. The patient was hyperventilating, with a progressive decline in end tidal CO_2 below 25 mm Hg (normal end tidal CO_2 >35 mm Hg). The decline in end tidal CO_2 was also associated with a decline in CBFv (48% uncorrected, 28% corrected declline in mean CBFv for declline in mean CBFv end tidal CO_2 at the end of the tilt).

progressively dizzy at about minute 5 of the tilt and later experienced chest tightness, chest pain, and severe shortness of breath. She was hyperventilating both during the supine position and even more during the tilt and was unable to control her breathing rate due severe shortness of breath.

TREATMENT AND FOLLOW-UP

- Cerebral vasoreactivity study.
- Calcium channel blockers may dilate the cerebral vessels and improve cerebral perfusion.
- Clinical workup for neuropathy revealed elevated acetylcholine receptor antibodies, both modulating (28%, normal 0–20%) and binding (0.05 nm/L, normal <0.02 nmol/L) and GAD65 antibody (0.04 nmol/L, normal ≤0.02). This patient therefore has probably autoimmune small fiber neuropathy and can benefit from immunomodulatory therapy.[2]

CAVEATS

- Autonomic testing may reveal multiple abnormalities, and therefore it is important to be familiar with criteria for respective syndromes or disorders.

REFERENCES

1. Novak P. Orthostatic cerebral hypoperfusion syndrome. *Front Aging Neurosci*. 2016;8:22. doi:10.3389/fnagi.2016.00022.
2. Klein CM, Vernino S, Lennon VA, et al. The spectrum of autoimmune autonomic neuropathies. *Ann Neurol*. 2003;53(6):752–758. doi:10.1002/ana.10556.

85.

CASE 80: VITAMIN B_{12} DEFICIENCY

Chief complaint: Dizziness.

Case presentation: A 36-year-old women presents with a history of severe fatigue since age 15 following mononucleosis. She complained of orthostatic intolerance and was briefly treated with β-blockers that were stopped because of hypotension. She was still able to exercise. More recently she developed severe disabling fatigue, worsening of orthostatic symptoms, and palpitations within 1 year after the birth of her daughter. Stress test, cardiology evaluation, sleep study, and orthostatic vital signs at the office were normal.

Past medical history: Vitamin B_{12} deficiency.

Current medication: Vitamin B_{12} supplements.

Assessment plan: Functional autonomic tests and skin biopsy.

AUTONOMIC TESTING EVALUATION

See Table 85.1.

Heart rate: Supine heart rate was normal. Heart rate responses to deep breathing were normal. Heart rate increment during the tilt (6 BPM) was reduced.

Blood pressure:

Valsalva maneuver: Blood pressure responses were normal.

Tilt: Supine blood pressure was normal. Blood pressure responses to tilt were normal.

Sudomotor evaluation: Electrochemical skin conductance was normal at hands and normal at feet.

Respiratory system: Respiratory frequency and end tidal CO_2 were normal in supine position and during the tilt.

Cerebral blood flow velocity (CBFv): CBFv in middle cerebral artery was normal in supine position. CBFv in middle cerebral artery was stable during the tilt.

Skin biopsy (sensory-epidermal): Epidermal nerve fiber density was abnormal (reduced to 76.5% of normal limit) at proximal leg and abnormal (reduced to 75.1% of normal limit) at distal leg.

Skin biopsy (sweat glands): Sweat gland nerve fiber density was abnormal (reduced to 54.5% of normal limit) at distal leg.

Patient-reported symptoms during testing: Dizziness during the Valsalva maneuver.

Patient-reported symptoms for past 2 weeks:

Lightheadedness or dizziness: Occasionally
Dry eyes or mouth: Occasionally
Pale feet: None
Cold feet: None
Reduced sweating: None

TABLE 85.1 **RESULTS OF AUTONOMIC TESTING**

Blood pressure evaluation					
Test: Valsalva maneuver					
Pressure [mmHg]	Baseline	Phase 2			Phase 4
		Early	End		
Systolic	64	58	73		
Mean	53.3	51.3	62.3	n/a	
Diastolic	48	48	57	n/a	

Heart rate evaluation	
Test: Deep breathing	
Results	Norm*
26.1	≥12
Test: Valsalva ratio	
1.52	≥1.5
* adjusted for a gender and age	

(continued)

TABLE 85.1 CONTINUED

Test: Tilt test										
Position		HR [BPM]	Blood pressure [mmHg]		MCA Blood flow velocity [cm/s]				Respiratory frequency [breaths/min]	End tidal CO_2 [mmHg]
			Systolic	Diastolic	Systolic	Mean	Mean drop [%]	Diastolic		
Supine		77	110	71	107	68.3		49	19	35
Tilt [min]	1	77	135	78	105	69.7	-2	52	15	36
	2	71	112	76						
	3	77	114	77						
	4	83	112	75						
	5	77	108	73	108	73.3	-7.3	56	13	33
	6	81	107	74						
	7	79	112	74						
	8	83	112	76						
	9	80	108	74						
	10	82	109	72	101	69.7	-2	54	17	38
	15									
	20									
	30									
	40									

Sudomotor evaluation - functional

Test: Quantitative sudomotor axon reflex test (QSART)				
Location	Site (l/r)	Latency [min]	Volume [µl]	Norm [µl]*
Forearm				≥0.08
Prox. leg				≥0.14
Distal leg				≥0.15
Foot				≥0.07

* Normative data are adjusted for gender and age of patient.

Test: Electrochemical skin conductance (ESC)				
Location	Left [µS]	Right [µS]	Average [µS/k]	Norm [µS/kg]
Hand	80	82	1.19	≥1.03
Feet	89	91	1.34	≥1.14
Forehead				

For grading uses ESC [µS] adjusted for weight [µS/k].

TABLE 85.1 CONTINUED

Small fiber (sensory + sudomotor) evaluation - morphological					
Test: Skin biopsy					
Location	Site (l/r)	Nerve fibers			
		Epidermal*		Sweat glands	
		Density	Norm	Density	Norm
Proximal leg – thigh	Right	6.35	≥8.3		≥37.8
Distal leg - calf	Right	6.17	≥8.22	19.9	≥36.5
Foot	Right		≥3.11		≥34.8

*Normative data for distal leg are adjusted for gender and age of patient.

QASAT*										
Heart rate		**BP**		**CBFv**		**ET-CO2**		**Sudomotor**		**Total QASAT score**
S. bradycardia	0	Low supine	0	Low supine	0	Low supine	0	QSART		
S. tachycardia	0	High supine	0	High supine	0	High supine	0	ESC	0	
Increase tilt	0	OH	0	Tilt response	0	Tilt low	0			
Decrease tilt	1	OHTN	0	CA	0	Tilt high	0	**Skin biopsy**		6
Deep breathing	0	VM	0	CVR	0			Epidermal	2	
VR	0			VM	0			Sweat gland	3	
Total	1	Total	0	Total	0	Total	0			

*QASAT. See Novak. Quantitative Scale for Grading of Cardiovascular Autonomic Reflex Tests and Small Fibers from Skin Biopsies. *J Neurol Disord* 2015;3:2.

S, supine; Increase tilt, increased response to tilt; Decrease tilt, decreased response to tilt; BP, blood pressure; VM, Valsalva maneuver; CBFv, cerebral blood flow velocity; CA, cerebral autoregulation; MCA, middle cerebral artery; VR, Valsalva ratio; CVR, cerebral vasoreactivity.

Reduced sweating after exercise: None
Increased sweating: Occasionally
Nausea: Occasionally
Diarrhea: Occasionally
Constipation: Occasionally
Urinary leaks: None
Current pain severity: 0
Aching pain: Occasionally, mild
Allodynia: Occasionally, severe
Burning pain: None
Lancinating pain: Occasionally, moderate
Numbness: Occasionally, moderate
Prickling sensation: Occasionally, moderate

AUTONOMIC TESTING INTERPRETATION

- Small fiber neuropathy, mixed, length-dependent.

COMMENT

The testing showed small fiber neuropathy but essentially normal autonomic functions (Figure 85.1). Reduced heart rate responses to the tilt can be seen in minimal parasympathetic dysfunction of questionable clinical significance.

Further clinical workup for small fiber neuropathy was unrevealing, therefore the patient's small

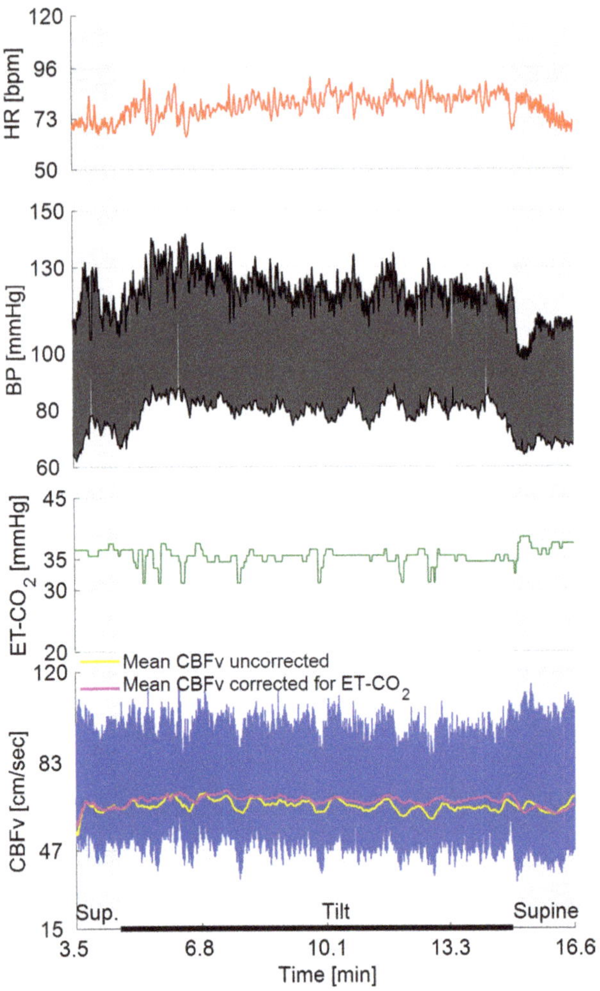

Figure 85.1 The cardiovascular and cerebrovascular responses to tilt were normal.

fiber neuropathy is likely related to B_{12} deficiency.[1] Women of reproductive age are at higher risk of B_{12} deficiency.[2] Patient may suffer from postpartum depression and deconditioning which may amplify orthostatic intolerance.

TREATMENT AND FOLLOW-UP

- Continue B_{12} supplementation.

CAVEATS

- Vitamin B_{12} deficiency is associated with small fiber neuropathy.

REFERENCES

1. Franques J, Verschueren A. [Metabolic neuropathies: overview in 2011]. *Rev Neurol (Paris)*. 2012;168(12):979–982. doi:10.1016/j.neurol.2012.09.004.
2. Green R, Allen LH, Bjørke-Monsen A-L, et al. Vitamin B_{12} deficiency. *Nat Rev Dis Primer*. 2017;3:17040. doi:10.1038/nrdp.2017.40.

86.

CASE 81: HYPOVOLEMIA IN VALSALVA MANEUVER

Chief complaint: Dizziness.

Case presentation: A 47-year-old woman presents with episodic dizziness for 3 years. She suddenly gets dizzy, typically while standing or sitting. There has been no change in dizziness with vestibular therapy or meclizine. The patient also reports numbness and burning sensation in the extremities, more pronounced in the feet. Neurologic examination, nerve conduction studies, MRI, and magnetic resonance angiography (MRA) of the brain and neck were normal. She was referred for suspected orthostatic intolerance and small fiber neuropathy.

Past medical history: Hypothyroidism, migraine, attention deficit disorder, celiac disease, depression, chronic daily headache, Hashimoto's thyroiditis, gastroesophageal reflux, hip dysplasia, iron deficiency anemia, sinus surgery ×3, knee surgery ×3, tonsillectomy.

Current medication: Levothyroxine.

Assessment plan: Functional autonomic tests and skin biopsy.

AUTONOMIC TESTING EVALUATION

See Table 86.1.

Heart rate: Supine heart rate was normal. Heart rate responses to deep breathing were normal. Heart rate increment during the tilt (17 BPM) was normal.

Blood pressure:

Valsalva maneuver: Blood pressure responses were normal.

Tilt: Supine blood pressure was normal. Mean blood pressure during the tilt was normal.

Sudomotor evaluation: Electrochemical skin conductance was abnormal (reduced to 75.6% of normal limit) at hands and normal at feet.

Respiratory system: Respiratory frequency was normal in supine position and during the tilt. End tidal CO_2 was minimally reduced in supine position and was further reduced during the tilt.

Cerebral blood flow velocity (CBFv): CBFv in middle cerebral artery was reduced in supine position and was further reduced the tilt.

Skin biopsy (sensory-epidermal): Epidermal nerve fiber density was normal at proximal leg and abnormal (reduced to 74.9% of normal limit) at distal leg.

Skin biopsy (sweat glands): Sweat gland nerve fiber density was normal at proximal leg and normal at distal leg.

Patient-reported symptoms during testing: Headache, shortness of breath, feeling to be close to passing out during the tilt test.

Patient-reported symptoms for past 2 weeks:

Lightheadedness or dizziness: Occasionally
Dry eyes or mouth: Occasionally
Pale feet: Yes, minor annoyance

TABLE 86.1 **RESULTS OF AUTONOMIC TESTING**

Blood pressure evaluation					
Test: Valsalva maneuver					
Pressure [mmHg]	Baseline	Phase 2			Phase 4
		Early	End		
Systolic	102	69	84		
Mean	75.3	64.3	76	n/a	
Diastolic	62	62	72	n/a	

Heart rate evaluation	
Test: Deep breathing	
Results	Norm*
24	≥10
Test: Valsalva ratio	
2.4	≥1.51
* adjusted for a gender and age	

(continued)

TABLE 86.1 **CONTINUED**

Test: Tilt test										
Position		HR [BPM]	Blood pressure [mmHg]		MCA Blood flow velocity [cm/s]				Respiratory frequency [breaths/min]	End tidal CO2 [mmHg]
			Systolic	Diastolic	Systolic	Mean	Mean drop [%]	Diastolic		
Supine		76	111	72	74	48		35	6	34
Tilt [min]	1	79	113	70	64	40	16.7	28	18	23
	2	77	104	68						
	3	79	103	62						
	4	85	104	70						
	5	79	93	63	64	41.3	14	30	8	34
	6	82	93	66						
	7	86	106	72						
	8	93	115	74						
	9	88	104	70						
	10	90	103	69	63	40.3	16	29	13	29
	15									
	20									
	30									
	40									

Sudomotor evaluation - functional

Test: Quantitative sudomotor axon reflex test (QSART)				
Location	Site (l/r)	Latency [min]	Volume [µl]	Norm [µl]*
Forearm				≥0.08
Prox. leg				≥0.14
Distal leg				≥0.15
Foot				≥0.07

* Normative data are adjusted for gender and age of patient.

Test: Electrochemical skin conductance (ESC)				
Location	Left [µS]	Right [µS]	Average [µS/k]	Norm [µS/kg]
Hand	54	53	0.78	≥1.03
Feet	86	84	1.23	≥1.14
Forehead				

For grading uses ESC [µS] adjusted for weight [µS/k].

TABLE 86.1 CONTINUED

Small fiber (sensory + sudomotor) evaluation - morphological					
Test: Skin biopsy					
Location	Site (l/r)	Nerve fibers			
		Epidermal*		Sweat glands	
		Density	Norm	Density	Norm
Proximal leg – thigh	Right	9.04	≥8.3	43.6	≥37.8
Distal leg - calf	Right	5.5	≥7.34	36.8	≥36.5
Foot	Right		≥3.11		≥34.8

*Normative data for distal leg are adjusted for gender and age of patient.

QASAT*										
Heart rate		**BP**		**CBFv**		**ET CO2**		**Sudomotor**		**Total QASAT score**
S. bradycardia	0	Low sup.	0	Low sup.	1	Low sup.	1	QSART		
S. tachycardia	0	High sup.	0	High sup.	0	High sup.	0	ESC	1	10
Increase. tilt	0	OH	0	Tilt resp.	3	Tilt low	3			
Decreas. tilt	0	OHTN	0	CA	0	Tilt high	0	**Skin biopsy**		
Deep breath	0	VM	0	CVR	0			Epidermal	1	
VR	0			VM	0			Sweat gland	0	
Total	0	Total	0	Total	4	Total	4			

*QASAT. See Novak. Quantitative Scale for Grading of Cardiovascular Autonomic Reflex Tests and Small Fibers from Skin Biopsies. *J Neurol Disord* 2015;3:2.

S, supine; Increase tilt, increased response to tilt; Decrease tilt, decreased response to tilt; BP, blood pressure; VM, Valsalva maneuver; CBFv, cerebral blood flow velocity; CA, cerebral autoregulation; MCA, middle cerebral artery; VR, Valsalva ratio; CVR, cerebral vasoreactivity.

Cold feet: Occasionally
Reduced sweating: Occasionally
Reduced sweating after exercise: Occasionally
Increased sweating: None
Nausea: Often
Diarrhea: None
Constipation: Often
Urinary leaks: Occasionally
Current pain severity: 3
Aching pain: Often, moderate
Allodynia: None
Burning pain: Occasionally, mild
Lancinating pain: Occasionally, mild
Numbness: Often, mild
Prickling sensation: Often, moderate

AUTONOMIC TESTING INTERPRETATION

- Small fiber neuropathy, length-dependent, affecting mainly sensory fibers.
- No evidence of autonomic failure.
- Low cerebral blood flow velocity (CBFv) due to hypovolemia.[1]

COMMENT

Pulse pressure collapse during the Valsalva maneuver can be seen in volume depletion (Figure 86.1).[2]

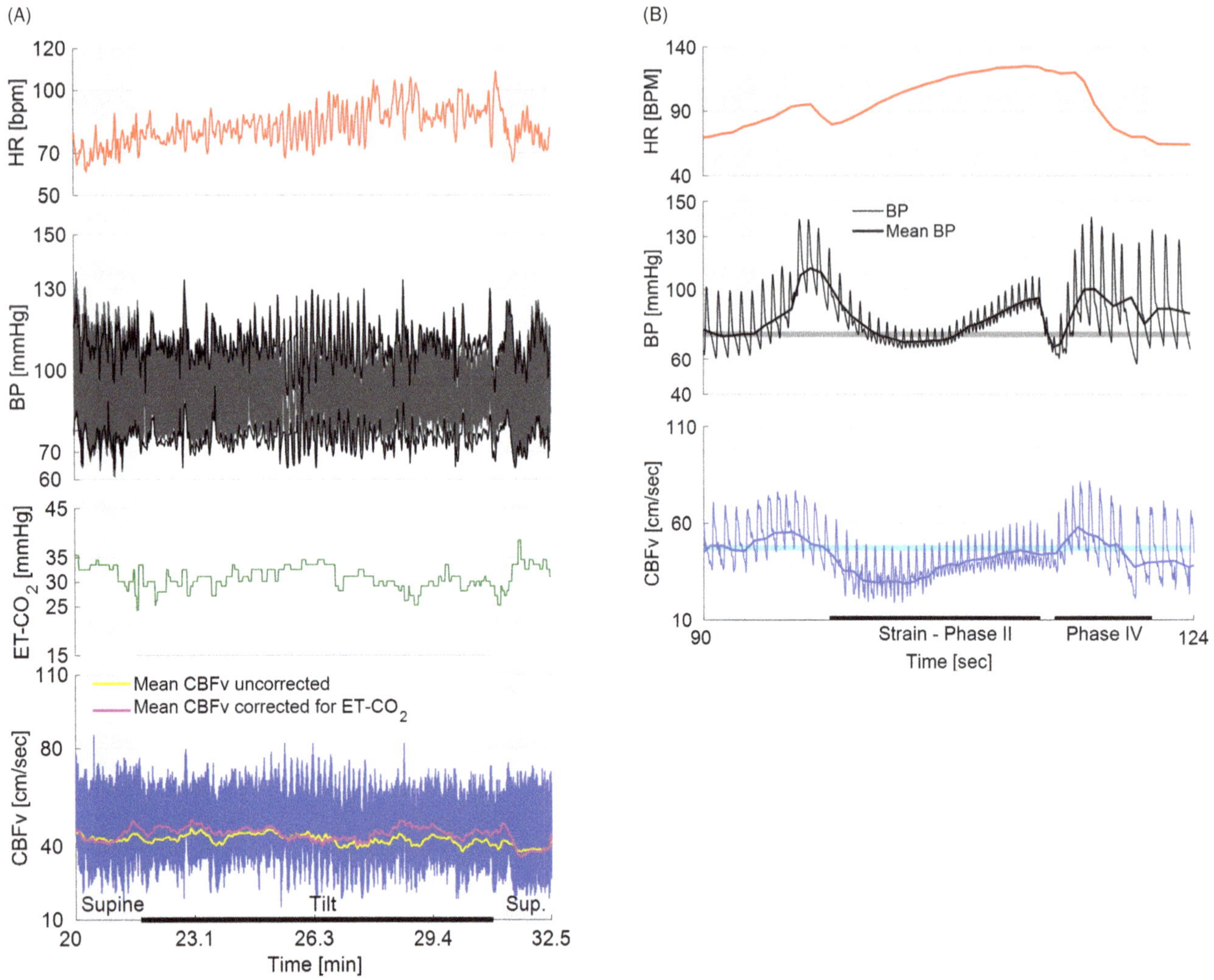

Figure 86.1 The tilt test showed normal responses in heart rate and blood pressure (A). Cerebral blood flow velocity (CBFv) was reduced in supine position patient's average supine velocity was 48.2 cm/s, normal ≥ 53.7 cm/s. Note also large oscillations in blood pressure and CBFv around minute 26.3. Valsalva maneuver showed normal recovery at the end of Phase 2 in blood pressure (B). However, there was prominent (>50%) pulse pressure collapse (difference between systolic and diastolic blood pressure) in the middle of Phase 2. CBFv in Valsalva maneuver was abnormal and showed very low diastolic CBFv.

TREATMENT AND FOLLOW-UP

- Clinical workup for neuropathy.
- Volume expansion with high fluid and high salt intake.
- Endocrine evaluation for hypovolemia.

CAVEATS

- Volume depletion can be associated with low CBFv.

REFERENCES

1. Novak P. Cerebral blood flow, heart rate, and blood pressure patterns during the tilt test in common orthostatic syndromes. *Neurosci J.* 2016;2016:6127340. doi:10.1155/2016/6127340.
2. Low PA, Tomalia VA, Park K-J. Autonomic function tests: some clinical applications. *J Clin Neurol Seoul Korea.* 2013;9(1):1–8. doi:10.3988/jcn.2013.9.1.1.

87.

CASE 82: POSTURAL TACHYCARDIA SYNDROME AND HYPOVOLEMIA

Chief complaint: Fatigue.

Case presentation: A 43-year-old woman presents with disabling fatigue. She was diagnosed with rheumatoid arthritis at age 22 and complex partial seizures at age 23. She experienced persistent fatigue since the diagnosis of seizures. About 2 years ago, she began to experience presyncopal and syncopal episodes. At this time, she is unable to exercise and feels dizzy most of the time. She cannot drive since exposure to bright light exacerbates dizziness. Additional complaints include headaches, tremors, stuttering, chest pain, shortness of breath, and headaches. Lumbar puncture was done twice and showed normal cells and protein, glucose, immunoglobulin G index, and absent oligoclonal bands. MRI of the brain and electroencephalogram were unrevealing. Electromyogram and nerve conduction studies were normal. She is treated with hydrochloroquine, prednisone, and intravenous immunoglobulins for rheumatoid arthritis but she responds poorly to therapy. She was referred for evaluation of suspected autonomic failure.

Past medical history: Rheumatoid arthritis, complex partial seizures, migraine.

Current medication: Oxcarbazepine, hydrochloroquine, prednisone (on hold for a week).

Assessment plan: Functional autonomic testing and skin biopsy.

AUTONOMIC TESTING EVALUATION

See Table 87.1.

Heart rate: Heart rate was within normal range in supine position. Heart rate responses to deep breathing were normal. Heart rate increment during the tilt (50 BPM) was exaggerated and exceeded 120 BPM.

Blood pressure:

Valsalva maneuver: Mean blood pressure failed to return to baseline at the end of Phase 2 by 15 mm Hg (i.e., 83% of baseline).

Tilt: Supine blood pressure was within normal range. Blood pressure responses to tilt were abnormal with noticeable prominent slow oscillations.

Sudomotor evaluation: Electrochemical skin conductance was abnormal (reduced to 75.3% of normal limit) at hands and abnormal (reduced to 86.7% of normal limit) at feet.

Respiratory system: End tidal CO_2 was reduced during supine and during the tilt.

Cerebral blood flow velocity (CBFv): CBFv in middle cerebral artery was normal in supine position. CBFv in middle cerebral artery was mildly reduced during the tilt test.

Skin biopsy (sensory-epidermal): Epidermal nerve fiber density was normal at proximal leg and normal at distal leg.

TABLE 87.1 **RESULTS OF AUTONOMIC TESTING**

Blood pressure evaluation					
Test: Valsalva maneuver					
Pressure [mmHg]	Baseline	Phase 2			Phase 4
		Early	End		
Systolic	105	45	98		
Mean	69.7	48.3	78.7	n/a	
Diastolic	52	50	69	n/a	

Heart rate evaluation	
Test: Deep breathing	
Results	Norm*
10	≥10
Test: Valsalva ratio	
1.76	≥1.51
* adjusted for a gender and age	

(continued)

TABLE 87.1 **CONTINUED**

Test: Tilt test										
Position		HR [BPM]	Blood pressure [mmHg]		MCA Blood flow velocity [cm/s]				Respiratory frequency [breaths/min]	End tidal CO_2 [mmHg]
			Systolic	Diastolic	Systolic	Mean	Mean drop [%]	Diastolic		
Supine		84	121	80	105	69		51	12	29
Tilt [min]	1	101	95	62	103	65.7	4.8	47	13	28
	2	124	114	84						
	3	109	109	81						
	4	116	113	81						
	5	120	106	77	91	57.7	16.4	41	12	26
	6	122	119	84						
	7	116	113	80						
	8	116	126	85						
	9	129	129	84						
	10	113	115	87	91	57.7	16.4	41	17	25
	15									
	20									
	30									
	40									

Sudomotor evaluation - functional

Test: Quantitative sudomotor axon reflex test (QSART)				
Location	Site (l/r)	Latency [min]	Volume [μl]	Norm [μl]*
Forearm				≥0.08
Prox. leg				≥0.14
Distal leg				≥0.15
Foot				≥0.07

* Normative data are adjusted for gender and age of patient.

Test: Electrochemical skin conductance (ESC)				
Location	Left [μS]	Right [μS]	Average [μS/k]	Norm [μS/kg]
Hand	54	49	0.78	≥1.03
Feet	64	67	1.02	≥1.14
Forehead				

For grading uses ESC [μS] adjusted for weight [μS/k].

TABLE 87.1 CONTINUED

Small fiber (sensory + sudomotor) evaluation - morphological					
Test: Skin biopsy					
Location	Site (l/r)	Nerve fibers			
		Epidermal*		Sweat glands	
		Density	Norm	Density	Norm
Proximal leg – thigh	Right	9.07	≥8.3	14	≥37.8
Distal leg - calf	Right	7.59	≥7.5		≥36.5
Foot	Right		≥3.11		≥34.8

*Normative data for distal leg are adjusted for gender and age of patient.

QASAT*											
Heart rate		**BP**		**CBFv**		**ET-CO2**		**Sudomotor**			**Total QASAT score**
S. bradycardia	0	Low supine	0	Low supine	0	Low supine	1	QSART			
S. tachycardia	0	High supine	0	High supine	0	High supine	0	ESC	1		
Increase tilt	4	OH	1	Tilt response	2	Tilt low	5				
Decrease tilt	0	OHTN	0	CA	0	Tilt high	0	**Skin biopsy**			18
Deep breathing	0	VM	0	CVR	0			Epidermal	0		
VR	0			VM	0			Sweat gland	4		
Total	4	Total	1	Total	2	Total	6				

*QASAT. See Novak. Quantitative Scale for Grading of Cardiovascular Autonomic Reflex Tests and Small Fibers from Skin Biopsies. *J Neurol Disord* 2015;3:2.

S, supine; Increase tilt, increased response to tilt; Decrease tilt, decreased response to tilt; BP, blood pressure; VM, Valsalva maneuver; CBFv, cerebral blood flow velocity; CA, cerebral autoregulation; MCA, middle cerebral artery; VR, Valsalva ratio; CVR, cerebral vasoreactivity.

Skin biopsy (sweat glands): Sweat gland nerve fiber density was abnormal (reduced to 37% of normal limit) at proximal leg.

Patient-reported symptoms during testing: Dizziness during the tilt test.

Patient-reported symptoms for past 2 weeks:

Lightheadedness or dizziness: Often
Dry eyes or mouth: Occasionally
Pale feet: Yes, minor annoyance
Cold feet: Occasionally
Reduced sweating: None
Reduced sweating after exercise: None
Increased sweating: None
Nausea: Occasionally
Diarrhea: None
Constipation: Occasionally
Urinary leaks: Occasionally
Current pain severity: 5
Aching pain: Continuous, severe
Allodynia: Occasionally, mild
Burning pain: Often, moderate
Lancinating pain: Often, moderate
Numbness: Occasionally, mild
Prickling sensation: Occasionally, mild

AUTONOMIC TESTING INTERPRETATION

- Postural tachycardia syndrome (POTS), mild, hypovolemic form.
- No evidence of autonomic failure.
- Initial orthostatic hypotension.
- Small fiber neuropathy.

COMMENT

Although the patient had many complaints indicative of dysautonomia, the autonomic testing showed postural tachycardia with essentially normal autonomic functions. The testing also revealed initial orthostatic hypotension, which is a self-limiting benign syndrome (Figure 87.1).[1] The pattern seen in the tilt is consistent with hypovolemia. Large

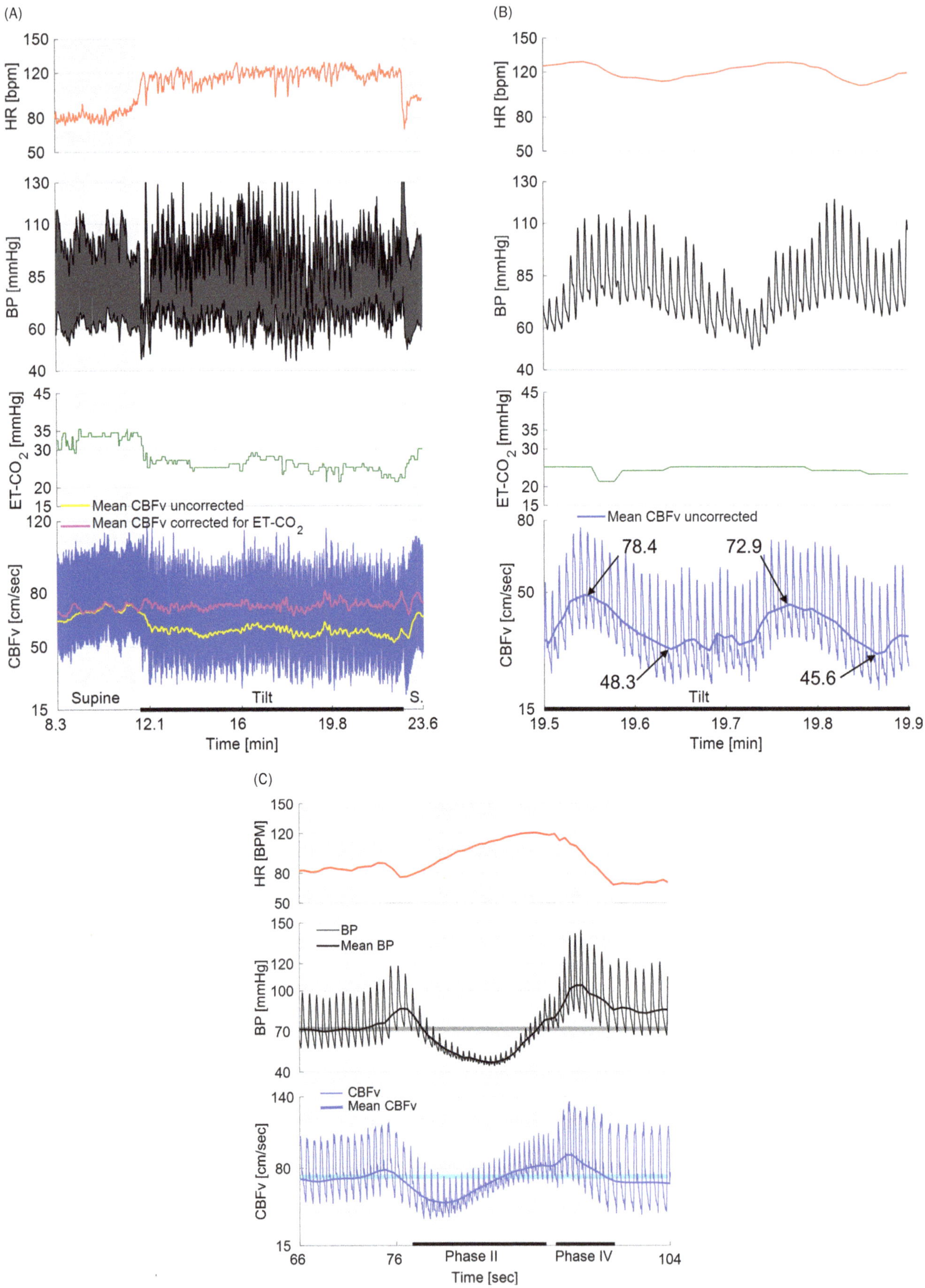

Figure 87.1 The tilt provoked immediate decline in blood pressure with recovery within a minute, which was consistent with initial orthostatic hypotension. Heart rate responses to tilt were exaggerated, and mean heart rate was close to 120 BPM during the tilt. Blood pressure and cerebral blood flow velocity (CBFv) showed prominent oscillations during the tilt. The patient was hyperventilating (end tidal CO_2 <35 mm Hg), and, as a consequence, mean CBFv declined due to vasoconstrictive effect of hypocapnia (A). Panel B shows details of prominent blood pressure and CBFv oscillations. Patient felt dizzy, weak, and short of breath during the tilt. The Valsalva maneuver showed pulse collapse (difference between systolic and diastolic values), but the end of Phase 2 exceeded the baseline (C).

fluctuations with periods of about 1 minute in blood pressure and in CBFv reflect sympathetic compensatory activation in response to hypovolemia. Responses in the Valsalva maneuver were also consistent with hypovolemia, showing pulse collapse in Phase 2 and normal Phase 2 and Phase 4.[2,3] Hypovolemia is recognized as one of the cause of orthostatic intolerance.[4] Small fiber neuropathy is likely due to rheumatoid arthritis.[5]

TREATMENT AND FOLLOW-UP

- Volume expansion through with fluid and high salt intake. Consider therapy with fludrocortisone which may improve orthostatic tolerance.[6]
- Endocrine evaluation for hypovolemia.

CAVEATS

- Autonomic testing is useful to rule out severe dysautonomia, as in this case.

REFERENCES

1. Wieling W, Krediet CTP, van Dijk N, Linzer M, Tschakovsky ME. Initial orthostatic hypotension: review of a forgotten condition. *Clin Sci Lond Engl 1979*. 2007;112(3):157–165. doi:10.1042/CS20060091.
2. Low PA, Tomalia VA, Park K-J. Autonomic function tests: some clinical applications. *J Clin Neurol Seoul Korea*. 2013;9(1):1–8. doi:10.3988/jcn.2013.9.1.1.
3. Low PA. Composite autonomic scoring scale for laboratory quantification of generalized autonomic failure. *Mayo Clin Proc.* 1993;68(8):748–752.
4. Jacob G, Robertson D, Mosqueda-Garcia R, Ertl AC, Robertson RM, Biaggioni I. Hypovolemia in syncope and orthostatic intolerance role of the renin-angiotensin system. *Am J Med*. 1997;103(2):128–133.
5. Syngle V, Syngle A, Garg N, Krishan P, Verma I. Predictors of autonomic neuropathy in rheumatoid arthritis. *Auton Neurosci Basic Clin*. 2016;201:54–59. doi:10.1016/j.autneu.2016.07.008.
6. Grigoriou E, Boris JR, Dormans JP. Postural orthostatic tachycardia syndrome (POTS): association with Ehlers-Danlos syndrome and orthopaedic considerations. *Clin Orthop*. 2015;473(2):722–728. doi:10.1007/s11999-014-3898-x.

PART X

PAROXYSMAL ABNORMALITIES

88.

CASE 83: SMALL FIBER NEUROPATHY AND PRELOAD FAILURE

Chief complaint: Dyspnea.

Case presentation: A 53-year-old man presents with progressive dyspnea on exertion for the past 3 years. He also noted postural dizziness, fatigue, and leg pain. Invasive cardiopulmonary exercise test was consistent with preload failure.[1]

Past medical history: Deep vein thrombosis, pulmonary embolism, asthma.

Current medication: Fondaparinux, gabapentin.

Assessment plan: Functional autonomic tests and skin biopsy.

AUTONOMIC TESTING EVALUATION

See Table 88.1.

Heart rate: Supine heart rate was normal. Heart rate responses to deep breathing were reduced to 79.7% of normal value. Heart rate increment during the tilt (24 BPM) was normal.

Blood pressure:

Valsalva maneuver: Mean blood pressure failed to return to baseline at the end of Phase 2 by 7.7 mm Hg (i.e., 91.2% of baseline).

Tilt: Supine blood pressure was normal. Blood pressure responses to tilt were normal.

Sudomotor evaluation: Electrochemical skin conductance was abnormal (reduced to 71.3% of normal limit) at hands and abnormal (reduced to 68.7% of normal limit) at feet.

Respiratory system: Respiratory frequency was normal in supine position and during the tilt. End tidal CO_2 was reduced in supine position and during the tilt.

Cerebral blood flow velocity (CBFv): CBFv in middle cerebral artery was normal in supine position but was severely reduced during the tilt.

Skin biopsy (sensory-epidermal): Epidermal nerve fiber density was abnormal (reduced to 15.7% of normal limit) at distal leg.

Skin biopsy (sweat glands): Sweat gland nerve fiber density was abnormal (reduced to 16.7% of normal limit) at distal leg.

Patient-reported symptoms during testing: Dizziness and shortness of breath during the tilt.

Patient-reported symptoms for past 2 weeks:

Lightheadedness or dizziness: Often
Dry eyes or mouth: None
Pale feet: Often
Cold feet: Often
Reduced sweating: Occasionally
Reduced sweating after exercise: Occasionally
Increased sweating: Occasionally
Nausea: Occasionally
Diarrhea: Occasionally
Constipation: Occasionally

TABLE 88.1 RESULTS OF AUTONOMIC TESTING

Blood pressure evaluation					
Test: Valsalva maneuver					
Pressure [mmHg]	Baseline	Phase 2			Phase 4
		Early	End		
Systolic	119	82	92		
Mean	87.7	74	80	n/a	
Diastolic	72	70	74	n/a	

Heart rate evaluation	
Test: Deep breathing	
Results	Norm*
7.17	≥9
Test: Valsalva ratio	
1.55	≥1.36
* adjusted for a gender and age	

(continued)

TABLE 88.1 **CONTINUED**

Test: Tilt test										
Position		HR [BPM]	Blood pressure [mmHg]		MCA Blood flow velocity [cm/s]				Respiratory frequency [breaths/min]	End tidal CO_2 [mmHg]
			Systolic	Diastolic	Systolic	Mean	Mean drop [%]	Diastolic		
Supine		73	135	84	75	48.3		35	14	26
Tilt [min]	1	95	128	92	54	31.3	35.2	20	9	25
	2	86	140	88						
	3	96	139	90						
	4	96	140	84						
	5	97	144	92	53	35.7	26.1	27	14	22
	6	92	142	89						
	7	89	138	93						
	8	85	140	86						
	9	86	132	90						
	10	85	141	93	56	34	29.6	23	11	30
	15									
	20									
	30									
	40									

Sudomotor evaluation – functional

Test: Quantitative sudomotor axon reflex test (QSART)				
Location	Site (l/r)	Latency [min]	Volume [μl]	Norm [μl]*
Forearm				≥0.3
Prox. leg				≥0.23
Distal leg				≥0.23
Foot				≥0.27

* Normative data are adjusted for gender and age of patient.

Test: Electrochemical skin conductance (ESC)				
Location	Left [μS]	Right [μS]	Average [μS/k]	Norm [μS/kg]
Hand	79	74	0.73	≥1.03
Feet	80	82	0.79	≥1.14
Forehead				

For grading uses ESC [μS] adjusted for weight [μS/k].

TABLE 88.1 CONTINUED

Small fiber (sensory + sudomotor) evaluation – morphological					
Test: Skin biopsy					
Location	Site (l/r)	Nerve fibers			
		Epidermal*		Sweat glands	
		Density	Norm	Density	Norm
Proximal leg – thigh	Right		≥8.3		≥37.8
Distal leg - calf	Right	0.87	≥5.525	6.1	≥36.5
Foot	Right		≥3.11		≥34.8

*Normative data for distal leg are adjusted for gender and age of patient.

QASAT*										
Heart rate		BP		CBFv		ET-CO2		Sudomotor		Total QASAT score
S. bradycardia	0	Low supine	0	Low supine	0	Low supine	1	QSART		
S. tachycardia	0	High supine	0	High supine	0	High supine	0	ESC	2	
Increase tilt	0	OH	0	Tilt response	7	Tilt low	3			
Decrease tilt	0	OHTN	0	CA	0	Tilt high	0	**Skin biopsy**		23
Deep breathing	1	VM	1	CVR	0			Epidermal	4	
VR	0			VM	0			Sweat gland	4	
Total	1	Total	1	Total	7	Total	4			

*QASAT. See Novak. Quantitative Scale for Grading of Cardiovascular Autonomic Reflex Tests and Small Fibers from Skin Biopsies. *J Neurol Disord* 2015;3:2.

S, supine; Increase tilt, increased response to tilt; Decrease tilt, decreased response to tilt; BP, blood pressure; VM, Valsalva maneuver; CBFv, cerebral blood flow velocity; CA, cerebral autoregulation; MCA, middle cerebral artery; VR, Valsalva ratio; CVR, cerebral vasoreactivity.

Urinary leaks: Often
Aching pain: Continuous, severe
Allodynia: Often, moderate
Burning pain: Continuous, severe
Lancinating pain: Often, moderate
Numbness: Continuous, severe
Prickling sensation: Continuous, severe

AUTONOMIC TESTING INTERPRETATION

- Small fiber neuropathy, severe, mixed, length-dependent.
- Severe hypocapnic cerebral hypoperfusion (HYCH).
- Autonomic dysfunction, mild.

COMMENT

The testing showed severe mixed small fiber neuropathy and severe HYCH (Figure 88.1). Patient experienced dizziness and shortness of breath during the tilt. Shortness of breath resulted in severe hypocapnic hyperventilation, which in turn reduced CBFv (HYCH syndrome), likely resulting in signs of cerebral hypoperfusion. There were prominent blood pressure fluctuations usually mediated by the sympathetic system due to hypovolemia. Blood pressure fluctuations were also transmitted to CBFv fluctuations, which likely exacerbates orthostatic intolerance.

Invasive cardiopulmonary exercise testing showed reduced cardiac output associated with lower biventricular filling pressures and blunted stroke volume augmentation during exercise.[1] The reduced filling pressure was attributed to inadequate vasoconstriction of capacitance vessels causing preload failure. Interestingly, postural tachycardia syndrome (POTS) is associated with dyspnea, and several POTS patients were found to have preload failure.[1]

Although the patient presented in this chapter does not have POTS, he has severe small fiber neuropathy which in theory may be associated with denervation of capacitance vessels leading to a preload failure.

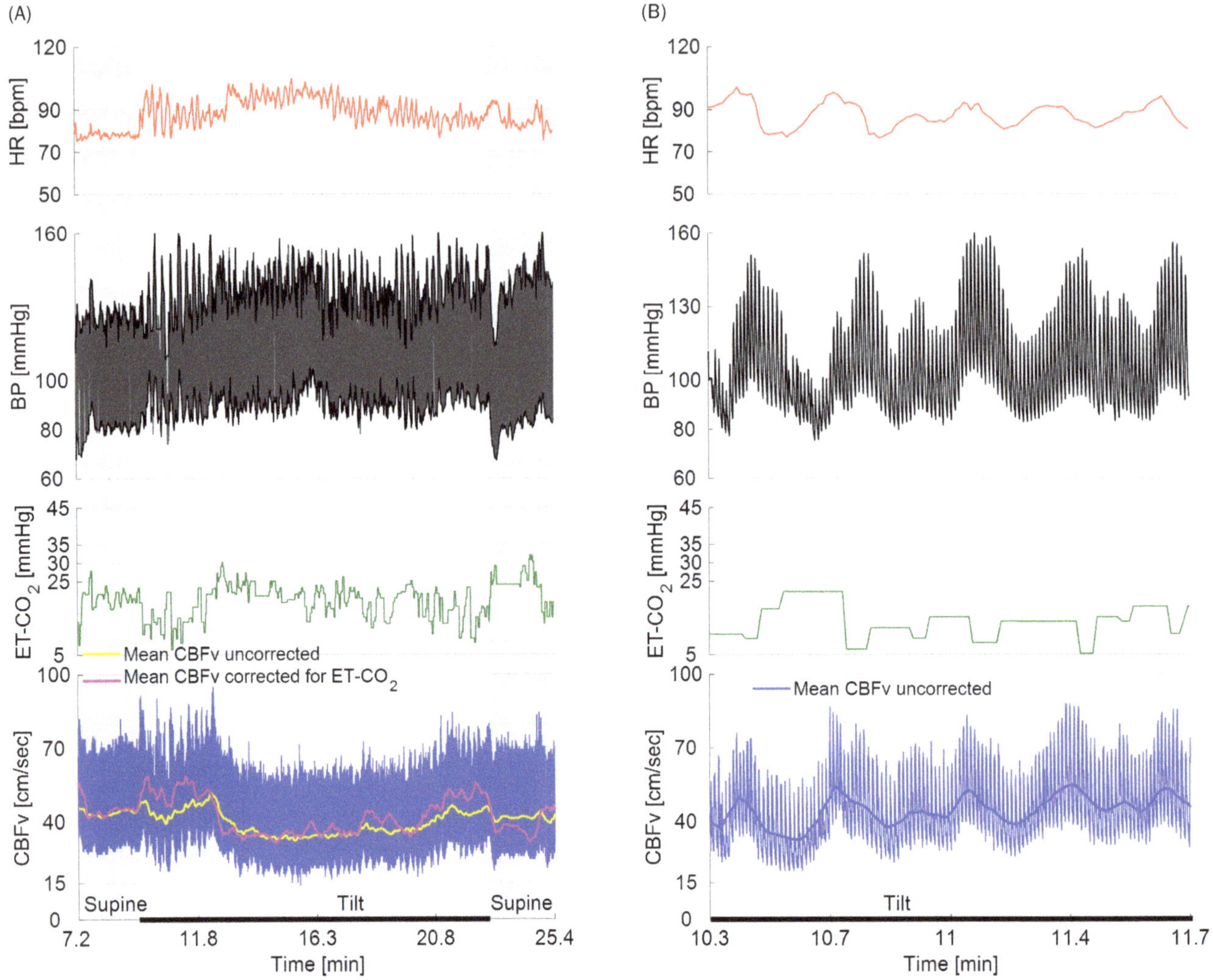

Figure 88.1 Mean heart rate and blood pressure responses to tilt were normal (A). There was supine and orthostatic hypocapnia. Cerebral blood flow velocity (CBFv) was reduced during the tilt. Blood pressure showed prominent fluctuations with about a 1-minute period that were transmitted into heart rate and CBFv (B). Patient was extremely short of breath but oxygen saturation remained above 98% throughout the testing.

TREATMENT AND FOLLOW-UP

- Clinical workup for neuropathy.
- Volume expansion with high fluid and high salt intake.

CAVEATS

- Sympathetically medicated blood pressure oscillations are typical for hypovolemia and can be associated with catecholamine surge. They are also transmitted into CBFv, which may contribute to fluctuating perfusion and symptoms of dizziness.

REFERENCE

1. Oldham WM, Lewis GD, Opotowsky AR, Waxman AB, Systrom DM. Unexplained exertional dyspnea caused by low ventricular filling pressures: results from clinical invasive cardiopulmonary exercise testing. *Pulm Circ.* 2016;6(1):55–62. doi:10.1086/685054.

89.

CASE 84: INTERMITTENT CONFUSION

Chief complaint: Intermittent confusion.

Case presentation: A 45-year-old woman presents with intermittent dizziness, shortness of breath, confusion, and fatigue for 5 years. Most of her complaints are exacerbated by standing and relieved by sitting or lying down. She also has history of chronic back pain with multiple failed surgeries and pain medications. She has chronic constipation that was attributed to opiates, which she receives via an intrathecal pump. The intermittent complaints started before pump insertion. Detailed cardiology, pulmonary, and neurology evaluations were unrevealing. She was referred for evaluation of orthostatic intolerance.

Past medical history: Lumbar radiculopathy, chronic pain syndromes, failed back surgery syndrome.

Current medication: Sertraline, promethazine, intrathecal morphine.

Assessment plan: Functional autonomic tests and skin biopsy.

AUTONOMIC TESTING EVALUATION

See Table 89.1.

Heart rate: Supine heart rate was normal. Heart rate responses to deep breathing were normal. Heart rate increment during the tilt (24 BPM) was normal.

Blood pressure:

Valsalva maneuver: Blood pressure responses were normal. Supine blood pressure was normal.

Tilt: Blood pressure responses to tilt were normal.

Sudomotor evaluation: Electrochemical skin conductance was normal at hands and normal at feet.

Respiratory system: Respiratory frequency was normal in supine position. Respiratory frequency during the tilt was fluctuating with short episodes of hyperventilation and irregular breathing. End tidal CO_2 was normal in supine position. End tidal CO_2 was fluctuating from 25 mm Hg to 35 mm Hg due to an irregular breathing pattern.

Cerebral blood flow velocity (CBFv): CBFv in middle cerebral artery was normal in supine position. CBFv during the tilt was fluctuating intermittently up 20%.

Skin biopsy (sensory-epidermal): Epidermal nerve fiber density was normal at proximal leg and normal at distal leg.

Skin biopsy (sweat glands): Sweat gland nerve fiber density was normal at distal leg.

Patient-reported symptoms during testing: Dizziness during the tilt.

TABLE 89.1 RESULTS OF AUTONOMIC TESTING

Blood pressure evaluation					
Test: Valsalva maneuver					
Pressure [mmHg]	Baseline	Phase 2			Phase 4
		Early	End		
Systolic	97	84	101		
Mean	75.7	74	89.7	n/a	
Diastolic	65	69	84	n/a	

Heart rate evaluation	
Test: Deep breathing	
Results	Norm*
21.57	≥10
Test: Valsalva ratio	
1.39	≥1.51
* adjusted for a gender and age	

(continued)

TABLE 89.1 **CONTINUED**

Test: Tilt test										
Position		HR [BPM]	Blood pressure [mmHg]		MCA Blood flow velocity [cm/s]				Respiratory frequency [breaths/min]	End tidal CO_2 [mmHg]
			Systolic	Diastolic	Systolic	Mean	Mean drop [%]	Diastolic		
Supine		70	111	75	102	62		42	9	31
Tilt [min]	1	94	108	77	78	52	16.1	39	22	30
	2	82	117	82						
	3	73	115	82						
	4	87	118	84						
	5	82	116	78	82	52.7	15	38	26	34
	6	86	117	80						
	7	75	113	81						
	8	85	123	78						
	9	83	113	79						
	10	80	116	82	82	58	6.5	46	13	19
	15									
	20									
	30									
	40									

Sudomotor evaluation - functional

Test: Quantitative sudomotor axon reflex test (QSART)				
Location	Site (l/r)	Latency [min]	Volume [µl]	Norm [µl]*
Forearm				≥0.08
Prox. leg				≥0.14
Distal leg				≥0.15
Foot				≥0.07

Test: Electrochemical skin conductance (ESC)				
Location	Left [µS]	Right [µS]	Average [µS/k]	Norm [µS/kg]
Hand	80	79	1.12	≥1.03
Feet	89	86	1.22	≥1.14
Forehead				
For grading uses ESC [µS] adjusted for weight [µS/k].				

* normative data are adjusted for a gender and age of a patient

TABLE 89.1 **CONTINUED**

Small fiber (sensory + sudomotor) evaluation - morphological					
Test: Skin biopsy					
Location	Site (l/r)	Nerve fibers			
		Epidermal*		Sweat glands	
		Density	Norm	Density	Norm
Proximal leg – thigh	Right	19.81	≥8.3	53.8	≥37.8
Distal leg - calf	Right	8.22	≥7.5	70.6	≥36.5
Foot	Right		≥3.11		≥34.8

* normative data for distal leg are adjusted for a gender and age of a patient

QASAT*										
Heart rate		**BP**		**CBFv**		**ET-CO$_2$**		**Sudomotor**		**Total QASAT score**
S. bradycardia	0	Low supine	0	Low supine	0	Low supine	1	QSART		
S. tachycardia	0	High supine	0	High supine	0	High supine	0	ESC	0	
Increase tilt	0	OH	0	Tilt response	2	Tilt low	4			
Decrease tilt	0	OHTN	0	CA	0	Tilt high	0	**Skin biopsy**		8
Deep breathing	0	VM	0	CVR	0			Epidermal	0	
VR	1			VM	0			Sweat gland	0	
Total	1	Total	0	Total	2	Total	5			

*QASAT = Quantitative Scale for Grading of Cardiovascular Autonomic Reflex Tests and Small Fibers from Skin Biopsies, Novak, J Neurol Disord 2015, 3:2, S. = supine, Increase tilt = increased response to tilt, Decrease tilt = decreased response to tilt, BP = blood pressure, VM = Valsalva maneuver, CBFv = cerebral blood flow velocity; CA = cerebral autoregulation, VR = Valsalva ratio, CVR = cerebral vasoreactivity.

Patient-reported symptoms for past 2 weeks:

Lightheadedness or dizziness: Often
Dry eyes or mouth: None
Pale feet: Occasionally
Cold feet: Occasionally
Reduced sweating: None
Reduced sweating after exercise: None
Increased sweating: None
Nausea: Occasionally
Diarrhea: None
Constipation: Occasionally
Urinary leaks: None
Current pain severity: 0
Aching pain: None
Allodynia: None
Burning pain: None
Lancinating pain: None
Numbness: Occasionally, mild
Prickling sensation: Occasionally, mild

AUTONOMIC TESTING INTERPRETATION

- Orthostatic cerebral hypoperfusion syndrome (OCHOS).
- Mild autonomic dysfunction.

COMMENT

The tilt provoked typical this patient's short episodes of confusion, dizziness, and shortness of breath (Figure 89.1). These episodes were associated with an

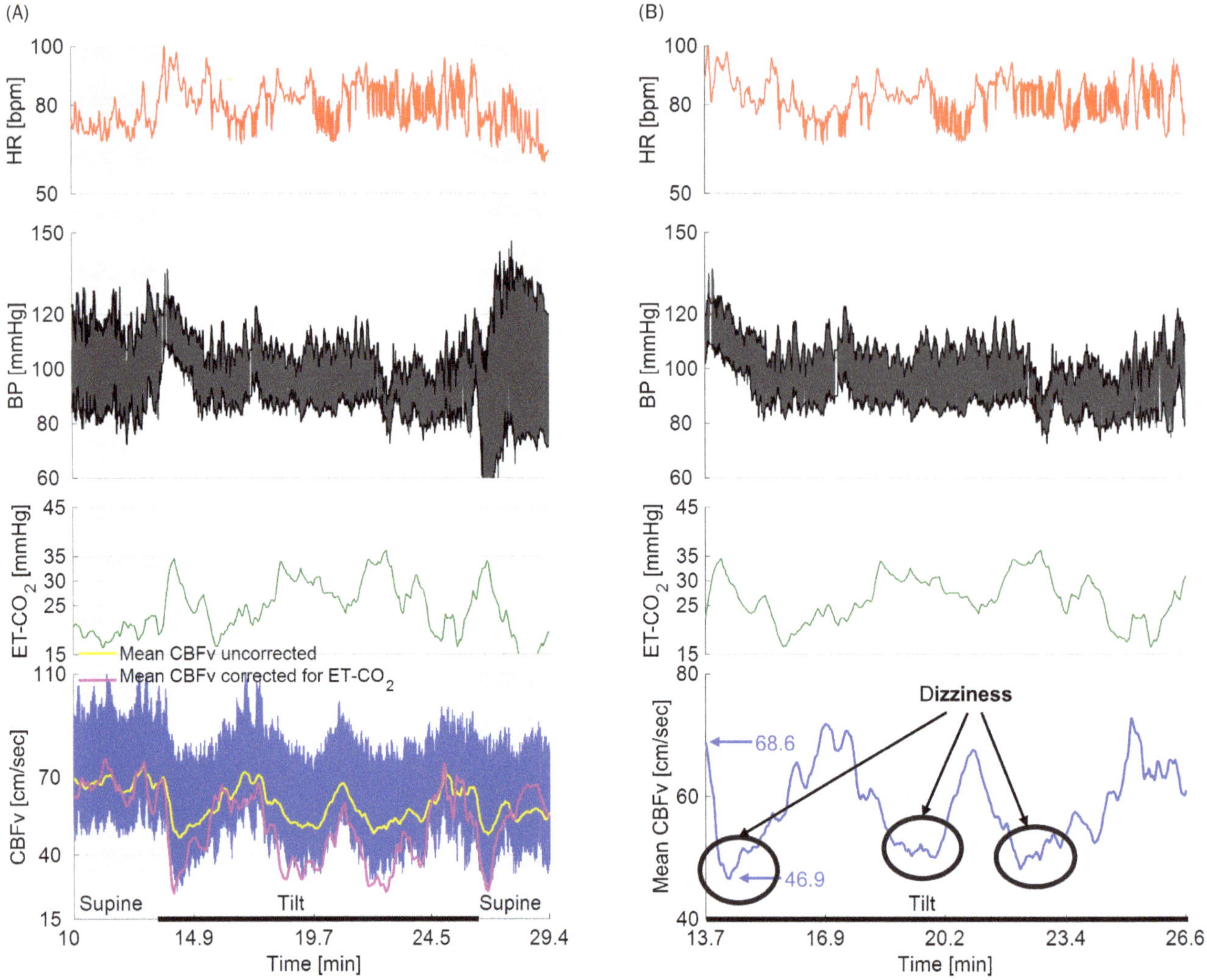

Figure 89.1 Heart rate and blood pressure responses to tilt were normal (A). Breathing pattern was irregular and end tidal CO_2 fluctuating. Cerebral blood flow velocity (CBFv) was fluctuating as well and occasionally reached very low values comparable to presyncope, with a diastolic CBFv of close to 20 cm/s. The decline in CBFv was not synchronized with end tidal CO_2 fluctuations and was out of proportion of the effect of hypocapnia since even CBFv adjusted for end tidal CO_2 was intermittently reduced (A, B). The patient became very dizzy during these episodes. Panel B shows uncorrected mean CBFv.

intermittent decline in CBFv without orthostatic hypotension or decline in end tidal CO_2, thus satisfying OCHOS criteria.[1] The decline in CBFv reflects abnormal cerebral vasoconstriction due to cerebral autoregulatory failure.[1]

TREATMENT AND FOLLOW-UP

- Volume expansion may change the set point of cerebral autoregulation and stabilize the cerebral blood flow.
- If ineffective, consider low-dose calcium channel blockers that dilate cerebral vessels and, in theory, may improve cerebral perfusion.[2]

CAVEATS

- OCHOS can be associated with intermittent confusion.

REFERENCES

1. Novak P. Orthostatic cerebral hypoperfusion syndrome. *Front Aging Neurosci.* 2016;8:22. doi:10.3389/fnagi.2016.00022.
2. Lavine SD, Wang M, Etu JJ, Meyers PM, Joshi S. Augmentation of cerebral blood flow and reversal of endothelin-1-induced vasospasm: a comparison of intracarotid nicardipine and verapamil. *Neurosurgery.* 2007;60(4):742–748; discussion 748–749. doi:10.1227/01.NEU.0000255404.30904.CE.

90.

CASE 85: RHYTHMIC DIZZINESS

Chief complaint: Dizziness.

Case presentation: A 48-year-old woman presents with postural dizziness. The dizziness began 7 years ago. She suddenly felt lightheaded while driving. Since then, she has had occasional short spells of lightheadedness. A year ago, again while driving, she became severely lightheaded, had to pull over, and was in the hospital for several days. Evaluations for cerebrovascular accident were unrevealing She was told her blood pressure was low and her heart rate was slow. She had about 20 spells while sitting and standing. The onset of spells is quick: she suddenly feels her body is draining, her heart is pounding. She also noted headache typically afterward. Typical spell duration is seconds to minutes. Electroencephalogram was normal. She wore a Holter heart monitor, but it did not record the spells. Current complaints include shortness of breath, fatigue, palpitations, and weakness. She was referred for evaluation of dizziness.

Past medical history: Migraine, biliary atresia, multiple ventral hernia repairs.

Current medication: None.

Assessment plan: Functional autonomic tests and skin biopsy.

AUTONOMIC TESTING EVALUATION

See Table 90.1.

Heart rate: Supine heart rate was normal. Heart rate responses to deep breathing were reduced to 78% of normal value. Heart rate increment during the tilt (18 BPM) was normal.

Blood pressure:

Valsalva maneuver: Blood pressure responses were normal.

Tilt: Supine blood pressure was normal. Blood pressure responses to tilt were normal.

Sudomotor evaluation: Electrochemical skin conductance was abnormal (reduced to 54.5% of normal limit) at hands and normal at feet.

Respiratory system: Respiratory frequency and end tidal CO_2 were normal in supine position and during the tilt.

Cerebral blood flow velocity (CBFv): CBFv in middle cerebral artery was normal in supine position but was moderately reduced during the tilt.

Skin biopsy (sensory-epidermal): Epidermal nerve fiber density was normal at proximal leg and normal at distal leg.

Skin biopsy (sweat glands): Sweat gland nerve fiber density was normal at proximal leg and normal at distal leg.

Patient-reported symptoms during testing: Dizziness, leg weakness during the tilt.

Patient-reported symptoms for past 2 weeks:

Lightheadedness or dizziness: Often
Dry eyes or mouth: Occasionally
Pale feet: None
Cold feet: Occasionally

TABLE 90.1 **RESULTS OF AUTONOMIC TESTING**

Blood pressure evaluation					
Test: Valsalva maneuver					
Pressure [mmHg]	Baseline	Phase 2			Phase 4
		Early	End		
Systolic	122	79	118		
Mean	84	73.7	102	n/a	
Diastolic	65	71	94	n/a	

Heart rate evaluation	
Test: Deep breathing	
Results	Norm*
7.8	≥10
Test: Valsalva ratio	
2.73	≥1.51
* adjusted for a gender and age	

(continued)

TABLE 90.1 CONTINUED

Test: Tilt test										
Position		HR [BPM]	Blood pressure [mmHg]		MCA Blood flow velocity [cm/s]				Respiratory frequency [breaths/min]	End tidal CO_2 [mmHg]
			Systolic	Diastolic	Systolic	Mean	Mean drop [%]	Diastolic		
Supine		63	128	82	101	66.3		49	15	35
Tilt [min]	1	77	132	85	91	61.7	6.9	47	14	34
	2	68	133	89						
	3	77	135	89						
	4	71	135	89						
	5	79	138	93	81	50.3	24.1	35	9	36
	6	73	134	88						
	7	81	147	93						
	8	74	133	92						
	9	76	136	90						
	10	75	134	91	86	56	15.5	41	11	35
	15									
	20									
	30									
	40									

Sudomotor evaluation - functional

Test: Quantitative sudomotor axon reflex test (QSART)				
Location	Site (l/r)	Latency [min]	Volume [µl]	Norm [µl]*
Forearm				≥0.08
Prox. leg				≥0.14
Distal leg				≥0.15
Foot				≥0.07

* Normative data are adjusted for gender and age of patient.

Test: Electrochemical skin conductance (ESC)				
Location	Left [µS]	Right [µS]	Average [µS/k]	Norm [µS/kg]
Hand	43	41	0.56	≥1.03
Feet	91	92	1.23	≥1.14
Forehead				

For grading uses ESC [µS] adjusted for weight [µS/k].

TABLE 90.1 **CONTINUED**

Small fiber (sensory + sudomotor) evaluation - morphological					
Test: Skin biopsy					
Location	Site (l/r)	Nerve fibers			
		Epidermal*		Sweat glands	
		Density	Norm	Density	Norm
Proximal leg – thigh	Right	12.28	≥8.3	62.5	≥37.8
Distal leg - calf	Right	10.35	≥7.26	47.8	≥36.5
Foot	Right		≥3.11		≥34.8

*Normative data for distal leg are adjusted for gender and age of patient.

QASAT*											
Heart rate		**BP**		**CBFv**		**ET-CO2**		**Sudomotor**			**Total QASAT score**
S. bradycardia	0	Low supine	0	Low supine	0	Low supine	0	QSART			
S. tachycardia	0	High supine	0	High supine	0	High supine	0	ESC	0		4
Increase tilt	0	OH	0	Tilt response	3	Tilt low	0				
Decrease tilt	0	OHTN	0	CA	0	Tilt high	0	**Skin biopsy**			
Deep breathing	1	VM	0	CVR	0			Epidermal	0		
VR	0			VM	0			Sweat gland	0		
Total	1	Total	0	Total	3	Total	0				

*QASAT. See Novak. Quantitative Scale for Grading of Cardiovascular Autonomic Reflex Tests and Small Fibers from Skin Biopsies. *J Neurol Disord* 2015;3:2.

S, supine; Increase tilt, increased response to tilt; Decrease tilt, decreased response to tilt; BP, blood pressure; VM, Valsalva maneuver; CBFv, cerebral blood flow velocity; CA, cerebral autoregulation; MCA, middle cerebral artery; VR, Valsalva ratio; CVR, cerebral vasoreactivity.

Reduced sweating: None
Reduced sweating after exercise: None
Increased sweating: None
Nausea: Occasionally
Diarrhea: None
Constipation: None
Urinary leaks: Occasionally
Current pain severity: 8
Aching pain: Often, moderate
Allodynia: Occasionally, moderate
Burning pain: None
Lancinating pain: Often, moderate
Numbness: Occasionally, moderate
Prickling sensation: Occasionally, mild

AUTONOMIC TESTING INTERPRETATION

- Episodic decrease in CBFv triggered by deep breaths associated with dizziness.
- Mild parasympathetic dysfunction.

COMMENT

The tilt test showed transient drops in CBFv consistent with deep breaths and dizziness, thus establishing that the dizziness is related to cerebral blood flow changes (Figure 90.1).

Respiratory activity has a profound effect on cerebral blood flow.[1] Even a simple deep breath or yawning can trigger dizziness and a decline in CBFv. The episodic drops in CBFv with normal cardiovascular parameters are not well explained and may be related to several potential mechanisms, ranging from abnormal cerebral autoregulation to potential internal carotid fluctuating thrombus,[2] apneustic breathing,[3] migraine-like patterns,[4] or central dysautonomic as seen in Alzheimer's disease.[5] Follow-up assessment of the internal carotid artery vascular bed may useful.

TREATMENT AND FOLLOW-UP

- Vascular imaging study of the neck and brain.
- Respiratory breathing therapy.
- Trial of buspirone.[6]

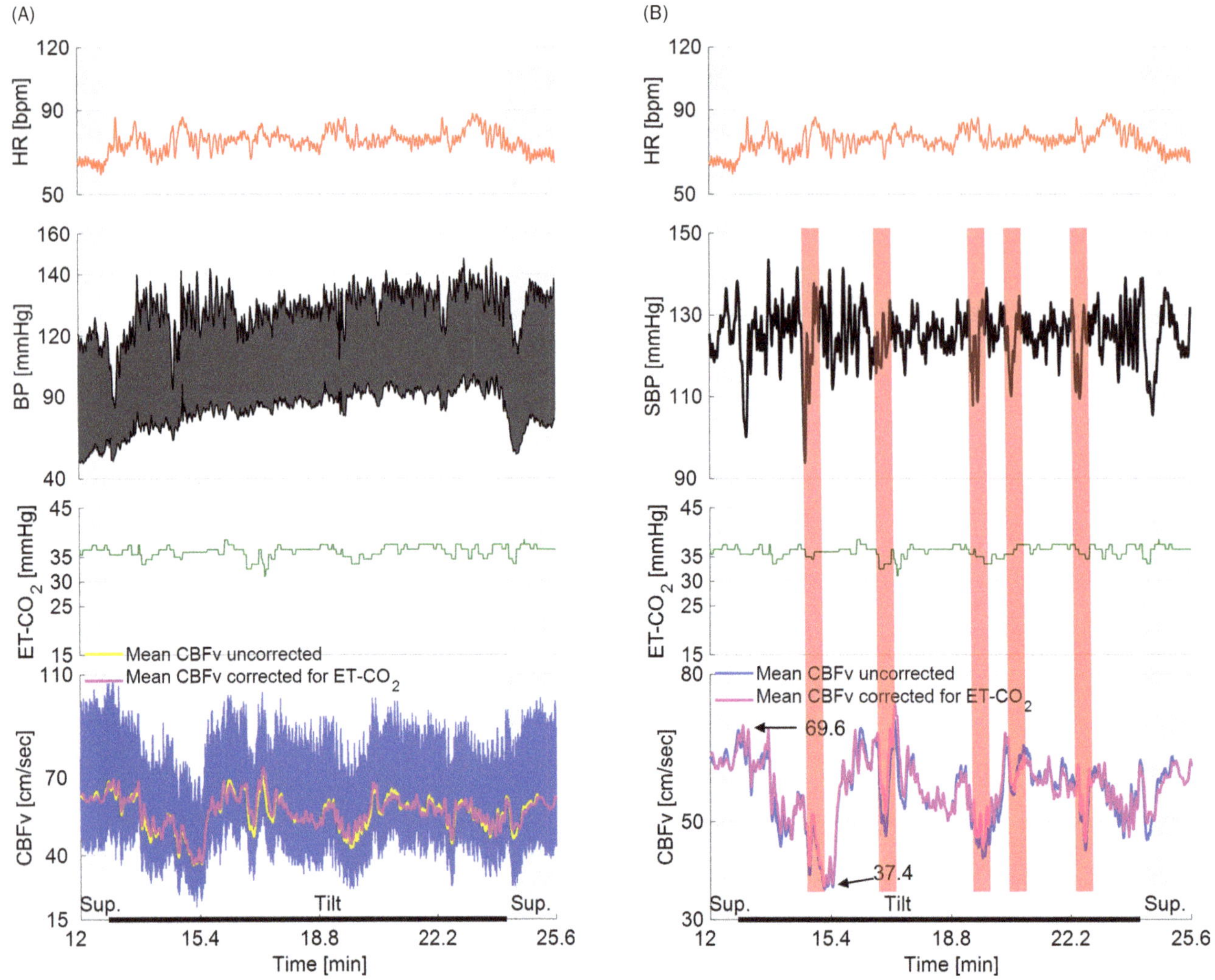

Figure 90.1 Cardiovascular responses to tilt were normal (A). The patient became dizzy several times during the tilt (B). These episodes demarkated by pink columns, were synchronous with a transient drop of blood pressure, cerebral blood flow velocity, and deep breaths.

CAVEATS

- Even a single deep breath can trigger a decline in cerebral blood flow and dizziness.

REFERENCES

1. Czosnyka M, Richards H, Kirkpatrick P, Pickard J. Assessment of cerebral autoregulation with ultrasound and laser Doppler wave forms: an experimental study in anesthetized rabbits. *Neurosurgery.* 1994;35(2):287–292; discussion 292–293.
2. Samii C, Diehl RR, Berlit P. Intermittent drop in blood flow velocity in the internal carotid artery and its branches. *J Clin Ultrasound JCU.* 2002;30(2):98–102.
3. Foster GE, Brugniaux JV, Pialoux V, et al. Cardiovascular and cerebrovascular responses to acute hypoxia following exposure to intermittent hypoxia in healthy humans. *J Physiol.* 2009;587(Pt 13):3287–3299. doi:10.1113/jphysiol.2009.171553.
4. Friberg L, Olesen J, Iversen HK, Sperling B. Migraine pain associated with middle cerebral artery dilatation: reversal by sumatriptan. *Lancet Lond Engl.* 1991;338(8758):13–17.
5. Novak P, Novak V, Li Z, Remillard G. Time-frequency analysis of slow cortical activity and cardiovascular fluctuations in a case of Alzheimer's disease. *Clin Auton Res Off J Clin Auton Res Soc.* 1994;4(3):141–148.
6. Wilken B, Lalley P, Bischoff AM, et al. Treatment of apneustic respiratory disturbance with a serotonin-receptor agonist. *J Pediatr.* 1997;130(1):89–94.

91.

CASE 86: PAROXYSMAL DYSAUTONOMIA

Chief complaint: Spells of altered consciousness.

Case presentation: A 56-year-old man presents with unexplained spells. In a typical spell, he suddenly becomes weak and shaky. He describes the sensation as a "blood rush" in his head; he feels "heart in his throat" and that his "head will fall off." These spells occur daily and last from seconds to minutes. His wife noted reduced responsiveness during the spells. Neurologic examination was entirely normal. MRI of the brain, magnetic resonance angiography (MRA) of the brain and neck, and electroencephalogram were normal. Cardiologic evaluation including Holter monitor was unrevealing. Autonomic testing showed small fiber neuropathy, mixed, length-dependent, affecting sensory and autonomic fibers and generalized but mild autonomic failure. There was no evidence of orthostatic hypotension. Orthostatic cerebral blood flow velocity (CBFv) was reduced by 29% and was felt to be due orthostatic cerebral hypoperfusion syndrome (OCHOS). However, no typical spell occurred during the autonomic testing. A week after testing, the patient experienced increased frequency of the spells, occurring several times per day. Therefore, a repeat tilt test was arranged with the goal to record and characterize the spells.

Past medical history: Hypertension.

Current medication: Amlodipine.

Assessment plan: Functional autonomic tests and skin biopsy.

AUTONOMIC TESTING EVALUATION

See Table 91.1.

Heart rate: Supine heart rate was normal. Heart rate responses to deep breathing were reduced to 75% of normal value. Heart rate increment during the tilt (21 BPM) was normal.

Blood pressure:

Valsalva maneuver: Mean blood pressure failed to return to baseline at the end of Phase 2 by 19.6 mm Hg (i.e., 82.9% of baseline).

Tilt: Supine blood pressure was elevated. Blood pressure responses to tilt were normal.

Sudomotor evaluation: Electrochemical skin conductance was abnormal (reduced to 78.5% of normal limit) at hands and abnormal (reduced to 75.5% of normal limit) at feet.

Respiratory system: Respiratory frequency was normal in supine position but was increased during the tilt. End tidal CO_2 was reduced in supine position and during the tilt.

Cerebral blood flow velocity (CBFv): CBFv in middle cerebral artery was normal in supine position but was reduced during the tilt.

Skin biopsy (sensory-epidermal): Epidermal nerve fiber density was normal at proximal leg and abnormal (reduced to 32.8% of normal limit) at distal leg.

TABLE 91.1 **RESULTS OF AUTONOMIC TESTING**

Blood pressure evaluation					
Test: Valsalva maneuver					
Pressure [mmHg]	Baseline	Phase 2			Phase 4
		Early	End		
Systolic	147	96	116		
Mean	114.3	86	94.7	n/a	
Diastolic	98	81	84	n/a	

Heart rate evaluation	
Test: Deep breathing	
Results	Norm*
6.75	≥9
Test: Valsalva ratio	
1.33	≥1.36
* adjusted for a gender and age	

(continued)

TABLE 91.1 **CONTINUED**

Test: Tilt test										
Position		HR [BPM]	Blood pressure [mmHg]		MCA Blood flow velocity [cm/s]				Respiratory frequency [breaths/min]	End tidal CO_2 [mmHg]
			Systolic	Diastolic	Systolic	Mean	Mean drop [%]	Diastolic		
Supine		61	152	93	73	47.7		35	16	34
Tilt [min]	1	66	152	97	72	45.3	5	32	18	32
	2	77	161	106						
	3	79	154	113						
	4	82	138	100						
	5	82	165	123	55	33.7	29.4	23	22	32
	6	80	146	103						
	7	81	164	99						
	8	77	147	103						
	9	75	159	100						
	10	76	160	98	60	37.3	21.8	26	22	31
	15									
	20									
	30									
	40									

Sudomotor evaluation - functional

Test: Quantitative sudomotor axon reflex test (QSART)				
Location	Site (l/r)	Latency [min]	Volume [µl]	Norm [µl]*
Forearm				≥0.3
Prox. leg				≥0.23
Distal leg				≥0.23
Foot				≥0.27

* Normative data are adjusted for gender and age of patient.

Test: Electrochemical skin conductance (ESC)				
Location	Left [µS]	Right [µS]	Average [µS/k]	Norm [µS/kg]
Hand	80	74	0.81	≥1.03
Feet	81	83	0.87	≥1.14
Forehead				

For grading uses ESC [µS] adjusted for weight [µS/k].

TABLE 91.1 CONTINUED

Small fiber (sensory + sudomotor) evaluation - morphological					
Test: Skin biopsy					
Location	Site (l/r)	Nerve fibers			
		Epidermal*		Sweat glands	
		Density	Norm	Density	Norm
Proximal leg – thigh	Right	13.47	≥8.3		≥37.8
Distal leg - calf	Right	1.74	≥5.3	14.7	≥36.5
Foot	Right		≥3.11		≥34.8

*Normative data for distal leg are adjusted for gender and age of patient.

QASAT*											
Heart rate		BP		CBFv		ET-CO2		Sudomotor			Total QASAT score
S. bradycardia	0	Low supine	0	Low supine	0	Low supine	1	QSART			
S. tachycardia	0	High supine	1	High supine	0	High supine	0	ESC	1		
Increase tilt	0	OH	0	Tilt response	3	Tilt low	1				
Decrease tilt	0	OHTN	0	CA	0	Tilt high	0	**Skin biopsy**			18
Deep breathing	1	VM	2	CVR	0			Epidermal	3		
VR	1			VM	0			Sweat gland	4		
Total	2	Total	3	Total	3	Total	2				

*QASAT. See Novak. Quantitative Scale for Grading of Cardiovascular Autonomic Reflex Tests and Small Fibers from Skin Biopsies. *J Neurol Disord* 2015;3:2.

S, supine; Increase tilt, increased response to tilt; Decrease tilt, decreased response to tilt; BP, blood pressure; VM, Valsalva maneuver; CBFv, cerebral blood flow velocity; CA, cerebral autoregulation; MCA, middle cerebral artery; VR, Valsalva ratio; CVR, cerebral vasoreactivity.

Skin biopsy (sweat glands): Sweat gland nerve fiber density was abnormal (reduced to 40.3% of normal limit) at distal leg.

Patient-reported symptoms during testing: Dizziness during the tilt.

Patient-reported symptoms for past 2 weeks:

Lightheadedness or dizziness: Occasionally
Dry eyes or mouth: Yes, minor annoyance
Pale feet: Occasionally
Cold feet: Yes, minor annoyance
Reduced sweating: Yes, minor annoyance
Reduced sweating after exercise: Yes, minor annoyance
Increased sweating: Yes, minor annoyance
Nausea: Yes, minor annoyance
Diarrhea: Yes, minor annoyance
Constipation: Occasionally
Urinary leaks: Yes, minor annoyance
Erection problems: Yes, minor annoyance
Current pain severity: 0
Aching pain: Occasionally, mild
Allodynia: None
Burning pain: None
Lancinating pain: Occasionally, mild
Numbness: Occasionally, mild
Prickling sensation: Occasionally, moderate

AUTONOMIC TESTING INTERPRETATION

- Paroxysmal autonomic overactivity.
- Orthostatic cerebral hypoperfusion syndrome (OCHOS) was diagnosed during the first tilt test.
- Generalized but mild autonomic failure without evidence of orthostatic hypotension.

COMMENT

The second tilt provoked a typical patient's spell (Figures 91.1 and 91.2). About 1 minute after the tilt onset, the patient became less responsive, disoriented, weak, and tearful. There was a full-body, coarse, high-frequency tremor. During the spell, blood pressure became elevated (systolic 174 mm Hg, supine baseline 165 mm Hg). The patient was severely hyperventilating (end tidal CO_2 ~17 mmHg [normal ≥ 35 mmHg] and respiratory frequency >35 breaths per minute [normal < 20 breaths per minute]) which was associated with a drop in CBFv to 50/15 cm/s (baseline 74/35 cm/s). Duration of the spell was about 2 minutes (Figures 91.1 and 91.2). After the spell resolved, vitals normalized within seconds. Patient never lost completely consciousness.

Hyperventilation (2 minutes) in supine position (Figure 91.3) provoked another spell with a similar pattern (low end tidal CO_2 and low CBFv, high blood pressure, and tachycardia). The blood pressure pattern of the spell was opposite to neurally mediated syncope or cardiovagal reaction, in which the blood pressure is reduced. The CBFv was very low, which was consistent with hypocapnic cerebral vasoconstriction. This finding is consistent with hypocapnic cerebral hypoperfusion (HYCH), which is combined with an underlying OCHOS with reduced orthostatic cerebral perfusion associated with hypertension. The spells resemble an anxiety reaction or a response to a surge of catecholamines. Patient was tested twice for levels of catecholamines, both supine and standing. The standing norepinephrine levels were not elevated but they were obtained without the presence of a spell.

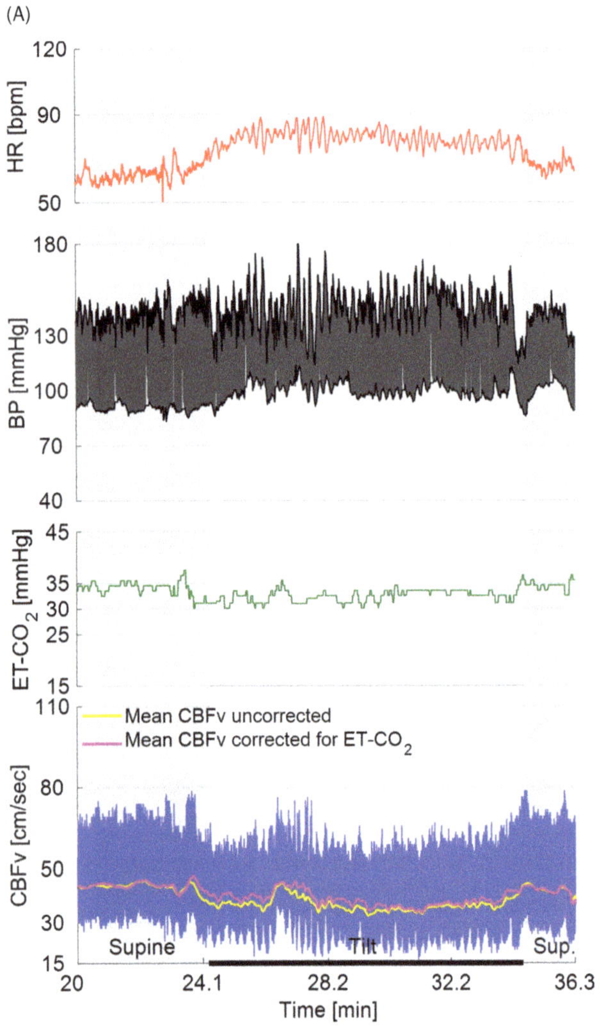

Figure 91.1 The first tilt test was consistent with orthostatic cerebral hypoperfusion syndrome (OCHOS, A, B). Blood pressure and heart rate responses to tilt were normal. Orthostatic cerebral blood flow velocity (CBFv) was reduced intermittently by 23% compared to the supine baseline. Although there was mild hypocapnia, CBFv corrected for end tidal CO_2 was similar to the uncorrected level (B).

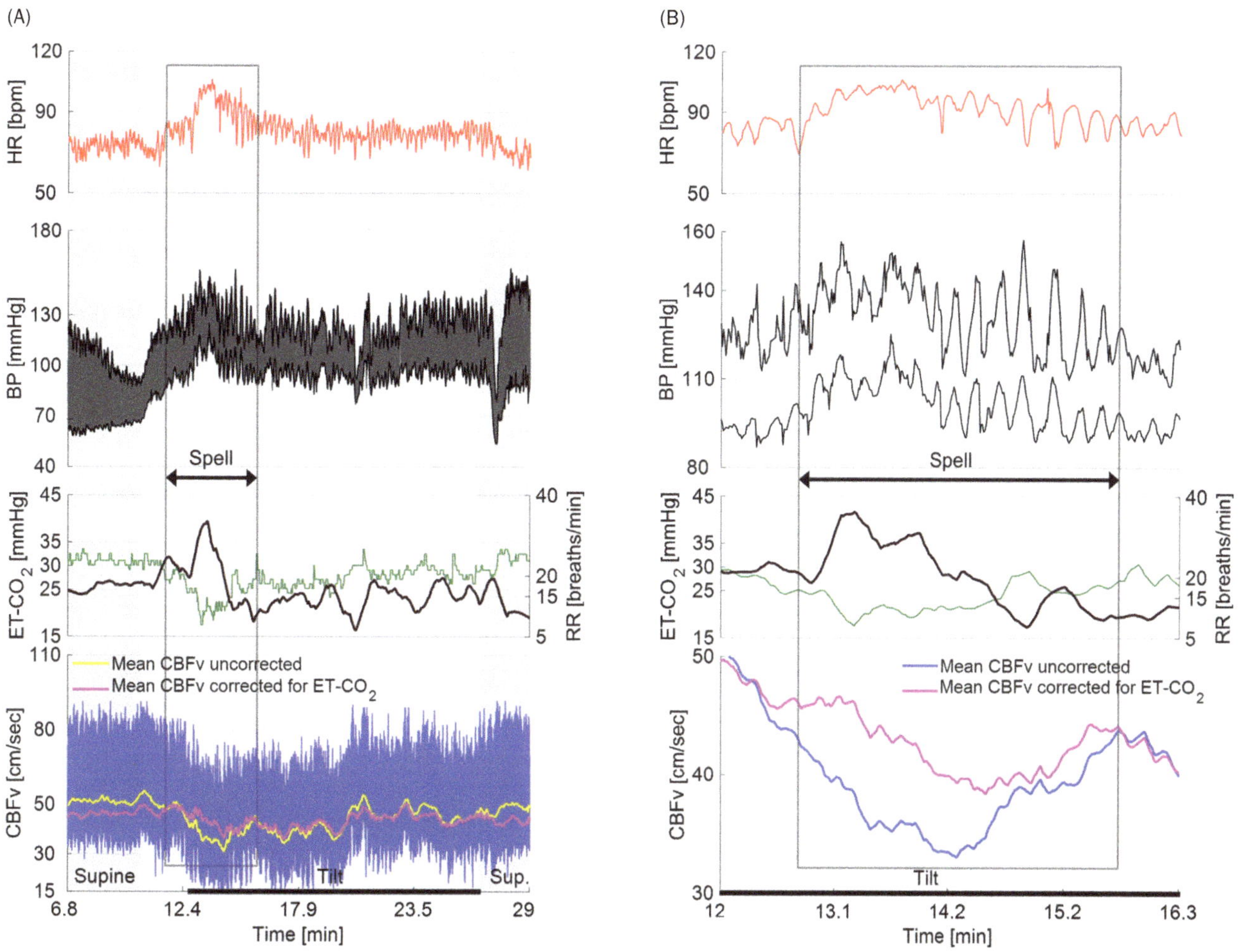

Figure 91.2 The second tilt test provoked the patient's characteristic spell (A–D). Patient became restless, confused, disoriented, and tearful. During the spell, there was profound decline in cerebral blood flow velocity associated with tachypnea and low end tidal CO_2. Blood pressure and heart rate were elevated during the spell.

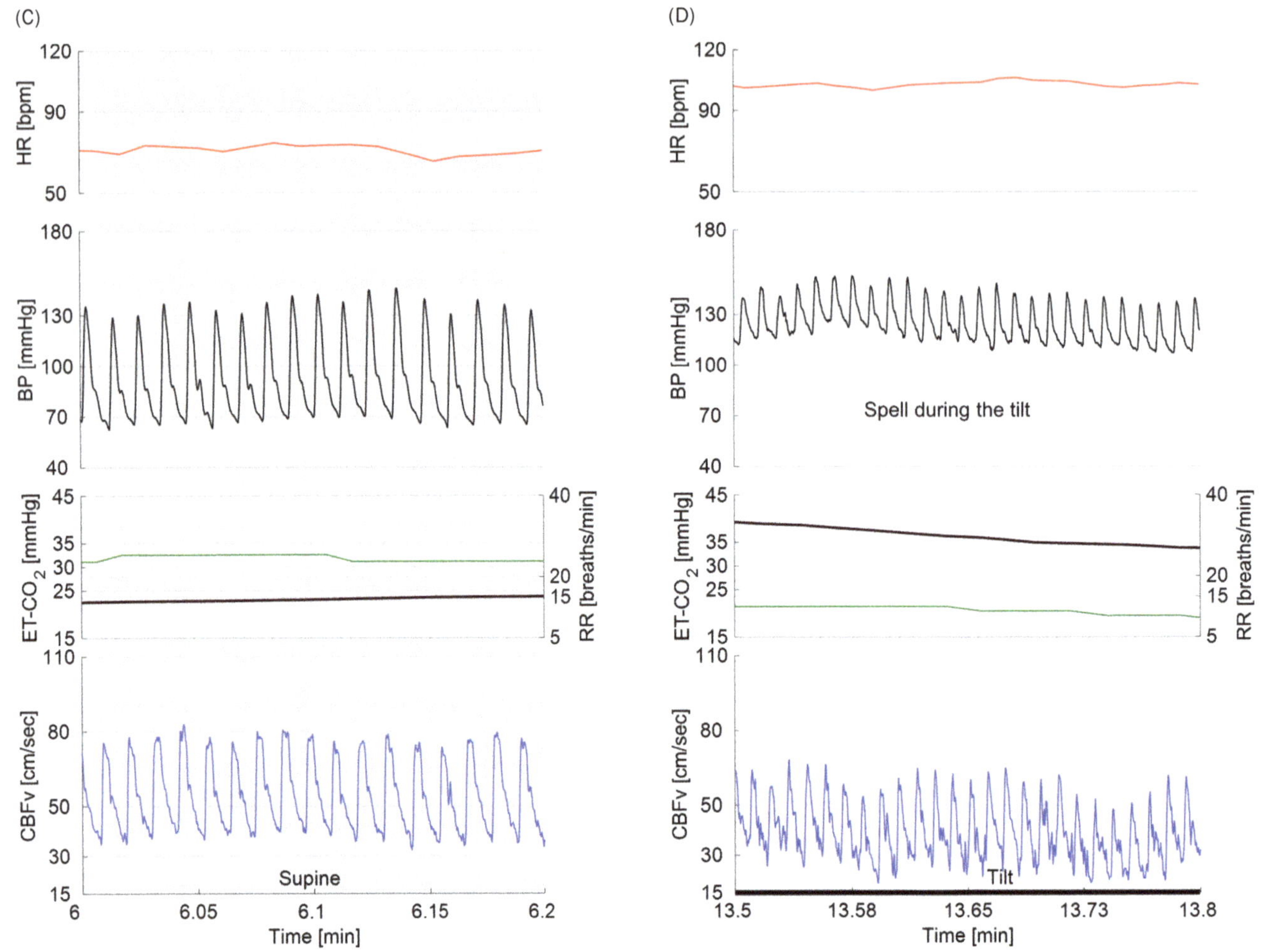

Figure 91.2 Continued

Paroxysmal sympathetic hyperactivity (PHS) is a poorly understood syndrome which can be seen after traumatic brain injury[1,2] or pheochromocytoma or that has a psychological basis.[3] Typical signs and symptoms are elevated heart rate, blood pressure, respiratory rate, temperature, and motor posturing.[1,2] The treatment is supportive, usually by combining pharmaceutical and nonpharmaceutical treatments. In the presented case, anxiety may play a role.

TREATMENT AND FOLLOW-UP

- Combined pharmacological and psychological therapy.[3]

CAVEATS

- Paroxysmal dysautonomia, hyperventilation, and hypocapnic cerebral hypoperfusion can underlie spells of altered consciousness.

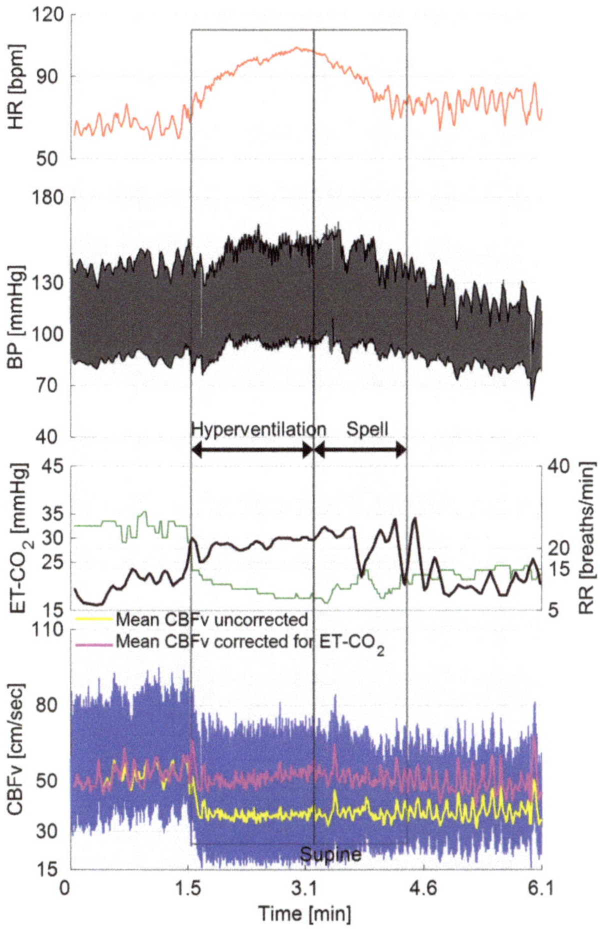

Figure 91.3 Hyperventilation in supine position provoked the patient's typical spell. The spell had characteristics similar to the spell recorded during the tilt, with a short decline in cerebral blood flow due to hyperventilation.

REFERENCES

1. Thomas A, Greenwald BD. Paroxysmal sympathetic hyperactivity and clinical considerations for patients with acquired brain injuries: a narrative review. *Am J Phys Med Rehabil.* June 2018. doi:10.1097/PHM.0000000000000990.
2. Meyfroidt G, Baguley IJ, Menon DK. Paroxysmal sympathetic hyperactivity: the storm after acute brain injury. *Lancet Neurol.* 2017;16(9):721–729. doi:10.1016/S1474-4422(17)30259-4.
3. Mann SJ. Severe paroxysmal hypertension (pseudopheochromocytoma). *Curr Hypertens Rep.* 2008;10(1):12–18.

92.

CASE 87: INTERMITTENT SUPINE HYPOTENSION

Chief complaint: Dizziness.

Case presentation: A 62-year-old man presents with intermittent dizziness and limb pain. His typical dizzy spell lasts from seconds to minutes; it can be postural but is not always. Skin biopsy assessment of small epidermal fibers was done at another institution and was consistent with small fiber neuropathy. Otolaryngology evaluation was normal. Electroencephalogram and MRI of the brain were normal. Patient was referred for evaluation of autonomic failure.

Past medical history: Dyslipidemia, small fiber neuropathy, anemia, scoliosis, lumbar arthritis, idiopathic urticaria.

Current medication: Atorvastatin, cetirizine.

Assessment plan: Functional autonomic tests.

AUTONOMIC TESTING EVALUATION

See Table 92.1.

Heart rate: Supine heart rate was normal. Heart rate responses to deep breathing were reduced to 44.3% of normal value. Heart rate increment during the tilt (15 BPM) was normal.

Blood pressure:

Valsalva maneuver: Blood pressure responses were normal.

Tilt: Supine blood pressure was fluctuating, but mean blood pressure was normal. Blood pressure responses to tilt were normal.

Sudomotor evaluation: Electrochemical skin conductance was abnormal (reduced to 96.3% of normal limit) at hands and normal at feet.

Respiratory system: Respiratory frequency and end tidal CO_2 were was normal in supine position and during the tilt.

Cerebral blood flow velocity (CBFv): CBFv in middle cerebral artery was fluctuating, but mean CBFv normal in supine position. CBFv in middle cerebral artery was stable during the tilt.

Skin biopsy (sensory-epidermal): N/A

Skin biopsy (sweat glands): N/A

Patient-reported symptoms during testing: Dizziness during the tilt.

Patient-reported symptoms for past 2 weeks:

Lightheadedness or dizziness: Occasionally
Dry eyes or mouth: Occasionally
Pale feet: Occasionally
Cold feet: Often

TABLE 92.1 **RESULTS OF AUTONOMIC TESTING**

Blood pressure evaluation					
Test: Valsalva maneuver					
Pressure [mmHg]	Baseline	Phase 2			Phase 4
		Early	End		
Systolic	124	72	72		
Mean	84	84.7	84.7	n/a	
Diastolic	64	91	91	n/a	

Heart rate evaluation	
Test: Deep breathing	
Results	Norm*
3.1	≥7
Test: Valsalva ratio	
1.62	≥1.29
* adjusted for a gender and age	

TABLE 92.1 **CONTINUED**

Test: Tilt test										
Position		HR [BPM]	Blood pressure [mmHg]		MCA Blood flow velocity [cm/s]				Respiratory frequency [breaths/min]	End tidal CO_2 [mmHg]
			Systolic	Diastolic	Systolic	Mean	Mean drop [%]	Diastolic		
Supine		69	128	78	108	66.7		46	10	39
Tilt [min]	1	69	118	73	102	68.7	-3	52	8	36
	2	78	120	80						
	3	78	117	79						
	4	77	114	76						
	5	75	142	77	112	72.7	-9	53	9	38
	6	77	114	79						
	7	78	120	80						
	8	79	123	84						
	9	79	125	81						
	10	84	122	83	111	71.7	-7.5	52	11	37
	15									
	20									
	30									
	40									

Sudomotor evaluation - functional

Test: Quantitative sudomotor axon reflex test (QSART)				
Location	Site (l/r)	Latency [min]	Volume [μl]	Norm [μl]*
Forearm				≥0.3
Prox. leg				≥0.23
Distal leg				≥0.23
Foot				≥0.27

* Normative data are adjusted for gender and age of patient.

Test: Electrochemical skin conductance (ESC)				
Location	Left [μS]	Right [μS]	Average [μS/k]	Norm [μS/kg]
Hand	73	71	0.99	≥1.03
Feet	86	83	1.14	≥1.14
Forehead				

For grading uses ESC [μS] adjusted for weight [μS/k].

(continued)

TABLE 92.1 CONTINUED

Small fiber (sensory + sudomotor) evaluation - morphological					
Test: Skin biopsy					
Location	Site (l/r)	Nerve fibers			
		Epidermal*		Sweat glands	
		Density	Norm	Density	Norm
Proximal leg – thigh	Right		≥8.3		≥37.8
Distal leg - calf	Right		≥4.85		≥36.5
Foot	Right		≥3.11		≥34.8

*Normative data for distal leg are adjusted for gender and age of patient.

QASAT*											
Heart rate		**BP**		**CBFv**		**ET-CO2**		**Sudomotor**			**Total QASAT score**
S. bradycardia	0	Low supine	0	Low supine	0	Low supine	0	QSART			
S. tachycardia	0	High supine	0	High supine	0	High supine	0	ESC	1		
Increase tilt	0	OH	0	Tilt response	0	Tilt low	0				
Decrease tilt	0	OHTN	0	CA	0	Tilt high	0	**Skin biopsy**			3
Deep breathing	2	VM	0	CVR	0			Epidermal			
VR	0			VM	0			Sweat gland			
Total	2	Total	0	Total	0	Total	0				

*QASAT. See Novak. Quantitative Scale for Grading of Cardiovascular Autonomic Reflex Tests and Small Fibers from Skin Biopsies. *J Neurol Disord* 2015;3:2.

S, supine; Increase tilt, increased response to tilt; Decrease tilt, decreased response to tilt; BP, blood pressure; VM, Valsalva maneuver; CBFv, cerebral blood flow velocity; CA, cerebral autoregulation; MCA, middle cerebral artery; VR, Valsalva ratio; CVR, cerebral vasoreactivity.

Reduced sweating: None
Reduced sweating after exercise: Occasionally
Increased sweating: None
Nausea: Often
Diarrhea: None
Constipation: None
Urinary leaks: Occasionally
Erection problems: None
Current pain severity: 9
Aching pain: Continuous, severe
Allodynia: None
Burning pain: Continuous, severe
Lancinating pain: Often, severe
Numbness: Often, moderate
Prickling sensation: Often, moderate

AUTONOMIC TESTING INTERPRETATION

- Paroxysmal dysautonomia associated with blood pressure and CBFv decline.

COMMENT

Patient was intermittently dizzy during the supine position but not during the tilt test (Figure 92.1). The dizziness was associated with severe decline in CBFv, up 42% (Figure 92.1D)

Usually, orthostatic blood pressure or CBFv changes are related to dizziness caused by cerebral hypoperfusion. However, this case demonstrates that even a supine decline in blood pressure and CBFv can result in dizziness.

Intermittent decline in blood pressure and CBFv can reflect abnormal central autonomic rhythms.[1]

TREATMENT AND FOLLOW-UP

- Patient was reassured that he does not have severe autonomic failure.
- This patient was started on a low dose of lisinopril that increases CBFv in patients with hypertension[2] and also may reduce blood pressure fluctuations by altering the cardiovascular feedback loops.

CAVEATS

- Even in the supine position, intermittent fluctuations in blood pressure and CBFv can results in dizziness.

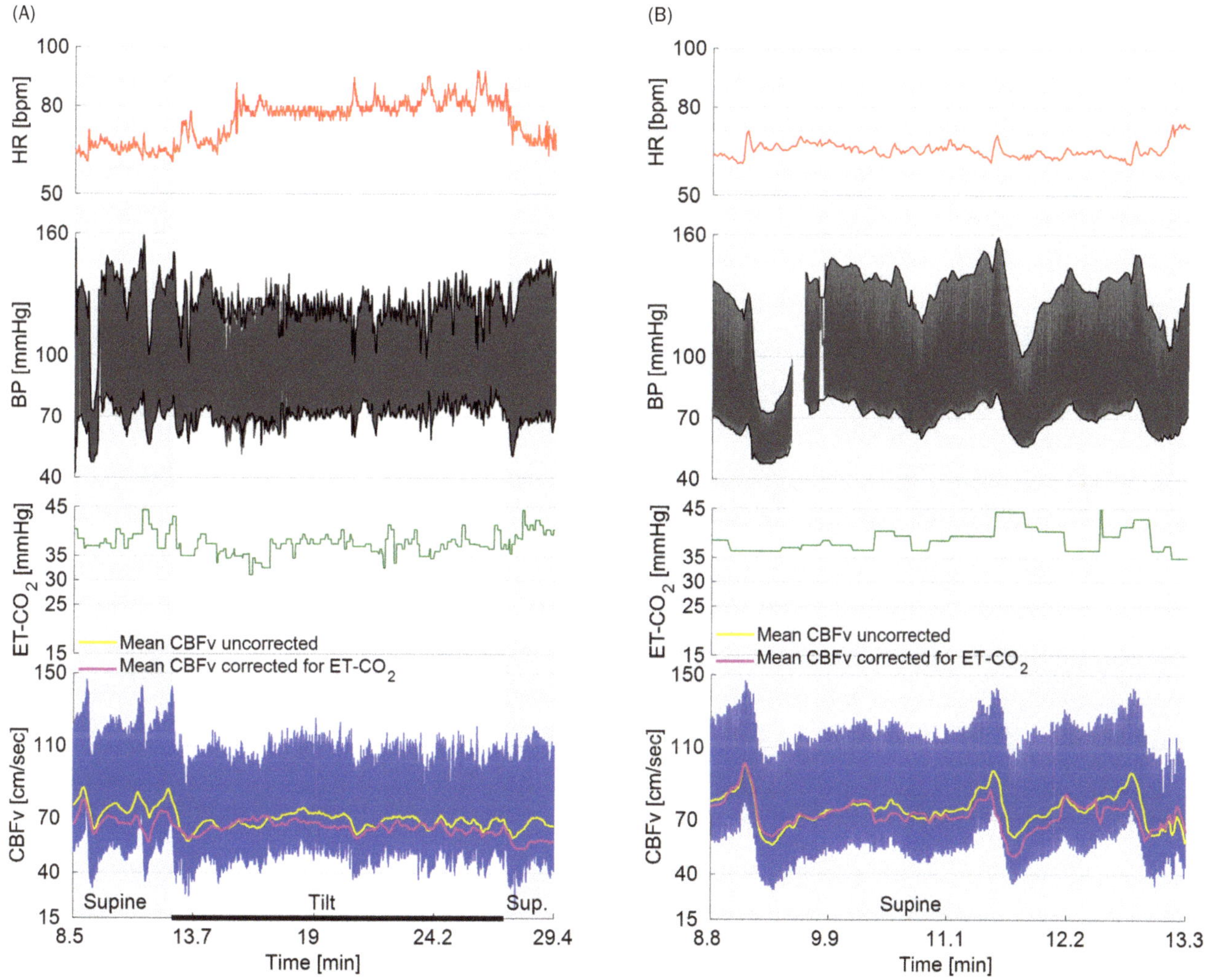

Figure 92.1 Blood pressure and cerebral blood flow velocity (CBFv) were fluctuating in supine position (A–D). Patient was very dizzy during each decline in CBFv. All orthostatic responses were normal. Details of two episodes of dizziness are in panels C and D showing severe decline in CBFv during each episode by 42% and 35%.

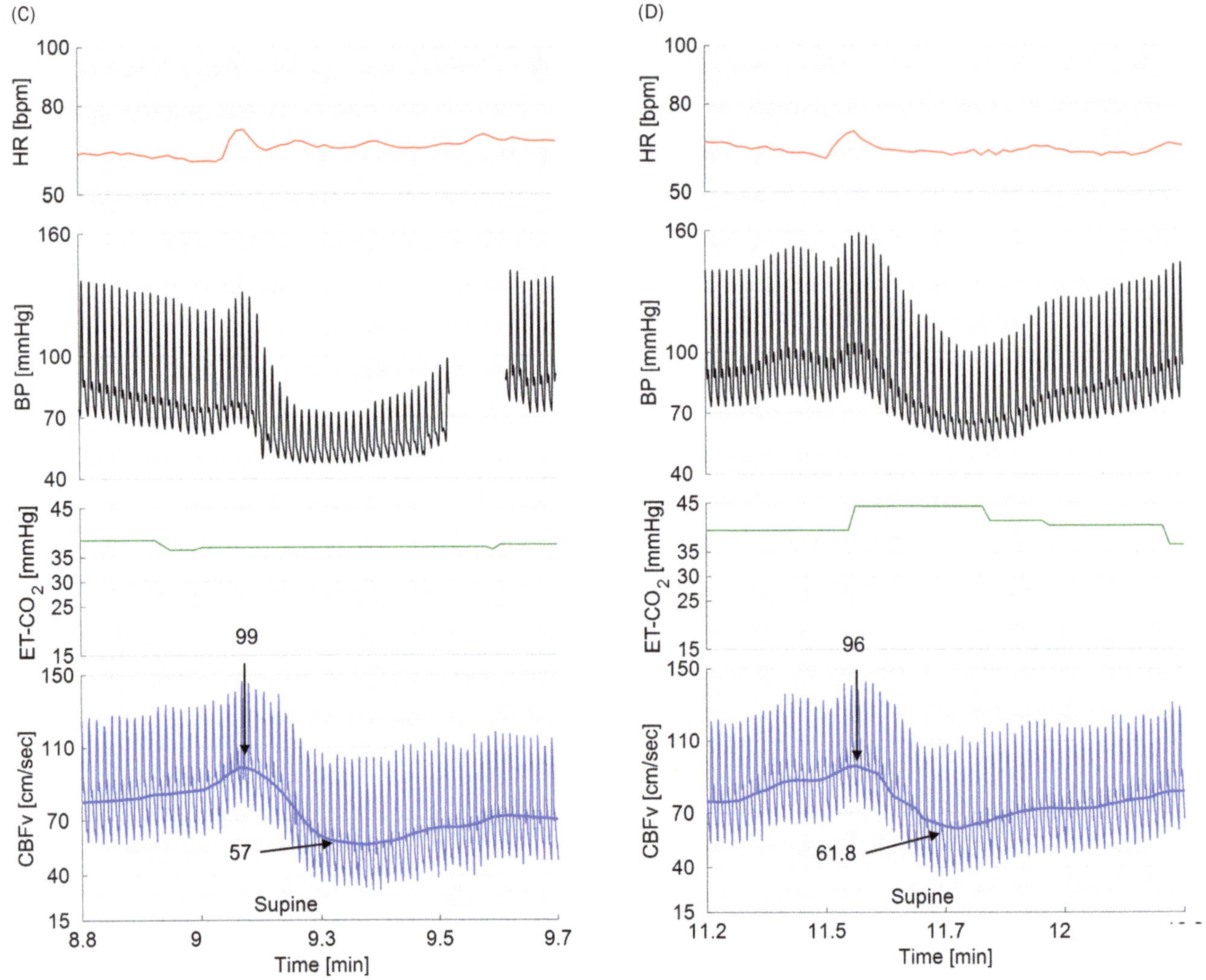

Figure 92.1 Continued

REFERENCES

1. Novak P, Novak V, Li Z, Remillard G. Time-frequency analysis of slow cortical activity and cardiovascular fluctuations in a case of Alzheimer's disease. *Clin Auton Res Off J Clin Auton Res Soc.* 1994;4(3):141–148.
2. Lipsitz LA, Gagnon M, Vyas M, et al. Antihypertensive therapy increases cerebral blood flow and carotid distensibility in hypertensive elderly subjects. *Hypertens Dallas Tex 1979.* 2005;45(2):216–221. doi:10.1161/01.HYP.0000153094.09615.11.

93.

CASE 88: INTERMITTENT VISION LOSS AFTER CERVICAL SPINE INJURY

Chief complaint: Intermittent vision loss.

Case presentation: A 22-year-old woman has a history of traumatic C5 vertebral body fracture resulting in severe spinal stenosis, status post C5 corpectomy and C4–C6 anterior cervical discectomy and fusion. Since the neck injury, she experienced orthostatic dizziness associated with blood pressure fluctuations, gait problems, and right-sided weakness attributed to hemicord injury. She also experiences intermittent visual changes: typically, when she stands up or performs strenuous exercises, she experiences "blacking out" and "darkening" but denies passing out. She is able to abort the visual problems by either lying down or stopping the physical activity. Electromyogram and nerve conduction study were normal. Repeated imaging of the cervical spine ruled out cervical compression. She was referred for autonomic testing to assess if the visual symptoms are due to autonomic failure.

Past medical history: Attention deficit disorder.

Current medication: None.

Assessment plan: Functional autonomic tests.

AUTONOMIC TESTING EVALUATION

See Table 93.1.

Heart rate: Supine heart rate was normal. Heart rate increment during the tilt (47 BPM) was exaggerated and exceeded 120 BPM.

Blood pressure:

Valsalva maneuver: Mean blood pressure failed to return to baseline at the end of Phase 2 by 20.7 mm Hg (i.e., 80.7% of baseline).

Tilt: Supine blood pressure was elevated. Blood pressure fluctuated during the tilt, but mean blood pressure was stable.

Sudomotor evaluation: Electrochemical skin conductance was normal at hands and normal at feet.

Respiratory system: Respiratory frequency was normal in supine position and during the tilt. End tidal CO_2 was reduced in supine position and declined further during the tilt.

Cerebral blood flow velocity (CBFv): CBFv in middle cerebral artery was increased in supine position. CBFv in middle cerebral artery was severely reduced during the tilt.

Skin biopsy (sensory-epidermal): Epidermal nerve fiber density was normal at proximal leg and normal at distal leg.

Skin biopsy (sweat glands): Sweat gland nerve fiber density was normal at proximal leg and abnormal (reduced to 60% of normal limit) at distal leg.

Patient-reported symptoms during testing: Dizziness during the tilt.

Patient-reported symptoms for past 2 weeks:

Lightheadedness or dizziness: Occasionally
Dry eyes or mouth: Occasionally
Pale feet: Occasionally

TABLE 93.1 **RESULTS OF AUTONOMIC TESTING**

Blood pressure evaluation					
Test: Valsalva maneuver					
Pressure [mmHg]	Baseline	Phase 2			Phase 4
		Early	End		
Systolic	147	98	103		
Mean	107	80.7	86.3	n/a	
Diastolic	87	72	78	n/a	

Heart rate evaluation	
Test: Deep breathing	
Results	Norm*
27.17	≥14
Test: Valsalva ratio	
2.23	≥1.46
* adjusted for a gender and age	

TABLE 93.1 **CONTINUED**

Test: Tilt test										
Position		HR [BPM]	Blood pressure [mmHg]		MCA Blood flow velocity [cm/s]				Respiratory frequency [breaths/min]	End tidal CO_2 [mmHg]
			Systolic	Diastolic	Systolic	Mean	Mean drop [%]	Diastolic		
Supine		99	142	92	135	95		75	9	30
Tilt [min]	1	140	134	93	111	71.7	24.5	52	12	30
	2	146	137	94						
	3	130	123	87						
	4	136	135	90						
	5	138	128	91	93	58.3	38.6	41	10	24
	6	139	134	88						
	7	132	143	106						
	8	125	131	98						
	9	127	126	93						
	10	135	141	98	97	65.7	30.8	50	13	22
	15	127	129	91						
	20									
	30									
	40									

Sudomotor evaluation - functional

Test: Quantitative sudomotor axon reflex test (QSART)				
Location	Site (l/r)	Latency [min]	Volume [μl]	Norm [μl]*
Forearm				≥0.08
Prox. leg				≥0.14
Distal leg				≥0.24
Foot				≥0.09

* Normative data are adjusted for gender and age of patient.

Test: Electrochemical skin conductance (ESC)				
Location	Left [μS]	Right [μS]	Average [μS/k]	Norm [μS/kg]
Hand	78	69	1.48	≥1.03
Feet	91	92	1.86	≥1.14
Forehead				

For grading uses ESC [μS] adjusted for weight [μS/k].

TABLE 93.1 CONTINUED

Small fiber (sensory + sudomotor) evaluation - morphological					
Test: Skin biopsy					
Location	Site (l/r)	Nerve fibers			
		Epidermal*		Sweat glands	
		Density	Norm	Density	Norm
Proximal leg – thigh	Right	16.5	≥8.3	43.3	≥37.8
Distal leg - calf	Right	11.65	≥9.34	21.9	≥36.5
Foot	Right		≥3.11		≥34.8

*Normative data for distal leg are adjusted for gender and age of patient.

QASAT*										
Heart rate		**BP**		**CBFv**		**ET-CO2**		**Sudomotor**		**Total QASAT score**
S. bradycardia	0	Low supine	0	Low supine	0	Low supine	1	QSART		
S. tachycardia	0	High supine	1	High supine	1	High supine	0	ESC	0	
Increase tilt	8	OH	0	Tilt response	7	Tilt low	5			
Decrease tilt	0	OHTN	0	CA	0	Tilt high	0	**Skin biopsy**		28
Deep breathing	0	VM	2	CVR	0			Epidermal	0	
VR	0			VM	0			Sweat gland	3	
Total	8	Total	3	Total	8	Total	6			

*QASAT. See Novak. Quantitative Scale for Grading of Cardiovascular Autonomic Reflex Tests and Small Fibers from Skin Biopsies. *J Neurol Disord* 2015;3:2.

S, supine; Increase tilt, increased response to tilt; Decrease tilt, decreased response to tilt; BP, blood pressure; VM, Valsalva maneuver; CBFv, cerebral blood flow velocity; CA, cerebral autoregulation; MCA, middle cerebral artery; VR, Valsalva ratio; CVR, cerebral vasoreactivity.

Cold feet: Often
Reduced sweating: Occasionally
Reduced sweating after exercise: Occasionally
Increased sweating: Occasionally
Nausea: None
Diarrhea: Yes, minor annoyance
Constipation: None
Urinary leaks: Yes, minor annoyance
Current pain severity: 0
Aching pain: Often, moderate
Allodynia: Occasionally, mild
Burning pain: Often, moderate
Lancinating pain: None
Numbness: Often, moderate
Prickling sensation: Occasionally, mild

AUTONOMIC TESTING INTERPRETATION

- Autonomic dysreflexia.
- Postural tachycardia syndrome (POTS), neuropathic form.
- Small fiber autonomic neuropathy.
- Visual changes are likely a cerebral blood flow-related phenomenon as the Valsalva maneuver reproduced the visual symptoms.

COMMENT

Autonomic testing, in addition to showing and autonomic neuropathy (Figure 93.1), was positive for two additional findings: (1) it reproduced the visual changes, and (2) it showed signs of sympathetic overactivity to cold stimulation. Prominent blood pressure oscillations with about a 1-minute period, are due to exaggerated sympathetic outflow. Cerebral autoregulation was intact. Patient noted black-out for about 5 seconds during Phase 2 of the Valsalva maneuver, exactly at the nadir of CBFv. This was reproduced twice during the testing. Patient has a history of cervical spine injury, which can result in autonomic dysreflexia.[1–3]

Autonomic dysreflexia is a form of autonomic overactivity that may occur after a spinal cord injury above the T5 level. It includes spells of elevated heart rate and blood pressure, sweating, and bowel and bladder problems. The spells usually have a trigger, the most common being bladder or bowel distension. Management involves appropriate bladder and bower care, avoidance of triggers, and low-dose β-blockers. POTS can result from trauma.

TREATMENT AND FOLLOW-UP

- Physical therapy.
- Low-dose β-blocker, which may help with both autonomic dysreflexia and POTS.

CAVEATS

- Cervical injury is associated with autonomic dysreflexia and POTS.
- Visual changes may reflect low cerebral blood flow.

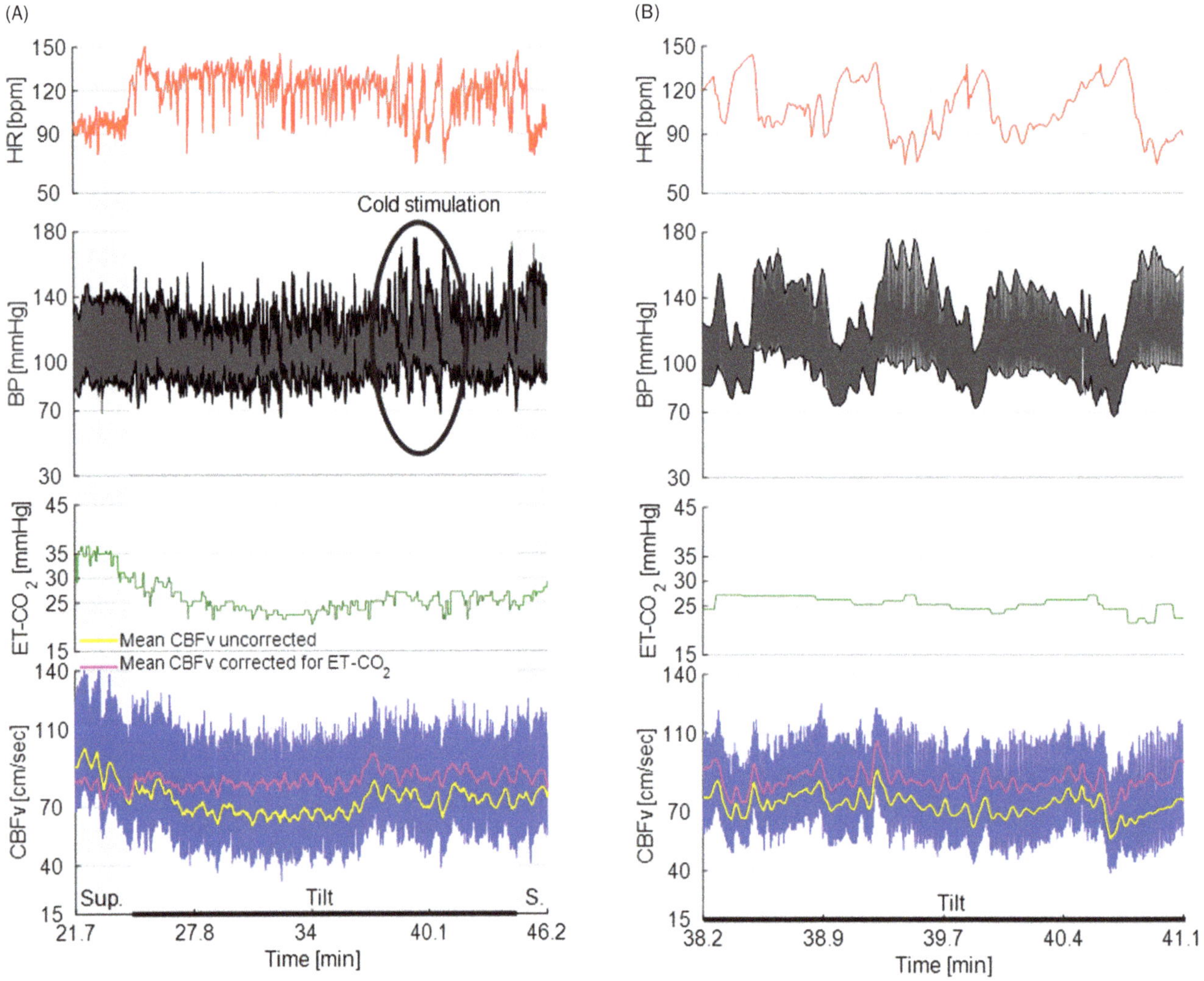

Figure 93.1 The tilt test showed exaggerated heart rate responses to the tilt while the mean blood pressure was stable (A). Cold stimulation with ice below the injury at the lower chest provoked marked fluctuations in heart rate and blood pressure and to a lesser extent in cerebral blood flow velocity (CBFv; A–C). Damped fluctuations in CBFv indicate intact cerebral autoregulation. Valsalva maneuver reproduced the patient symptoms: patient experienced darkening of vision exactly at the nadir of CBFv during Phase 2 (D).

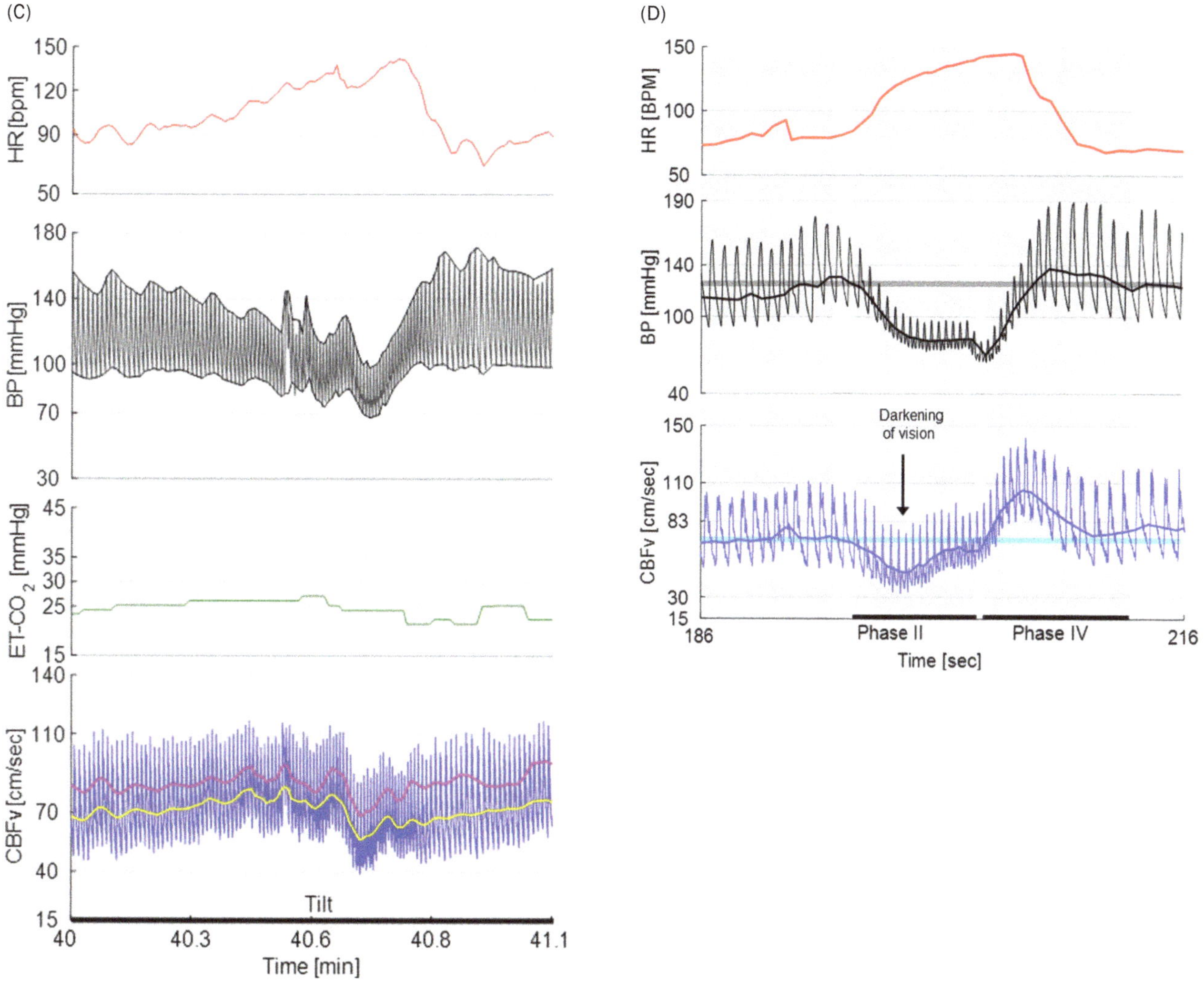

Figure 93.1 Continued

REFERENCES

1. Eldahan KC, Rabchevsky AG. Autonomic dysreflexia after spinal cord injury: Systemic pathophysiology and methods of management. *Auton Neurosci Basic Clin*. 2018;209:59–70. doi:10.1016/j.autneu.2017.05.002.
2. Karlsson A-K. Autonomic dysfunction in spinal cord injury: clinical presentation of symptoms and signs. *Prog Brain Res*. 2006;152:1–8. doi:10.1016/S0079-6123(05)52034-X.
3. Grigorean VT, Sandu AM, Popescu M, et al. Cardiac dysfunctions following spinal cord injury. *J Med Life*. 2009;2(2):133–145.

94.

CASE 89: PERIODIC APNEA

Chief complaint: Orthostatic intolerance.

Case presentation: A 20-year-old woman presents with orthostatic intolerance. She had several concussions from playing soccer. She was in good health until she had acute appendicitis at age 11 years. After the surgery, she noted headaches, nausea, hives, flashing, brain fog, fatigue, and body temperature changes. She had autonomic testing 3 years ago that was consistent with postural tachycardia syndrome (POTS). Nevertheless, in spite of POTS therapy (diet, exercise; she could not tolerate fludrocortisone, propranolol, and proamatine), she continues to have frequent, short dizzy spells while standing. MRI of the brain showed a small venous angioma at the right parietal lobe.

Past medical history: Concussions, POTS.

Current medication: None.

Assessment plan: Functional autonomic tests and skin biopsy.

AUTONOMIC TESTING EVALUATION

See Table 94.1.

Heart rate: Supine heart rate was normal. Heart rate responses to deep breathing were normal. Heart rate increment during the tilt (29 BPM) was normal.

Blood pressure:

Valsalva maneuver: Blood pressure responses were normal.

Tilt: Supine blood pressure was normal. Blood pressure responses to tilt were normal.

Sudomotor evaluation: Electrochemical skin conductance was normal at hands and normal at feet.

Respiratory system: Respiratory frequency was normal in supine position and during the tilt. End tidal CO_2 was minimally reduced in supine position but was normal during the tilt.

Cerebral blood flow velocity (CBFv): CBFv in middle cerebral artery was increased in supine position. CBFv in middle cerebral artery was stable during the tilt.

Skin biopsy (sensory-epidermal): Epidermal nerve fiber density was normal at proximal leg and normal at distal leg.

Skin biopsy (sweat glands): Sweat gland nerve fiber density was normal at proximal leg and normal at distal leg.

Patient-reported symptoms during testing: Dizziness in supine position, no symptoms during the tilt.

Patient-reported symptoms for past 2 weeks:

Lightheadedness or dizziness: Often
Dry eyes or mouth: Occasionally
Pale feet: Often
Cold feet: Often
Reduced sweating: Often
Reduced sweating after exercise: Often
Increased sweating: Occasionally
Nausea: Often
Diarrhea: None

TABLE 94.1 **RESULTS OF AUTONOMIC TESTING**

Blood pressure evaluation					
Test: Valsalva maneuver					
Pressure [mmHg]	Baseline	Phase 2			Phase 4
		Early	End		
Systolic	124	110	124		
Mean	94.7	86	100	n/a	
Diastolic	80	74	88	n/a	

Heart rate evaluation	
Test: Deep breathing	
Results	Norm*
22.5	≥14
Test: Valsalva ratio	
1.79	≥1.46
* adjusted for a gender and age	

TABLE 94.1 CONTINUED

Test: Tilt test										
Position		HR [BPM]	Blood pressure [mmHg]		MCA Blood flow velocity [cm/s]				Respiratory frequency [breaths/min]	End tidal CO_2 [mmHg]
			Systolic	Diastolic	Systolic	Mean	Mean drop [%]	Diastolic		
Supine		74	136	78	141	91.7		67	18	32
Tilt [min]	1	95	141	96	132	89.3	2.6	68	13	34
	2	95	142	92						
	3	94	137	95						
	4	94	125	86						
	5	93	132	95	132	89.3	2.6	68	20	33
	6	92	129	90						
	7	99	146	100						
	8	95	145	95						
	9	103	139	90						
	10	98	128	89	128	84	8.4	62	15	33
	15									
	20									
	30									
	40									

Sudomotor evaluation - functional

Test: Quantitative sudomotor axon reflex test (QSART)				
Location	Site (l/r)	Latency [min]	Volume [μl]	Norm [μl]*
Forearm				≥0.08
Prox. leg				≥0.14
Distal leg				≥0.24
Foot				≥0.09

* Normative data are adjusted for gender and age of patient.

Test: Electrochemical skin conductance (ESC)				
Location	Left [μS]	Right [μS]	Average [μS/k]	Norm [μS/kg]
Hand	82	80	1.15	≥1.03
Feet	87	91	1.29	≥1.14
Forehead				

For grading uses ESC [μS] adjusted for weight [μS/k].

(continued)

TABLE 94.1 CONTINUED

Small fiber (sensory + sudomotor) evaluation - morphological						
Test: Skin biopsy						
Location	Site (l/r)	Nerve fibers				
		Epidermal*			Sweat glands	
		Density	Norm		Density	Norm
Proximal leg – thigh	Right	17.43	≥8.3		63.1	≥37.8
Distal leg - calf	Right	13.86	≥9.5		59.2	≥36.5
Foot	Right		≥3.11			≥34.8

*Normative data for distal leg are adjusted for gender and age of patient.

QASAT*											
Heart rate		BP		CBFv		ET-CO2		Sudomotor			Total QASAT score
S. bradycardia	0	Low supine	0	Low supine	0	Low supine	1	QSART			
S. tachycardia	0	High supine	0	High supine	1	High supine	0	ESC	0		
Increase tilt	0	OH	0	Tilt response	0	Tilt low	0				
Decrease tilt	0	OHTN	0	CA	0	Tilt high	0	Skin biopsy			2
Deep breathing	0	VM	0	CVR	0			Epidermal	0		
VR	0			VM	0			Sweat gland	0		
Total	0	Total	0	Total	1	Total	1				

*QASAT. See Novak. Quantitative Scale for Grading of Cardiovascular Autonomic Reflex Tests and Small Fibers from Skin Biopsies. *J Neurol Disord* 2015;3:2.

S, supine; Increase tilt, increased response to tilt; Decrease tilt, decreased response to tilt; BP, blood pressure; VM, Valsalva maneuver; CBFv, cerebral blood flow velocity; CA, cerebral autoregulation; MCA, middle cerebral artery; VR, Valsalva ratio; CVR, cerebral vasoreactivity.

Constipation: Occasionally
Urinary leaks: Occasionally
Current pain severity: 5
Aching pain: Occasionally, mild
Allodynia: None
Burning pain: Occasionally, mild
Lancinating pain: Continuous, severe
Numbness: Continuous, severe
Prickling sensation: Often, moderate

AUTONOMIC TESTING INTERPRETATION

- Recurrent apnea in inspiration.
- No evidence of POTS, autonomic failure, or small fiber neuropathy.

COMMENTS

The testing showed recurrent supine apnea associated with dizziness (Figure 94.1). According to the patient, the dizziness experienced during the testing was her typical dizziness. During supine position, there was a periodic decline in blood pressure (systolic by ~60 mm Hg), tachycardia (BPM increase ~30 BPM), and reduced CBFv (by 38%) associated with apnea.(Figure 94.1). Patient was very dizzy, had feeling of passing out during the spells. The average duration of the each spell was 0.5 seconds, and the spells repeated itself with an average period of 1 minute. This pattern likely represents abnormal brainstem activity because it mimics the 1minute brainstem rhythm.

Apneusis is an abnormal respiratory pattern characterized by an apneustic pause in inspiration. It has been reported after insult to the respiratory network within the brainstem and

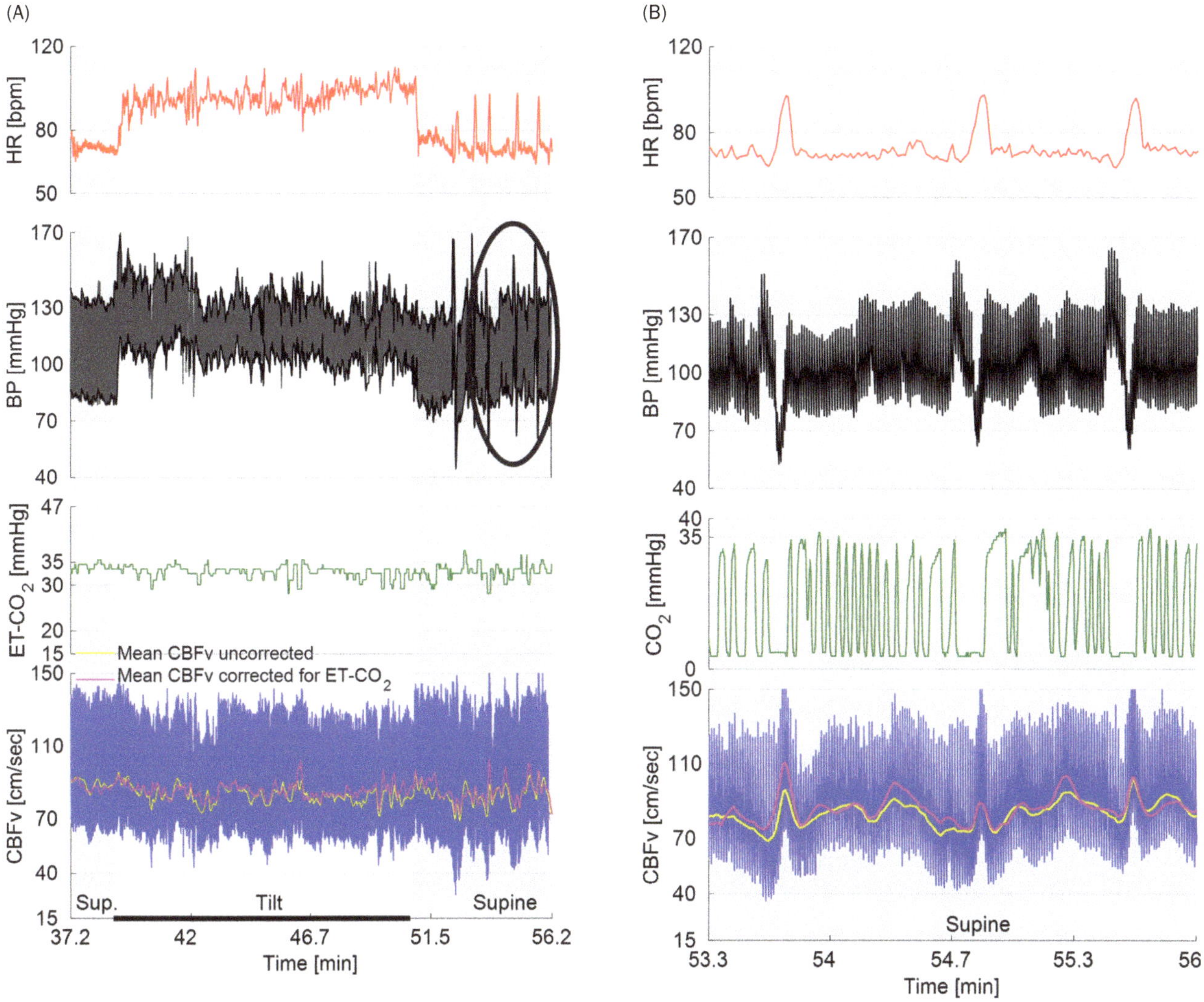

Figure 94.1 Tilt test showed normal mean heart rate, blood pressure, and cerebral blood flow (A, B). The patient reported intermittent dizziness in supine period after the tilt (Black oval). The dizziness was associated with intermittent apnea associated with blood pressure fluctuations occurring in 1-minute intervals (B, C). Details of event showed an apnea in inspiration and a sigmoid blood pressure (elevation followed by a decline), inverse response in cerebral blood flow velocity (decline followed by an increase), and tachycardia are in panel C.

(C)

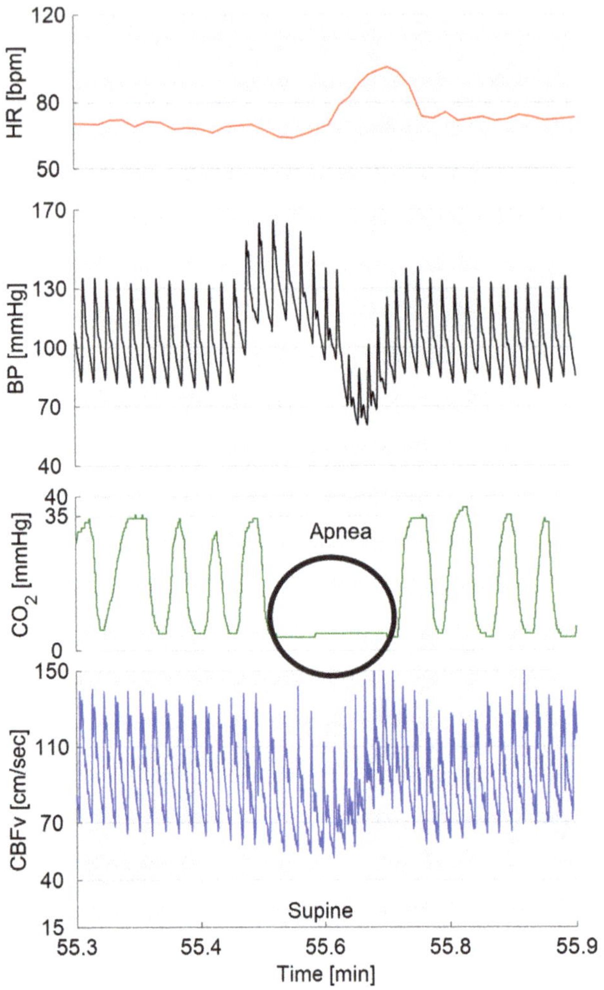

Figure 94.1 Continued

pons from an overdose of central nervous system depressants, blockade of glutamate receptors, asphyxia, hypoxia, or ischemia.[1] Apneustic patterns can be converted to normal by the administration of serotonin type 1A (5-HT1A) receptor agonists, including buspirone.

TREATMENT AND FOLLOW-UP

- Trial of buspirone.[1]
- Reason for apnea is unclear; it can be related to traumatic brain injury associated with concussion.

CAVEATS

- Apneusis can be associated with dizzy spells.

REFERENCE

1. Wilken B, Lalley P, Bischoff AM, et al. Treatment of apneustic respiratory disturbance with a serotonin-receptor agonist. *J Pediatr.* 1997;130(1):89–94.

CASE 90: REPETITIVE DIZZINESS

Chief complaint: Dizziness.

Case presentation: A 39-year-old woman presents with dizziness and palpitations. At age 18, she experienced constant headaches for a year. She was found to have a Chiari I malformation and was treated with surgical decompression and C4–C5 fusion. At age 28, she had tethered cord surgery. After the surgery, she experienced dizziness upon standing, and she has fainted twice. She was seen by cardiology and diagnosed with postural tachycardia syndrome (POTS). At age 35, she had a spinal cord stimulator implanted for chronic pain. For the past 10 years, she has had intermittent postural dizziness. She did not respond to propranolol, nortriptyline, or meclizine. She was referred for evaluation of POTS versus autonomic failure.

Past medical history: Ehlers-Danlos syndrome hypermobile type, Chiari I malformation, Lyme disease.

Current medication: None.

Assessment plan: Functional autonomic tests and skin biopsy.

AUTONOMIC TESTING EVALUATION

See Table 95.1.

Heart rate: Supine heart rate was normal. Heart rate responses to deep breathing were normal. Heart rate increment during the tilt (11 BPM) was normal.

Blood pressure:

Valsalva maneuver: Mean blood pressure failed to return to baseline at the end of Phase 2 by 6.7 mm Hg (i.e., 92.9% of baseline).

Tilt: Supine blood pressure was normal. Blood pressure responses to tilt were normal.

Sudomotor evaluation: N/A due to technical reasons.

Respiratory system: Respiratory frequency was normal in supine position and during the tilt. End tidal CO_2 was reduced in supine position and during the tilt.

Cerebral blood flow velocity (CBFv): CBFv in middle cerebral artery was normal in supine position but was mildly reduced during the tilt.

Skin biopsy (sensory-epidermal): Epidermal nerve fiber density was normal at proximal leg and normal at distal leg.

Skin biopsy (sweat glands): Sweat gland nerve fiber density was normal at distal leg.

Patient-reported symptoms during testing: Short episodic dizziness during the tilt.

Patient-reported symptoms for past 2 weeks:

Lightheadedness or dizziness: Occasionally
Dry eyes or mouth: Occasionally
Pale feet: Yes, minor annoyance
Cold feet: Occasionally
Reduced sweating: Yes, minor annoyance

TABLE 95.1 **RESULTS OF AUTONOMIC TESTING**

Blood pressure evaluation					
Test: Valsalva maneuver					
Pressure [mmHg]	Baseline	Phase 2			Phase 4
		Early	End		
Systolic	140	98	110		
Mean	94.7	76.7	88	n/a	
Diastolic	72	66	77	n/a	

Heart rate evaluation	
Test: Deep breathing	
Results	Norm*
17.17	≥12
Test: Valsalva ratio	
1.67	≥1.5
* adjusted for a gender and age	

(continued)

TABLE 95.1 CONTINUED

Test: Tilt test											
Position		HR [BPM]	Blood pressure [mmHg]		MCA Blood flow velocity [cm/s]				Respiratory frequency [breaths/min]	End tidal CO_2 [mmHg]
			Systolic	Diastolic	Systolic	Mean	Mean drop [%]	Diastolic		
Supine		80	137	86	94	64		49	7	33
Tilt [min]	1	77	121	84	85	53.7	16.1	38	11	28
	2	77	121	86						
	3	77	116	82						
	4	75	127	84						
	5	80	125	85	88	54.7	14.5	38	12	29
	6	79	115	82						
	7	86	125	84						
	8	86	123	84						
	9	86	128	85						
	10	91	123	86	97	65.7	-2.7	50	13	27
	15									
	20									
	30									
	40									

Sudomotor evaluation - functional

Test: Quantitative sudomotor axon reflex test (QSART)				
Location	Site (l/r)	Latency [min]	Volume [μl]	Norm [μl]*
Forearm				≥0.08
Prox. leg				≥0.14
Distal leg				≥0.15
Foot				≥0.07

* Normative data are adjusted for gender and age of patient.

Test: Electrochemical skin conductance (ESC)				
Location	Left [μS]	Right [μS]	Average [μS/k]	Norm [μS/kg]
Hand				≥1.03
Feet				≥1.14
Forehead				
For grading uses ESC [μS] adjusted for weight [μS/k].				

TABLE 95.1 CONTINUED

Small fiber (sensory + sudomotor) evaluation - morphological					
Test: Skin biopsy					
Location	Site (l/r)	Nerve fibers			
		Epidermal*		Sweat glands	
		Density	Norm	Density	Norm
Proximal leg – thigh	Right	11.55	≥8.3		≥37.8
Distal leg - calf	Right	8.06	≥7.98	40.1	≥36.5
Foot	Right		≥3.11		≥34.8

*Normative data for distal leg are adjusted for gender and age of patient.

QASAT*												
Heart rate		BP		CBFv		ET-CO2		Sudomotor			Total QASAT score
S. bradycardia	0	Low supine	0	Low supine	0	Low supine	1	QSART			
S. tachycardia	0	High supine	0	High supine	0	High supine	0	ESC			
Increase tilt	0	OH	0	Tilt response	2	Tilt low	2				
Decrease tilt	0	OHTN	0	CA	0	Tilt high	0	**Skin biopsy**			6
Deep breathing	0	VM	1	CVR	0			Epidermal	0		
VR	0			VM	0			Sweat gland	0		
Total	0	Total	1	Total	2	Total	3				

*QASAT. See Novak. Quantitative Scale for Grading of Cardiovascular Autonomic Reflex Tests and Small Fibers from Skin Biopsies. *J Neurol Disord* 2015;3:2.

S, supine; Increase tilt, increased response to tilt; Decrease tilt, decreased response to tilt; BP, blood pressure; VM, Valsalva maneuver; CBFv, cerebral blood flow velocity; CA, cerebral autoregulation; MCA, middle cerebral artery; VR, Valsalva ratio; CVR, cerebral vasoreactivity.

Reduced sweating after exercise: Yes, minor annoyance
Increased sweating: Yes, minor annoyance
Nausea: Occasionally
Diarrhea: Yes, minor annoyance
Constipation: Yes, minor annoyance
Urinary leaks: Yes, minor annoyance
Current pain severity: 6
Aching pain: Often, moderate
Allodynia: Occasionally, moderate
Burning pain: Occasionally, moderate
Lancinating pain: Occasionally, moderate
Numbness: Occasionally, mild
Prickling sensation: Occasionally, mild

AUTONOMIC TESTING INTERPRETATION

- Cerebral autoregulatory failure, dynamic.
- Mild adrenergic dysfunction.

COMMENT

The tilt test reproduces this patient's symptoms. The patient reported short, repetitive episodes of dizziness that were associated with a decline in CBFv (Figure 95.1) indicating abnormal vasodilation and vasoconstriction due to failure of dynamic autoregulation. Dynamic cerebral autoregulation refers to the brain's ability to keep cerebral blood flow constant despite fast changes in blood pressure.[1,2]

TREATMENT AND FOLLOW-UP

- Volume expansion through high fluid and high salt intake.

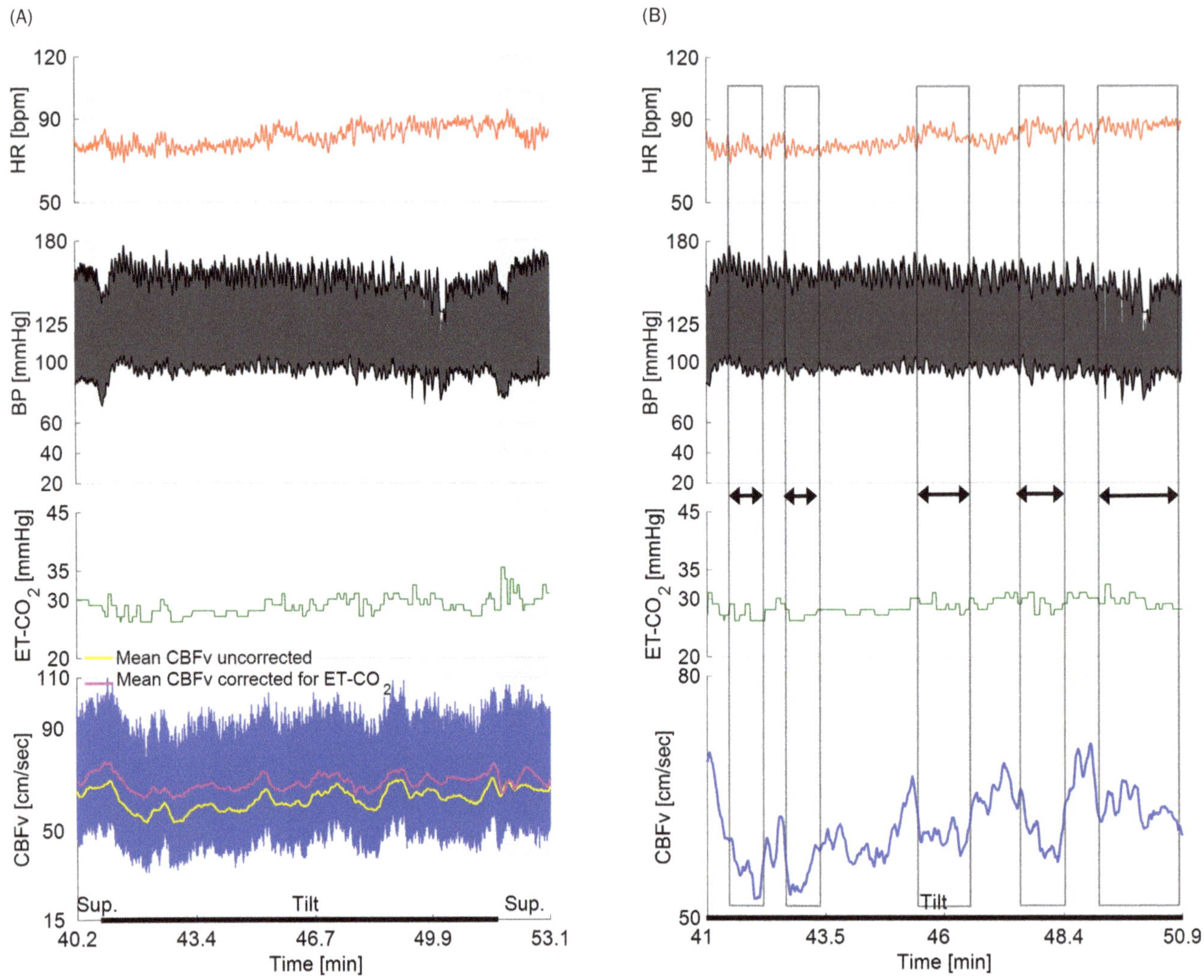

Figure 95.1 Heart rate and blood pressure responses to tilt were normal (A, B). End tidal CO_2 was mildly reduced (level ~30 mm Hg) but was stable during the tilt. Cerebral blood flow velocity (CBFv) was intermittently reduced (*black arrows*, B, C), which was associated with dizziness.

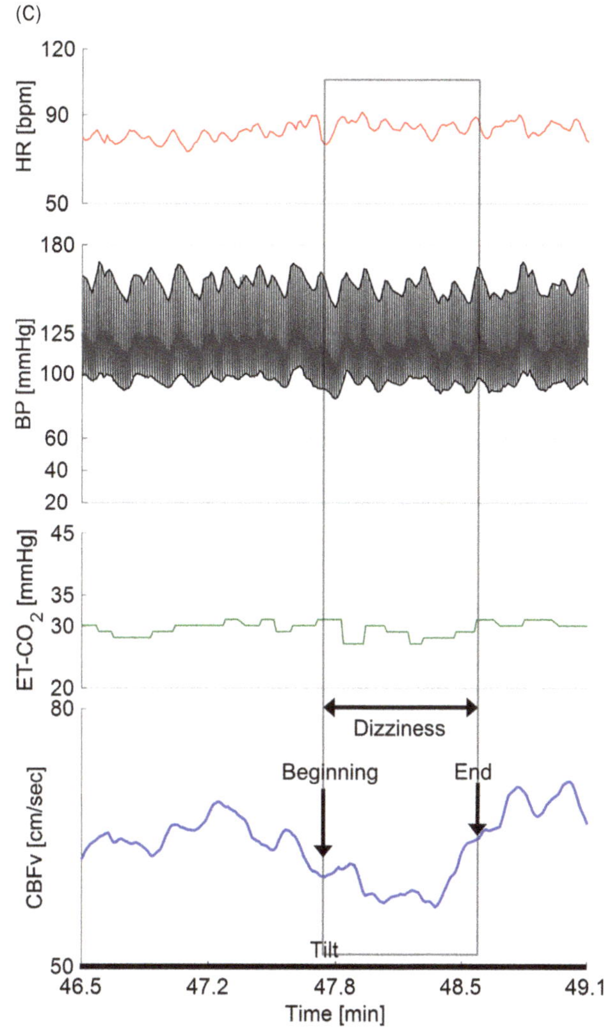

Figure 95.1 Continued

CAVEATS

- Repetitive dizziness can be related to CBFv fluctuations and likely represents episodic cerebral hypoperfusion.

REFERENCES

1. Czosnyka M, Richards H, Kirkpatrick P, Pickard J. Assessment of cerebral autoregulation with ultrasound and laser Doppler wave forms: an experimental study in anesthetized rabbits. *Neurosurgery*. 1994;35(2):287–292; discussion 292–293.
2. Czosnyka M, Brady K, Reinhard M, Smielewski P, Steiner LA. Monitoring of cerebrovascular autoregulation: facts, myths, and missing links. *Neurocrit Care*. 2009;10(3):373–386. doi:10.1007/s12028-008-9175-7.

96.

CASE 91: PRIMARY CEREBRAL AUTOREGULATORY FAILURE

Chief complaint: Dizziness.

Case presentation: A 54-year-old man presents with recurrent episodes of hypertensive crisis (>220/100 mm Hg) and chest tightness for the past 5 years. He has episodic hypertensive spells associated with tremor and deep pain once or twice per month. He fainted after taking clonidine and then when coughing vigorously. He also reports headaches, dizziness, fatigue, abdominal and chest pains. Thorough evaluation included MRI of the brain, computed tomography (CT) of the chest, nerve conduction study, electromyogram, repeated catecholamines level in serum and urine, toxicology screenings, hemoglobin A1C, gastrointestinal endoscopies, and positron emission tomography (PET) of the brain and of the adrenal glands. All tests were within normal limits or unrevealing. He was referred for suspected autonomic hyperactivity or abnormal cerebral blood flow.

Past medical history: Sarcoidosis, Lyme disease, hypertension.

Current medication: Fluoxetine, hydrochlorothiazide, omeprazole.

Assessment plan: Functional autonomic tests and skin biopsy.

AUTONOMIC TESTING EVALUATION

See Table 96.1.

Heart rate: Supine heart rate was normal. Heart rate responses to deep breathing were reduced to 77.8% of normal value. Heart rate increment during the tilt (20 BPM) was normal.

Blood pressure:

Valsalva maneuver: Mean blood pressure failed to return to baseline at the end of Phase 2 by 6.3 mm Hg (i.e., 92.3% of baseline).

Tilt: Supine blood pressure was normal. Blood pressure responses to tilt were normal.

Sudomotor evaluation: Electrochemical skin conductance was abnormal (reduced to 70.3% of normal limit) at hands and abnormal (reduced to 68.6% of normal limit) at feet.

Respiratory system: Respiratory frequency was normal in supine position and during the tilt. End tidal CO_2 was reduced in supine position but was stable during the tilt.

Cerebral blood flow velocity (CBFv): CBFv in middle cerebral artery was reduced in supine position and during the tilt.

Skin biopsy (sensory-epidermal): Epidermal nerve fiber density was normal at proximal leg and abnormal (reduced to 56% of normal limit) at distal leg.

Skin biopsy (sweat glands): Sweat gland nerve fiber density was abnormal (reduced to 18.6% of normal limit) at distal leg.

Patient-reported symptoms during testing: Dizziness during the tilt.

Patient-reported symptoms for past 2 weeks:

Lightheadedness or dizziness: Occasionally
Dry eyes or mouth: Occasionally

TABLE 96.1 **RESULTS OF AUTONOMIC TESTING**

Blood pressure evaluation					
Test: Valsalva maneuver					
Pressure [mmHg]	Baseline	Phase 2			Phase 4
		Early	End		
Systolic	126	81	99		
Mean	82	64.3	75.7	n/a	
Diastolic	60	56	64	n/a	

Heart rate evaluation	
Test: Deep breathing	
Results	Norm*
7	≥9
Test: Valsalva ratio	
1.45	≥1.36

* adjusted for a gender and age

TABLE 96.1 **CONTINUED**

Test: Tilt test										
Position		HR [BPM]	Blood pressure [mmHg]		MCA Blood flow velocity [cm/s]				Respiratory frequency [breaths/min]	End tidal CO_2 [mmHg]
			Systolic	Diastolic	Systolic	Mean	Mean drop [%]	Diastolic		
Supine		65	132	89	63	42.3		32	13	30
Tilt [min]	1	80	126	89	54	32.7	22.7	22	17	31
	2	80	120	85						
	3	85	133	92						
	4	78	123	87						
	5	77	136	83	60	37.3	11.8	26	12	31
	6	78	133	87						
	7	79	122	84						
	8	78	125	86						
	9	80	122	84						
	10	80	128	88	60	36.7	13.2	25	15	31
	15									
	20									
	30									
	40									

Sudomotor evaluation - functional

Test: Quantitative sudomotor axon reflex test (QSART)				
Location	Site (l/r)	Latency [min]	Volume [µl]	Norm [µl]*
Forearm				≥0.3
Prox. leg				≥0.23
Distal leg				≥0.23
Foot				≥0.27

* Normative data are adjusted for gender and age of patient.

Test: Electrochemical skin conductance (ESC)				
Location	Left [µS]	Right [µS]	Average [µS/k]	Norm [µS/kg]
Hand	86	88	0.72	≥1.03
Feet	94	94	0.78	≥1.14
Forehead				

For grading uses ESC [µS] adjusted for weight [µS/k].

(continued)

TABLE 96.1 **CONTINUED**

Small fiber (sensory + sudomotor) evaluation - morphological

Test: Skin biopsy

Location	Site (l/r)	Nerve fibers			
		Epidermal*		Sweat glands	
		Density	Norm	Density	Norm
Proximal leg – thigh	Right	13.43	≥8.3		≥37.8
Distal leg - calf	Right	3.05	≥5.45	6.8	≥36.5
Foot	Right		≥3.11		≥34.8

*Normative data for distal leg are adjusted for gender and age of patient.

QASAT*

Heart rate		BP		CBFv		ET-CO2		Sudomotor			Total QASAT score
S. bradycardia	0	Low supine	0	Low supine	1	Low supine	1	QSART			
S. tachycardia	0	High supine	0	High supine	0	High supine	0	ESC	2		
Increase tilt	0	OH	0	Tilt response	3	Tilt low	2				
Decrease tilt	0	OHTN	0	CA	0	Tilt high	0	**Skin biopsy**			18
Deep breathing	1	VM	1	CVR	0			Epidermal	3		
VR	0			VM	0			Sweat gland	4		
Total	1	Total	1	Total	4	Total	3				

*QASAT. See Novak. Quantitative Scale for Grading of Cardiovascular Autonomic Reflex Tests and Small Fibers from Skin Biopsies. *J Neurol Disord* 2015;3:2.

S, supine; Increase tilt, increased response to tilt; Decrease tilt, decreased response to tilt; BP, blood pressure; VM, Valsalva maneuver; CBFv, cerebral blood flow velocity; CA, cerebral autoregulation; MCA, middle cerebral artery; VR, Valsalva ratio; CVR, cerebral vasoreactivity.

Pale feet: Occasionally
Cold feet: Occasionally
Reduced sweating: None
Reduced sweating after exercise: None
Increased sweating: Occasionally
Nausea: Occasionally
Diarrhea: None
Constipation: None
Urinary leaks: Occasionally
Erection problems: Occasionally
Current pain severity: 2
Aching pain: Often, moderate
Allodynia: Occasionally, moderate
Burning pain: Often, moderate
Lancinating pain: Occasionally, moderate
Numbness: None
Prickling sensation: None

AUTONOMIC TESTING INTERPRETATION

- Primary cerebral autoregulatory failure.
- Mild autonomic failure. There was no evidence of autonomic overactivity.
- Small fiber neuropathy, mixed, length-dependent.

COMMENT

The main finding of the study was reduced CBFv in supine position and during the tilt (Figure 96.1), which is consistent with primary cerebral autoregulatory failure due to abnormal cerebral vasoconstriction.[1] Small vessel disease likely plays a role. Low CBFv may be associated with chronic cerebral hypoperfusion.

This patient has a history of hypertensive crisis of unclear cause. In theory, acute reduction in already very low cerebral blood flow may trigger a hypertensive episode by inducing endothelial injury with resulting ischemia that may release vasoactive substances.[2,3]

Hypertension-associated small vessel disease may lead to abnormal cerebral autoregulation with chronic vasoconstriction and hypoperfusion.[4] Antihypertensive therapy may increase cerebral blood flow.[4]

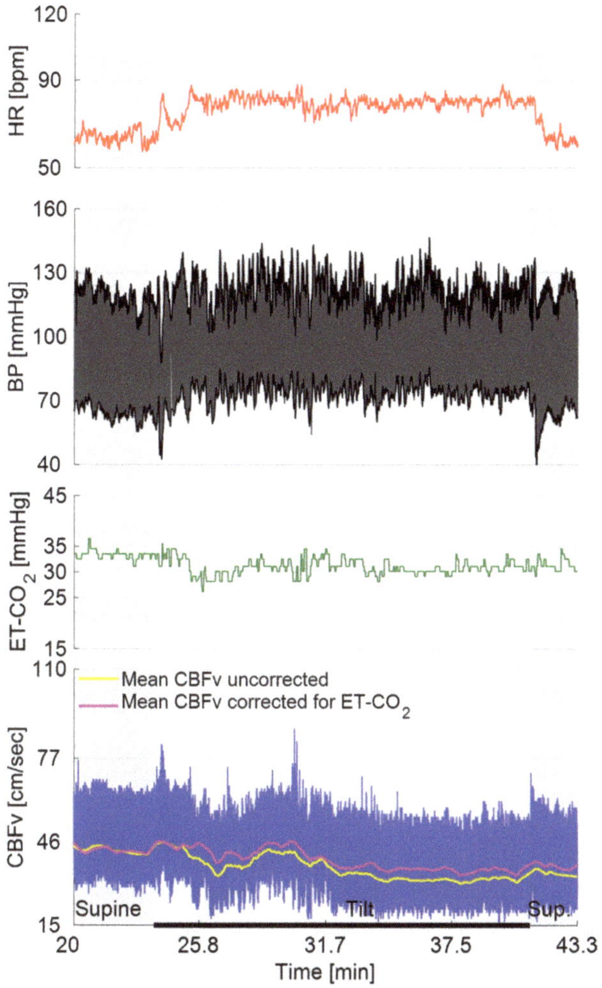

Figure 96.1 Cardiovascular responses to tilt were normal. Cerebral blood flow velocity was markedly reduced in supine baseline and during the tilt. End tidal CO_2 was normal.

Patient also has small fiber neuropathy that is likely due to sarcoidosis.[5]

TREATMENT AND FOLLOW-UP

- Consider switching antihypertensive therapy to angiotensin converting enzyme (ACE) inhibitors, which have been shown to improve cerebral autoregulation.

CAVEATS

- Primary cerebral autoregulatory failure may be associated with hypertensive crisis.

REFERENCES

1. Novak P. Cerebral blood flow, heart rate, and blood pressure patterns during the tilt test in common orthostatic syndromes. *Neurosci J.* 2016;2016:6127340. doi:10.1155/2016/6127340.
2. Arbe G, Pastor I, Franco J. Diagnostic and therapeutic approach to the hypertensive crisis. *Med Clin (Barc).* 2018;150(8):317–322. doi:10.1016/j.medcli.2017.09.027.
3. Martin JFV, Higashiama E, Garcia E, Luizon MR, Cipullo JP. Hypertensive crisis profile. Prevalence and clinical presentation. *Arq Bras Cardiol.* 2004;83(2):131–136; 125–130. doi:/S0066-782X2004001400004.
4. Lipsitz LA, Gagnon M, Vyas M, et al. Antihypertensive therapy increases cerebral blood flow and carotid distensibility in hypertensive elderly subjects. *Hypertens Dallas Tex 1979.* 2005;45(2):216–221. doi:10.1161/01.HYP.0000153094.09615.11.
5. Gorson KC, Herrmann DN, Thiagarajan R, et al. Non-length dependent small fibre neuropathy/ganglionopathy. *J Neurol Neurosurg Psychiatry.* 2008;79(2):163–169. doi:10.1136/jnnp.2007.128801.

PART XI

PSYCHOGENIC DISORDERS

97.

CASE 92: ANXIETY

Chief complaint: Dizziness.

Case presentation: A 35-year-old woman presents with anxiety. All problems started at college at the age 20. She began to experience stomach discomfort after each meal, including food regurgitation, nausea, bloating, and abdominal pain. Her symptoms improved after a switch to a low-fat diet. She started to wake up early in the mornings and notice pins-and-needles sensations in her feet and intermittent shortness of breath. She began to have neck pain and discomfort down both arms and, within weeks, also in her legs. She has been evaluated by rheumatology and diagnosed with fibromyalgia. About 3 years ago, she began to experience brain fog, fatigue, headaches and burning pain over her scalp, tachycardia, and excessive sweating. She transiently improved on physical therapy. Nevertheless, for the past few months, she has experienced elevated heart rate, dyspnea, and chest discomfort on standing. She had autonomic testing that, according to the patient, was consistent with postural tachycardia syndrome (POTS). However, she did not respond to β-blockers, fludrocortisone, or proamatine. She was referred for evaluation of small fiber neuropathy and orthostatic intolerance.

Past medical history: Anxiety, fibromyalgia.

Current medication: None.

Assessment plan: Functional autonomic tests, patient was offered skin biopsy, but declined.

AUTONOMIC TESTING EVALUATION

See Table 97.1.

Heart rate: Supine heart rate was normal. Heart rate responses to deep breathing were normal. Heart rate increment during the tilt (33 BPM) was exaggerated.

Blood pressure:

Valsalva maneuver: Mean blood pressure failed to return to baseline at the end of Phase 2 by 11.7 mm Hg (i.e., 89% of baseline).

Tilt: Supine blood pressure was normal. Blood pressure responses to tilt were normal.

Sudomotor evaluation: Electrochemical skin conductance was normal at hands and normal at feet.

Respiratory system: Respiratory frequency and end tidal CO_2 were normal in supine position and during the tilt.

Cerebral blood flow velocity (CBFv): CBFv in middle cerebral artery was reduced in supine position. CBFv in middle cerebral artery was stable during the tilt.

Skin biopsy (sensory-epidermal): N/A

Skin biopsy (sweat glands): N/A

Patient-reported symptoms during testing: Dizziness during the tilt.

TABLE 97.1 **RESULTS OF AUTONOMIC TESTING**

Blood pressure evaluation					
Test: Valsalva maneuver					
Pressure [mmHg]	Baseline	Phase 2			Phase 4
		Early	End		
Systolic	140	70	115		
Mean	106.7	58	95	n/a	
Diastolic	90	52	85	n/a	

Heart rate evaluation	
Test: Deep breathing	
Results	Norm*
23	≥12
Test: Valsalva ratio	
1.72	≥1.5
* adjusted for a gender and age	

(continued)

TABLE 97.1 **CONTINUED**

Test: Tilt test										
Position		HR [BPM]	Blood pressure [mmHg]		MCA Blood flow velocity [cm/s]				Respiratory frequency [breaths/min]	End tidal CO_2 [mmHg]
			Systolic	Diastolic	Systolic	Mean	Mean drop [%]	Diastolic		
Supine		88	125	84	74	50.7		39	13	37
Tilt [min]	1	121	126	91	82	52.7	-3.9	38	18	33
	2	84	119	85						
	3	94	118	85						
	4	94	129	88						
	5	95	123	88	83	57.7	-13.8	45	13	37
	6	95	122	87						
	7	82	115	81						
	8	88	122	85						
	9	89	110	78						
	10	95	122	88	84	59.3	-17	47	17	37
	15									
	20									
	30									
	40									

Sudomotor evaluation - functional

Test: Quantitative sudomotor axon reflex test (QSART)				
Location	Site (l/r)	Latency [min]	Volume [μl]	Norm [μl]*
Forearm				≥0.08
Prox. leg				≥0.14
Distal leg				≥0.15
Foot				≥0.07

* Normative data are adjusted for gender and age of patient.

Test: Electrochemical skin conductance (ESC)				
Location	Left [μS]	Right [μS]	Average [μS/k]	Norm [μS/kg]
Hand	81	77	1.29	≥1.03
Feet	84	83	1.36	≥1.14
Forehead				

For grading uses ESC [μS] adjusted for weight [μS/k].

TABLE 97.1 CONTINUED

Small fiber (sensory + sudomotor) evaluation - morphological					
Test: Skin biopsy					
Location	Site (l/r)	Nerve fibers			
		Epidermal*		Sweat glands	
		Density	Norm	Density	Norm
Proximal leg – thigh	Right		≥8.3		≥37.8
Distal leg - calf	Right		≥8.3		≥36.5
Foot	Right		≥3.11		≥34.8

*Normative data for distal leg are adjusted for gender and age of patient.

QASAT*

Heart rate		BP		CBFv		ET-CO2		Sudomotor			Total QASAT score
S. bradycardia	0	Low supine	0	Low supine	1	Low supine	0	QSART			
S. tachycardia	0	High supine	0	High supine	0	High supine	0	ESC	0		
Increase tilt	1	OH	0	Tilt response	0	Tilt low	0				
Decrease tilt	0	OHTN	0	CA	0	Tilt high	0	**Skin biopsy**			4
Deep breathing	0	VM	2	CVR	0			Epidermal			
VR	0			VM	0			Sweat gland			
Total	1	Total	2	Total	1	Total	0				

*QASAT. See Novak. Quantitative Scale for Grading of Cardiovascular Autonomic Reflex Tests and Small Fibers from Skin Biopsies. *J Neurol Disord* 2015;3:2.

S, supine; Increase tilt, increased response to tilt; Decrease tilt, decreased response to tilt; BP, blood pressure; VM, Valsalva maneuver; CBFv, cerebral blood flow velocity; CA, cerebral autoregulation; MCA, middle cerebral artery; VR, Valsalva ratio; CVR, cerebral vasoreactivity.

Patient-reported symptoms for past 2 weeks:

Lightheadedness or dizziness: Often
Dry eyes or mouth: Occasionally
Pale feet: Occasionally
Cold feet: Occasionally
Reduced sweating: None
Increased sweating: Occasionally
Nausea: Occasionally
Diarrhea: Occasionally
Constipation: None
Urinary leaks: None
Current pain severity: 7
Aching pain: Often, moderate
Allodynia: Continuous, severe
Burning pain: Continuous, mild
Lancinating pain: Often, moderate
Numbness: Often, mild
Prickling sensation: Often, moderate

AUTONOMIC TESTING INTERPRETATION

- Anxiety with mild orthostatic intolerance.
- There was no evidence of autonomic failure or POTS.

COMMENT

This patient had a transient increase of heart rate during the tilt up (Figure 97.1), which was associated with her typical complaints including shortness of breath, dizziness, feeling pins and needles at feet and hands, bloated stomach, and feeling extremely anxious. Excessive (>120 BPM) tachycardia at the tilt onset with resolution of tachycardia later during the tilt is typical of an anxiety reaction and is not consistent with POTS.[1]

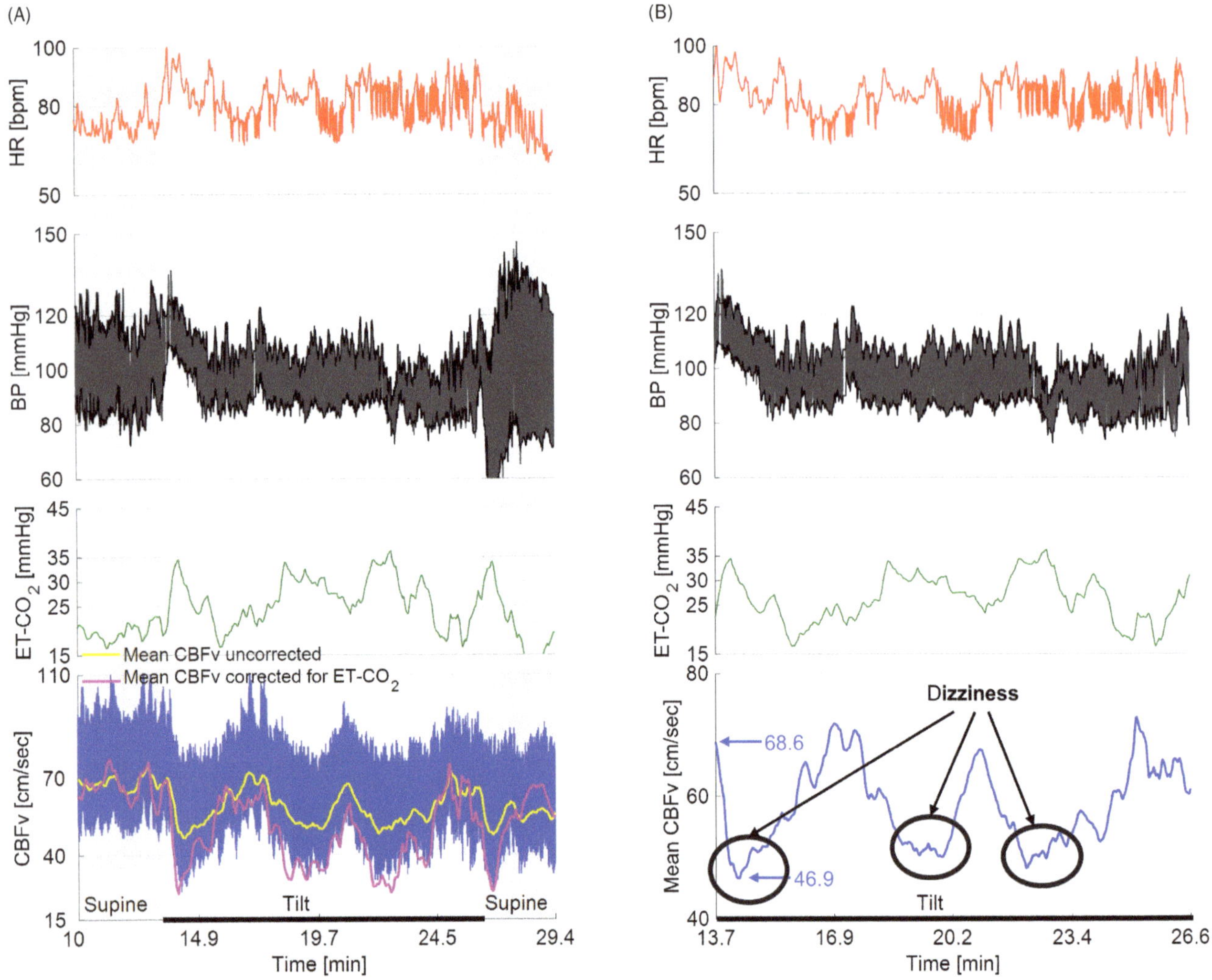

Figure 97.1 The tilt-up evoked a transient tachycardia and mild systolic blood pressure ([black vertical arrow] and cerebral blood flow velocity [CBFv, blue vertical arrow]) decline associated with several deep breaths and lower end tidal CO_2 (A, B). Both blood pressure and CBFv recovered within seconds. Almost immediately afterwards the patient experienced severe anxiety for about 1 minute (B). The anxiety was associated with tachycardia, mild hypocapnic hyperventilation, stable blood pressure and stable CBFv.

TREATMENT AND FOLLOW-UP

- Therapy for anxiety.

CAVEATS

- Anxiety can be associated with symptoms seen in orthostatic intolerance.[2]

REFERENCES

1. Novak P. Cerebral blood flow, heart rate, and blood pressure patterns during the tilt test in common orthostatic syndromes. *Neurosci J.* 2016;2016:6127340. doi:10.1155/2016/6127340.
2. Raj V, Opie M, Arnold AC. Cognitive and psychological issues in postural tachycardia syndrome. *Auton Neurosci Basic Clin.* March 2018. doi:10.1016/j.autneu.2018.03.004.

98.

CASE 93: ANXIETY MIMICKING POSTURAL TACHYCARDIA SYNDROME

Chief complaint: Dizziness.

Case presentation: A 51-year-old woman presents with dizziness and palpitations that started within 24–48 hours of receiving an influenza vaccine 5 years ago. Since then, she has had multiple episodes of dizziness, palpitations, and fluctuating paresthesia at distal legs. She had to reduce her office work to 3 days a week. She mostly has two types of episodic palpitations: (1) sudden onset and (2) a waxing and waning course. The episodes with a sudden onset are commonly triggered by eating and terminated by coughing or burping. An event monitor recorded the sudden onset periods of sinus tachycardia. The nature of the second type of episodes remains unclear. She was not able to tolerate multiple β-blockers and therefore she was referred for autonomic testing to evaluate palpitations.

Past medical history: Paroxysmal sinus tachycardia, borderline hypertension, migraine.

Current medication: Multivitamins.

Assessment plan: Functional autonomic tests and skin biopsy because of sensory complaints.

AUTONOMIC TESTING EVALUATION

See Table 98.1.

Heart rate: Supine heart rate was normal. Heart rate responses to deep breathing were normal. Heart rate increment during the tilt (44 BPM) was exaggerated.

Blood pressure:

Valsalva maneuver: Mean blood pressure failed to return to baseline at the end of Phase 2 by 17.3 mm Hg (i.e., 88% of baseline).

Tilt: Supine blood pressure was normal. Blood pressure was transiently elevated during the tilt.

Sudomotor evaluation: Electrochemical skin conductance was normal at hands and normal at feet.

Respiratory system: Respiratory frequency was normal in supine position and during the tilt. End tidal CO_2 was normal in supine position but was transiently reduced during the tilt.

Cerebral blood flow velocity (CBFv): CBFv in middle cerebral artery was normal in supine position but was transiently elevated during the tilt.

Skin biopsy (sensory-epidermal): Epidermal nerve fiber density was abnormal (reduced to 66.5% of normal limit) at proximal leg and abnormal (reduced to 45.2% of normal limit) at distal leg.

Skin biopsy (sweat glands): Sweat gland nerve fiber density was normal at proximal leg.

Patient-reported symptoms during testing: Anxiety and dizziness during the tilt.

Patient-reported symptoms for past 2 weeks:

Lightheadedness or dizziness: Occasionally
Dry eyes or mouth: Occasionally

TABLE 98.1 **RESULTS OF AUTONOMIC TESTING**

Blood pressure evaluation					
Test: Valsalva maneuver					
Pressure [mmHg]	Baseline	Phase 2			Phase 4
		Early	End		
Systolic	124	92	109		
Mean	96	76.7	83.0	n/a	
Diastolic	82	69	70	n/a	

Heart rate evaluation	
Test: Deep breathing	
Results	Norm*
10.2	≥9
Test: Valsalva ratio	
1.36	≥1.47
* adjusted for a gender and age	

(continued)

TABLE 98.1 CONTINUED

Test: Tilt test											
Position		HR [BPM]	Blood pressure [mmHg]		MCA Blood flow velocity [cm/s]				Respiratory frequency [breaths/min]	End tidal CO_2 [mmHg]
			Systolic	Diastolic	Systolic	Mean	Mean drop [%]	Diastolic		
Supine		87	122	79	78	55.3		44	7	38
Tilt [min]	1	125	142	78	91	57	-3.1	40	10	37
	2	100	130	86						
	3	95	126	84						
	4	94	117	83						
	5	92	116	83	88	58	-4.9	43	10	34
	6	101	125	85						
	7	105	123	88						
	8	104	134	88						
	9	102	129	93						
	10	131	139	91	92	65.3	-18.1	52	8	32
	15									
	20									
	30									
	40									

Sudomotor evaluation - functional

Test: Quantitative sudomotor axon reflex test (QSART)				
Location	Site (l/r)	Latency [min]	Volume [µl]	Norm [µl]*
Forearm				≥0.08
Prox. leg				≥0.14
Distal leg				≥0.07
Foot				≥0.05

* Normative data are adjusted for gender and age of patient.

Test: Electrochemical skin conductance (ESC)				
Location	Left [µS]	Right [µS]	Average [µS/k]	Norm [µS/kg]
Hand	68	71	1.38	≥1.03
Feet	88	87	1.74	≥1.14
Forehead				

For grading uses ESC [µS] adjusted for weight [µS/k].

TABLE 98.1 **CONTINUED**

Small fiber (sensory + sudomotor) evaluation - morphological					
Test: Skin biopsy					
Location	Site (l/r)	Nerve fibers			
		Epidermal*		Sweat glands	
		Density	Norm	Density	Norm
Proximal leg – thigh	Right	5.52	≥8.3	52.6	≥37.8
Distal leg - calf	Right	3.17	≥7.02		≥36.5
Foot	Right		≥3.11		≥34.8

*Normative data for distal leg are adjusted for gender and age of patient.

QASAT*											
Heart rate		**BP**		**CBFv**		**ET-CO2**		**Sudomotor**			**Total QASAT score**
S. bradycardia	0	Low supine	0	Low supine	0	Low supine	0	QSART			
S. tachycardia	0	High supine	0	High supine	0	High supine	0	ESC	0		
Increase tilt	2	OH	0	Tilt response	0	Tilt low	0				
Decrease tilt	0	OHTN	0	CA	0	Tilt high	0	**Skin biopsy**			8
Deep breathing	0	VM	2	CVR	0			Epidermal	3		
VR	1			VM	0			Sweat gland	0		
Total	3	Total	2	Total	0	Total	0				

*QASAT. See Novak. Quantitative Scale for Grading of Cardiovascular Autonomic Reflex Tests and Small Fibers from Skin Biopsies. *J Neurol Disord* 2015;3:2.

S, supine; Increase tilt, increased response to tilt; Decrease tilt, decreased response to tilt; BP, blood pressure; VM, Valsalva maneuver; CBFv, cerebral blood flow velocity; CA, cerebral autoregulation; MCA, middle cerebral artery; VR, Valsalva ratio; CVR, cerebral vasoreactivity.

Pale feet: Occasionally
Cold feet: Occasionally
Reduced sweating: Occasionally
Reduced sweating after exercise: Yes, minor annoyance
Increased sweating: Occasionally
Nausea: Yes, minor annoyance
Diarrhea: Yes, minor annoyance
Constipation: Occasionally
Urinary leaks: Occasionally
Current pain severity: 2
Aching pain: Continuous, severe
Allodynia: Occasionally, none
Burning pain: Occasionally, mild
Lancinating pain: Occasionally, mild
Numbness: Often, moderate
Prickling sensation: Continuous, mild

AUTONOMIC TESTING INTERPRETATION

- Anxiety.
- Mild adrenergic dysfunction of unclear clinical significance. There was no evidence of autonomic failure or postural tachycardia syndrome (POTS) that can explain this patient's orthostatic intolerance.
- Small fiber neuropathy affecting sensory fibers.

COMMENT

The tilt test provoked the patient's typical waxing and waning spell associated with palpitations and dizziness (Figure 98.1). The spells are associated with a characteristic anxiety pattern: transient elevation of heart rate, blood

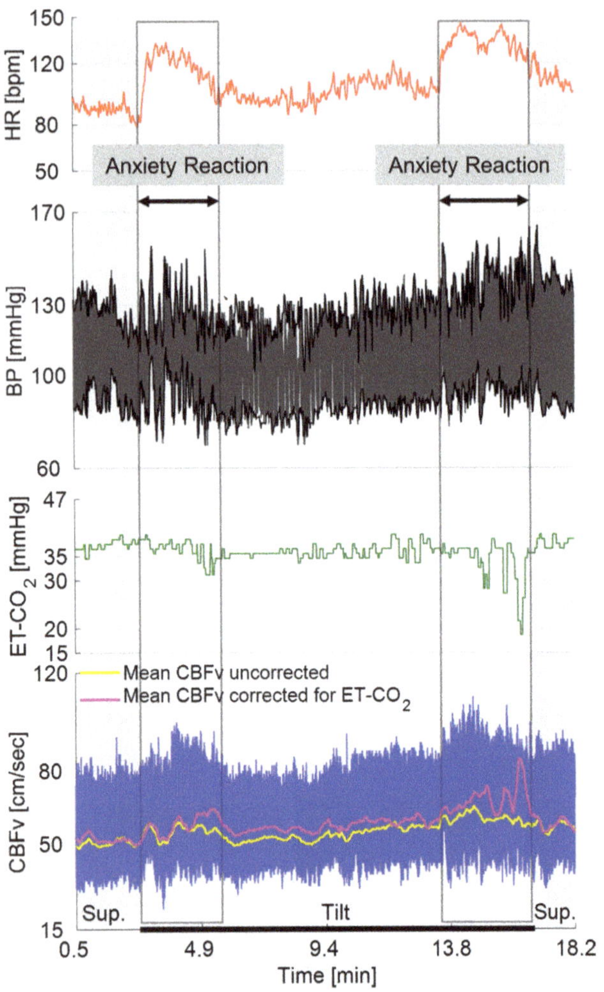

Figure 98.1 The tilt provoked transient elevation of heart rate, blood pressure, and cerebral blood flow velocity twice, which is consistent with anxiety response. Electrocardiogram showed sinus rhythm throughout the tilt test.

pressure, and CBFv.[1] The dizziness may result from sympathetic adrenergic overstimulation driven by release of catecholamines that underlie the spells. An alternative explanation of dizziness is the effect of hyperemia. The brain is sensitive to even miniscule changes in blood flow and therefore elevated CBFv during anxiety may be perceived as dizziness.

Small fiber neuropathy may underlie fluctuating paresthesia in the distal legs.[2]

TREATMENT AND FOLLOW-UP

- Anxiety treatment.
- Clinical workup for small fiber neuropathy.

CAVEATS

- Anxiety reaction has a distinct profile in the tilt and should be differentiated from POTS or inappropriate sinus tachycardia (IST).

REFERENCES

1. Novak P. Cerebral blood flow, heart rate, and blood pressure patterns during the tilt test in common orthostatic syndromes. *Neurosci J.* 2016;2016:6127340. doi:10.1155/2016/6127340.
2. de Greef BTA, Hoeijmakers JGJ, Gorissen-Brouwers CML, Geerts M, Faber CG, Merkies ISJ. Associated conditions in small fiber neuropathy—a large cohort study and review of the literature. *Eur J Neurol.* 2018;25(2):348–355. doi:10.1111/ene.13508.

99.

CASE 94: ANXIETY AND POSTURAL TACHYCARDIA SYNDROME

Chief complaint: Dizziness in the context of anxiety.

Case presentation: A 30-year-old woman presented with severe fluctuating dizziness. She had a concussion when playing basketball 16 years ago, which resulted in dizziness and anxiety treated with escitalopram. Anxiety markedly worsened with she became pregnant 4 years ago. About 3 years ago, she noted worsening of dizziness, typically exacerbated by bending forward or stretching the body. She often became disoriented when standing or when walking. She developed chronic fatigue and has to spend most of her time in bed. She cannot focus on simple tasks (e.g., running the household). She has also experienced pain in her legs, brain fog, floaters, and blurry vision. Thorough evaluations (neurology, cardiology, rheumatology, endocrinology) were positive only for mild vitamin B_{12} deficiency (B_{12} corrected at this time) and low platelets (123 K/μL, normal range 142–424 K/μL) without anemia in addition to anxiety disorder. MRI of the brain was normal, electroencephalogram was normal. She was referred for evaluation of dysautonomia.

Past medical history: Concussion, anxiety, vitamin B_{12} deficiency.

Current medication: Escitalopram.

Assessment plan: Functional autonomic tests and skin biopsy.

AUTONOMIC TESTING EVALUATION

See Table 99.1.

Heart rate: Supine heart rate was normal. There was supine tachycardia. Heart rate increment during the tilt (52 BPM) was exaggerated and exceeded 150 BPM.

Blood pressure:

Valsalva maneuver: Mean blood pressure failed to return to baseline at the end of Phase 2 by 22.2 mm Hg (i.e., 73.4% of baseline).

Tilt: Supine blood pressure was normal. Tilt showed two presyncopal reactions; it was terminated at minute 5 due to severe anxiety.

Sudomotor evaluation: Electrochemical skin conductance was normal at hands and normal at feet.

Respiratory system: Respiratory frequency was normal in supine position and during the tilt. End tidal CO_2 was normal in supine position but was severely reduced during the tilt.

Cerebral blood flow velocity (CBFv): CBFv in middle cerebral artery was normal in supine position but was severely reduced during the tilt.

Skin biopsy (sensory-epidermal): Epidermal nerve fiber density was abnormal (reduced to 38% of normal limit) at proximal leg and abnormal (reduced to 34.4% of normal limit) at distal leg.

TABLE 99.1 RESULTS OF AUTONOMIC TESTING

Blood pressure evaluation					
Test: Valsalva maneuver					
Pressure [mmHg]	Baseline	Phase 2			Phase 4
		Early	End		
Systolic	109	65.3	65.3		
Mean	83.6	61.4	61.4	n/a	
Diastolic	70.9	59.4	59.4	n/a	

Heart rate evaluation	
Test: Deep breathing	
Results	Norm*
9.5	≥12
Test: Valsalva ratio	
1.56	≥1.5
* adjusted for a gender and age	

(continued)

TABLE 99.1 **CONTINUED**

Test: Tilt test											
Position		HR [BPM]	Blood pressure [mmHg]		MCA Blood flow velocity [cm/s]				Respiratory frequency [breaths/min]	End tidal CO_2 [mmHg]
			Systolic	Diastolic	Systolic	Mean	Mean drop [%]	Diastolic		
Supine		114	125	69	118	76		55	13	37
Tilt [min]	1	150	119	77	103	62.3	18	42	12	28
	2	147	87	57						
	3	138	101	69						
	4	166	86	64						
	5	145	64	54	102	44.1	42	15.2	18	22
	6									
	7									
	8									
	9									
	10									
	15									
	20									
	30									
	40									

Sudomotor evaluation - functional

Test: Quantitative sudomotor axon reflex test (QSART)				
Location	Site (l/r)	Latency [min]	Volume [µl]	Norm [µl]*
Forearm				≥0.08
Prox. leg				≥0.14
Distal leg				≥0.15
Foot				≥0.07

* Normative data are adjusted for gender and age of patient.

Test: Electrochemical skin conductance (ESC)				
Location	Left [µS]	Right [µS]	Average [µS/k]	Norm [µS/kg]
Hand	81	84	1.42	≥1.03
Feet	94	93	1.61	≥1.14
Forehead				

For grading uses ESC [µS] adjusted for weight [µS/k].

Small fiber (sensory + sudomotor) evaluation - morphological					
Test: Skin biopsy					
Location	Site (l/r)	Nerve fibers			
		Epidermal*		Sweat glands	
		Density	Norm	Density	Norm
Proximal leg – thigh	Right	3.15	≥8.3	48.3	≥37.8
Distal leg – calf	Right	2.99	≥8.7	41.7	≥36.5
Foot	Right		≥3.11		≥34.8

*Normative data for distal leg are adjusted for gender and age of patient.

QASAT*											
Heart rate		BP		CBFv		ET-CO2		Sudomotor			Total QASAT score
S. bradycardia	0	Low supine	0	Low supine	0	Low supine	0	QSART			
S. tachycardia	0	High supine	0	High supine	0	High supine	0	ESC	0		
Increase tilt	5	OH	0	Tilt response	7	Tilt low	5				
Decrease tilt	0	OHTN	0	CA	0	Tilt high	0	**Skin biopsy**			25
Deep breathing	1	VM	2	CVR	0			Epidermal	4		
VR				VM	0			Sweat gland	0		
Total	7	Total	2	Total	7	Total	5				

*QASAT. See Novak. Quantitative Scale for Grading of Cardiovascular Autonomic Reflex Tests and Small Fibers from Skin Biopsies. *J Neurol Disord* 2015;3:2. QASAT requites at least 10 minutes of the tilt to grade orthostatic responses. In this case (the duration of the tilt was 5 minutes) the missing 5 minutes values were considered as normal.

S, supine; Increase tilt, increased response to tilt; Decrease tilt, decreased response to tilt; BP, blood pressure; VM, Valsalva maneuver; CBFv, cerebral blood flow velocity; CA, cerebral autoregulation; MCA, middle cerebral artery; VR, Valsalva ratio; CVR, cerebral vasoreactivity.

Skin biopsy (sweat glands): Sweat gland nerve fiber density was normal at proximal leg and normal at distal leg.

Patient-reported symptoms during testing: Dizziness during the tilt.

Patient-reported symptoms for past 2 weeks:

Lightheadedness or dizziness: Often
Dry eyes or mouth: Occasionally
Pale feet: Occasionally
Cold feet: Occasionally
Reduced sweating: None
Reduced sweating after exercise: None
Increased sweating: None
Nausea: None
Diarrhea: None
Constipation: None
Urinary leaks: None
Current pain severity: 0
Aching pain: Occasionally, mild
Allodynia: None
Burning pain: Occasionally, mild
Lancinating pain: Occasionally, mild
Numbness: Occasionally, mild
Prickling sensation: Occasionally, mild

AUTONOMIC TESTING INTERPRETATION

- Severe anxiety.
- Postural tachycardia syndrome (POTS).
- Small fiber neuropathy.

COMMENT

The tilt test showed severe anxiety and severe POTS associated with reduced CBFv (Figure 99.1), likely resulting in cerebral hypoperfusion.[1] In addition, the POTS pattern was combined with presyncopal reactions, potentially amplifying anxiety. In summary, both main syndromes—anxiety and dysautonomia (POTS + presyncope)—are likely contributing to the patient's disability and need to be addressed.

The testing also showed small fiber neuropathy that can be responsible for the distal leg pain. This patient has a history of vitamin B_{12} deficiency that can be associated with small fiber neuropathy.[2] Extensive evaluations for secondary causes of neuropathy, including evaluations for systemic autoimmunity, were unrevealing. The patient's current levels of B_{12} are normal, and sensory symptoms seem to be slowly improving.

TREATMENT AND FOLLOW-UP

- Volume expansion through high fluid and high salt intake, physical therapy with focus on reconditioning.
- Psychiatry therapy for anxiety.
- Evaluation by traumatic brain injury clinic.

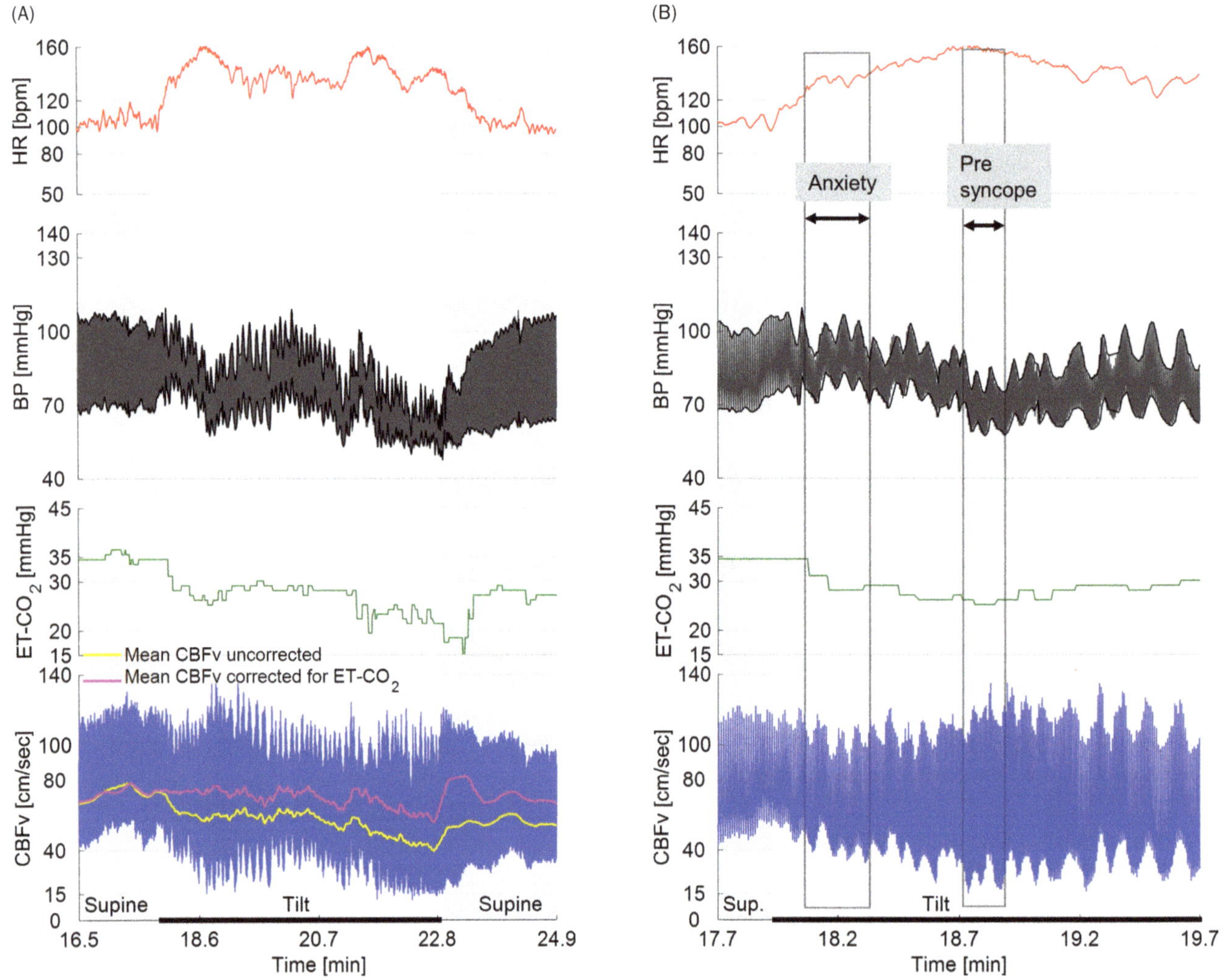

Figure 99.1 The tilt provoked anxiety reaction at the onset of the tilt and two presyncopal reactions. There was also severe supine and orthostatic tachycardia. Heart rate responses to tilt were exaggerated >150 BPM (A–C). Blood pressure declined with presyncope (B, C). Cerebral blood flow velocity declined due to hypocapnia. The patient became dizzy, confused, and anxious after minute 3 of the tilt. She requested the tilt to be terminated at minute 5; she felt like she was "going to die."

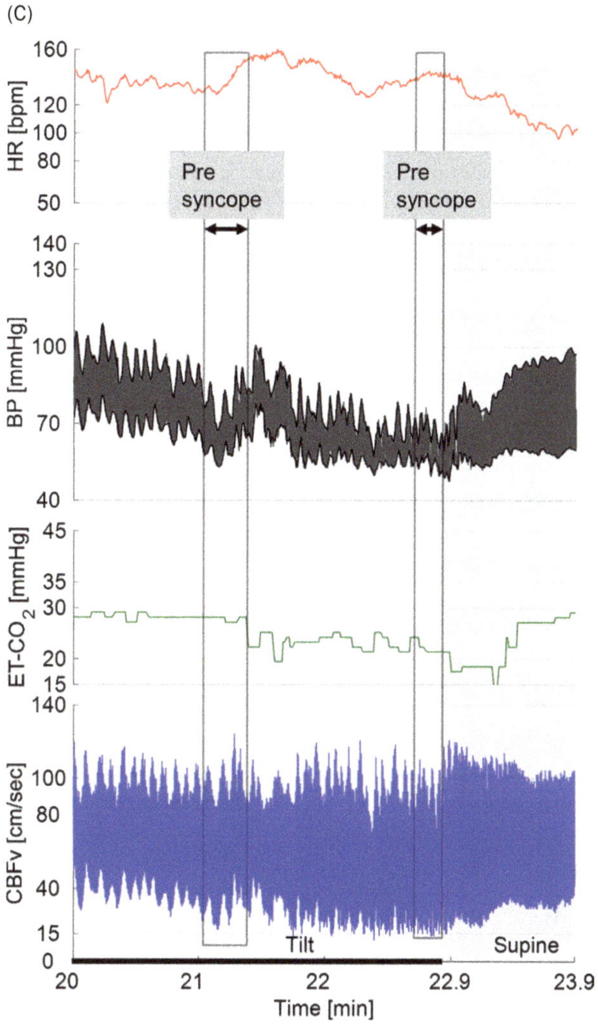

Figure 99.1 Continued

CAVEATS

- Severe anxiety and severe POTS may coexist, and both require adequate therapy.

REFERENCES

1. Novak P. Cerebral blood flow, heart rate, and blood pressure patterns during the tilt test in common orthostatic syndromes. *Neurosci J.* 2016;2016:6127340. doi:10.1155/2016/6127340.
2. Güneş HN, Bekircan-Kurt CE, Tan E, Erdem-Özdamar S. The histopathological evaluation of small fiber neuropathy in patients with vitamin B12 deficiency. *Acta Neurol Belg.* October 2017. doi:10.1007/s13760-017-0847-y.

100.

CASE 95: FLUCTUATING PSYCHOGENIC DIZZINESS

Chief complaint: Dizziness.

Case presentation: A 53-year-old woman presents with unexplained, usually orthostatic, dizziness for 3 years. Dizziness occurs in "waves" lasting from seconds to minutes and is usually associated with perception of unusual colors. She was treated for suspected epilepsy. However, the seizure medication has no effect on the dizziness and visual disturbances. She was referred for evaluation of orthostatic intolerance.

Past medical history: Epilepsy, insomnia.

Current medication: Lamotrigine, gabapentin, meclizine, multivitamins, melatonin, ibuprofen.

Assessment plan: Functional autonomic tests.

AUTONOMIC TESTING EVALUATION

See Table 100.1.

Heart rate: Supine heart rate was normal. Heart rate responses to deep breathing were reduced to 88.9% of normal value. Heart rate increment during the tilt (16 BPM) was normal.

Blood pressure:

Valsalva maneuver: Mean blood pressure failed to return to baseline at the end of Phase 2 by 32.3 mm Hg (i.e., 65.6% of baseline).

Tilt: Supine blood pressure was normal. Blood pressure responses to tilt were normal.

Sudomotor evaluation: Electrochemical skin conductance was abnormal (reduced to 76.8% of normal limit) at hands and normal at feet.

Respiratory system: Respiratory frequency and end tidal CO_2 were normal in supine position and during the tilt.

Cerebral blood flow velocity (CBFv): CBFv in middle cerebral artery was normal in supine position and was stable during the tilt.

Skin biopsy (sensory-epidermal): N/A

Skin biopsy (sweat glands): N/A

Patient-reported symptoms during testing: Waves of dizziness and seeing unusual colors during the tilt.

Patient-reported symptoms for past 2 weeks:

Lightheadedness or dizziness: Occasionally
Dry eyes or mouth: Often
Pale feet: Occasionally
Cold feet: Occasionally
Reduced sweating: None
Reduced sweating after exercise: None
Increased sweating: None
Nausea: Occasionally
Diarrhea: Yes, minor annoyance
Constipation: Often
Urinary leaks: None
Current pain severity: 0
Aching pain: Often, moderate
Allodynia: None
Burning pain: Often, severe

TABLE 100.1 RESULTS OF AUTONOMIC TESTING

Blood pressure evaluation

Test: Valsalva maneuver

Pressure [mmHg]	Baseline	Phase 2			Phase 4
		Early	End		
Systolic	136	69	71		
Mean	94	59.7	61.7	n/a	
Diastolic	73	55	57	n/a	

Heart rate evaluation

Test: Deep breathing	
Results	Norm*
8	≥9
Test: Valsalva ratio	
1.88	≥1.47

* adjusted for a gender and age

TABLE 100.1 **CONTINUED**

Test: Tilt test											
Position		HR [BPM]	Blood pressure [mmHg]		MCA Blood flow velocity [cm/s]				Respiratory frequency [breaths/min]	End tidal CO_2 [mmHg]
			Systolic	Diastolic	Systolic	Mean	Mean drop [%]	Diastolic		
Supine		73	126	86	97	63		46	11	42
Tilt [min]	1	83	113	78	86	60	4.8	47	8	41
	2	82	115	81						
	3	89	123	87						
	4	88	120	84						
	5	85	119	84	84	58	7.9	45	10	42
	6	84	117	78						
	7	87	119	83						
	8	85	114	79						
	9	86	112	78						
	10	86	110	76	82	56.7	10	44	14	41
	15									
	20									
	30									
	40									

Sudomotor evaluation - functional

Test: Quantitative sudomotor axon reflex test (QSART)				
Location	Site (l/r)	Latency [min]	Volume [μl]	Norm [μl]*
Forearm				≥0.08
Prox. leg				≥0.14
Distal leg				≥0.07
Foot				≥0.05

* Normative data are adjusted for gender and age of patient.

Test: Electrochemical skin conductance (ESC)				
Location	Left [μS]	Right [μS]	Average [μS/k]	Norm [μS/kg]
Hand	54	51	0.79	≥1.03
Feet	75	75	1.14	≥1.14
Forehead				

For grading uses ESC [μS] adjusted for weight [μS/k].

TABLE 100.1 CONTINUED

Small fiber (sensory + sudomotor) evaluation - morphological					
Test: Skin biopsy					
Location	Site (l/r)	Nerve fibers			
		Epidermal*		Sweat glands	
		Density	Norm	Density	Norm
Proximal leg – thigh	Right		≥8.3		≥37.8
Distal leg - calf	Right		≥6.86		≥36.5
Foot	Right		≥3.11		≥34.8

*Normative data for distal leg are adjusted for gender and age of patient.

QASAT*											
Heart rate		**BP**		**CBFv**		**ET-CO2**		**Sudomotor**			**Total QASAT score**
S. bradycardia	0	Low supine	0	Low supine	0	Low supine	0	QSART			
S. tachycardia	0	High supine	0	High supine	0	High supine	0	ESC	1		
Increase tilt	0	OH	0	Tilt response	0	Tilt low	0				
Decrease tilt	0	OHTN	0	CA	0	Tilt high	0	**Skin biopsy**			4
Deep breathing	1	VM	2	CVR	0			Epidermal			
VR	0			VM	0			Sweat gland			
Total	1	Total	2	Total	0	Total	0				

*QASAT. See Novak. Quantitative Scale for Grading of Cardiovascular Autonomic Reflex Tests and Small Fibers from Skin Biopsies. *J Neurol Disord* 2015;3:2.

S, supine; Increase tilt, increased response to tilt; Decrease tilt, decreased response to tilt; BP, blood pressure; VM, Valsalva maneuver; CBFv, cerebral blood flow velocity; CA, cerebral autoregulation; MCA, middle cerebral artery; VR, Valsalva ratio; CVR, cerebral vasoreactivity.

Lancinating pain: Occasionally, severe
Numbness: Continuous, moderate
Prickling sensation: Often, moderate

AUTONOMIC TESTING INTERPRETATION

- Generalized, but mild autonomic dysfunction (QASAT score total = 4). Orthostatic hypotension, a marker of more widespread autonomic adrenergic failure, was absent.
- Orthostatic CBFv was stable.

COMMENT

The tilt test reproduced the patient's symptoms including seeing of unusual colors (Figure 100.1). Although mild generalized dysautonomia has been detected in this study, the dysautonomia is unlikely responsible for the patient's symptoms since, during the occurrence of symptoms during the tilt, all vitals were stable. The fluctuating dizziness with color perception abnormalities is likely of psychogenic origin.

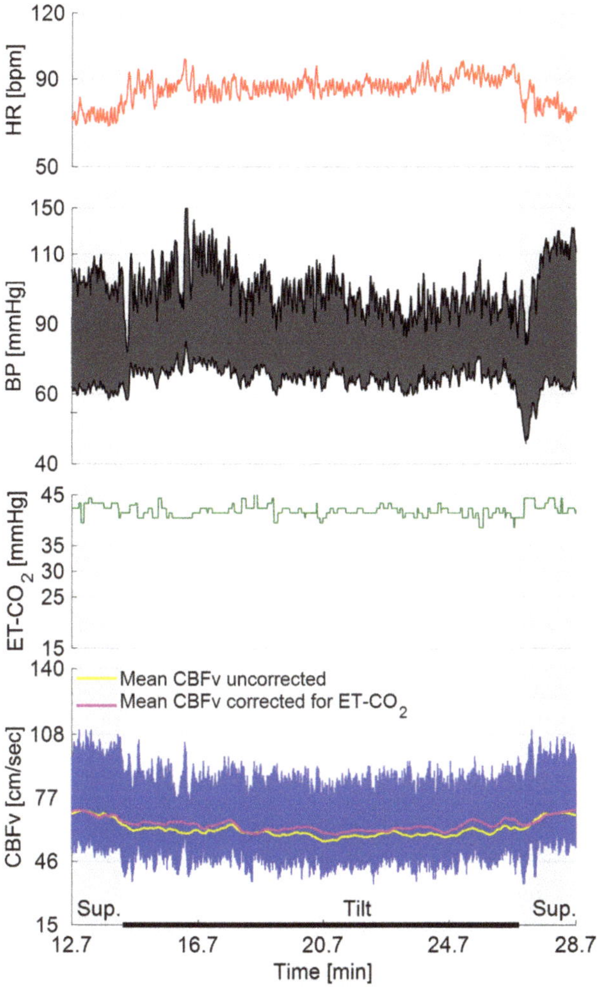

Figure 100.1 The tilt test showed normal heart rate, blood pressure, end tidal CO_2, and cerebral blood flow velocity. Patient experienced her typical symptoms during the tilt, including fluctuating dizziness and seeing unusual colors (>20 times), with each spell having a duration of seconds. Consciousness was unchanged. Patient denied headaches.

TREATMENT AND FOLLOW-UP

- Consider repeating autonomic testing in 1 year or later since generalized dysautonomia may be an early sign of more widespread neurodegenerative disorders such as synucleinopathy.[1]

CAVEATS

- The presence of mild dysautonomia does not necessary lead to orthostatic symptoms, particularly if the orthostatic hypotension is absent and orthostatic CBFv is stable.

REFERENCE

1. Iodice V, Sandroni P. Autonomic neuropathies. *Contin Minneap Minn.* 2014;20(5 Peripheral Nervous System Disorders):1373–1397. doi:10.1212/01.CON.0000455875.76179.b1.

CASE 96: FUNCTIONAL NEUROLOGIC DISORDER AND POSTURAL TACHYCARDIA SYNDROME

Chief complaint: Spells of altered consciousness.

Case presentation: A 22-year-old woman presented with multiple symptoms. Over the past several years, she has experienced episodic spells where she cannot move or talk without losing consciousness. The spells are associated with an electrical feeling throughout her body and are often been triggered by stress, fatigue, or her menstrual periods. The frequency of the spells varies from several per month to several per day. A behavioral neurologist diagnosed a functional neurological disorder, and the patient was doing well on amantadine. She also has a history of postural dizziness and was diagnosed postural tachycardia syndrome (POTS) on formal autonomic testing. She was doing well on droxidopa. She also has a history of chronic myofascial pain, joint pain, instability, and back and neck pain. She was diagnosed with hypermobile Ehlers-Danlos syndrome 2 years ago. The patient was referred for repeat autonomic testing because of an increased frequency of the episodic spells.

Past medical history: Anxiety, functional neurologic disorder, obstructive sleep apnea, POTS, Ehlers-Danlos syndrome hypermobility type.

Current medication: Fluoxetine, amantadine, droxidopa.

Assessment plan: Functional autonomic tests and skin biopsy.

AUTONOMIC TESTING EVALUATION

See Table 101.1.

Heart rate: Supine heart rate was normal. Heart rate responses to deep breathing were reduced to 50% of normal value. Heart rate increment during the tilt (44 BPM) was exaggerated.

Blood pressure:

Valsalva maneuver: Mean blood pressure failed to return to baseline at the end of Phase 2 by 7.3 mm Hg (i.e., 91.4% of baseline).

Tilt: Supine blood pressure was normal. Blood pressure responses to tilt were normal.

Sudomotor evaluation: Electrochemical skin conductance was abnormal (reduced to 87.9% of normal limit) at hands and abnormal (reduced to 85.5% of normal limit) at feet.

Respiratory system: Respiratory frequency was normal in supine position and during the tilt. End tidal CO_2 was normal in supine position but was mildly reduced during the tilt.

Cerebral blood flow velocity (CBFv): CBFv in middle cerebral artery was normal in supine position but was severely reduced during the tilt.

TABLE 101.1 RESULTS OF AUTONOMIC TESTING

Blood pressure evaluation					
Test: Valsalva maneuver					
Pressure [mmHg]	Baseline	Phase 2			Phase 4
		Early	End		
Systolic	116	93	98		
Mean	85.3	71.7	78	n/a	
Diastolic	70	61	68	n/a	

Heart rate evaluation	
Test: Deep breathing	
Results	Norm*
7	≥14
Test: Valsalva ratio	
1.52	≥1.46
* adjusted for a gender and age	

TABLE 101.1 **CONTINUED**

Test: Tilt test										
Position		HR [BPM]	Blood pressure [mmHg]		MCA Blood flow velocity [cm/s]				Respiratory frequency [breaths/min]	End tidal CO_2 [mmHg]
			Systolic	Diastolic	Systolic	Mean	Mean drop [%]	Diastolic		
Supine		72	119	80	89	60.3		46	20	35
Tilt [min]	1	103	120	84	73	51.7	14.3	41	10	31
	2	108	122	91						
	3	104	122	86						
	4	104	115	88						
	5	104	115	88	67	45	25.4	34	15	30
	6	104	115	88						
	7	116	134	83						
	8	121	120	78						
	9	108	114	80						
	10	103	132	82	71	47	22.1	35	14	34
	15									
	20									
	30									
	40									

Sudomotor evaluation - functional

Test: Quantitative sudomotor axon reflex test (QSART)				
Location	Site (l/r)	Latency [min]	Volume [μl]	Norm [μl]*
Forearm				≥0.08
Prox. leg				≥0.14
Distal leg				≥0.24
Foot				≥0.09

* Normative data are adjusted for gender and age of patient.

Test: Electrochemical skin conductance (ESC)				
Location	Left [μS]	Right [μS]	Average [μS/k]	Norm [μS/kg]
Hand	81	76	0.91	≥1.03
Feet	85	84	0.97	≥1.14
Forehead				

For grading uses ESC [μS] adjusted for weight [μS/k].

(continued)

TABLE 101.1 CONTINUED

Small fiber (sensory + sudomotor) evaluation - morphological					
Test: Skin biopsy					
Location	Site (l/r)	Nerve fibers			
		Epidermal*		Sweat glands	
		Density	Norm	Density	Norm
Proximal leg – thigh	Right	11.92	≥8.3		≥37.8
Distal leg - calf	Right	10.15	≥9.34	37.4	≥36.5
Foot	Right		≥3.11		≥34.8

*Normative data for distal leg are adjusted for gender and age of patient.

QASAT*										
Heart rate		**BP**		**CBFv**		**ET-CO2**		**Sudomotor**		**Total QASAT score**
S. bradycardia	0	Low supine	0	Low supine	0	Low supine	0	QSART		
S. tachycardia	0	High supine	0	High supine	0	High supine	0	ESC	1	
Increase tilt	1	OH	0	Tilt response	4	Tilt low	2			
Decrease tilt	0	OHTN	0	CA	0	Tilt high	0	**Skin biopsy**		10
Deep breathing	1	VM	1	CVR	0			Epidermal	0	
VR	0			VM	0			Sweat gland	0	
Total	2	Total	1	Total	4	Total	2			

*QASAT. See Novak. Quantitative Scale for Grading of Cardiovascular Autonomic Reflex Tests and Small Fibers from Skin Biopsies. *J Neurol Disord* 2015;3:2.

S, supine; Increase tilt, increased response to tilt; Decrease tilt, decreased response to tilt; BP, blood pressure; VM, Valsalva maneuver; CBFv, cerebral blood flow velocity; CA, cerebral autoregulation; MCA, middle cerebral artery; VR, Valsalva ratio; CVR, cerebral vasoreactivity.

Skin biopsy (sensory-epidermal): Epidermal nerve fiber density was normal at proximal leg and normal at distal leg.

Skin biopsy (sweat glands): Sweat gland nerve fiber density was normal at distal leg.

Patient-reported symptoms during testing: Dizziness, shortness of breath during the tilt.

Patient-reported symptoms for past 2 weeks:

Lightheadedness or dizziness: Often
Dry eyes or mouth: Occasionally
Pale feet: Yes, minor annoyance
Cold feet: Occasionally
Reduced sweating: Occasionally
Reduced sweating after exercise: Occasionally
Increased sweating: Occasionally
Nausea: Occasionally
Diarrhea: Occasionally
Constipation: Occasionally
Urinary leaks: Occasionally
Current pain severity: 2
Aching pain: Continuous, severe
Allodynia: Occasionally, moderate
Burning pain: Occasionally, mild
Lancinating pain: Often, severe
Numbness: Often, severe
Prickling sensation: Often, none

AUTONOMIC TESTING INTERPRETATION

- POTS, mild, neuropathic form.
- Psychogenic unresponsiveness.

COMMENT

This patient has a history of a typical functional neurologic disorder, and the tilt reproduced the spell of altered responsiveness. However, the CBFv was significantly reduced (25% at the first minute of tilt, normal <11%) and that reduction may induce signs of cerebral hypoperfusion (Figure 101.1). Nevertheless, the severity of the spells was out of proportion to CBFv changes. The decline in CBFv

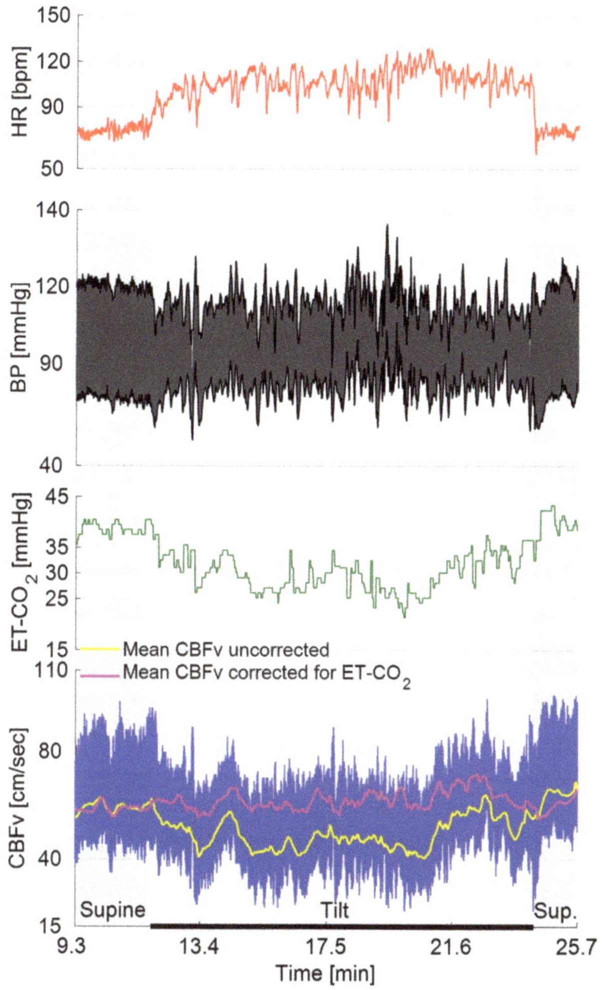

Figure 101.1 Heart rate showed exaggerated increment and postural tachycardia during the tilt. Cerebral blood flow velocity (CBFv) declined due to hyperventilation. The patient became dizzy and complained of shortness of breath. The tilt reproduced the patient's typical spell. At minute 4 of the tilt, she became confused, weaker, and could not talk but was able to communicate by gestures.

of similar magnitude (~20%) is seen in POTS or orthostatic cerebral hypoperfusion syndrome (OCHOS) and typically results in signs of orthostatic intolerance, including dizziness fatigue and shortness of breath but not in overt encephalopathy.[1]

TREATMENT AND FOLLOW-UP

- Volume expansion through high fluid and high salt intake.
- Increased dose of droxidopa.
- Behavioral therapy.

CAVEATS

- Functional neurological disorder and POTS may coexist.[2]

REFERENCES

1. Novak P. Orthostatic cerebral hypoperfusion syndrome. *Front Aging Neurosci*. 2016;8:22. doi:10.3389/fnagi.2016.00022.
2. Raj V, Opie M, Arnold AC. Cognitive and psychological issues in postural tachycardia syndrome. *Auton Neurosci Basic Clin*. March 2018. doi:10.1016/j.autneu.2018.03.004.

102.

CASE 97: UNUSUAL POSTURAL SPELLS

Chief complaint: Dizziness.

Case presentation: A 27-year-old woman presents with intermittent postural dizziness, fatigue, and spells associated with altered consciousness. During her spells, she becomes confused, "cannot see," and her whole body shakes. She rarely loses consciousness, but she had a number of spell-associated falls. She also complains of whole-body aches. Imaging and repeated electroencephalograms (EEGs) were unrevealing. She does not have a definite diagnosis. Differential diagnosis includes psychogenic movement disorder, nonepileptogenic seizures, and/or autonomic dysfunction. She was referred for evaluation of orthostatic intolerance.

Past medical history: Lyme disease, vitamin B_{12} deficiency, obstructive sleep apnea, myoclonus.

Current medication: Continuous positive airway pressure (CPAP), intravenous immune globulins.

Assessment plan: Functional autonomic tests and skin biopsy.

AUTONOMIC TESTING EVALUATION

See Table 102.1.

Heart rate: Supine heart rate was normal. Heart rate responses to deep breathing were reduced to 64.3% of normal value. Heart rate increment during the tilt (46 BPM) was exaggerated and exceeded 120 BPM.

Blood pressure:

Valsalva maneuver: Mean blood pressure failed to return to baseline at the end of Phase 2 by 0.3 mm Hg (i.e., 99.7% of baseline).

Tilt: Supine blood pressure was normal. Patient was tilted for 5 minutes; the tilt was aborted when the patient experienced syncope.

Sudomotor evaluation: Electrochemical skin conductance was abnormal (reduced to 83.3% of normal limit) at hands and abnormal (reduced to 79.6% of normal limit) at feet.

Respiratory system: Respiratory frequency was normal in supine position and during the tilt. End tidal CO_2 was reduced in supine position and was further severely reduced during the tilt.

Cerebral blood flow velocity (CBFv): CBFv in middle cerebral artery was normal in supine position but was severely reduced during the tilt.

Skin biopsy (sensory-epidermal): Epidermal nerve fiber density was normal at proximal leg and normal at distal leg.

Skin biopsy (sweat glands): Sweat gland nerve fiber density was normal at proximal leg and normal at distal leg.

Patient-reported symptoms during testing: "Black out" during the tilt.

Patient-reported symptoms for past 2 weeks:

Lightheadedness or dizziness: Occasionally
Dry eyes or mouth: Occasionally

TABLE 102.1 RESULTS OF AUTONOMIC TESTING

Blood pressure evaluation					
Test: Valsalva maneuver					
Pressure [mmHg]	Baseline	Phase 2			Phase 4
		Early	End		
Systolic	142	108	133		
Mean	109.3	84.7	109	n/a	
Diastolic	93	73	97	n/a	

Heart rate evaluation	
Test: Deep breathing	
Results	Norm*
9	≥14
Test: Valsalva ratio	
1.4	≥1.46
* adjusted for a gender and age	

TABLE 102.1 **CONTINUED**

Test: Tilt test										
Position		HR [BPM]	Blood pressure [mmHg]		MCA Blood flow velocity [cm/s]				Respiratory frequency [breaths/min]	End tidal CO_2 [mmHg]
			Systolic	Diastolic	Systolic	Mean	Mean drop [%]	Diastolic		
Supine		75	105	72	98	62.7		45	13	34
Tilt [min]	1	111	122	79	97	60.3	3.8	42	10	19
	2	120	109	72						
	3	116	101	68						
	4	121	107	74						
	5	121	107	74	75	39	37.8	21	19	15
	6									
	7									
	8									
	9									
	10									
	15									
	20									
	30									
	40									

Sudomotor evaluation - functional

Test: Quantitative sudomotor axon reflex test (QSART)				
Location	Site (l/r)	Latency [min]	Volume [µl]	Norm [µl]*
Forearm				≥0.08
Prox. leg				≥0.14
Distal leg				≥0.24
Foot				≥0.09

* Normative data are adjusted for gender and age of patient.

Test: Electrochemical skin conductance (ESC)				
Location	Left [µS]	Right [µS]	Average [µS/k]	Norm [µS/kg]
Hand	88	89	0.86	≥1.03
Feet	94	93	0.91	≥1.14
Forehead				

For grading uses ESC [µS] adjusted for weight [µS/k].

(continued)

TABLE 102.1 **CONTINUED**

Small fiber (sensory + sudomotor) evaluation - morphological					
Test: Skin biopsy					
Location	Site (l/r)	Nerve fibers			
		Epidermal*		Sweat glands	
		Density	Norm	Density	Norm
Proximal leg – thigh	Right	14.51	≥8.3	81.3	≥37.8
Distal leg - calf	Right	9.07	≥8.94	60.6	≥36.5
Foot	Right		≥3.11		≥34.8

*Normative data for distal leg are adjusted for gender and age of patient.

Heart rate		BP		CBFv		ET-CO2		Sudomotor		Total QASAT score
S. bradycardia	0	Low supine	0	Low supine	0	Low supine	1	QSART		
S. tachycardia	0	High supine	0	High supine	0	High supine	0	ESC	1	
Increase tilt		OH		Tilt response		Tilt low				
Decrease tilt		OHTN		CA	0	Tilt high		**Skin biopsy**		25
Deep breathing	1	VM	1	CVR	0			Epidermal	0	
VR	1			VM	0			Sweat gland	0	
Total	2	Total	1	Total	0	Total	1			

QASAT*

*QASAT. See Novak. Quantitative Scale for Grading of Cardiovascular Autonomic Reflex Tests and Small Fibers from Skin Biopsies. *J Neurol Disord* 2015;3:2. Orthostatic (tilt) responses were not graded since QASAT requires the duration of the tilt at least 10 minutes.

S, supine; Increase tilt, increased response to tilt; Decrease tilt, decreased response to tilt; BP, blood pressure; VM, Valsalva maneuver; CBFv, cerebral blood flow velocity; CA, cerebral autoregulation; MCA, middle cerebral artery; VR, Valsalva ratio; CVR, cerebral vasoreactivity.

Pale feet: Occasionally
Cold feet: Often
Reduced sweating: None
Reduced sweating after exercise: None
Increased sweating: None
Nausea: Occasionally
Diarrhea: None
Constipation: None
Urinary leaks: Occasionally
Current pain severity: 5
Aching pain: Occasionally, mild
Allodynia: None
Burning pain: None
Lancinating pain: Occasionally, severe
Numbness: Occasionally, moderate
Prickling sensation: Often, moderate

AUTONOMIC TESTING INTERPRETATION

- Postural tachycardia syndrome (POTS).
- Presyncope.
- Psychogenic pseudosyncope.
- Syncope with ischemic convulsions.
- Cerebral autoregulatory failure.

COMMENT

There was a strong suspicion of a psychogenic cause for this patient's problems. Although psychogenic syncope also called psychogenic pseudosyncope, was indeed observed during the tilt, there were several other abnormalities.

At the beginning of the tilt, when patient became agitated, there was a widening in the CBFv signal indicating cerebral vasodilation (Figure 102.1).[1] The vasodilation pattern is usually seen when the blood pressure drops as, for example, in syncope. However, blood pressure in this patient did not decline, which means that the vasodilation pattern was abnormal and is indicative of cerebral autoregulatory failure. This interpretation was confirmed by the hyperventilation test, when a similar pattern (vasodilation) was induced by hyperventilation instead of a normal vasoconstrictor pattern induced by hypocapnia.

The second striking abnormality was the tremor-associated signal changes during the tilt. The body tremor affecting both arms and trunk was of relatively high frequency, very close to the heart rate (150 BPM = 2.5 Hz). The initial impression was that the tremor was of psychogenic origin since the blood pressure and CBFv were elevated (blood pressure up to 190 mm Hg). However, closer inspection of the signal showed that the true blood pressure and CBFv were very low (Figure 102.1F,G). The spuriously elevated blood pressure and CBFv were likely due to a resonance phenomenon. Here a mechanical tremor of a body induced tremor of the electrocardiogram (ECG) leads . Lead tremor induced periodic electric current in all linked amplifiers (blood pressure, CBF and ECG) since they are all linked by a floating ground. Each systolic contractions trigger systolic CBFv and systolic blood pressure at the frequency of heart rate. Both sources of fluctuations (heart rate and external tremor) amplify each other since there are a similar frequency with the net effect being an increase of CBFv amplitude.

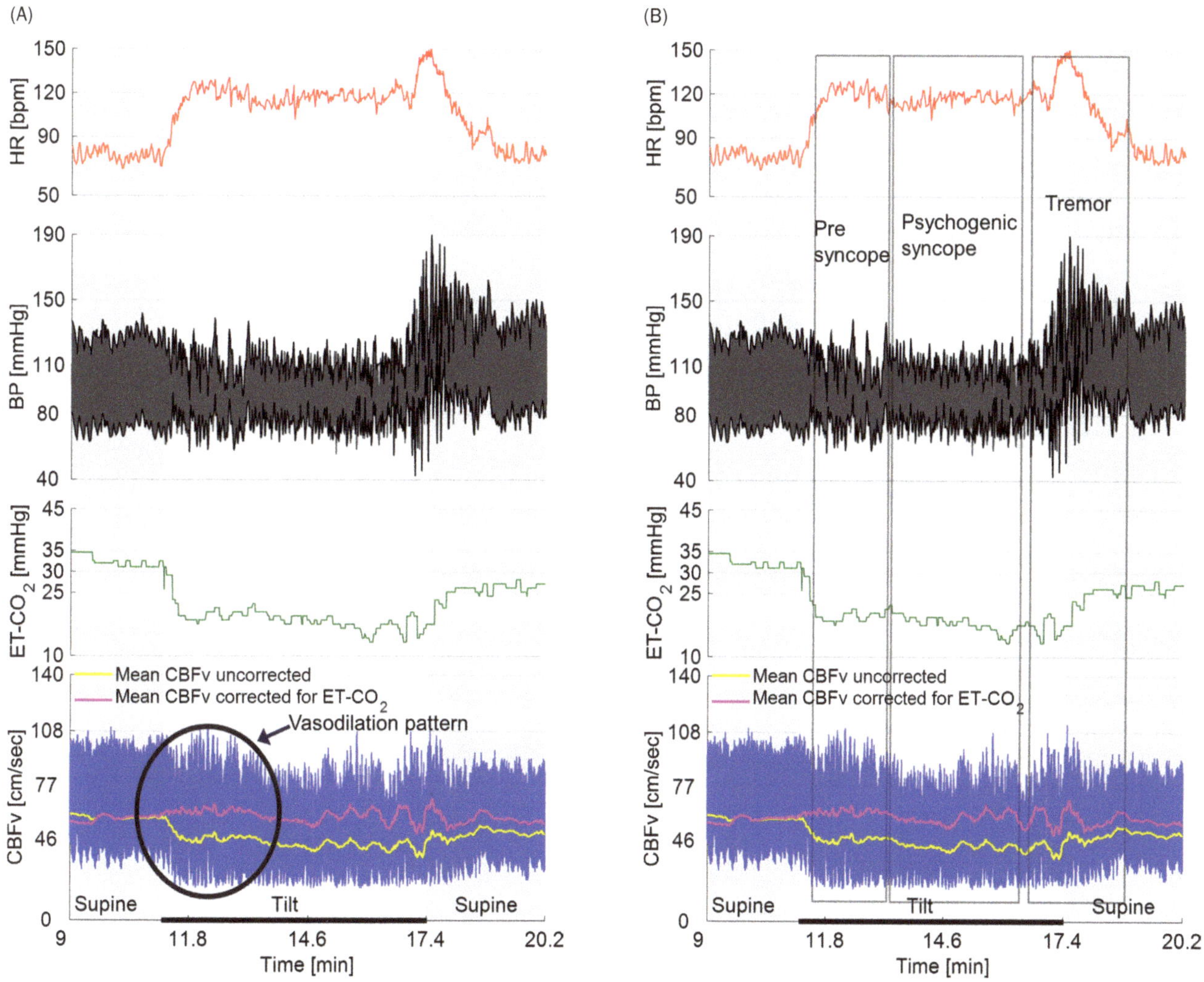

Figure 102.1 Three patterns were observed during the tilt test: (1) presyncope, (2) psychogenic syncope, and (3) syncope with ischemic convulsions. The patient became dizzy and agitated at the onset of the tilt, which was associated with tachycardia (heart rate ~150 BPM), modest decline in blood pressure (does not satisfy criteria for orthostatic hypotension), and a cerebral vasodilation pattern (A, E). These findings are consistent with presyncope. Patient became less agitated after 3 minutes of the tilt and felt better, complaining only “not feeling well.” Then she became unresponsive (B). During that time, her vitals were stable. This episode was consistent with psychogenic syncope. She “regained consciousness” at about minute 4 of the tilt. Twenty seconds later, her whole body started to shake vigorously. Her mother that was present during the testing and confirmed that this was her typical spell. During the tremor, large artifacts obscured physiological signals. Blood pressure signal fluctuated between 40 and 190 mm Hg, and cerebral blood flow velocity (CBFv) signal also fluctuated widely (F). Careful inspection of signals showed that the blood pressure and CBFv was markedly reduced (G) indicating syncope with cerebral hypoperfusion. Hyperventilation in the supine position showed decline in blood pressure and a vasodilation pattern in cerebral blood flow (widening of signal due to increased difference between systolic and diastolic flow velocity, H).

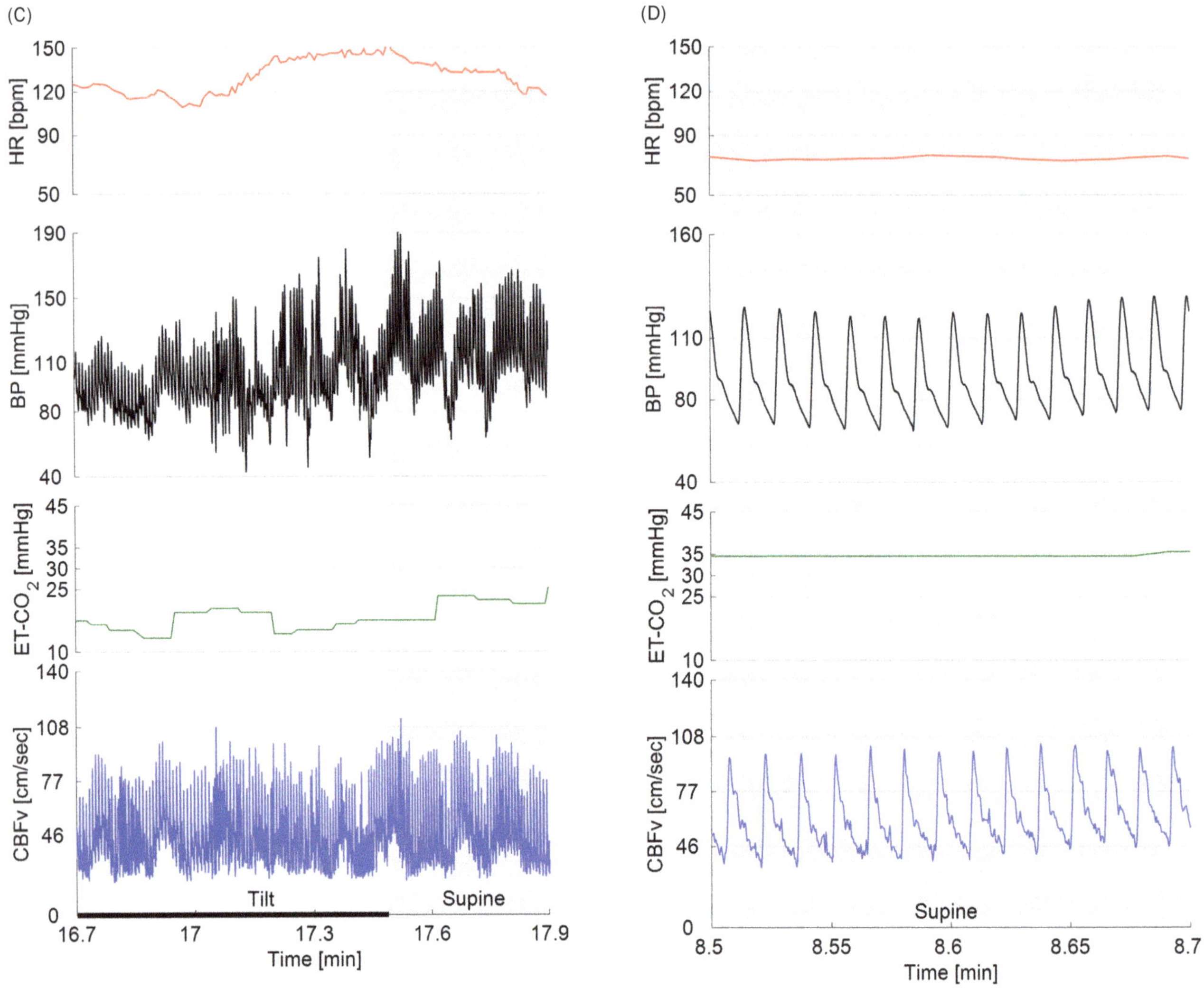

Figure 102.1 Continued

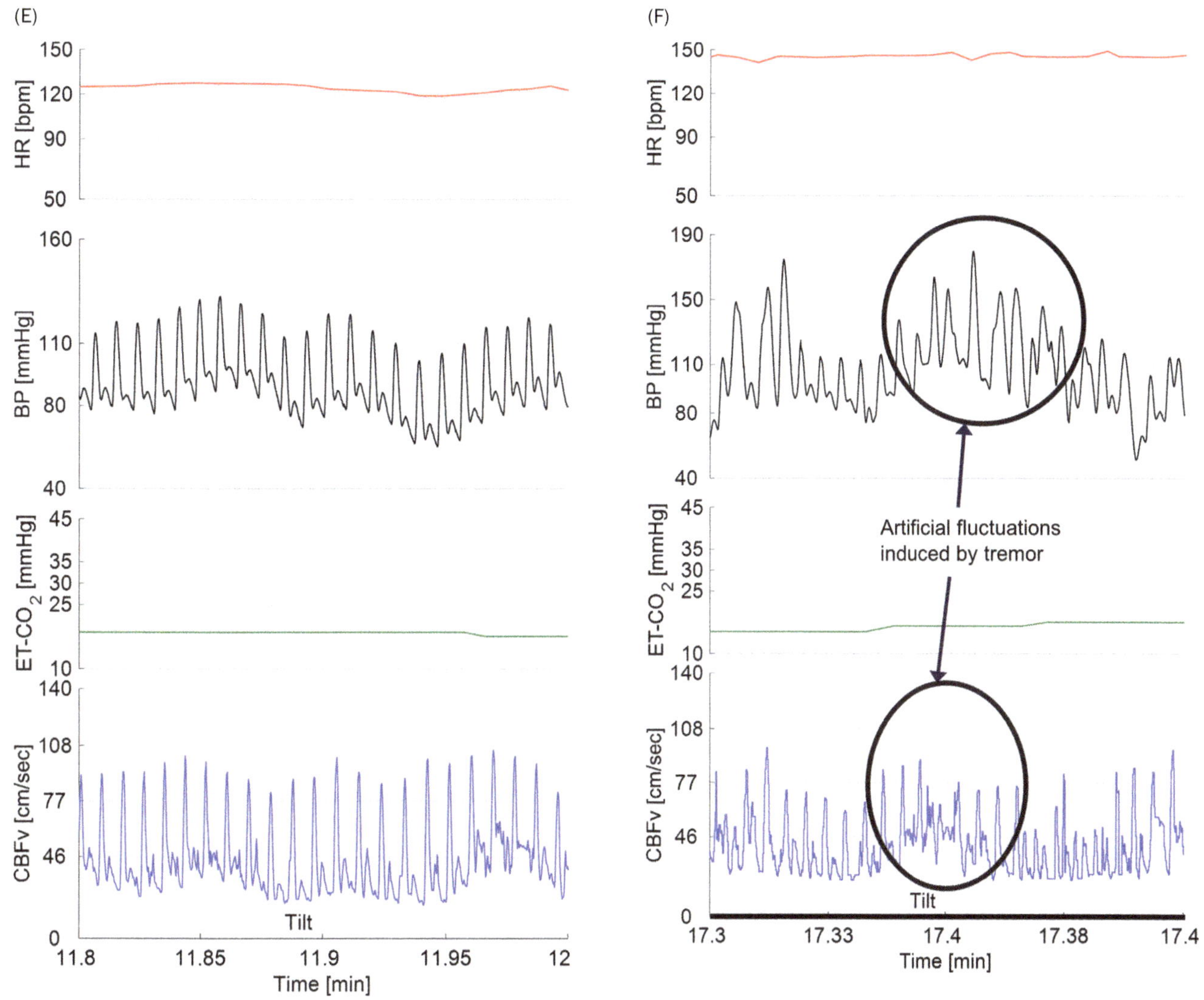

Figure 102.1 Continued

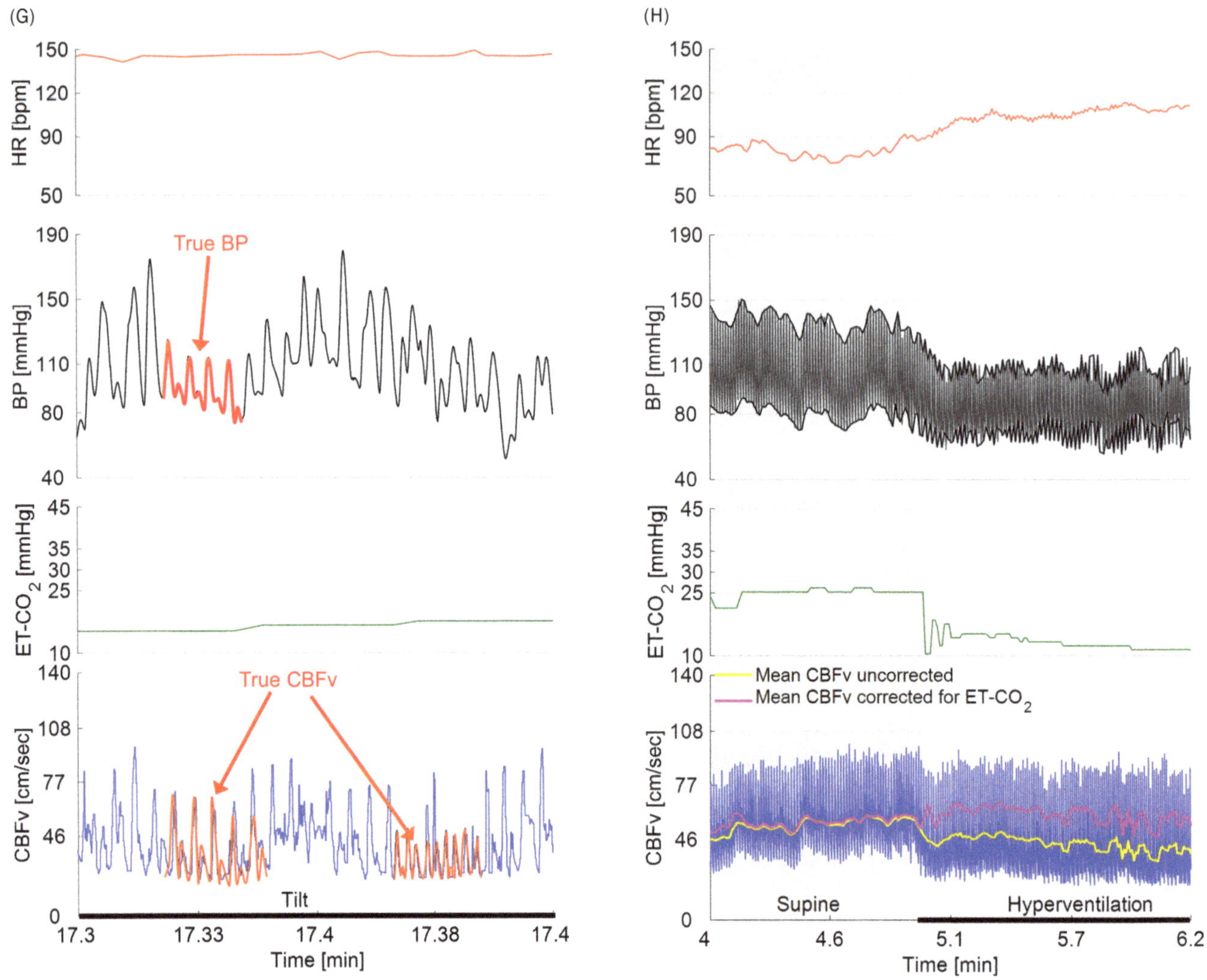

Figure 102.1 Continued

TREATMENT AND FOLLOW-UP

- POTS.
- Clinical workup for neuropathy and volume expansion through high fluid and high salt intake.
- Since baseline blood pressure is low, we recommend starting fludrocortisone for volume expansion, which also may reduce postural tachycardia.
- Consider β-blockers if tachycardia is suboptimally controlled.
- Cerebral autoregulatory failure. The intervention for POTS should also improve the cerebral blood flow and orthostatic tolerance.
- Psychiatric evaluation and therapy for psychogenic pseudosyncope.

CAVEATS

- Tremor or any other abnormal movement may induce artifacts in signals.
- POTS, presyncope, syncope, and psychogenic pseudosyncope may coexist, but they represent different pathophysiological entities.[1]

REFERENCE

1. Novak P. Cerebral blood flow, heart rate, and blood pressure patterns during the tilt test in common orthostatic syndromes. *Neurosci J.* 2016;2016:6127340. doi:10.1155/2016/6127340.

103.

CASE 98: REPETITIVE PSYCHOGENIC PSEUDOSYNCOPE

Chief complaint: Multiple episodes of loss of consciousness.

Case presentation: A 27-year-old woman presents with multiple episodes of loss of consciousness. She has had syncopal episodes "all her life." In addition, she is always tired, does not sweat, and cannot tolerate temperature changes. After each meal, she experiences nausea. She also has chronic leg pain, loose joints, and a history of large joints dislocations. She was diagnosed with hypermobile Ehlers-Danlos syndrome. She had tethered cord surgery a year ago that improved leg pain, but she continues to have episodes of loss of consciousness. She had a tilt test that, according to the patient, was positive for syncope. She did not respond to any intervention including hydration, compression stockings, pressor medications, or β-blockers. She was referred for reevaluation of syncope.

Past medical history: Ehlers-Danlos syndrome hypermobility type, interstitial cystitis, migraine.

Current medication: Sertraline.

Assessment plan: Functional autonomic tests.

AUTONOMIC TESTING EVALUATION

See Table 103.1.

Heart rate: Supine heart rate was normal. Heart rate responses to deep breathing were normal. Heart rate increment during the tilt (40 BPM) was exaggerated.

Blood pressure:

Valsalva maneuver: Mean blood pressure failed to return to baseline at the end of Phase 2 by 13 mm Hg (i.e., 80.1% of baseline).

Tilt: Supine blood pressure was normal. Blood pressure responses to tilt were normal.

Sudomotor evaluation: Sweat output was abnormal (reduced to 48.8% of lower limit) at forearm, normal at proximal leg, normal at distal leg, and abnormal (reduced to 61.1% of lower limit) at foot.

Respiratory system: Respiratory frequency and end tidal CO_2 were normal in supine position and during the tilt.

Cerebral blood flow velocity (CBFv): CBFv in middle cerebral artery was normal in supine position. CBFv in middle cerebral artery was stable during the tilt.

Skin biopsy (sensory-epidermal): Epidermal nerve fiber density was normal at proximal leg and normal at distal leg.

Skin biopsy (sweat glands): Sweat gland nerve fiber density was normal at proximal leg and normal at distal leg.

Patient-reported symptoms during testing: Dizziness, nausea, shortness of breath during the tilt.

Patient-reported symptoms for past 2 weeks:

Lightheadedness or dizziness: Often
Dry eyes or mouth: Often

TABLE 103.1 **RESULTS OF AUTONOMIC TESTING**

Blood pressure evaluation					
Test: Valsalva maneuver					
Pressure [mmHg]	Baseline	Phase 2			Phase 4
		Early	End		
Systolic	96	59	59		
Mean	65.3	52.3	52.3	n/a	
Diastolic	50	49	49	n/a	

Heart rate evaluation	
Test: Deep breathing	
Results	Norm*
14.4	≥14
Test: Valsalva ratio	
1.73	≥1.46
* adjusted for a gender and age	

(continued)

TABLE 103.1 **CONTINUED**

Test: Tilt test										
Position		HR [BPM]	Blood pressure [mmHg]		MCA Blood flow velocity [cm/s]				Respiratory frequency [breaths/min]	End tidal CO_2 [mmHg]
			Systolic	Diastolic	Systolic	Mean	Mean drop [%]	Diastolic		
Supine		65	93	61	100	59.3		39	12	39
Tilt [min]	1	96	103	73	89	55.7	6.1	39	17	38
	2	90	108	74						
	3	90	95	69						
	4	90	101	71						
	5	95	104	73	88	53.3	10.1	36	19	37
	6	93	95	69						
	7	98	100	72						
	8	104	101	72						
	9	99	99	69						
	10	105	106	77	88	53.3	10.1	36	17	37
	15									
	20									
	30									
	40									

Sudomotor evaluation - functional

Test: Quantitative sudomotor axon reflex test (QSART)				
Location	Site (l/r)	Latency [min]	Volume [μl]	Norm [μl]*
Forearm	l	2.36	0.039	≥0.08
Prox. leg	l	1.54	0.171	≥0.14
Distal leg	l	2.19	0.325	≥0.24
Foot	l	2.18	0.055	≥0.09

* Normative data are adjusted for gender and age of patient.

Test: Electrochemical skin conductance (ESC)				
Location	Left [μS]	Right [μS]	Average [μS/k]	Norm [μS/kg]
Hand				≥1.03
Feet				≥1.14
Forehead				

For grading uses ESC [μS] adjusted for weight [μS/k].

Small fiber (sensory + sudomotor) evaluation - morphological					
Test: Skin biopsy					
Location	Site (l/r)	Nerve fibers			
		Epidermal*		Sweat glands	
		Density	Norm	Density	Norm
Proximal leg – thigh	Right	14.32	≥8.3	48.1	≥37.8
Distal leg - calf	Right	12.59	≥8.94	57.4	≥36.5
Foot	Right		≥3.11		≥34.8

*Normative data for distal leg are adjusted for gender and age of patient.

QASAT*											
Heart rate		BP		CBFv		ET-CO2		Sudomotor			Total QASAT score
S. bradycardia	0	Low supine	0	Low supine	0	Low supine	0	QSART	2		
S. tachycardia	0	High supine	0	High supine	0	High supine	0	ESC			
Increase tilt	1	OH	0	Tilt response	0	Tilt low	0				
Decrease tilt	0	OHTN	0	CA	0	Tilt high	0	**Skin biopsy**			5
Deep breathing	0	VM	2	CVR	0			Epidermal	0		
VR	1			VM	0			Sweat gland	0		
Total	1	Total	2	Total	0	Total	0				

*QASAT. See Novak. Quantitative Scale for Grading of Cardiovascular Autonomic Reflex Tests and Small Fibers from Skin Biopsies. *J Neurol Disord* 2015;3:2.

S, supine; Increase tilt, increased response to tilt; Decrease tilt, decreased response to tilt; BP, blood pressure; VM, Valsalva maneuver; CBFv, cerebral blood flow velocity; CA, cerebral autoregulation; MCA, middle cerebral artery; VR, Valsalva ratio; CVR, cerebral vasoreactivity.

Pale feet: Often
Cold feet: Often
Reduced sweating: Often
Reduced sweating after exercise: Often
Increased sweating: Yes, minor annoyance
Nausea: Occasionally
Diarrhea: None
Constipation: Often
Urinary leaks: Occasionally
Current pain severity: 5
Aching pain: Occasionally, mild
Allodynia: Occasionally, ,mild
Burning pain: Occasionally, moderate
Lancinating pain: Often, moderate
Numbness: Often, moderate
Prickling sensation: Often, moderate

AUTONOMIC TESTING INTERPRETATION

- Psychogenic pseudosyncope.
- Autonomic dysfunction, mild, affecting sympathetic adrenergic and sudomotor systems. There was no evidence of orthostatic hypotension or postural tachycardia syndrome (POTS). Medication effect can contribute to sudomotor dysfunction.
- Cerebral blood flow was normal in supine position. Orthostatic cerebral blood flow was stable.
- Respiratory functions were normal; there was no evidence of hyperventilation or hypoventilation.

COMMENT

The tilt test showed repetitive episodes of unresponsiveness associated with stable cardiovascular and respiratory signals and symptoms resolved with reassurance (Figure 103.1). These patterns are consistent with psychogenic pseudosyncope defined by an apparent loss of consciousness without global cerebral hypoperfusion.[1] CBFv appears to be a reasonable proxy for cerebral perfusion, and stable

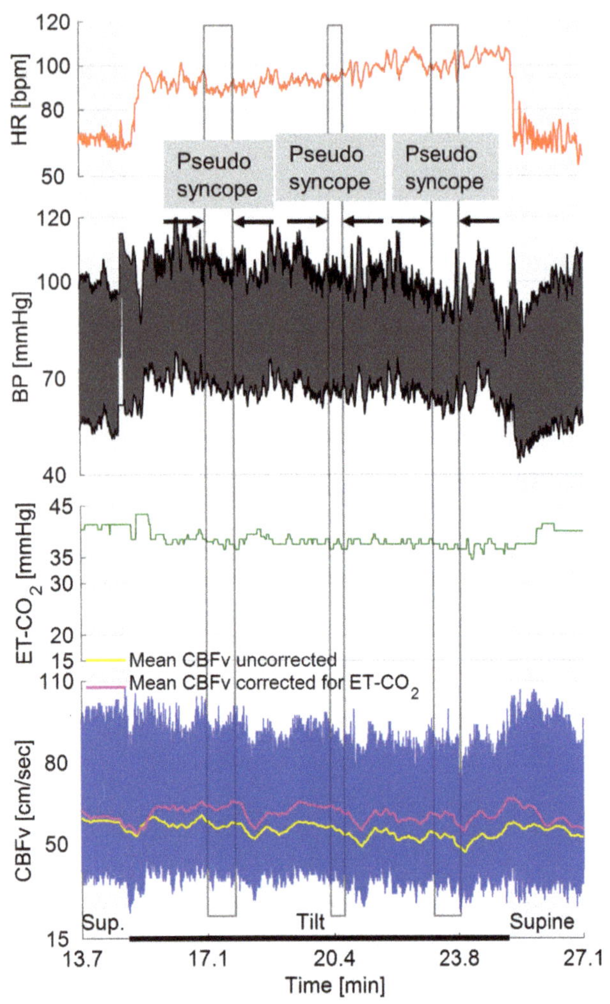

Figure 103.1 The tilt showed normal responses in all signals. Heart rate increment to tilt was exaggerated (40 BPM) but <120 BPM. Patient became unresponsive several times during the tilt; these were marked as pseudosyncope.

CBFv supports diagnosis of pseudosyncope in the context of loss of consciousness.[2] If there is clinical evidence of seizure activity (e.g., the presence of abnormal movement), then additional electroencephalogram monitoring should be performed. The tilt test showed exaggerated heart rate responsive to tilt, however the orthostatic heart rate usually exceeds 120 BPM in POTS.[3]

TREATMENT AND FOLLOW-UP

- Referral to psychiatry.

CAVEATS

- CBFv monitoring can be useful to diagnose psychogenic pseudosyncope.

REFERENCES

1. Task Force for the Diagnosis and Management of Syncope, European Society of Cardiology (ESC), European Heart Rhythm Association (EHRA), et al. Guidelines for the diagnosis and management of syncope (version 2009). *Eur Heart J*. 2009;30(21):2631–2671. doi:10.1093/eurheartj/ehp298.
2. Novak P. Cerebral blood flow, heart rate, and blood pressure patterns during the tilt test in common orthostatic syndromes. *Neurosci J*. 2016;2016:6127340. doi:10.1155/2016/6127340.
3. Low PA, Sandroni P, Joyner M, Shen W-K. Postural tachycardia syndrome (POTS). *J Cardiovasc Electrophysiol*. 2009;20(3):352–358. doi:10.1111/j.1540-8167.2008.01407.x.

104.

CASE 99: MIXED TILT PATTERNS IN RHEUMATOID ARTHRITIS

Chief complaint: Dizziness.

Case presentation: A 32-year-old woman was healthy until 2.5 years ago, at which point she experienced the sudden onset of diffuse joint and muscle pain with several tender points. She had a slipped disk 3 months before pain onset. Later, she noted constant nausea, alternating diarrhea and constipation, orthostatic dizziness, and cold/heat intolerance. She passed out twice. She was diagnosed with fibromyalgia and rheumatoid arthritis by rheumatology. She tested negative for diabetes, vitamin B_{12} deficiency, Sjögren's syndrome, lupus, and thyroid disorders. She could not tolerate the nerve conduction studies, but neurological examination showed normal deep tendon reflexes. She was referred for autonomic testing for suspected dysautonomia.

Past medical history: Inflammatory arthritis, fibromyalgia, hypothyroidism.

Current medication: Methotrexate, thyroid replacement, montelukast, nortriptyline, pyridostigmine, cyclobenzaprine, duloxetine (Cymbalta), prednisone, isoniazid, birth control pills.

Assessment plan: Functional autonomic tests and skin biopsy.

AUTONOMIC TESTING EVALUATION

See Table 104.1.

Heart rate: Supine heart rate was normal. Heart rate responses to deep breathing were normal. Heart rate increment during the tilt (53 BPM) was exaggerated.

Blood pressure:

Valsalva maneuver: Mean blood pressure failed to return to baseline at the end of Phase 2 by 7 mm Hg (i.e., 86% of baseline).

Tilt: Supine blood pressure was within normal range. Blood pressure was reduced during the tilt consistent with severe orthostatic hypotension. The tilt was aborted at minute 4 per patient request.

Sudomotor evaluation: Electrochemical skin conductance was abnormal (reduced to 64.2% of normal limit) at hands and abnormal (reduced to 67.7% of normal limit) at feet.

Respiratory system: Respiratory frequency was normal during supine and during the tilt. End tidal CO_2 was reduced in supine position and declined further during the tilt.

TABLE 104.1 **RESULTS OF AUTONOMIC TESTING**

Blood pressure evaluation					
Test: Valsalva maneuver					
Pressure [mmHg]	Baseline	Phase 2			Phase 4
		Early	End		
Systolic	58	49	49		
Mean	50	43	43	n/a	
Diastolic	46	40	40	n/a	

Heart rate evaluation	
Test: Deep breathing	
Results	Norm*
13.5	≥12
Test: Valsalva ratio	
1.55	≥1.5
* adjusted for a gender and age	

(continued)

TABLE 104.1 **CONTINUED**

Test: Tilt test										
Position		HR [BPM]	Blood pressure [mmHg]		MCA Blood flow velocity [cm/s]				Respiratory frequency [breaths/min]	End tidal CO_2 [mmHg]
			Systolic	Diastolic	Systolic	Mean	Mean drop [%]	Diastolic		
Supine		88	112	75	93	59		42	12	31
Tilt [min]	1	114	110	64	66	44	25.4	33	17	19
	2	123	115	75						
	3	138	91	67						
	4	141	69	54	64	36.7	37.8	23	16	16
	5									
	6									
	7									
	8									
	9									
	10									
	15									
	20									
	30									
	40									

Sudomotor evaluation - functional

Test: Quantitative sudomotor axon reflex test (QSART)				
Location	Site (l/r)	Latency [min]	Volume [µl]	Norm [µl]*
Forearm				≥0.08
Prox. leg				≥0.14
Distal leg				≥0.15
Foot				≥0.07

* Normative data are adjusted for gender and age of patient.

Test: Electrochemical skin conductance (ESC)				
Location	Left [µS]	Right [µS]	Average [µS/k]	Norm [µS/kg]
Hand	49	47	0.66	≥1.03
Feet	57	56	0.77	≥1.14
Forehead				

For grading uses ESC [µS] adjusted for weight [µS/k].

TABLE 104.1 **CONTINUED**

Small fiber (sensory + sudomotor) evaluation - morphological					
Test: Skin biopsy					
Location	Site (l/r)	Nerve fibers			
		Epidermal*		Sweat glands	
		Density	Norm	Density	Norm
Proximal leg – thigh	Right	13.98	≥8.3	66.5	≥37.8
Distal leg - calf	Right	6.25	≥8.54		≥36.5
Foot	Right		≥3.11		≥34.8

*Normative data for distal leg are adjusted for gender and age of patient.

QASAT*										
Heart rate		**BP**		**CBFv**		**ET-CO2**		**Sudomotor**		**Total QASAT score**
S. bradycardia	0	Low supine	0	Low supine	0	Low supine	1	QSART		
S. tachycardia	0	High supine	0	High supine	0	High supine	0	ESC	3	
Increase tilt		OH		Tilt response		Tilt low				
Decrease tilt		OHTN		CA		Tilt high		**Skin biopsy**		7
Deep breathing	0	VM	2	CVR	0			Epidermal	1	
VR	0			VM	0			Sweat gland	0	
Total	0	Total	2	Total	0	Total	1			

*QASAT. See Novak. Quantitative Scale for Grading of Cardiovascular Autonomic Reflex Tests and Small Fibers from Skin Biopsies. *J Neurol Disord* 2015;3:2. Orthostatic (tilt) responses were not graded since QASAT requires the duration of the tilt at least 10 minutes.

S, supine; Increase tilt, increased response to tilt; Decrease tilt, decreased response to tilt; BP, blood pressure; VM, Valsalva maneuver; CBFv, cerebral blood flow velocity; CA, cerebral autoregulation; MCA, middle cerebral artery; VR, Valsalva ratio; CVR, cerebral vasoreactivity.

Cerebral blood flow velocity (CBFv): CBFv in middle cerebral artery was normal in supine position but was severely reduced during the tilt test.

Skin biopsy (sensory-epidermal): Epidermal nerve fiber density was normal at proximal leg and abnormal (reduced to 73.2% of normal limit) at distal leg.

Skin biopsy (sweat glands): Sweat gland nerve fiber density was normal at proximal leg.

Patient-reported symptoms during testing: Dizziness, dizziness, agitation, shortness of breath during the tilt.

Patient-reported symptoms for past 2 weeks:

Lightheadedness or dizziness: Occasionally
Dry eyes or mouth: Occasionally
Pale feet: Occasionally
Cold feet: Often
Reduced sweating: Occasionally
Reduced sweating after exercise: Occasionally
Increased sweating: Occasionally
Nausea: Occasionally
Diarrhea: Occasionally
Constipation: Occasionally
Urinary leaks: None
Current pain severity: 2
Aching pain: Often, moderate
Allodynia: Occasionally, mild
Burning pain: None
Lancinating pain: Occasionally, mild
Numbness: Occasionally, mild
Prickling sensation: Occasionally, mild

AUTONOMIC TESTING INTERPRETATION

- Initial orthostatic hypotension (IOH).
- Orthostatic hypotension due to a combination of volume depletion and adrenergic failure.
- Presyncope, with prominent vasodepressor component.
- Small fiber neuropathy, mixed, length-dependent.

COMMENT

The autonomic testing showed several patterns (Figure 104.1). IOH triggered a decline in CBFv that resulted in severe dizziness which persisted throughout the tilt. IOH partially recovered, but blood pressure remained low and satisfied criteria for orthostatic hypotension (OH). The OH was due both volume depletion (as indicated by collapse of the pulse pressure) and due to mild adrenergic failure (as indicated by abnormal Valsalva maneuver). Patient experienced signs of cerebral hypoperfusion throughout the tilt that correlated with low diastolic CBFv. There were also large fluctuations in CBFv that can also contribute to dizziness because the brain is very sensitive to any changes in cerebral blood flow. CBFv decline was due to the combined effect of hypocapnia and to OH since even CBFv corrected for the effect of hypocapnia declined. Patient was progressively hyperventilating throughout the tilt.

The cause of small fiber neuropathy in this patient is likely rheumatoid arthritis since other causes of neuropathy including diabetes were ruled out and rheumatoid arthritis is known to be associated with small fiber neuropathy.[1]

TREATMENT AND FOLLOW-UP

- Complex therapy for orthostatic intolerance including diet control, physical therapy, and pressor medications.
- Consider antiinflammatory therapy for rheumatoid arthritis, which also may improve small fiber neuropathy.[2,3]

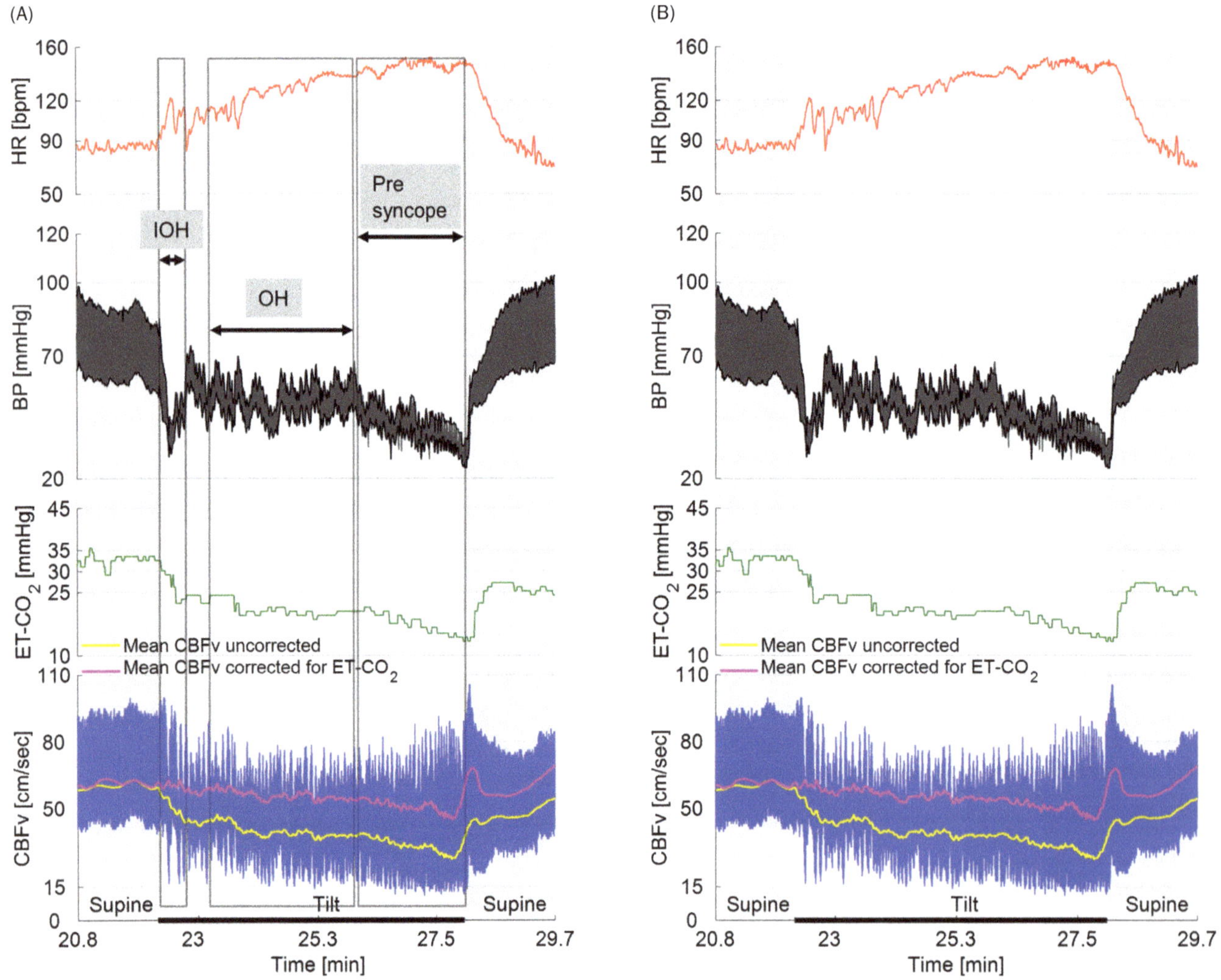

Figure 104.1 The tilt showed combination of initial orthostatic hypotension (IOH; A–C), orthostatic hypotension, and presyncope (A–D). The patient became dizzy immediately after the tilt onset and remained dizzy throughout the tilt. The tilt was aborted at minute 4 since patient became agitated and requested the testing stop. She never lost consciousness despite very low cerebral blood flow velocity.

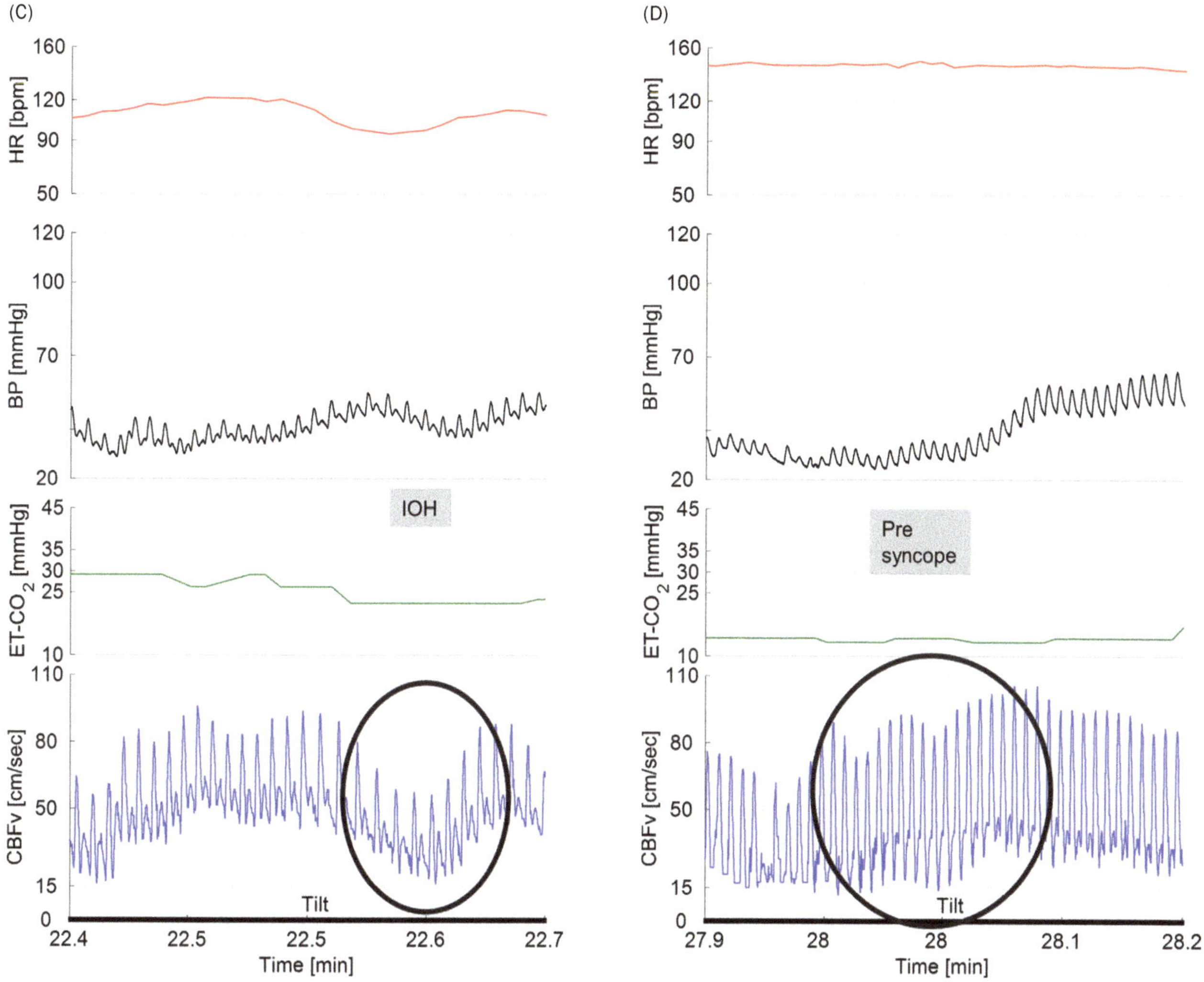

Figure 104.1 Continued

CAVEATS

- IOH, OH, and presyncope may coexist.
- Small fiber neuropathy that underlies the autonomic failure is likely due to rheumatoid arthritis.

REFERENCES

1. Birnbaum J, Bingham CO. Non-length-dependent and length-dependent small-fiber neuropathies associated with tumor necrosis factor (TNF)-inhibitor therapy in patients with rheumatoid arthritis: expanding the spectrum of neurological disease associated with TNF-inhibitors. *Semin Arthritis Rheum*. 2014;43(5):638–647. doi:10.1016/j.semarthrit.2013.10.007.
2. Syngle A, Verma I, Krishan P, Garg N, Syngle V. Disease-modifying anti-rheumatic drugs improve autonomic neuropathy in arthritis: DIANA study. *Clin Rheumatol*. 2015;34(7):1233–1241. doi:10.1007/s10067-014-2716-x.
3. Liu X, Treister R, Lang M, Oaklander AL. IVIg for apparently autoimmune small-fiber polyneuropathy: first analysis of efficacy and safety. *Ther Adv Neurol Disord*. 2018;11. doi:10.1177/1756285617744484.

105.

CASE 100: DIZZINESS AFTER CONCUSSION

Chief complaint: Dizziness.

Case presentation: A 75-year-old woman presents with disabling dizziness. The dizziness started after the head injury a year ago. More recently, the dizziness has worsened and become postural or provoked by changes in position, lasting seconds to minutes without any clear pattern. Patient was referred for an evaluation of dizziness and possible autonomic failure.

Past medical history: Hypothyroidism, hypertension, dyslipidemia, postconcussion syndrome.

Current medication: Levothyroxine, olmesartan, sertraline, ibuprofen.

Assessment plan: Functional autonomic tests.

AUTONOMIC TESTING EVALUATION

See Table 105.1.

Heart rate: Supine heart rate was normal. Heart rate responses to deep breathing were reduced to 51.4% of normal value. Heart rate increment during the tilt (6 BPM) was minimally reduced.

Blood pressure:

Valsalva maneuver: Mean blood pressure failed to return to baseline at the end of Phase 2 by 13.6 mm Hg (i.e., 87.7% of baseline).

Tilt: Supine blood pressure was elevated. Blood pressure responses to tilt were abnormal and consistent with mild and transient orthostatic hypotension.

Sudomotor evaluation: Electrochemical skin conductance was normal at hands and normal at feet.

Respiratory system: Respiratory frequency was normal in supine position and during the tilt. The end tidal CO_2 was minimally reduced during supine position and was further reduced during the tilt test.

Cerebral blood flow velocity (CBFv): CBFv in middle cerebral artery was normal in supine position. CBFv in middle cerebral artery was stable during the tilt.

Skin biopsy (sensory-epidermal): N/A

Skin biopsy (sweat glands): N/A

Patient-reported symptoms during testing: Dizziness during the tilt.

Patient-reported symptoms for past 2 weeks:

Lightheadedness or dizziness: Occasionally
Dry eyes or mouth: None
Pale feet: None
Cold feet: None
Reduced sweating: None
Reduced sweating after exercise: None
Increased sweating: None
Nausea: None
Diarrhea: None

TABLE 105.1 RESULTS OF AUTONOMIC TESTING

Blood pressure evaluation					
Test: Valsalva maneuver					
Pressure [mmHg]	Baseline	Phase 2			Phase 4
		Early	End		
Systolic	167	150	150		
Mean	110.3	96.7	96.7	n/a	
Diastolic	82	70	70	n/a	

Heart rate evaluation	
Test: Deep breathing	
Results	Norm*
3.6	≥7
Test: Valsalva ratio	
1.42	≥1.39
* adjusted for a gender and age	

TABLE 105.1 **CONTINUED**

Test: Tilt test										
Position		HR [BPM]	Blood pressure [mmHg]		MCA Blood flow velocity [cm/s]				Respiratory frequency [breaths/min]	End tidal CO_2 [mmHg]
			Systolic	Diastolic	Systolic	Mean	Mean drop [%]	Diastolic		
Supine		64	144	71	107	63		41	13	32
Tilt [min]	1	70	113	71	97	57.7	8.4	38	18	26
	2	68	118	76						
	3	67	125	70						
	4	65	120	77						
	5	68	120	77	94	57.3	9	39	15	35
	6	67	127	80						
	7	66	119	76						
	8	68	121	81						
	9	70	119	75						
	10	68	128	81	92	56.7	10	39	18	33
	15									
	20									
	30									
	40									

Sudomotor evaluation - functional

Test: Quantitative sudomotor axon reflex test (QSART)				
Location	Site (l/r)	Latency [min]	Volume [µl]	Norm [µl]*
Forearm				≥0.08
Prox. leg				≥0.14
Distal leg				≥0.07
Foot				≥0.05

* Normative data are adjusted for gender and age of patient.

Test: Electrochemical skin conductance (ESC)				
Location	Left [µS]	Right [µS]	Average [µS/k]	Norm [µS/kg]
Hand	69	77	1.33	≥1.03
Feet	71	71	1.29	≥1.14
Forehead				

For grading uses ESC [µS] adjusted for weight [µS/k].

(continued)

TABLE 105.1 CONTINUED

Small fiber (sensory + sudomotor) evaluation - morphological					
Test: Skin biopsy					
Location	Site (l/r)	Nerve fibers			
		Epidermal*		Sweat glands	
		Density	Norm	Density	Norm
Proximal leg – thigh	Right		≥8.3		≥37.8
Distal leg - calf	Right		≥5.1		≥36.5
Foot	Right		≥3.11		≥34.8

*Normative data for distal leg are adjusted for gender and age of patient.

QASAT*											
Heart rate		BP		CBFv		ET-CO2		Sudomotor			Total QASAT score
S. bradycardia	0	Low supine	0	Low supine	0	Low supine	1	QSART			
S. tachycardia	0	High supine	1	High supine	0	High supine	0	ESC	0		9
Increase tilt	0	OH	1	Tilt response	0	Tilt low	2				
Decrease tilt	1	OHTN	0	CA	0	Tilt high	0	**Skin biopsy**			
Deep breathing	1	VM	2	CVR	0			Epidermal			
VR	0			VM	0			Sweat gland			
Total	2	Total	4	Total	0	Total	3				

*QASAT. See Novak. Quantitative Scale for Grading of Cardiovascular Autonomic Reflex Tests and Small Fibers from Skin Biopsies. *J Neurol Disord* 2015;3:2.

S, supine; Increase tilt, increased response to tilt; Decrease tilt, decreased response to tilt; BP, blood pressure; VM, Valsalva maneuver; CBFv, cerebral blood flow velocity; CA, cerebral autoregulation; MCA, middle cerebral artery; VR, Valsalva ratio; CVR, cerebral vasoreactivity.

Constipation: None
Urinary leaks: None
Aching pain: None
Allodynia: None
Burning pain: None
Lancinating pain: None
Numbness: None
Prickling sensation: None

AUTONOMIC TESTING INTERPRETATION

- Autonomic failure, generalized, associated with mild orthostatic hypotension.
- Cerebral blood flow was normal in supine position. Orthostatic cerebral blood flow was stable except for a transient decline at tilt onset, which was associated with hypocapnia. The transient decline was due to hypocapnia-induced cerebral vasoconstriction.
- Hypocapnic hyperventilation in supine position and during the tilt.

COMMENT

Although the testing showed generalized autonomic failure with orthostatic hypotension (Figure 105.1), the orthostatic hypotension was compensated and was associated with stable CBFv; therefore, autonomic failure is unlikely responsible for this patient's dizziness.

Dizziness is common after concussion.[1] In a majority of patients, dizziness is often multifactorial and involves oculomotor control and cervical spine pathways. Postural dizziness can be related to cerebral hypoperfusion and

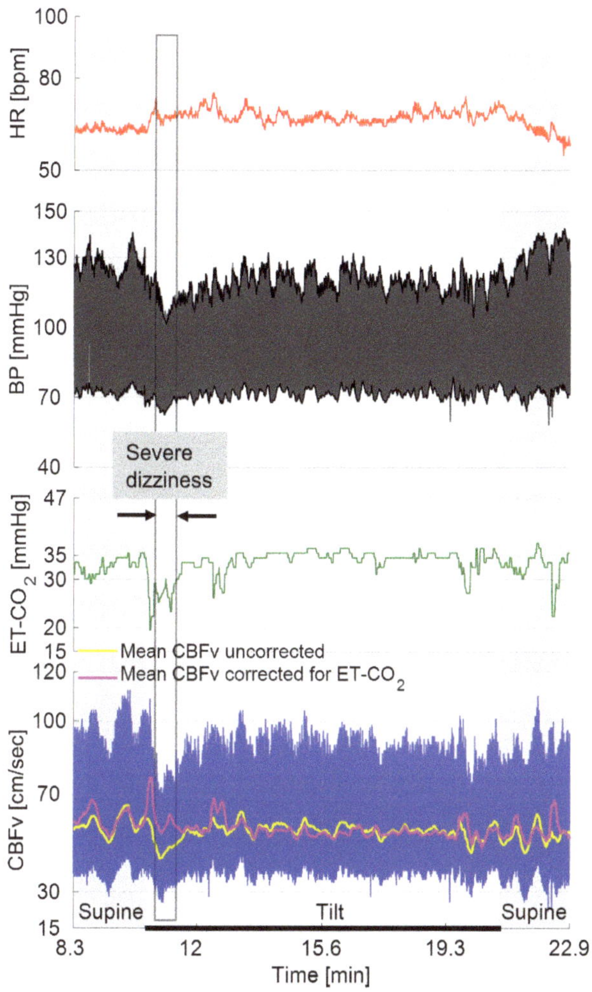

Figure 105.1 The tilt test showed decline in blood pressure, end tidal CO_2, and cerebral blood flow velocity (CBFv) by 29% at the beginning of the tilt. The patient became dizzy. Heart rate responses were normal. The decline in CBFv was due to a decline in end tidal CO_2 and not due to a decline in blood pressure since the orthostatic CBFv corrected for the level of end tidal CO_2 was stable.

autonomic dysfunction. In this patient, the dizziness was reproduced by the tilt and was shown to be a cerebral blood flow-related phenomenon.

TREATMENT AND FOLLOW-UP

- Adequate hydration, compressions stockings, blood pressure control.
- Referral to traumatic brain and concussion clinic.

CAVEATS

- Low CBFv can cause cerebral hypoperfusion with dizziness after concussion.
- The tilt test with CBFv monitoring can be helpful to differentiate causes of dizziness.

REFERENCE

1. Reneker JC, Cheruvu VK, Yang J, James MA, Cook CE. Physical examination of dizziness in athletes after a concussion: A descriptive study. *Musculoskelet Sci Pract*. 2017;34:8–13. doi:10.1016/j.msksp.2017.11.012.

INDEX

Tables and figures are indicated by an italic *t* and *f* following the page number.

E

Q

R

T

W

www.ingramcontent.com/pod-product-compliance
Lightning Source LLC
LaVergne TN
LVHW070845210926
848482LV00016B/869
* 9 7 8 0 1 9 0 8 8 9 2 2 7 *